DOROTHY B. VILLEE, M.D.

Department of Pediatrics;
Harvard Medical School
Boston, Massachusetts

HUMAN ENDOCRINOLOGY

A Developmental Approach

W. B. SAUNDERS COMPANY
Philadelphia, London, Toronto 1975

W. B. Saunders Company: West Washington Square
Philadelphia, PA 19105

12 Dyott Street
London, WC1A 1DB

833 Oxford Street
Toronto, Ontario M8Z 5T9, Canada

Library of Congress Cataloging in Publication Data

Villee, Dorothy B

Human endocrinology.

1. Endocrinology. 2. Developmental biology. I. Title.

QP187.V57 1975 612'.4 73–91280

ISBN 0–7216–9041–6

Human Endocrinology ISBN 0-7216-9041-6

Last digit is the print number: 9 8 7 6 5 4 3 2 1

To Claude

PREFACE

The regulation of biological phenomena by hormones is a complex subject not readily reduced to a single volume of modest size. Of special interest in recent years has been the incredible increase in our knowledge of endocrine regulation in the fetus and newborn, a subject which often receives short shrift in standard textbooks. There was a clear need for an overview of the subject in which human development would be treated as a sequence of events regulated in part by genetic expression, in part by nutritional milieu, and in part by the circulating hormones. Such an approach would of necessity emphasize aspects of development such as differentiation, growth, homeostasis, maturation, and senescence rather than simply discuss the individual endocrine glands, their secretions, and what goes wrong when there is too much or too little of each hormone. This book attempts to present a cohesive story, unfolding in logical sequence from procreation to death.

The book is designed for the student of endocrinology, but it could also serve as a useful guide for the student of development. The progression of normal events is highlighted by contrast with examples of aberrations from the norm. These "experiments of nature" are considered in detail in order to illustrate alterations in the normal regulatory processes. Specific clinical entities are presented after the normal processes have been discussed.

The first portion of the book deals with early human development. A full chapter is devoted to the placenta and its special role as an endocrine organ in pregnancy. The cooperation of the placenta and the fetus in the formation of steroid hormones is emphasized in a detailed discussion of the "fetoplacental unit." Chapter Three is devoted to the embryonic development and function of the endocrine glands. Their origins from the primary germ layers, the evidence of hormone secretion during fetal life, and the role of these hormones in differentiation and growth are described. This chapter should serve the student as an introduction to each of the endocrine glands and their hormones.

Several succeeding chapters are devoted to the endocrine disorders of the newborn, with special emphasis on disorders of glucose metabolism and on sexual anomalies. In each case the basic concepts are presented and discussed before deviations from the norm are described.

Chapters on homeostasis, growth, maturation, and senescence follow a logical developmental sequence. Each new concept is supported with biochemical and physiological data wherever possible. In particular, the concepts of hormone receptors, mechanisms of hormone action involving genetic derepression or adenyl cyclase activation, and prohormone formation within endocrine glands are given detailed attention. The metabolism of carbohydrates, lipids, and proteins and the endocrine regulation of these processes are discussed in those portions of the book where it seemed most appropriate. Thus there is no one chapter on biochemical endocrinology; rather, the chemical concepts are distributed wherever appropriate throughout the book. The student who approaches biochemistry with reluctance may find this more palatable. The biochemically oriented student is provided with additional reading material to supplement the discussions presented.

By and large, biological phenomena are not regulated by a single hormone or endocrine gland but by many hormones and glands acting in concert. I have attempted to discuss the entire endocrine system as a regulatory unit and not just as the sum of the individual parts of the system. The student who wishes to read about a specific endocrine gland can use the index and cross-references in the text to locate all of the discussions relevant to that subject.

Therapy for endocrine disorders is discussed in general terms; obviously, details of therapy must be learned during a clinical clerkship. A number of endocrine diseases have been left unmentioned (or only briefly sketched) either because they were too esoteric or because they were not germane. For example, neoplasms of the endocrine glands have not been discussed in depth; the student interested in this subject should consult a standard textbook for detailed information.

The goal of this book is to present in concise and readable form an overview of developmental endocrinology. With this background of information, supplemented with examples of clinical disorders, the medical student should be prepared for a clinical clerkship in endocrinology.

In preparing such a book as this I was fortunate to have advice and help from my clinical colleagues. Portions of the manuscript were read by Dr. Melvin Grumbach, University of California Medical Center, Dr. John Parks, University of Pennsylvania Medical School, and Dr. Leslie Rose, Harvard Medical School. Their helpful comments were deeply appreciated. Clinical illustrations were provided by my colleagues at Harvard Medical School: Dr. Shirley Driscoll, Boston Hospital for Women, Dr. Leslie Rose, Peter Bent Brigham Hospital, and Dr. John Crigler, Children's Hospital Medical Center. I am very grateful for their efforts in behalf of the book. I wish also to thank Frank Fancher for preparing the drawings for the book, Miss Kathleen Callinan for typing the manuscript, and my daughter, Suzanne, for helping in the preparation of the index. Few authors have had such constant support and encouragement as I, thanks to my husband Claude's firm belief in the value of such a book. Without his help and the encouragement of the staff at Saunders, especially Brian Decker, it would not have been possible to complete the manuscript.

DOROTHY B. VILLEE

CONTENTS

PART ONE

THE FETUS

PART FIVE

THE ADULT

PART ONE

THE FETUS

CHAPTER ONE

The First Weeks of Life

The classic puzzle "which came first—the chicken or the egg?" points up the difficulty in assigning a beginning to the cyclic process of development. Arbitrarily, then, we shall adopt the view that development begins with the union of male and female pronuclei at fertilization. At this point a new diploid organism is formed and will develop, mature, and undergo senescence at a predictable rate. Cetainly it is no longer acceptable to set the birth of the newborn as the time of onset of development.

As our knowledge of early human development increases we are impressed with the complexity of molecular controls, many of which are hormonally engendered. To understand the development of the endocrine system we must consider the events of early embryonic life. It is not enough to say that the human fetal adrenal cortex arose from coelomic epithelium without our first acquiring knowledge of the coelom and its mesodermal covering. A firm basis in embryology permits, in addition, an understanding of various endocrine developmental aberrations, such as adrenal cell tumors in the gonads. Therefore, though we know least about the controls of very early life, let us start there and proceed systematically through the life span of the individual, mapping the metabolic events and endocrine controls as we know them.

FERTILIZATION

Sexual reproduction involves two functional processes: a special kind of nuclear division, *meiosis,* that reduces the chromosome number from diploid (normal number of chromosomes) to haploid (half the diploid number of chromosomes), and *fertilization,* the fusion of two

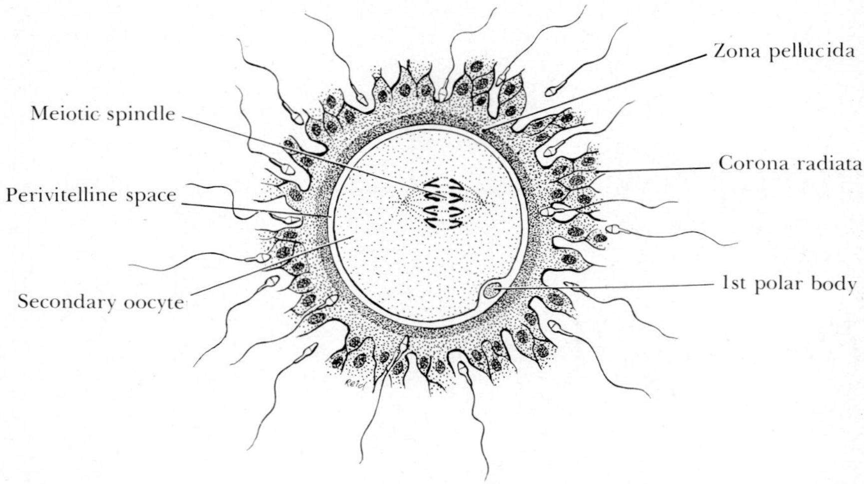

FIGURE 1–1. Secondary oocyte in late metaphase of the second meiotic division. Only 4 of the 23 chromosome pairs are shown. (From Moore, K. *The Developing Human.* Philadelphia: W. B. Saunders Company, 1973, p. 24.)

haploid gametes to form a diploid zygote. Fertilization involves not only the penetration of the egg by the sperm but also the union of egg and sperm nuclei and the activation of the egg to undergo cleavage and development.

During follicular development (p. 358), the oocyte acquires a jelly-like membrane, the *zona pellucida* (Figure 1–1). This membrane probably is secreted by the follicle cells and consists of mucopolysaccharide and trypsin-digestible material which stains with the periodic-acid Schiff (PAS) reaction. At midcycle ovulation occurs; the released egg is surrounded by the *corona radiata,* a layer of granulosa cells (p. 358) which are in close contact with the zona pellucida. Nutrient material passes from these cells by way of tubular processes through the zona pellucida into the *perivitelline space* (Figure 1–1) immediately surrounding the developing egg. The cytoplasm of the ovum itself contains some food reserves, but the human ovum will die within 12 to 24 hours unless fertilized.

Just before ovulation, the first meiotic division is completed, probably triggered by the midcycle surge of luteinizing hormone (LH) from the pituitary gland. The first polar body is found in the perivitelline space next to the ovum. Ovulation occurs in most mammals when the oocyte has reached the metaphase of the second meiotic division (Figure 1–1). The ovum enters the fallopian tube, in the distal third of which fertilization usually occurs.

The sperm move rapidly up the fallopian tube. This fact, plus the enormous number of sperm and the relatively large size of the egg, increases the probability of encounter. There is no evidence that chemotaxis is involved in the meeting of human egg and sperm. In the course of their stay in the female reproductive tract sperm undergo certain changes before they can actually engage in fertilization. The first change is known as *capacitation* and requires about 7 hours in the human. The nature of capacitation is unknown, beyond the fact that it must occur in order for the spermatozoan to penetrate the egg coats. After capacitation the sperm undergo a change in the structure of the acrosome *(acrosome reaction)*. In the process of this alteration the plasma membrane which overlies the acrosome fuses at certain points with the outer membrane of the acrosome. Fusion leads to the formation of openings into the cavity of the acrosome. In this manner acrosomal contents (largely hyaluronidase and a trypsin-like enzyme) can reach the jelly part of the egg coat and dissolve it, thus permitting the spermatozoan to reach the surface of the zona pellucida. The zona pellucida of mammals reacts to sperm penetration so that only one, or at most a few, sperm enter the egg. Passage through the zona pellucida does not seem to involve the actual release of enzymes. A lysin firmly attached to the acrosomal membrane liquefies the zona material, permitting passage of the spermatozoan into the perivitelline space where it fuses with the plasma membrane of the egg. As in other mammals, the whole sperm enters the human egg and may be seen intact for a short time in the egg cytoplasm.

Penetration of the egg by sperm *activates* the egg. Experiments with eggs of sea urchins and other lower animal forms indicate that oxygen consumption increases following fertilization, as does protein synthesis and the activity of the hexose monophosphate shunt (p. 77). The egg cytoplasm becomes violently active, with resulting far-reaching displacements of the cytoplasmic constituents. Sperm penetration also stimulates formation by the egg of the second polar body (second meiotic division). Fusion of egg and sperm nuclei can occur only after the egg nucleus has completed the two meiotic divisions.

Inside the egg the sperm head swells and becomes converted into the male pronucleus. Within about 12 hours the male and female pronuclei meet near the center of the ovum and their nuclear membranes disintegrate. At this time cytoplasm and nucleoplasm communicate with one another and, since the nucleoli disappear at this time, some nucleolar material apparently escapes. There is now considerable evidence that genetic function in lower forms is repressed during very early development. No RNA synthesis can be detected during fertilization; protein synthesis must depend, therefore, upon "long-lived" messenger RNA formed in the oocyte before ovulation. When fertilization is complete, the diploid state is established again and the resulting zygote is ready to divide in the ordinary mitotic way.

CLEAVAGE

The single cell—the fertilized ovum, or zygote—must now be transformed into the multicellular organism. The early cell divisions are called *cleavage* and are characterized by progressive transformation of cytoplasmic substances into nuclear material. This takes place with no change in size or shape of the embryo. At the end of cleavage the ratio of nucleus to cytoplasm, which was very low in the fertilized egg, reaches the value found in ordinary somatic cells.

The first cleavage division in the human egg, forming two approximately equal blastomeres, is not completed until about 30 hours after fertilization. However, once cleavage begins it accelerates as the cells become smaller. The human 4-cell stage is reached about 40 hours after fertilization, and at about 50 to 60 hours the organism consists of a cluster of cells shaped like a mulberry, called a *morula.* These cleavage divisions occur during the three-day period in which the embryo is traversing the fallopian tube.

The number of nuclei, of course, doubles with each cell division. This increase is accompanied by a large increase in DNA, since the amount of DNA per nucleus is constant. Unquestionably, most of the DNA is synthesized from precursors in the cytoplasm. In the normal adult cell there is a period of rest (G1 period) just before DNA synthesis. Studies with mouse embryos have shown that this characteristic G1 period cannot be detected before the 8- to 16-cell stage. Thus in the first cleavage divisions each mitotic division is followed immediately by DNA synthesis in the two daughter cells.

The fact that the embryo does not increase in size during early cleavage divisions does not imply that protein synthesis is halted. Ribosomal RNA is synthesized early in mammalian development, possibly during the first cleavage division. Certainly by the morula stage all cells are making ribosomal RNA rapidly. The ribosomes are important for protein synthesis and some of the protein is used for growth as the morula develops further.

No qualitative changes have been discovered in the chemical composition of developing embryos during cleavage. Obviously, however, the distribution of various cytoplasmic constituents may differ from cell to cell. Experiments with lower animal forms, such as the sea urchin or frog, in which an animal and a vegetal pole can be distinguished, have shown that cytoplasmic substances in the egg are distributed to the daughter cells in relation to local differences in the egg cortex. Therefore the egg cortex provides a pattern for future development of the embryo. We do not know if a similar process of differentiation obtains for the human embryo. In his beautiful studies on early human embryos Hertig has noted differences in the size and appearance of cells as early as the 5-cell stage. He suggests that these differences represent the differentiation of the future embryonic and trophoblastic cells.

By the fourth day the embryo has reached the uterine cavity. Fluid collects within the center of the morula. The whole embryo becomes bloated, and the outer layer of cells, the *chorion,* projects away from all but one of the sides of the *inner cell mass.* A mammalian embryo at this stage is called a *blastocyst* (Figure 1–2). Some of the cells of the blastocyst

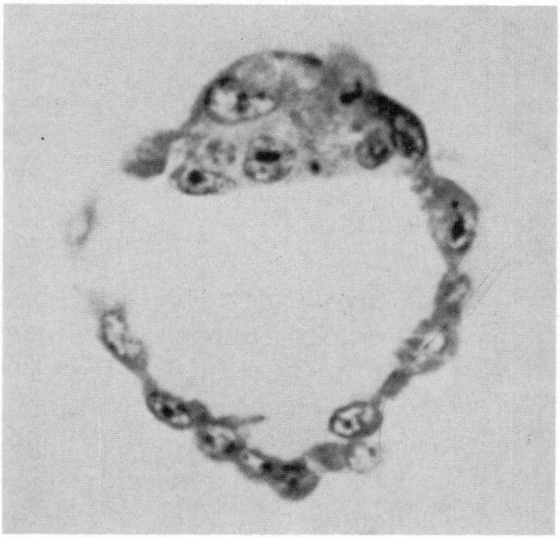

FIGURE 1–2. Photomicrograph of a human blastocyst. (From Reid, D. E. *Principles of Obstetrics.* Philadelphia: W. B. Saunders Company, 1962.)

lie in direct contact with the inner surface of the zona pellucida. Nutrients and oxygenated fluid can pass through the zona pellucida to these cells. Over the following day or two these cells close to the zona pellucida send out cytoplasmic processes in preparation for attachment to the uterine wall. The function of this enveloping layer of cells (chorion) is to form a connection with the maternal uterus and to supply the embryo with nourishment. The cells constituting the chorion at this stage are known as *trophoblastic cells.* These rather specialized cells are large and flattened, with numerous microvilli. Under the electron microscope they are seen as closely spaced cells with membranes linked by tight junctions. This adhesiveness of the trophoblastic cells is in contrast to the cells of the inner cell mass, which are small, round, rapidly dividing cells with minimal mutual adhesion. The inner cell mass is destined to form the embryo and to contribute to the formation of certain of the placental membranes, namely, the amnion and the yolk sac.

Our understanding of the differentiation of the trophoblast and inner cell mass has been enhanced by the study of embryonic development in vitro. The work with mouse embryos has shown that if one cell of a 2-cell embryo is destroyed, the surviving blastomere can give rise to a normal blastocyst; however, only half the usual number of cells is present. The reverse is also possible; that is, two mouse embryos (usually 8-cell) can be fused. Such a double embryo gives rise to a single blastocyst containing twice the normal number of cells. Experiments such as these suggest that there is no special type of cell which is destined from the beginning of cleavage to become the trophoblast (which has been suggested in the preformationist hypothesis). Rather, it appears that environmental influences may be far more important. In the morula stage some cells are in the middle and are surrounded by cells, while other cells are at the periphery and are in contact with the external milieu. Experiments with fused embryos have shown clearly that cells on the "inside" develop into embryonic cells while those on the periphery develop into trophoblastic cells.

IMPLANTATION

As the egg moves down the fallopian tube, the endometrium of the uterus undergoes changes controlled by steroid hormones of the ovaries. As soon as ovulation has occurred, the wall of the ruptured ovarian follicle collapses and the remaining follicular cells are gradually vascularized by vessels growing in from the periphery. The follicular cells then begin to hypertrophy, become polyhedral, and develop a yellowish pigment in a process called *luteinization*. The yellowish luteal cells constitute the *corpus luteum* and secrete progesterone. The latter, together with the estrogenic hormones produced by the theca cells (p. 362) and surrounding ovarian tissue, brings the uterine mucosa to its progestational stage in preparation for implantation of the blastocyst.

If the ovum is fertilized, the trophoblast secretes a peptide hormone, chorionic gonadotropin (p. 23), which prevents the degeneration of the corpus luteum. The corpus luteum of pregnancy grows considerably, some two- to threefold, and remains functional for eight to ten weeks after implantation. It may then disappear slowly or remain throughout the duration of pregnancy with a diminished secretory role, ending finally as a *corpus albicans*.

Progesterone is bound to the uterus, probably by a specific progesterone-binding protein, and its influence on the secretory activity of the endometrium can be observed as early as two to three days after ovulation. The epithelial cells lining the glands show active secretion and discharge their products, including mucin and glycogen, into the lumen. This provides a source of nourishment for the blastocyst. Like the endometrial glands, the arteries become very tortuous and are known as *spiral arteries*. The endometrium itself becomes highly edematous and is usually pale in color as a result of the accumulation of intercellular fluid. The corpus luteum of pregnancy ensures that the secretory activity of the endometrium will continue to increase. The uterine mucosa is then ready to receive the blastocyst.

The precise course of implantation is not known, but it is undoubtedly under the control of a delicate balance between estrogen and progesterone. In the rat, in which delayed implantation may be produced experimentally by castration followed by daily injections of progesterone, only a minute single dose of estrogen is required to induce implantation. In the human, hormones are probably maternal in origin; human blastocysts ($5\frac{1}{2}$ days) maintained in organ culture were unable to produce detectable amounts of estradiol, progesterone, 17α-

hydroxyprogesterone, or chorionic gonadotropin. The blastocyst almost always implants close to a maternal vessel, as though some type of tropism toward maternal blood were involved.

The human blastocyst is ready to implant on the sixth or seventh day after ovulation. The youngest attached human blastocyst described to date has an ovulation age estimated to be not more than 7½ days and is already partially implanted in the endometrium. One might consider the process of implantation as a kind of lying down of the blastocyst on the endometrial surface, with the inner cell mass closest to the endometrium. In response to the attaching blastocyst the uterus undergoes a reaction in which specialized stromal cells increase in size and number and surround the invading embryo. These cells (decidual cells) accumulate glycogen and lipid. The cellular changes, together with the vascular and glandular alterations, are referred to as the *decidual reaction.* Although initially confined to the area around the conceptus, this reaction soon is evident throughout the endometrium.

By the time the blastocyst is definitely attached to the endometrium the zona pellucida disappears in its entirety. The trophoblastic cells then begin to ingest portions of the uterine lining, penetrating into the endometrium. A protease, under the control of progesterone, has been isolated from rabbit blastocysts. This enzyme undoubtedly aids in the penetration of the endometrium. Implantation in the human is interstitial, and in the course of the period between the seventh and twelfth days after ovulation, the blastocyst becomes completely embedded in the uterine endometrium. The trophoblastic shell varies in thickness, that portion below the embryo being thickest.

By 7½ days two types of trophoblastic cells can be distinguished (Figure 1–3). An inner layer of pale, discrete, mononucleate cells constitutes the *cytotrophoblast.* The outer, multinucleate, darker zone is called the *syncytium* and is composed of *syncytiotrophoblastic cells.* The cytotrophoblastic cells are mitotically active, whereas the syncytium never shows mitotic activity. Various studies have shown clearly that nuclei and cytoplasm of the syncytium are derived from cytotrophoblastic precursors, through an intermediary cell type. Presumably, daughter cells of dividing cytotrophoblastic cells fuse to constitute the syncytium. The cytoplasm of the syncytiotrophoblastic cells is highly complex, containing an enormous number of vacuoles, lipid droplets, and ribosomes. The maternal surface of the syncytium is endowed with a complex microvillous structure that increases the exchange surface immensely.

As the cells on the surface of the endometrium dissociate during implantation, the epithelium of the lateral endometrial surfaces begins immediately to cover over the defect caused by the invading blastocyst. Often a small coagulum is formed at the invasion site and implantation bleeding may occur. By the twelfth day the endometrial defect has been closed and the entire embryo is surrounded by endometrium.

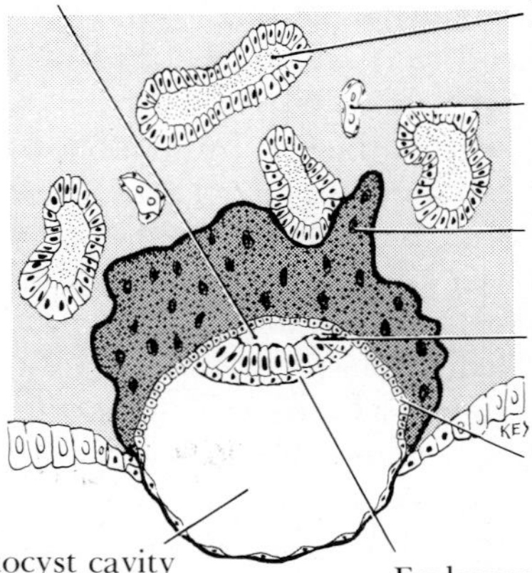

FIGURE 1–3. Drawing of a section through an 8-day blastocyst partially implanted in the endometrium. (From Moore, K. *The Developing Human.* Philadelphia: W. B. Saunders Company, 1973, p. 31.)

DIFFERENTIATION OF THE BLASTOCYST

The first sign of differentiation of the inner cell mass is the appearance of somewhat flattened cells which separate from its inner surface to form the *embryonic endoderm* (Figure 1–3). The remaining cells of the inner cell mass, arranged as a layer of high columnar cells, form the *embryonic ectoderm* Concurrently, stellate mesenchymal cells differentiate from the inner surface of the trophoblastic cells lining the blastocyst cavity. Proliferation of these mesenchymal cells gives rise to the extraembryonic mesoderm, which encroaches on and reduces the relative size of the blastocyst cavity. The cavity has now been converted into a *primitive yolk sac* The inner aspect of the mesenchymal cells forms a membrane, termed *Heuser's membrane* or the *exocoelomic membrane* (Figure 1–4), which is continuous with the embryonic endoderm. Cells from the embryonic endoderm soon grow round the inner aspect of Heuser's membrane, converting the primitive yolk sac into a *definitive yolk sac.*

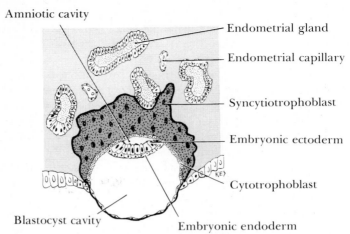

By the eighth day of life small spaces appear between the ectodermal layer of the inner cell mass and the outer covering trophoblast. These spaces coalesce to form the *amniotic cavity* (Figure 1–4). At this early stage the amniotic cavity is much smaller than the yolk sac cavity; however, as gestation proceeds the yolk sac cavity diminishes in size, whereas the amniotic cavity increases until it envelops the entire fetus.

In the succeeding days spaces (lacunae) form within the trophoblast, creating an intercommunicating lacunar network (Figure 1–4). The trophoblastic cells invade the endometrium and erode maternal blood vessels. Maternal blood then seeps into the trophoblastic lacunae, establishing a primitive *uteroplacental circulation.*

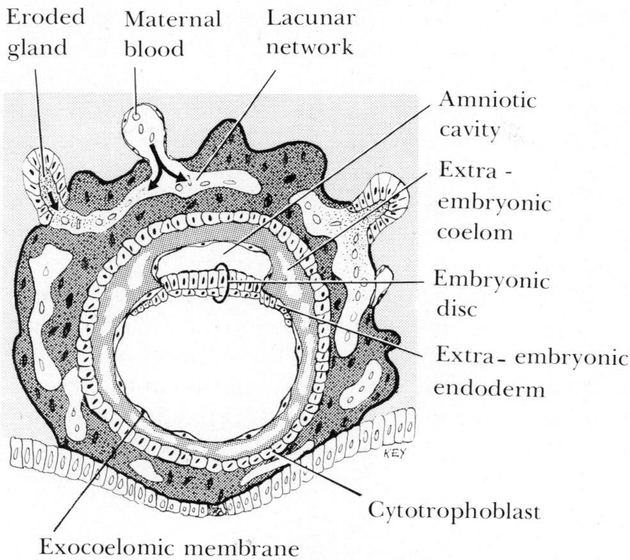

FIGURE 1–4. A completely implanted blastocyst at 12 days gestation. (From Moore, K. *The Developing Human.* Philadelphia: W. B. Saunders Company, 1973, p. 32.)

From mesenchymal cells within the blastocyst cavity connective tissue cells proliferate in finger-like projections into the trophoblast columns, thus providing the fibrous mesodermal core of the future placental villi. At about this time hematopoietic activity commences. Blood vessels and blood cells develop in the primitive yolk sac, while small capillaries differentiate within the mesodermal cores of the trophoblastic villi. The two portions of the fetal vascular system fuse about the twenty-fourth day after fertilization to become the future villous circulation.

The primitive extra-embryonic mesoderm shortly acquires small spaces which coalesce to form the *exocoel* or *extra-embryonic coelom* (Figure 1–4). The extra-embryonic coelom splits the extra-embryonic mesoderm into two layers, an outer somatic layer lining the trophoblast and an inner splanchnic layer covering the yolk sac.

PRIMITIVE STREAK

The next important phase in the development of the embryonic disc is the formation of its *mesodermal germ layer.* At the end of the second week, and becoming more evident by the beginning of the third week, ectodermal cells in the caudal region of the germ disc become spherical, begin to proliferate, and migrate toward the midline. These changes result in the formation of a thickened band of embryonic ectoderm, the *primitive streak,* and within it a narrow groove, the *primitive groove.* The bulging ridges on either side of the primitive groove are clearly visible in a 15- to 16-day-old embryo (Figure 1–5). When fully developed, the primitive streak extends along the posterior half of the embryo. Modified ectodermal cells move toward and migrate into the region of the primitive streak and then leave the basal layer of the primitive streak to move laterally and anteriorly between the ectodermal and endodermal germ layers (Figure 1–6). These cells (mesenchymal cells) form a new intermediate cell layer. This mesodermal germ layer is the last embryonic layer to develop.

As the surface cells are added to the mesodermal germ layer, the layer spreads laterally and eventually becomes continuous with the extra-embryonic mesoderm covering the amnion and yolk sac. Other cells of the intra-embryonic mesoderm migrate anteriorly on each side of the midline until they meet in the most cephalic part of the germ disc in front of the *prechordal plate* (an area in the cephalic region where the

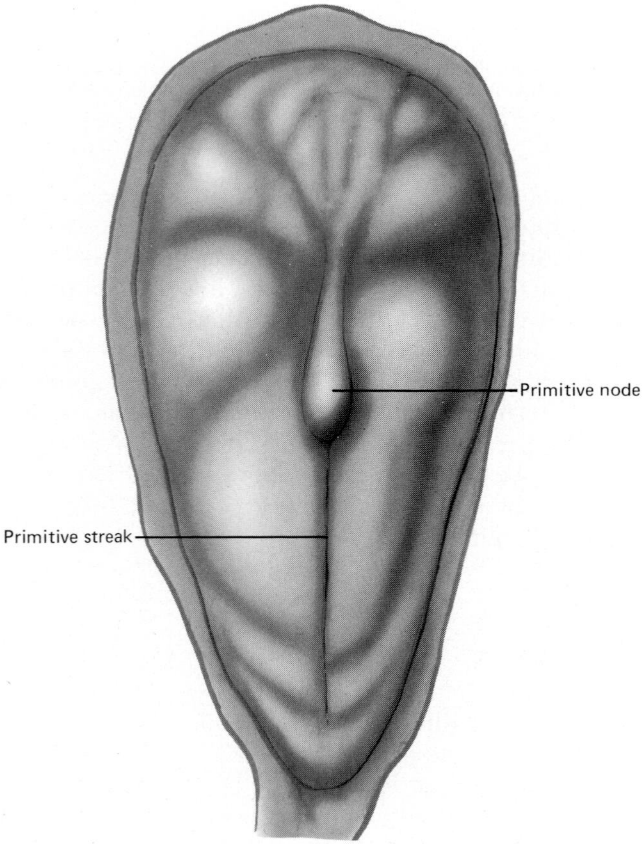

FIGURE 1–5. A dorsal view of a 16-day-old embryonic disc, showing the primitive streak and the primitive node. (From Page, E., Villee, C., and Villee, D. *Human Reproduction.* Philadelphia: W. B. Saunders Company, 1972, p. 226.)

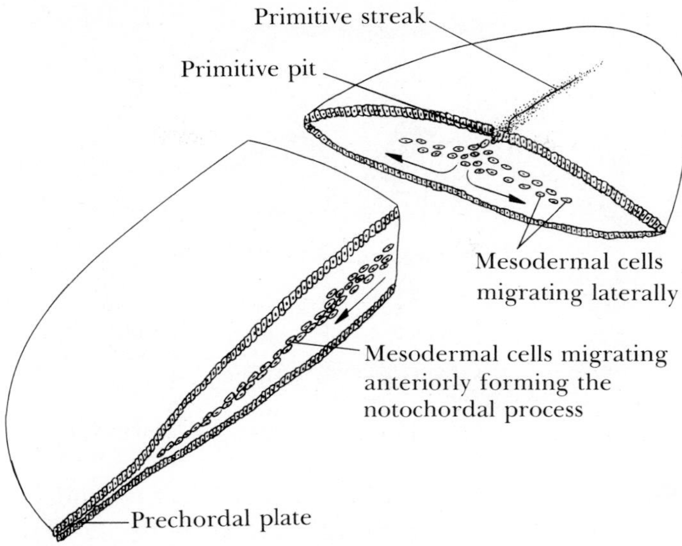

FIGURE 1–6. Perspective view of human embryo at primitive streak stage, showing sagittal and transverse sections.

endoderm is thickened, shown in Figure 1–6). As the primitive streak elongates by addition of cells at its caudal end, its cranial end thickens to form the *primitive node*, containing a small, central, *primitive pit*. The primitive pit is believed to be caused by the invagination of surface cells which then migrate cephalically along the midline until they reach the prechordal plate. Cells migrating from the primitive node to the prechordal plate form a midline cord known as the *notochordal process*. The ectodermal and endodermal layers are so tightly adherent at the prechordal plate that the forward migration of the cells cannot proceed. In 17-day-old embryos the notochordal process extending from the primitive node to the prechordal plate is clearly distinguishable (Figure 1–6). This forms the basis for the axial skeleton of the embryo.

Although the primitive streak regresses caudally after the nineteenth day of development, surface cells continue to invaginate and migrate anteriorly and laterally, forming mesenchyme until the end of the fourth week. At that stage the primitive streak and primitive node show regressive changes and rapidly diminish in size.

Initially the mesodermal cells arising from the primitive streak form a thin sheet of loose tissue on each side of the midline. By about the seventeenth day of development, however, the cells in the cephalic part of the embryo immediately lateral to the notochord proliferate and form a thickened mass of tissue known as the *paraxial mesoderm*. By the end of the third week the paraxial mesoderm forms a bilateral, thickened, longitudinal strip of solid tissue which gradually becomes segmented into blocks of epithelioid cells, the *somites* (Figure 1–7). The first pair of somites appears in the cephalic part of the embryo just caudal to the tip

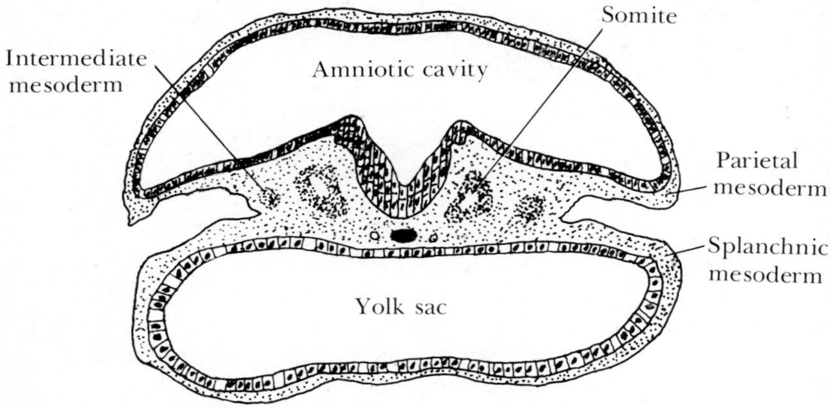

FIGURE 1–7. Transverse section of early human embryo.

of the notochord. Additional somites appear in craniocaudal sequence, and, by the end of the first month, approximately 40 pairs are present. Their formation molds the contours of the embryo, giving it a segmented appearance.

While the paraxial mesoderm is undergoing segmentation, that portion of mesoderm lateral to it *(lateral plate)* becomes split into two layers: an external layer in contact with the ectoderm and known as the *parietal mesoderm* (Figure 1–7), and another layer continuous with the mesoderm covering the yolk sac, known as the *splanchnic mesoderm* (Figure 1–7). Together, these layers line the newly formed intra-embryonic coelomic cavity, which on each side of the embryo is continuous with the extra-embryonic coelomic cavity.

The tissue initially connecting the paraxial mesoderm and the lateral plate, the *intermediate mesoderm* (Figure 1–7), differentiates in a manner entirely unlike that of the somites. In the cervical and upper thoracic regions it forms segmentally arranged cell clusters, whereas more caudally it forms an unsegmented mass of tissue known as the *nephrogenic cord* (p. 59).

The cardiovascular system, an important organ system derived from the mesodermal layer, arises at about the middle of the third week. At that time mesodermal cells located in front and on each side of the most cephalic part of the embryo differentiate into blood and vessel-forming cells which become arranged in isolated clusters of angiogenic cells. These clusters later become canalized, giving rise to centrally located primitive blood cells and peripheral endothelial cells. These *blood islands* eventually fuse to form small blood vessels.

THE FOLDED EMBRYO

During development to this stage the embryo has consisted of a flat, elongated disc; however, as the somites form and the nervous system develops (p. 44), the embryonic disc begins to bulge into the amniotic cavity. The head and tail of the embryo bend toward one another and the amniotic cavity becomes C-shaped (Figure 1–8). This process pinches off the gut from the yolk sac by a narrow neck, the *yolk stalk* (Figure 1–8). When folding is completed the three regions of the gut can be distinguished. The foregut lies cranial to the yolk stalk while the mid- and hindguts lie opposite and caudal respectively, to the yolk stalk. The embryonic disc also undergoes a lateral folding, hence the foregut and hindgut become blind tubes lined with endoderm.

As the embryo folds, an invagination of ectoderm appears at the cranial end, forming the stomodeum (Figure 1–8). The stomodeal ectoderm and the endoderm of the foregut come into contact and fuse to form the *pharyngeal membrane* (Figure 1–8). No mesoderm penetrates between ectoderm and endoderm of the pharyngeal membrane. The latter separates the stomodeum (oral cavity) from the cranial end of the foregut, which now expands to form the pharynx. Then, at the end of the third week, the pharyngeal membrane ruptures, thereby establishing an open connection between the stomodeum and the foregut.

Besides giving rise to part of the oral epithelium, the stomodeal invagination furnishes the cells which give rise to the *adenohypophysis* (p. 37). A solid bud of cells, or a small pocket, *Rathke's pouch,* appears just cranial to the stomodeum and in front of the pharyngeal membrane. This pouch burrows into the mesodermal tissues underlying the forebrain. Rathke's pouch is visible at three weeks as a distinct evagination of the stomodeum. By the end of the second month it loses its connection with the oral cavity and comes into close contact with the infundibulum.

THE *thyroid gland* appears at the seventeenth day of development (the early somite stage) as an epithelial proliferation in the floor of the pharynx between the tuberculum impar (medial swelling which forms part of the tongue) and the copula (a second medial swelling). Shortly thereafter (at 19 days) the thyroid primordium penetrates the underly-

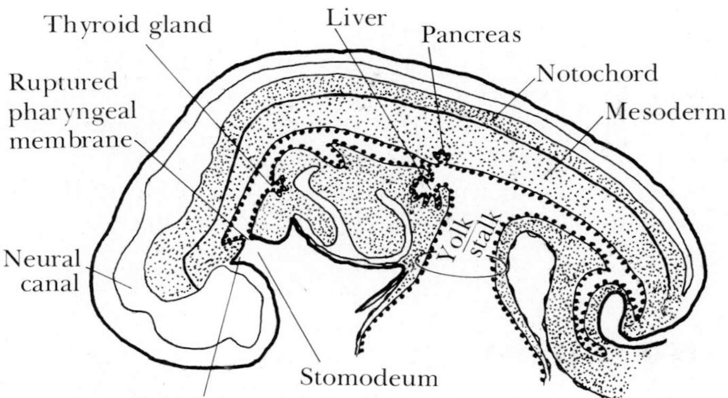

FIGURE 1–8. Diagrammatic longitudinal section of a 4-week-old human embryo.

ing mesoderm and descends in front of the pharynx as a bilobed diverticulum. At first the heart (at this stage the two endocardial tubes have fused to a single endocardial tube) and the pericardium lie immediately ventral to the floor of the pharynx. The thyroid rudiment, growing from the pharyngeal endoderm, comes into close contact with the aortic sac. As the heart and sac draw away from the pharynx so as to leave a mobile neck between the head and the thorax, the thyroid follows for part of the way. It reaches its final position in front of the trachea in the seventh week. The solid stalk of the thyroid rudiment is drawn out to form the *thyroglossal duct,* while the rudiment itself forms two lobes joined by a narrow isthmus. The thyroglossal duct disappears at 7 weeks; however, the lower portion of the duct may contribute to an upward extension of the thyroid gland at the isthmus. This extension is called the *pyramidal lobe* and is present in about half the thyroid glands examined.

In sum, in these first few weeks of development the supply line to the fetus (the placenta) is being formed, the definitive germ layers of the embryo differentiate, and the rudiments of the circulatory system, digestive tract, neural tube, and certain endocrine glands are established. Rathke s pouch has pushed upward from the stomodeum and the cells of the future adenohypophysis are well on their way to joining their neural partners, the forerunners of the posterior pituitary. The pharyngeal diverticulum of the thyroid has formed and is beginning its descent to the trachea. The pharynx itself is undergoing rapid differentiation with the formation of the pharyngeal pouches (see Chapter Three), which eventually contribute to the primordia of the parathyroid glands, the ultimobranchial bodies, and the thymus. Later (at about 26 days) the primordia of the fetal pancreas and liver will develop from the gut. The nephrogenic ridge formed from the intermediate mesoderm has appeared and, as we shall see, plays an important role in the formation of the adrenals and gonads (Chapter Three).

We know little or nothing of the controls of growth and differentiation in the human during this period. There is considerable evidence from lower forms that hormone-like substances from one tissue may induce differentiation of an adjacent tissue. These substances, however, are probably not part of the hormonal regulation seen in the adult organism. Since the endocrine organs of the early embryo have not yet formed, we must suppose that if there are any hormones reaching the embryo, they are maternal or placental in origin. The development of the placenta and its endocrine function will be considered in the following chapter, and the endocrine changes in the mother will be discussed in Chapter Five.

SUGGESTED READING

An Introduction to Embryology, B. I. Balinsky, W. B. Saunders Co., Philadelphia, 1970.
An excellent text, with a particularly good discussion of the details of fertilization and

cleavage. For the student who wants more information on comparative embryology this is probably the best source.

The Developing Human: Clinically-oriented Embryology, Keith L. Moore, W. B. Saunders Co., Philadelphia, 1973.

A very readable, well-illustrated account of human embryology. Clinical examples of aberrations in development are discussed and illustrated. An excellent reference text.

Illustrated Human Embryology, Vol. I, Embryogenesis, H. Tuchmann-Duplessis, P. Haegel (translated by L. S. Hurley), Springer-Verlag, New York, 1972.

This book is available in three volumes *(Vol. II, Organogenesis; Vol. III, Nervous System and Endocrine Glands)* and is an excellent aid for the student of human embryology. The emphasis is on visual presentation. The diagrams and photomicrographs are extremely clear and the text is informative.

Reproduction in Mammals, Book 1, Germ Cells and Fertilization, edited by C. R. Austin and R. V. Short, Cambridge University Press, New York, 1972.

The five books in this series are individually available and provide an excellent survey of reproduction in mammals. In Book 1 details are given of oogenesis, spermatogenesis, ovulation and fertilization. The illustrations are well done and are quite helpful.

CHAPTER TWO

The Placenta

The placenta is an organ consisting of both fetal and maternal tissues. In the human placenta, as in many other mammals, the fetal and maternal components are interdigitated in such a manner as to provide an extensive surface between the two tissues. The basic structural design provides for extensive exchanges of gases and nutrients between maternal blood in the intervillous space and the capillaries of the fetal villi. The chorionic villi, the functional units of the placenta, begin to form at day eleven to twelve, when finger-like projections of masses of trophoblast push out into the lacunae. By day thirteen the chorionic villi contain cores of mesoblastic and angioblastic cells. Once primary villi contain mesenchymal cores, they become "secondary villi." Finally, by the appearance within their mesenchymal cores of embryonic blood vessels, the "secondary villi" are gradually transformed into "tertiary villi" with developing trophoblastic lacunae. The villi begin to branch at about day sixteen. A large volume of blood in the fetal capillaries is brought into juxtaposition with the maternal blood in the intervillous space, but there is no mixing of the two circulations. The two circulations are separated by the endothelium of the fetal capillary with its basement membrane, the stroma of the villi, the trophoblastic basement membrane, the cytotrophoblast, and the syncytiotrophoblast. With advancing gestational age the fetal capillaries invade further and come to lie closer to the syncytiotrophoblast.

In the fourth week of life villi are present over the entire surface of the chorionic sac. All of the villi contain a layer of cytotrophoblast covered with a continuous layer of syncytium. Well-developed blood vessels are found in many of the mesenchymal cores of the villi in the basal and equatorial regions. The decidua can now be divided into three parts. The endometrial lining of the uterus (called the *decidua parietalis*) is about 6 to 8 mm thick at this stage, except at the site of implantation.

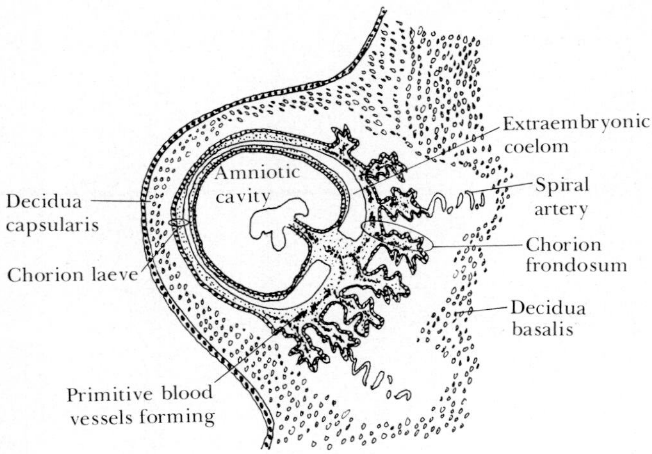

FIGURE 2–1. Diagrammatic sketch to show the interrelationships of fetus, placenta, and endometrium.

The portion of the endometrium underlying the conceptus is called the *decidua basalis,* and that overlying the conceptus the *decidua capsularis* (Figure 2–1).

In the early weeks of development the entire surface of the chorion is covered with villi, but as pregnancy advances only those villi over the embryonic pole continue to grow and expand, giving rise to the *chorion frondosum* Those on the abembryonic pole gradually degenerate, and by the third month this side of the chorion is smooth and is known as the chorion laeve (Figure 2–1).

The placenta has two components: (1) a fetal portion formed by the chorion frondosum and (2) a maternal portion formed by the decidua basalis. On the fetal side the placenta is bordered by the extra-embryonic mesoderm of the chorion (chorionic plate); on its maternal side it is bordered by the decidua basalis, composed of the compact and spongy layers of the endometrium. The portion most closely incorporated into the placenta is the *decidual plate.* Between the chorionic and decidual plates are the intervillous spaces, filled with maternal blood and lined with syncytium of fetal origin. The villous trees grow into these intervillous chorionic blood lakes.

During the fourth and fifth months the decidua basalis forms a number of decidual septa which project into the intervillous spaces but do not reach the chorionic plate. These septa have a core of maternal tissue, but their surface is covered by a layer of trophoblast. The appearance of these septa divides the placenta into a number of compartments or *cotyledons.*

The manner in which the cotyledons receive their blood supply has been a matter of much discussion. It is now generally accepted that the spiral arteries pierce the decidual plate and enter the intervillous spaces at more or less regular intervals. The pressure in these arteries forces the blood well into the intervillous spaces and bathes the numerous small villi of the villous tree with oxygenated blood. Venous openings draining the intervillous spaces are found over the entire surface of the decidual plate, and the blood from the intervillous lakes drains back into the maternal circulation through these openings.

Under normal conditions, at term the intervillous spaces contain approximately 150 ml of blood, which is replenished about three or four times per minute. This blood moves along the chorionic villi; estimates of the surface area of these villi range from 4 to 14 square meters. It must be remembered, however, that placental exchange will take place only in those villi in which the fetal vessels are in intimate contact with the covering syncytial membrane.

METABOLISM OF THE PLACENTA

Establishing a surface for exchange of gases and nutrients is just one of the many functions of the placenta. The trophoblast synthesizes and stores glycogen, and under appropriate stimuli the cells can break down the glycogen, releasing glucose for energy needs. Glycogen synthesis in the placenta (and in muscle and the liver) is enhanced in the presence of insulin. This effect was studied by Demers, who showed that insulin supplementation of the organ culture medium consistently caused an increase in the activity of glycogen synthetase I. This in effect activates the glycogen synthetase enzyme system by shifting from the D (inactive form) to the I (active form) of the enzyme (p. 236). The total amount of synthetase—I plus D forms—was unchanged by insulin. The effect of insulin on glycogen synthetase in the placenta took place irrespective of the glucose concentration in the medium, suggesting a direct effect on the enzyme itself. In addition, insulin has been shown to enhance the transport of glucose into placental tissue under in vitro conditions. It is of special interest that even immature placentas (11 weeks gestation) are responsive to insulin. Actually, immature placentas have significantly higher amounts of total synthetase enzyme than do term placentas. This observation is consistent with a decreased capacity for glycogen synthesis which has been found in the human placenta in the latter stages of pregnancy. Thus, until the fetal liver is mature enough to perform these tasks, the placenta can serve as a source of stored carbohydrate, but as the fetal liver becomes less hematopoietic and more glycogenic the placental stores of glycogen decrease.

In several animal species and probably the human as well, the placenta transfers free fatty acids from mother to fetus. The placenta is capable of incorporating fatty acids and the carbons of glucose into placental triglyceride. It also contains a lipoprotein lipase which is capable of removing free fatty acids from circulating maternal triglycerides. These free fatty acids can be oxidized by placental tissue. It is of interest that although fatty acids are incorporated rapidly into placental glycerides, the actual concentration of triglyceride in the placenta is rather low, suggesting rapid turnover.

The control of triglyceride formation in the placenta is fairly intriguing. The concentration of glucose in the medium has little effect on incorporation of fatty acids into triglyceride in vitro. This may be of some importance in diabetic pregnancies (p. 127). Another point of interest is that lipid synthesis from either pyruvate or glucose in vitro occurs as efficiently under anaerobic as under aerobic conditions, and incorporation of free fatty acids into placental triglyceride is only minimally reduced even by severe anaerobiosis (produced by cyanide). In contrast, adipose tissue is very vulnerable to cyanide. The placenta is dependent on glycolysis to provide α-glycerophosphate (p. 231) for triglyceride synthesis. Agents which inhibit glycolysis, e.g., fluoride, also inhibit triglyceride synthesis.

In addition to serving as a source of stored energy (glycogen, triglyceride), the placenta is involved in the transport of a variety of substances to the fetus. Perhaps most important are glucose for energy and amino acids for growth, but other materials, including drugs, reach the fetus and may exert profound effects on fetal metabolism. The role of the placenta in the transfer of so many materials cannot be covered in detail and will be referred to only as it appears appropriate to the endocrine system.

Human endometrium is capable of synthesizing prostaglandins, and it is entirely possible that the placenta can make this transformation also, since portions of the placenta are derived from endometrium. Prostaglandins have been isolated from human decidua and are present in high concentrations in human umbilical cord blood. Since prostaglandins can cause constriction of placental blood vessels, their release at birth (p. 109) may contribute to the constriction of the umbilical vessels. In contrast to the effects of insulin on glycogen in human placenta, prostaglandin E_2 (p. 83) evoked a glycogenolytic effect in immature placental villi in Demers' in vitro studies. The effect was produced by activation of the enzyme phosphorylase (p. 236), presumably via cyclic AMP (p. 84), since an increase in the concentration of this nucleotide was noted upon exposure of placenta to prostaglandin E_2.

Most interesting of all, from the viewpoint of the endocrinologist, is the ability of the trophoblast of the placenta to synthesize protein hormones and to modify steroid precursors to form large quantities of progesterone and estrogens. Letulle and Larrier, in 1901, were the first to refer to the secretory functions of the placenta. Four years later Halban made a number of observations based on the "active substances" possessed by the placenta. Estrogens were first extracted from the placenta by Laqueur in 1927, followed in 1932 by Mazer and Goldstein's work with progestins. Thus knowledge of the placenta as an endocrine organ is a fairly recent one.

PROTEIN HORMONES OF THE PLACENTA

At the present time only three protein hormones have been demonstrated to be formed by the human placenta: human chorionic gonadotropin, placental lactogen, and placental thyrotropin. The first two have been well characterized and will be discussed in some detail.

HUMAN CHORIONIC GONADOTROPIN (HCG)

Human chorionic gonadotropin has been detected very early in gestation (7 days) and is often used as a diagnostic test of pregnancy. This hormone is a glycoprotein (that is, it contains carbohydrate) and, like the other glycoprotein hormones (follicle-stimulating hormone, luteinizing hormone, and thyrotropin), it consists of two nonidentical subunits. The molecular weight of the entire molecule is about 36,000. The two subunits can be dissociated by incubation either with 10M urea or with 1M propionic acid. The α-subunit of hCG has been found to be a glycoprotein consisting of 92 amino acids which has two sites for carbohydrate attachment; in addition, its amino acid sequence has been determined. When the polypeptide chain of the α-subunit of hCG is aligned with the cysteine residues of the α-subunits of ovine luteinizing hormone and bovine thyrotropin, 72 percent of the amino acid residues of the three hormones are identical.

The larger, β-subunit of hCG is the hormone-specific unit. Unlike the entire hCG molecule, the individual subunits are not concentrated by the ovary and possess no biological activity. A sizeable portion (30 percent) of the hCG molecule is carbohydrate, and the sialic acid moiety is essential for biological activity. The high proline content of the molecule may explain the lack of any extensive α-helical structure.

Another placental glycoprotein hormone, human chorionic thyrotropin, has been described and characterized. Although little is known about the structure of the hormone, it may well be that the human placenta synthesizes two glycoprotein hormones with close structural relationships to their pituitary counterparts.

The concentration of hCG in both maternal blood and urine rises to a maximum during the first trimester and declines thereafter to a low level for the latter portion of pregnancy (Figure 2–2). Very little hCG can be detected in fetal fluids, suggesting that the placenta secretes the hormone primarily to the mother. This does not rule out the possible influence of this hormone on fetal development, particularly at the period of peak production.

Many of the biological effects of hCG are similar but not identical to those of pituitary luteinizing hormone (LH). hCG is capable of inducing ovulation of follicles previously primed by follicle-stimulating hormone (FSH) and LH. Follicular cells are luteinized under the influence of

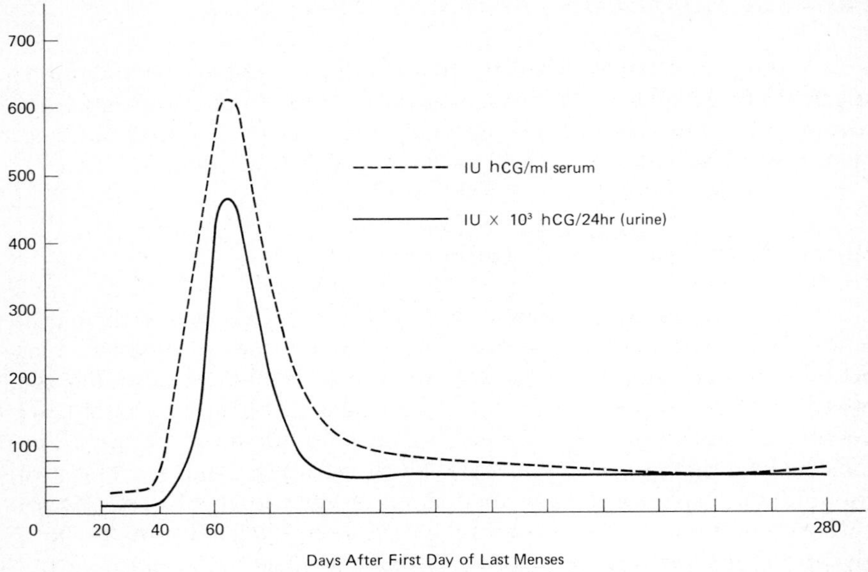

FIGURE 2–2. The concentrations of human chorionic gonadotropin (hCG) in serum and in urine as a function of the length of gestation. (From Page, E., Villee, C., and Villee, D. *Human Reproduction.* Philadelphia: W. B. Saunders Company, 1972, p. 236. The figure is a redrawing of data presented by Albert and Berkson, 1951.)

hCG, and the corpus luteum formed during the menstrual cycle or in pregnancy is stimulated to produce more progesterone when hCG is added in vitro or in vivo. The actual lifespan of the corpus luteum is extended beyond its usual duration by hCG. In the testis, a comparable LH-like stimulation of interstitial cells occurs under the influence of hCG. This latter effect is of importance when considering the role of hCG in the development of the fetal testis (see Chapter 3).

The molecular basis of these gonadal effects is not fully known. Some effects of hCG are abolished by inhibitors of RNA and protein synthesis, suggesting a locus of action involving protein (enzyme) synthesis. Cyclic AMP, LH, and hCG raise luteal progesterone production, and this increase is associated with expanded RNA and protein synthesis. Thus cyclic AMP may be an intracellular messenger for LH and hCG. Certainly a major consequence of the effect of hCG on gonads is increased steroid production, but at what phase of the biosynthetic pathway this effect occurs is still unknown. There is some evidence which suggests an effect on one of the steps in the conversion of cholesterol to pregnenolone (p. 157).

Cedard has found a stimulation of estrogen synthesis in the perfused placenta as a result of the addition of hCG (or LH) to the perfusion fluid. She postulates that LH or hCG stimulates adenyl cyclase (p. 361), increasing the intracellular cyclic AMP, which in turn increases the amount of active phosphorylase kinase (p. 236). Such an effect would increase the breakdown of glycogen, yielding more glucose-6-phosphate. The latter, by its metabolism via the pentose pathway (p. 77), produces increased amounts of NADPH. The hydrogen from NADPH would be available for steroid hydroxylation and aromatization. In the placental perfusion system of Cedard, cyclic AMP mimicks the effects of LH or hCG on estrogen synthesis.

Recently hCG was shown to stimulate the incorporation of ^{14}C-adenine into ^{14}C-cyclic AMP in the term placenta, further implicating adenyl cyclase as a site of action. Such a stimulation of adenyl cyclase by hCG is in agreement with the findings of Demers. He determined that hCG (50 to 250 IU/ml) caused an acute glycogenolytic response in placental tissue in vitro, coupled with a decrease in placental glycogen concentration and an increase in placental cyclic AMP concentration. Demers studied the inactive and active glycogen phosphorylases (p. 236) and noted a shift from the inactive to active form of the enzyme with hCG stimulation. This would be compatible with Cedard's theory of an effect of cyclic AMP on the phosphorylase phosphokinase (p. 236).

Thus the placental hormone hCG, perhaps via adenyl cyclase, enhances the synthesis of steroids in the gonads as well as in its own cells. The possibility that the placenta controls its own steroid synthesis is an intriguing one but so little is known that we can only speculate at present. By means of its gonadal effects, hCG prolongs the life span of the corpus luteum and possibly exerts an influence on the developing fetal gonads.

In addition to the normal trophoblast of pregnancy, trophoblastic tumors can form hCG. These tumors vary from the relatively benign *hydatidiform mole* to the locally invasive *chorioadenoma destruens* or the malignant *choriocarcinoma.* An elevated titer of hCG, exceeding 50,000 IU in the early weeks of pregnancy or values of 20,000 to 100,000 IU after the ninetieth day of pregnancy, is highly suggestive of hydatidiform mole. Both malignant and benign tumors are capable of metastasis. The most definitive diagnosis of a molar pregnancy is obtained by the use of intrauterine radiopaque material. A "motheaten" or "honeycomb" pattern of the roentgenogram is suggestive of the disease. The uterus is usually large for the stage of pregnancy and the fetus cannot be detected on x-ray examination. A roentgenogram of the chest may reveal metastases.

The hydatidiform molar tissues must be promptly removed from the uterus, but for several days prior to removal of the tumor, prophylactic chemotherapy with methotrexate (a folic acid antagonist) is used. The therapeutic use of methotrexate is based on the observation that uterine growth in response to estrogen administration fails to occur in the absence of folic acid. Fetal tissues are even more sensitive to the lack of folic acid; therefore, trophoblastic tissue might be expected to respond to doses of antagonists which are not harmful to other tissues.

This is indeed the case, and the use of methotrexate in conjunction with careful weekly assays for gonadotropins and frequent chest x-rays is the accepted therapeutic regimen and will bring about a remission and probable cure of metastatic disease in over 90 percent of patients. Actinomycin D is another effective agent, and in patients with hepatic dysfunction it is the preferred chemotherapeutic agent. Whatever chemotherapy is used, after the mole is removed the patient is observed at frequent intervals. Urinary or serum hCG should be negative within six weeks after removal of the molar tissue. If hCG can be detected in blood or urine after this period, invasive trophoblastic disease must be considered.

Human placental lactogen (hPL)

In contrast to hCG, hPL does not appear to have a carbohydrate moiety. It is a polypeptide of 191 amino acids with a molecular weight of about 20,000. Its amino acid composition and primary structure are very similar to those of growth hormone and prolactin. It is not surprising, therefore, that hPL has both growth-promoting and lactogenic properties. Preparations of the hormone can cause lactation in pseudopregnant rats and positive reactions in assays of the pigeon crop-sac (an analogue of the mammalian breast). The experiments of Turkington have shown that hPL (in combination with insulin and cortisol) stimulates the synthesis of casein and other proteins in cultures of mammary epithelial cells.

In hypophysectomized rats, the width of the tibeal epiphyseal cartilage increases after administration of hPL; however, this growth-promoting action of hPL is much weaker than that evoked by comparable doses of growth hormone. Mammotropic and luteotropic actions of hPL have also been documented.

A variety of metabolic changes in pregnancy have been ascribed to the action of hPL. Its administration in vivo increases the rate of lipolysis and the concentration of free fatty acids in the plasma. Experiments with rats in vivo and in vitro have shown that hPL has the following biological characteristics: strong lipolytic action, acceleration of insulin secretion, promotion of glucose uptake by the fat pad, and activation of hormone-sensitive lipase and lipoprotein lipase in the fat pad. These results could be mimicked with cyclic AMP, suggesting that hPL exerts its lipolytic action by stimulating adenyl cyclase. It has been postulated that by shifting maternal metabolism to the utilization of fat, hPL enhances the availability of glucose and amino acids to the fetus.

There seems no doubt that hPL and hCG are synthesized solely by trophoblastic tissue. In vitro cultures of placental fragments can form labeled hormone from ^{14}C-labeled amino acids. By immunofluorescent techniques, the syncytiotrophoblast has been implicated in the synthesis of these hormones. Moreover, hPL is present in hydatidiform moles and in choriocarcinomas.

Very little is known about the factors which regulate the synthesis and secretion of hPL. In several studies, the concentration of hPL in maternal serum could be correlated with placental weight, whereas in other studies no correlation was found. As there is considerable variation in different placental fragments in the synthesis of hPL in vitro, factors within the trophoblastic cells may govern hPL production. Recently, Tyson and his associates showed that the concentration of hPL in maternal serum was consistently higher in mothers undergoing prolonged food deprivation than that in mothers on complete diets. Prolonged fasting can be mimicked in vitro by adjusting the culture medium. Friesen and his colleagues found that under such conditions the synthesis and secretion of hPL increased. This effect of starvation on hPL concentration would lead to enhanced fat mobilization in the calorically deprived mother.

The concentration of hPL in maternal serum rises throughout pregnancy and attains values of 7000 to 8000 ng/ml (Figure 2–3). In con-

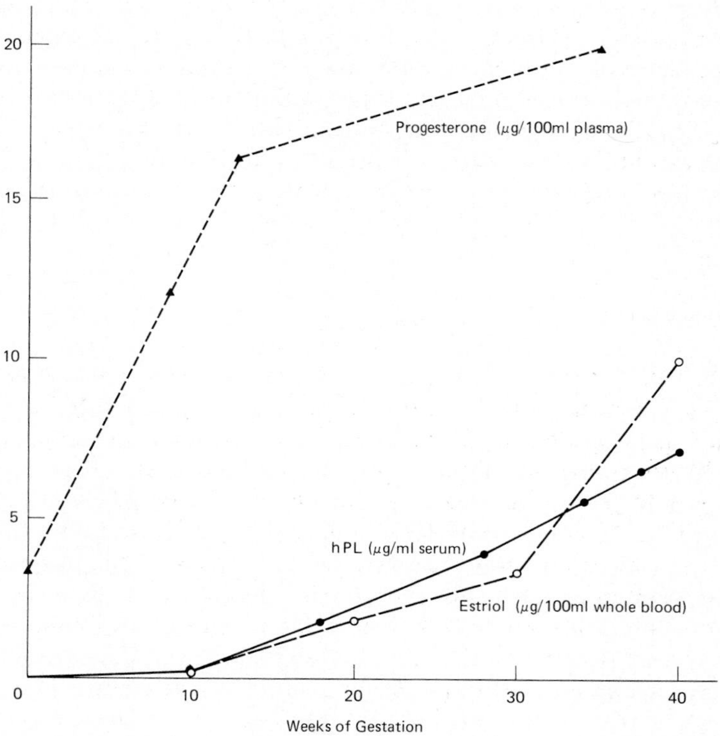

FIGURE 2–3. Concentration of progesterone, estriol and human placental lactogen (hPL) in blood or serum as a function of the length of gestation. (From Page, E., Villee, C., and Villee, D. *Human Reproduction.* Philadelphia: W. B. Saunders Company, 1972, p. 238. The figure is a redrawing of data presented by Selenkow, 1969.)

trast, the concentration in amniotic fluid is much lower, and very little hPL can be detected in cord blood. The hormone disappears rapidly from maternal blood postpartum.

So far, placental lactogen has been isolated and purified from placentas of primates only. Its increased concentration in the serum of pregnant monkeys as gestation proceeds is quite comparable to the condition in humans.

At the present time there is no convincing evidence for the formation of other protein hormones in the placenta. Extracts of placental tissue possess slight corticotropic activity; however, there is no real indication that the placenta synthesizes an ACTH-like hormone. Nevertheless, the synthesis of hCG (LH-like), hCT (thyrotropin-like), and hPL (growth hormone-like) by the placenta should suggest the possibility that other protein hormones related to the hormones of the adenohypophysis may also be produced by placental tissue.

STEROID HORMONES OF THE PLACENTA

There is a dramatic rise in the production of estrogens and progestins in pregnancy (Figure 2–3). There is little doubt that the placenta plays a major role in the production of these steroid hormones. However, since total synthesis of either progesterone or the estrogens occurs to a very limited and probably insignificant extent, the placenta is considered an incomplete steroidogenic organ. It apparently puts the "finishing touches" on steroid precursors arriving from the mother or the fetus.

PROGESTERONE

The role of the placenta in the production of progesterone in pregnancy has been suspected for some time. During pregnancy increasing amounts of progesterone are found in placental tissue as well as in maternal blood and urine (Figure 2–3). Zander has shown that there is a steady rise in the progesterone content of the whole placenta in pregnancy, while the concentration per microgram of tissue is constant between the fourth and tenth months of pregnancy. The progesterone concentration in maternal blood and urine declines after delivery of the placenta, suggesting a placental origin for progesterone. Progesterone is elevated in pregnancy even in the absence of pituitary, ovary, and adrenals—again suggesting placental origin. Measurements of progesterone show that its concentration is higher in effluent blood leaving the placenta than it is in maternal or fetal blood. Even after death or delivery of the fetus, progesterone concentrations in maternal blood and urine do not fall, but rather remain elevated until delivery of the placenta.

At this point, before we begin discussing the synthesis of progesterone, it might be helpful to review some aspects of steroid biochemistry. Steroids represent a group of tetracyclic compounds which are sterol-like in structure. The sterols are secondary alcohols containing 27 to 30 carbon atoms which differ from other alcohols in that they are crystalline solids (Gr. *stereos,* solid). The only major sterol of higher animals is cholesterol, a monounsaturated sterol with the formula $C_{27}H_{45}OH$. It is a constituent of all normal tissues; the total amount present in a man weighing 80 kg is about 240 g. It is present in part as the free alcohol and in part esterified with long chain fatty acids.

Cholesterol can be synthesized from acetate by a variety of tissues including liver, adrenal, gonads, and placenta; however, it must be remembered that cholesterol can also be derived from the diet. The actual biosynthesis of cholesterol takes place primarily in the liver and is a stepwise process using acetyl coenzyme A as the precursor. By labeling either the carboxyl or methyl carbons of acetate (which is converted to acetyl CoA), it was possible to trace the assemblage of this complex sterol in the liver. One of the early intermediates in the biosynthetic sequence (Figure 2–4), *mevalonic acid,* was actually discovered by Folkers and his colleagues as a growth factor for *Lactobacillus acidophilus.* This six-carbon compound is formed by the condensation of three molecules of acetyl CoA, which yields β-hydroxy-β-methyl glutaryl CoA (Figure 2–4). This in turn is reduced, by reactions requiring NADPH, to mevalonic acid. This step (hydroxymethylglutaryl reductase) is the "committed" step in cholesterol synthesis, at which point those dietary and other factors controlling the overall rate at which cholesterol is synthesized now act (p. 426).

Mevalonic acid is phosphorylated in three steps by ATP and then decarboxylated to yield isopentenyl pyrophosphate, a five-carbon compound (Figure 2–4). The latter is the active *isoprene unit* which condenses with another isopentenyl unit, 3,3-dimethylallyl pyrophosphate, to yield the ten-carbon compound *geranyl pyrophosphate.* The condensation of geranyl pyrophosphate with another isopentenyl pyrophosphate yields *farnesyl pyrophosphate* with fifteeen carbons. The condensation of two fifteen-carbon intermediates yields the thirty-carbon compound *squalene.*

Squalene, a *triterpene* originally found in shark oil, is known to be present in a variety of mammalian tissues. It can be cyclized ("zipped up") to *lanosterol* by an interesting reaction that requires molecular oxygen and NADPH and is catalyzed by squalene oxidocyclase (Figure 2–4). "Activated" oxygen makes an electrophilic attack on the carbon that will become carbon 3 in the sterol and forms an epoxide. This is followed by a series of interactions of electrophilic centers with the electrons of certain double bonds, which leads to the formation of carbon-carbon bonds and the production of the tetracyclic nucleus without any intermediate products being isolatable.

The conversion of lanosterol to cholesterol involves the removal of three angular methyl groups, the saturation of the double bonds in the

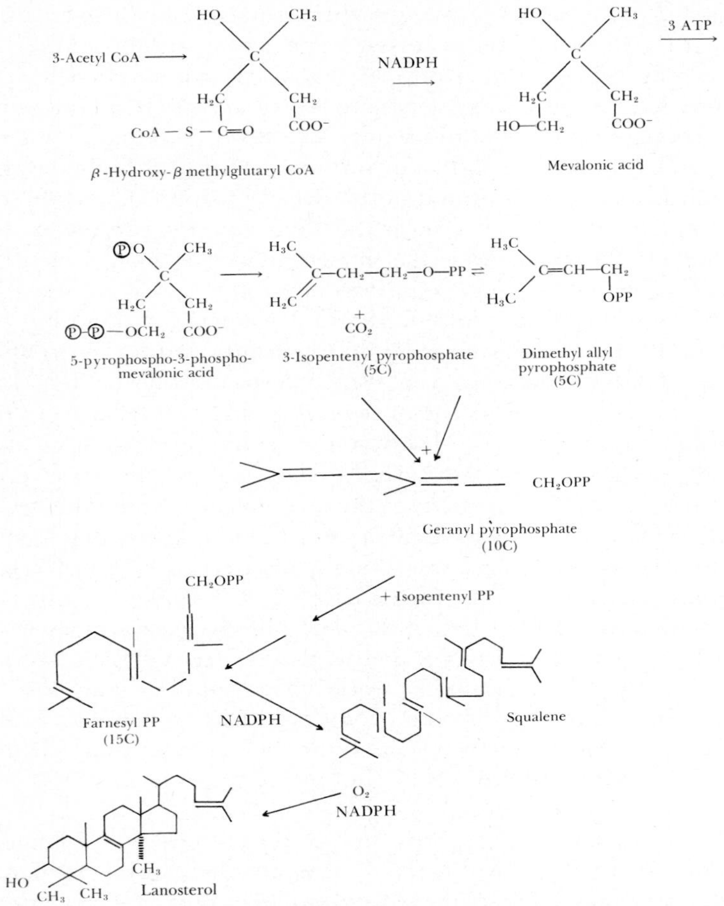

FIGURE 2–4. The synthesis of the sterol nucleus from acetyl coenzyme A by reactions involving the condensation of six molecules of isopentenyl pyrophosphate. (Adapted from Page, E., Villee, C., and Villee, D. *Human Reproduction.* Philadelphia, W. B. Saunders Company, 1972, p. 49.)

side chain and at the juncture of rings B and C, and the introduction of a double bond at position 5,6. These several processes apparently may occur in almost any order.

Although the placenta possesses the enzymes needed for the biosynthesis of cholesterol from acetate, the extent of transformation is very small, and it has been shown in vivo that maternal blood cholesterol is used in preference to endogenous cholesterol for the synthesis of progesterone in the placenta. In contrast, the gonads and adrenal glands synthesize considerable amounts of cholesterol.

In order to remove the side chain from cholesterol to form the steroid *pregnenolone*, the carbon atoms at positions 20 and 22 must first be hydroxylated (Figure 2–5). Enzymes which hydroxylate steroids are specific for each carbon atom of the steroid skeleton, and indeed are specific for carbon bonds above the plane of the molecule or below the plane of the molecule. Since the entire steroid skeleton (the four rings) is relatively flat, substitutents such as hydroxyl groups (OH) or methyl groups (CH_3) may be in either position. The two methyl groups of cholesterol on the steroid nucleus, for instance, lie above the plane of the molecule and are depicted conventionally as solid lines projecting from carbons 10 and 13 (Figure 2–5). The methyl carbons themselves become carbons 18 and 19 of the steroid nucleus. By convention all other substituents are referred to the methyl carbon 19. This, the reference carbon, is designated as β, and substituents also projecting up from the plane of the molecule (on the same side or *cis*) are termed β. Those projecting to the opposite side of the molecule *(trans)* are termed α. Ring fusions may be cis (substituents on same side) or trans (substituents on opposite side). In all natural steroids the fusions between rings B and C and between

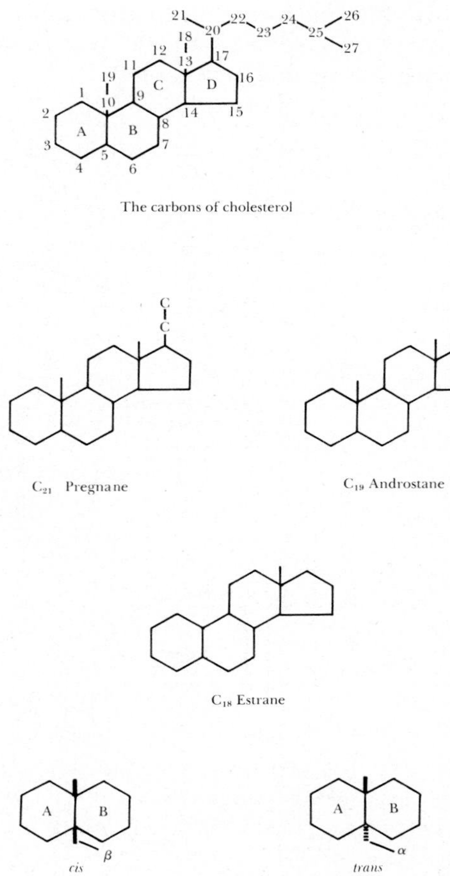

FIGURE 2–5. The numbering system of the carbons in the sterol molecule and the structures of the parent compounds, pregnane, androstane, and estrane.

rings C and D are trans, whereas the fusion between rings A and B may be either cis or trans (Figure 2–5).

The enzyme 20α-hydroxylase catalyzes the hydroxylation of carbon 20 of cholesterol. A separate enzyme, 22-hydroxylase, catalyzes the hydroxylation of cholesterol at carbon 22. Either 20α-hydroxycholesterol or 22-hydroxycholesterol may be converted to 20α,22-dihydroxycholesterol. The latter undergoes a cleavage of the 20-22 carbon-to-carbon bond (catalyzed by C20,22-desmolase), yielding a ketone (pregnenolone) and an aldehyde (isocaproic aldehyde). Pregnenolone is a precursor for all the steroid hormones. It is a twenty-one-carbon steroid of the pregnane series (Figure 2–5). Because of the presence of a double bond at the 5,6 position the suffix *-ene* is used instead of *-ane* (the latter designates a completely saturated molecule). In addition pregnenolone has a ketone group denoted by the suffix *-one* and an alcohol group denoted by the suffix *-ol*. Thus the correct chemical name for pregnenolone is pregn-5-ene-3β-ol-20-one. The position of the alcohol group may also be designated by the prefix "hydroxy"; thus pregnenolone may be termed 3β-hydroxy-pregn-5-ene-20-one. It may be oxidized to progesterone by the 3β-hydroxysteroid dehydrogenase-isomerase enzyme system (Figure 2–6). Progesterone also belongs to the pregnane series (pregn-4-ene-3,20-dione).

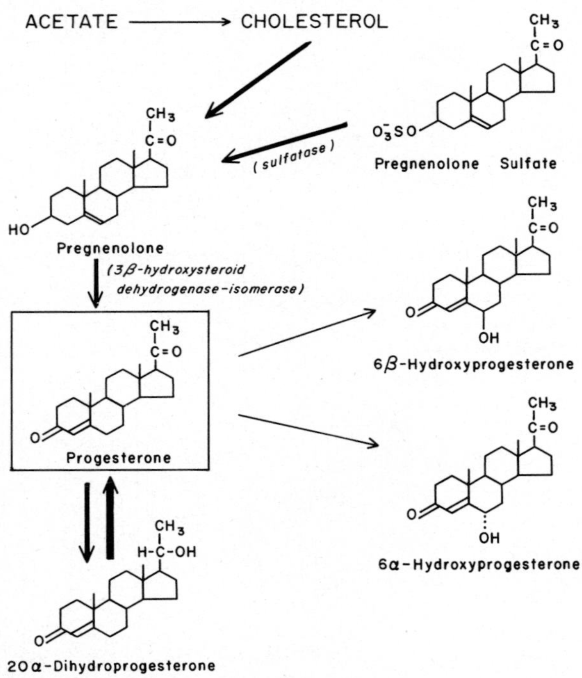

FIGURE 2–6. The synthesis and metabolism of progesterone in the human placenta. (From Page, E., Villee, C., and Villee, D. *Human Reproduction.* Philadelphia: W. B. Saunders Company, 1972, p. 239.)

Many investigations have shown that the human placenta can convert cholesterol or pregnenolone to progesterone in large yield. Following perfusion of mid-term placentas in situ with pregnenolone, 85 percent of the substrate was converted to progesterone. Judging from in vitro incubations, cholesterol appears to be an efficient precursor of progesterone also. Thus the following enzymes are undoubtedly present in placenta: 20α-hydroxylase, 22-hydroxylase, C20,22-desmolase, 3β-hydroxysteroid dehydrogenase, and 5-4 isomerase. The latter enzyme is involved in the shift of the double bond of pregnenolone from the 5,6 position (Δ5) to the 4,5 position (Δ4) as seen in progesterone (Figure 2–6). In the intact feto-maternal-placental unit the source of the cholesterol or pregnenolone is probably maternal blood.

In many tissues progesterone can be hydroxylated by 17α-hydroxylase and the resulting 17α-hydroxyprogesterone can undergo side chain cleavage (C17-20-desmolase) to form the nineteen-carbon androgen androstenedione (androstane series, Figure 2–5). However, our present evidence indicates that the human placenta has little or no 17α-hydroxylase or C17-20-desmolase. The placenta does have a very active 20α-hydroxysteroid dehydrogenase which can catalyze the reduction of progesterone to 20α-dihydroprogesterone (Figure 2–6). This reaction is a reversible oxidation-reduction and progesterone can be reformed from 20α-dihydroprogesterone.

ESTROGENS

Estrogens are eighteen-carbon steroid hormones. They are formed ordinarily from twenty-one-carbon precursors via nineteen-carbon androgens. Since the human placenta has little or no 17α-hydroxylase or C17-20-desmolase, the estrogens formed in the placenta cannot be produced from twenty-one-carbon precursors. This is documented by in vitro studies which have shown that estrogens can be formed in placental tissue only if nineteen-carbon precursors are provided. Dehydroepiandrosterone (Figure 2–7) serves as an excellent precursor of estrone and estradiol. Similarly, either androstenedione or testosterone (farther along the estrogen pathway) can serve as precursors of estrone and estradiol respectively. None of these nineteen-carbon precursors, however, is converted to estriol in the placenta. In order to form estriol, estradiol or a nineteen-carbon precursor must be hydroxylated at the 16 position. The placenta lacks 16α-hydroxylase and can form estriol only when supplied with precursors already hydroxylated at carbon 16. If 16α-hydroxydehydroepiandrosterone, 16α-hydroxyandrostenedione, or 16α-hydroxytestosterone are used as substrates in placental incubations, estriol is formed in good yield (Figure 2–7).

The estrogen precursors used by the placenta to synthesize estrogens arrive in that tissue in the form of sulfo-conjugates. The placenta is rich in sulfatases and the sulfate group is readily removed from

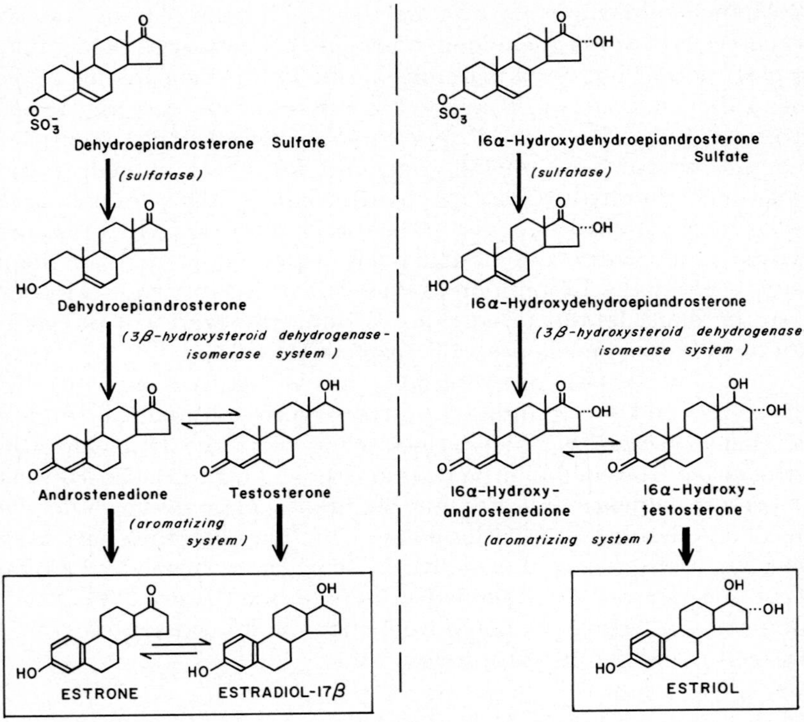

FIGURE 2–7. Diagram of the reactions by which estrogens are synthesized in the human placenta. Note the absence of 16α-hydroxylase in the human placenta. (From Page, E., Villee, C., and Villee, D. *Human Reproduction.* Philadelphia: W. B. Saunders Company, 1972, p. 241.)

the steroid molecule. For example, dehydroepiandrosterone sulfate is rapidly converted to free dehydroepiandrosterone (Figure 2–7), which can undergo conversion to estrone or estradiol. Steroids with the Δ5-3β-hydroxy configuration are usually conjugated in the 3 position; therefore, pregnenolone, 17-hydroxypregnenolone, and dehydroepiandrosterone usually reach the placenta as 3-sulfates. Though the placenta can remove sulfate groups, it has no sulfokinase to catalyze the conjugation of free steroids.

As with the protein hormones, the placental steroids are elaborated in the cytoplasm of the syncytial trophoblast. That the production of estrogen and progesterone in these cells of the placenta begins after the fortieth day from the last menstrual period is inferred from the steep rise of steroids after this time and from hormone determinations after removal of both maternal ovaries in pregnancy. Before this time, ovariectomy results in decreased excretion of estrogen and pregnanediol (the excretory product of progesterone) and abortion frequently ensues.

SUMMARY

The placenta forms progesterone from maternal cholesterol or pregnenolone and estrogens from nineteen-carbon precursors. There is little or no evidence for 17α-hydroxylase, 16α-hydroxylase, C17-20-desmolase, or sulfokinase (which transfers a sulfate group from phosphoadenosine phosphosulfate to the OH group at carbon 3) in the human placenta. Attempts to isolate glucocorticoids after incubations of placenta with appropriate substrates suggest that 21- and 11β-hydroxylases are also lacking. The placenta does, however, metabolize progesterone, primarily to 20α-dihydroprogesterone and 6β-hydroxyprogesterone, with minor amounts of 6α-hydroxyprogesterone (Figure 2–6). There is no indication that any reduction of the double bond in ring A of progesterone occurs.

The unique capability of the human placenta to form *both* protein and steroid hormones, as well as its vital function in gas exchange and fetal nutrition, justifies the enormous interest in this reproductive organ. Just when in its very early development it assumes its endocrine role is unknown, but it is quite likely that the original trophoblastic cells of the blastocyst possess the enzymes required for the synthesis of placental hormones. As we shall see later (Chapter Five), the interplay between the placenta and fetus in steroid metabolism is extensive. The fetus supplies many of the precursors needed for estrogen synthesis and the placenta probably provides the fetus with progesterone for adrenal synthesis of the steroid hormone cortisol. The role of the placental protein hormones in the control of maternal metabolism and fetal development will be discussed in the same chapter.

SUGGESTED READING

The Human Placenta, J. D. Boyd and W. J. Hamilton, W. Heffer and Sons Ltd., Cambridge, England, 1970.

A superbly written and illustrated reference text on the development of the human placenta. The electron micrographs and illustrations are excellent. The emphasis is on morphology with an opening chapter giving a nice historical survey.

Scientific Foundations of Obstetrics and Gynecology, E. E. Philipp, J. Barnes, and M. Newton, F. A. Davis Co., Philadelphia, 1970.

Several chapters in this large reference text are devoted particularly to the placenta. In Section III there is an excellent chapter by W. D. Billington on the Trophoblast and another by Hamilton and Boyd on the Development of the Human Placenta. In the section on endocrinology (X), Amoroso and Porter cover the endocrine functions of the placenta. Their approach includes other species and provides the reader with an opportunity to compare placental hormones in different species. Relaxin, a hormone of pregnancy synthesized in ovaries and placentas of several mammalian species but not the human, is discussed also.

Human Reproduction, E. Page, C. Villee, and D. Villee, W. B. Saunders Co., Philadelphia, 1972.

Chapters 8 and 11 provide discussions of the morphology and endocrinology, respectively, of the human placenta. The reader may find this less exhaustive coverage of the subject easier to assimilate.

CHAPTER THREE

The Development of the Endocrine Glands of the Fetus

Once the conceptus is well implanted in the uterine endometrium and differentiation of the three embryonic layers has begun, the emergence of endocrine tissue can be traced. Glands of internal secretion are derived from all three germ layers: ectoderm, endoderm, and mesoderm. Endocrine derivatives of neuroectoderm (pituitary, pineal, hypothalamus, calcitonin-secreting cells, adrenal medulla) will be considered first.

ECTODERMAL ENDOCRINE TISSUE

THE ADENOHYPOPHYSIS

The adenohypophysis is made up of an anterior and an intermediate lobe. It is derived from the primitive oropharynx as an evagination called Rathke's pouch (Chapter One). It becomes separated from the oral cavity during early development and ultimately lies in apposition to the neural lobe of the pituitary (p. 48). This endocrine gland produces 10 different hormones, some of which control the secretory function of other endocrine glands (Figure 3–1). It is believed that most of the hormones of the anterior pituitary are produced by unique cell types; thus the cytology is very complex.

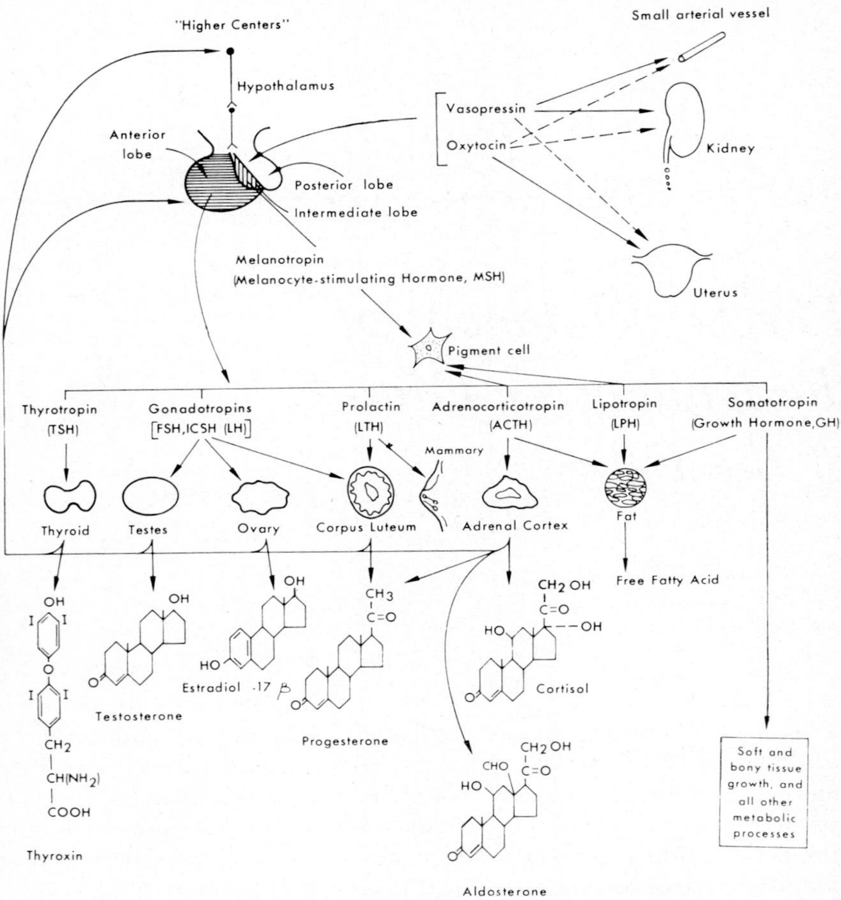

FIGURE 3–1. Diagrammatic summary of biological properties of pituitary hormones. (From Li, C. H. Proceedings of the American Philosophical Society, 1972, *116*: p. 366.)

Morphology

Cytologic differentiation of the anterior pituitary begins at about 8 weeks gestation; by the tenth week all specialized cell types are distinguishable. Studies of the ultrastructure of cells of the rat hypophysis showed that cells can be distinguished by the size and shape of their secretory granules. In addition, these granules show different affinities for histological stains. Some of the cells are basophilic (i.e., they show an affinity for basic dyes) while other pituitary cells are acidophilic (showing an affinity for acidic dyes). Two types of acidophilic cells in the adult pituitary can be distinguished by electron microscopy. One, which secretes growth hormone, is a rounded cell in which the cytoplasm is packed with dense, round acidophilic granules. These granules have been isolated by differential centrifugation and have been found to have a high content of growth hormone (GH). Another type of acidophil stains deeply with carmine and contains granules that are larger and more ovoid than are the granules in the GH-secreting cells. These cells, which probably secrete prolactin, are found in significant numbers only in pregnancy and in the postpartum period.

Other hormones of the anterior pituitary such as thyrotropin (thyroid-stimulating hormone, or TSH), follicle-stimulating hormone (FSH), and luteinizing hormone (LH) are elaborated in specific basophilic cells.

A number of cells in the anterior pituitary lack secretory granules and do not stain with either basic or acidic dyes. Some of these chromophobe cells, when examined under the electron microscope, show granules which are not detected under light microscopy. It is not certain whether adrenocorticotropic hormone (ACTH) is secreted by chromophobes or by basophils; hyperactivity of the adrenal gland has been noted in patients with chromophobe adenomas and in patients with basophilic adenomas. It is usually considered that ACTH and melanocyte-stimulating hormone (MSH) are secreted by basophilic cells. The cells which form MSH, however, are located in the intermediate lobe of the adenohypophysis.

Biochemistry

Growth Hormone. Human growth hormone, or somatotropin, is a single polypeptide chain consisting of 191 amino acids (Table 3–1). There are no carbohydrate residues. Much of the work elucidating the structure of GH was performed by C. H. Li and his coworkers. The molecule has two disulfide bridges which may result in a large and small loop in the chain. The true tertiary structure is not known as yet. Although the GH from other primates resembles human GH in many properties, there are immunologic differences which can be readily detected.

Growth hormones from pig, whale, sheep, and cow pituitaries are believed to have larger molecular weights than human GH. End group analyses suggest that bovine GH exists as a branched chain. The growth hormones of these species show little or no immunologic cross-reactivity with human GH and are biologically ineffective in the human. Li has suggested that the biologically active part of the molecule is located in the inner regions and is cloaked by amino acids which do not contribute to the biologic activity of this "core." This is supported by the fact that large portions of the bovine molecule can be removed without loss of its biologic activity (in rats).

GH has profound effects on many aspects of metabolism (p. 266). Its release from the pituitary can be triggered by stress, by a fall in blood glucose, or by a rise in the concentration of certain amino acids (particularly arginine) in the blood. The number of effects of GH is seemingly endless. As its name implies, this hormone plays an important role in

TABLE 3–1. Hormones of the Adenohypophysis

Hormone	Cell Type	Molecular Weight	Number of Amino Acids	Structural Characteristics	Effects
GH	Acidophil (350 nm* granules)	21,500	191	Two intramolecular disulfide bridges	↑ RNA synthesis ↑ Protein synthesis ↑ Transport of glucose and amino acids ↑ Lipolysis ↑ Somatomedin
ACTH	Basophil or chromophobe (200 nm granules)	4567	39	Single chain	↑ Adenyl cyclase in adrenal (increasing steroidogenesis)
βMSH		2734	22	Single chain	↑ Melanin synthesis
αMSH		1823	13	Single chain	↑ Melanin synthesis
βLPH		9500	90	Single chain	Lipolytic
αLPH		5810	58	Single chain	Lipolytic
TSH	Basophil (140 nm granules)	28,000	α 96 β 113	Glycoprotein; α and β subunits; intrachain disulfide bonds (5 in α, 6 in β)	↑ Adenyl cyclase in thyroid (increasing thyroid hormone synthesis)
LH	Basophil (200 nm granules)	30,000	α 96 β 119	Glycoprotein; α and β subunits; intrachain disulfide bonds (5 in α 6 in β)	↑ Adenyl cyclase in gonads (increasing steroidogenesis)
FSH	Basophil (200 nm granules)	32,000	α 96 β ?	Glycoprotein; α and β subunits	↑ Adenyl cyclase in gonads Follicle stimulation
Prolactin	Acidophil (600 nm granules)	22,500	198	Three intramolecular disulfide bridges	↑ Synthesis of milk proteins; luteotropic ↑ Growth of mammary gland

growth. Hypophysectomized rats grow poorly; however, with daily injections of GH, they begin to grow within a few days. This lag period and similar relatively long lag periods in studies of GH action in vitro have suggested to many investigators that the effects of GH on growth (particularly protein synthesis) may be secondary to an increase in the synthesis of RNA. Korner has shown that GH administration very rapidly increases the synthesis of all kinds of RNA. As a result of increased synthesis of messenger RNA, protein synthesis is stimulated. In addition to its effects on RNA synthesis and protein synthesis, GH has effects on the transport of glucose and amino acids and on the breakdown of fat in adipose tissue (p. 267). Many of the growth-promoting effects of GH are produced via an intermediate factor, called *somatomedin*, synthesized in the liver (p. 266).

At 7 weeks some fetal pituitaries contain GH, but most do not. By 9 weeks gestation all fetal pituitaries contain small amounts of GH (about 20 ng/gland), and as gestation proceeds, increasing amounts of GH are stored, reaching a value of about 40 μg/gland by 20 weeks. The concentration of GH in fetal cord blood is high also. Studies by Gitlin and his associates have shown that pituitary tissue from a 9-week-old fetus was capable of synthesizing labeled immunoreactive GH from labeled amino acids in vitro. Electron microscopy of fetal pituitaries has demonstrated that, at three months gestation, a major proportion of the granular cells (41 percent) are somatotrophs.

Although GH is formed in fetal pituitaries and is present in fetal blood, there is no indication that it is necessary for normal growth of the fetus. Anencephalic infants (lacking normal pituitary function) are born with roughly normal length and weight, if due allowance is made for cephalic underdevelopment.

Adrenocorticotropic Hormone (Corticotropin). In 1956, Sheppard determined the primary structure of ACTH (Figure 3–2), and subsequently Schwyzer and Sieber (1963) were able to synthesize the molecule. As the name implies, this hormone acts primarily on the adrenal cortex. It produces profound changes in adrenal cortical structure, chemical composition, and enzymatic activity, in addition to stimulating the release of cortical steroid hormones. Many extra-adrenal effects of ACTH have been demonstrated, such as its powerful lipolytic action in rats.

The first basophilic cells appear in the fetal pituitary at 8 weeks gestation, and ACTH has been detected by the tenth week of gestation. In fetal conditions where the pituitary fails to develop normally (as in anencephaly), the fetal adrenals are atrophic, suggesting that ACTH plays a role in the development of the fetal adrenal. In two anencephalic infants the concentration of ACTH in umbilical venous plasma at term was below the normal range and was much lower than the plasma ACTH of their respective mothers. In one infant a dramatic rise in plasma ACTH from less than 60 pg/ml to 350 pg/ml occurred following parenteral injection of a large dose of vasopressin (p. 51). This suggests that the

ACTH in cord blood is of fetal origin. In normal newborn offspring, the mean fetal plasma concentration has been found to be 226 pg/ml (range 53 to 570 pg/ml). Maternal plasma ACTH showed no significant correlation with fetal ACTH. On the basis of such studies it seems likely that (1) the normal fetus forms and secretes ACTH, and (2) the decrease in ACTH and the atrophy of the fetal adrenal found in anencephaly are secondary to lack of corticotropin releasing hormone (p. 51).

Thyrotropin. TSH is a glycoprotein with a molecular weight of about 28,000. TSH, hCG, and the gonadotropins share a common α-subunit but have different β-subunits (p. 23). TSH increases the size and vascularity of the thyroid. Examination of the thyroid gland microscopically reveals that after the administration of TSH, the height of the epithelial cells of the follicles is increased, and the amount of colloid within the follicles is reduced. The hormone is apparently bound at the cell surface, probably by hormone-specific binding sites, and it probably acts by stimulating adenyl cyclase on the inner side of the cell membrane. The adenyl cyclase then catalyzes the transformation of ATP to cyclic AMP. Intracellular cyclic AMP activates various enzymes and thus produces the hormonal effects (p. 274).

The cell involved in TSH secretion, the thyrotroph, cannot be demonstrated histochemically in the fetal pituitary until 13 weeks gestation; however, electron microscopy has shown that this cell represents about 10 percent of the granular cells of the pituitary at 12 weeks gestation. TSH is found in fetal serum at 11 weeks, and extracts of fetal pituitaries contain biologically active TSH as early as 12 weeks. There is also evidence that the fetal pituitary can synthesize labeled TSH from labeled amino acids in vitro at about this same age. The exact role of fetal TSH in fetal thyroid function is uncertain at the present time; however, conditions which inhibit the production of fetal thyroxine (goitrogenic agents given to the mother) can cause goiters to form in the fetus, presumably via stimulation of TSH secretion by the fetal pituitary.

Gonadotropins. The gonadotropins, FSH and LH, belong to that family of glycoprotein hormones which contain identical α-subunits and hormone-specific β-subunits. As the name implies, FSH stimulates growth of ovarian follicles. In the male it is concerned with gametogenesis. LH is involved in the maturation of the follicle and its subsequent ovulation. The granulosa cells of the emptied follicle undergo luteinization under the influence of LH. The interstitial or Leydig cells of the testis are similarly stimulated by LH, and the hormone may also be called interstitial cell-stimulating hormone (ICSH). In both luteinized granulosa cells and Leydig cells, LH increases the synthesis of their respective steroid hormones, progesterone and testosterone.

Studies by Gitlin and his associates have shown that the fetal pituitary is capable of forming gonadotropins in vitro. The amounts of FSH and LH in pituitaries of fetuses from 12 to 20 weeks gestation range from 3800 to 44,000 mIU/gland for LH and 56 to 260 mIU/gland for FSH, with no obvious sex differences. Gonadotropic cells account for about 11 percent of all granular cells in the pituitary at 12 weeks gestation.

The roles of FSH and LH in fetal development are unclear. Presumably, LH may be important in steroidogenesis in fetal Leydig cells, but solid evidence for this is lacking. Male anencephalic infants undergo normal male differentiation, suggesting that fetal LH may not be involved in fetal testicular function.

Prolactin. Prolactin consists of a single polypeptide chain of 198 amino acids. Like GH it affects many tissues, but its primary function in mammals is undoubtedly the regulation of lactation. It is capable of initiating and sustaining lactation (p. 114), but the mammary gland must first be "prepared" by the actions of insulin, estrogens, progestins, GH, and corticosteroids. Although prolactin can be formed in the fetal pituitary, its role in development is unknown.

Melanocyte-Stimulating Hormone. Both α-MSH and β-MSH are small peptides (Table 3–1) which are very similar in structure to the first portion of the ACTH molecule (Figure 3–2). Although both forms of MSH have effects on the darkening of skin and on lipolysis, only α-MSH has some corticotropic activity. The similarity in structure of MSH and ACTH suggests that they may have evolved from some common original peptide. The role of MSH in fetal development is unknown.

Lipotropic Hormone. Two lipolytic peptides have been isolated in pure form: β-LPH and α-LPH. The former contains 90 amino acids (Figure 3–2), the first 58 of which are identical to α-LPH. The heptapeptide Met-Glu-His-Phe-Arg-Try-Gly is common to ACTH, MSH, and LPH and possesses both melanotropic and lipolytic activities. LPH has not yet been reported in the human fetus.

Hypothalamic Extracts and the Fetal Pituitary. Recently Siler and coworkers reported culturing human fetal pituitaries for periods up to 11 months. They used radioimmunoassay to study the synthesis and release of GH, prolactin, LH, FSH, TSH, ACTH, and MSH. Pituitary anlage from embryos as early as 5 weeks gestation released hormones in vitro, whereas other tissues did not. Hypothalamic extracts increased GH, FSH, and LH release and inhibited prolactin release.

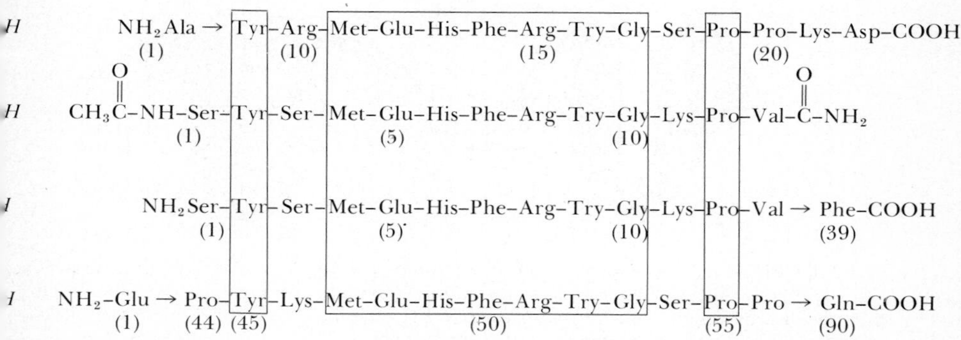

FIGURE 3–2. Comparison of amino acid sequences of ACTH, MSH, and LPH. The amino acid residues are denoted by number.

Effects of hypothalamic extracts on the fetal pituitary have been reported by several investigators, indicating not only that the fetal pituitary is capable of forming all the known pituitary hormones, but that it can also respond to hypothalamic controls. Indeed, it would seem that, with the possible exception of TSH, pituitary hormones cannot be formed unless the neuroendocrine control center is functioning. Anencephalic infants, lacking a hypothalamus, have active thyrotrophs in their pituitaries and appear to have fairly normal thyroid differentiation and some thyroxine synthesis.

Neuroendocrine tissues

Almost from the moment of its first appearance, the chordamesoderm (notochord) begins to induce changes in the ectoderm immediately overlying it. The ectoderm thickens and differentiates into a special *neuroectoderm,* extending from the caudal end of the buccopharyngeal membrane to a point just cephalic to Hensen's node as the *neural plate.* As Hensen's node and the buccopharyngeal membrane move apart, the notochord extends and the neural plate increases in length. Two longitudinal ridges, the *neural folds,* now appear as a result of the folding up of the neuroectoderm. By the end of the third week of life, the neural plate has the configuration of a V-shaped groove, which gradually deepens as the neural folds become elevated (Figure 3–3).

In the fourth week of life the neural folds fuse dorsally, forming a closed tube of neuroectoderm, the *neural tube.* The ectodermal wall of the neural tube forms the rudiment of the nervous system. As the

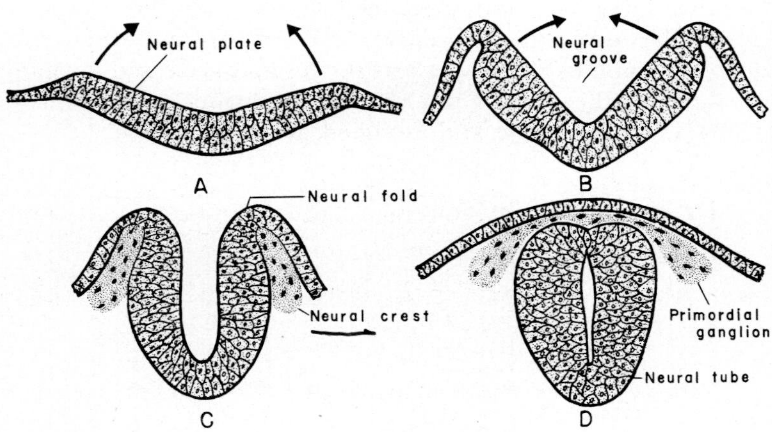

FIGURE 3–3. Cross sections of the ectoderm of human embryos at successively later stages to illustrate the origin of the neural tube and the neural crest, which forms the dorsal root ganglia and the sympathetic nerve ganglia. (From Villee, C. *Biology.* Philadelphia: W. B. Saunders Company, 1972, p. 606.)

neural plate develops further, a junctional zone appears between the neuroectoderm and the somatic ectoderm, which makes up the remainder of the surface of the embryonic disc. Some of the cells in this junctional region differentiate into *neural crest* cells. As the neural folds meet and fuse in the midline, the neural crest cells come to lie in the angle between the wall of the neural tube and the surface ectoderm (Figure 3–3). These cells eventually migrate ventrally down the sides of the neural tube to give rise to the spinal and cranial nerve ganglia, the ganglia of the sympathetic nervous system, and the adrenal medulla. Some of the neural crest cells migrate ventrally to become incorporated within the lateral margins of the last pharyngeal pouch. They become the calcitonin-secreting cells (C-cells) of the ultimobranchial body.

Diencephalon

The cranial and caudal ends of the neural folds are the last to close. Closure of the cranial end of the neural tube *(anterior neuropore)* occurs at the 18 to 20 somite stage (23 days), and closure of the *posterior neuropore* (caudal end) occurs at the 25 somite stage (25 days). The cephalic portion of the closed neural tube soon shows three distinct brain vesicles: the prosencephalon (forebrain), the mesencephalon (midbrain), and the rhombencephalon (hindbrain).

When the embryo is 5 weeks old the brain is divided further (Figure 3–4). The prosencephalon divides into an anterior *telencephalon,* which forms the cerebral cortex, and a posterior *diencephalon,* from which the optic vesicles arise. It is the diencephalon which is of special interest to the neuroendocrinologist, since it is the portion of the brain from which the pineal body, the hypothalamus, and the neurohypophysis arise. The brain cavity in the region of the diencephalon remains fairly large and is known as the third ventricle of the brain.

The greater part of the roof of the diencephalon becomes membranous and later does not contain any nerve cells at all. Instead, it is richly supplied with blood vessels and becomes the *choroid plexus* of the third ventricle. The choroid plexus is the pathway by which nutrients and oxygen are transported into the ventricles of the brain.

PINEAL GLAND

The most caudal portion of the roof plate does not participate in the formation of the choroid plexus but develops into the *pineal body.* This body initially appears as an epithelial thickening in the midline, but by the seventh week it begins to evaginate. Eventually it becomes a solid organ located on the roof of the mesencephalon.

The mammalian pineal differs significantly from the pineals (or epiphyses) of the lower vertebrates. In mammals the pineal has lost the direct photosensitivity of the lower forms, although the gland is influenced by environmental lighting indirectly via the sympathetic nervous system. Indeed, the pineal gland is innervated exclusively by sympathetic fibers. When stimulated, sympathetic nerves in the pineal

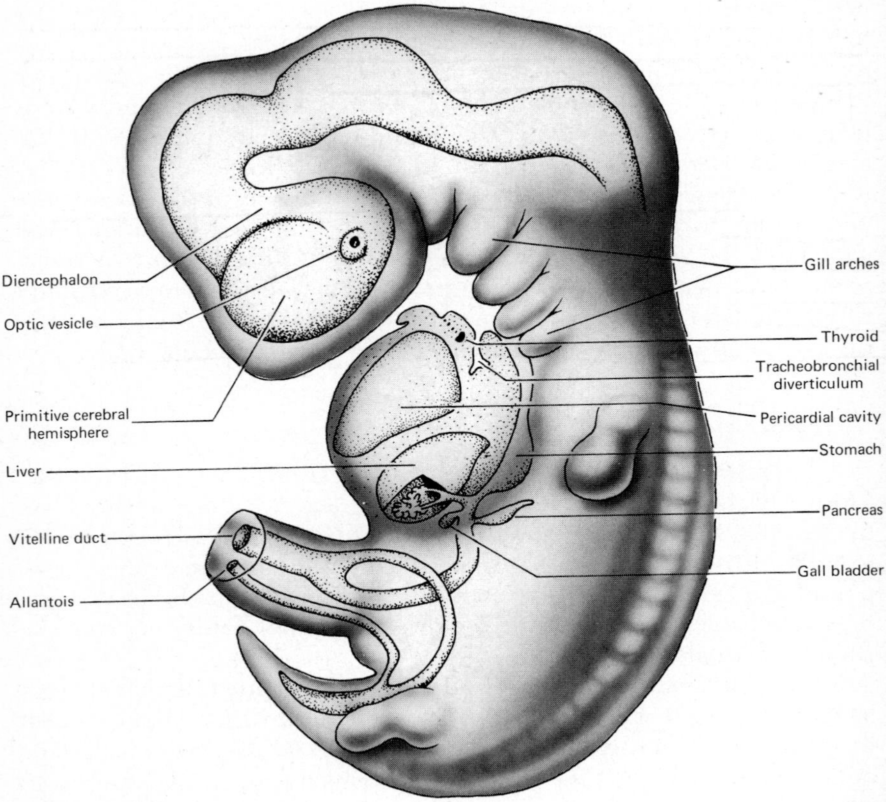

FIGURE 3–4. A lateral view of a 35-day-old human embryo, showing the development of the anterior portion of the nervous system and the gastrointestinal tract. (From Page, E., Villee, C., and Villee, D. *Human Reproduction.* Philadelphia: W. B. Saunders Company, 1972, p. 228.)

release norepinephrine, a powerful catecholamine which has the ability to increase the amount of cyclic AMP within pineal cells by stimulating adenyl cyclase. The increased cyclic AMP enhances the synthesis of N-acetyl serotonin from serotonin, which is found in the sympathetic nerve endings in the pineal. The N-acetyl-serotonin is methylated by the enzyme hydroxyindole-O-methyl transferase (HIOMT), found only in pineal cells in mammals. The product of the reaction is melatonin (Figure 3–5). The activity of HIOMT is dependent on sympathetic nerve supply. Exposure to darkness increases HIOMT activity, whereas activity is reduced under constant light conditions. Though HIOMT is not present in peripheral nerve, melatonin has been isolated from mammalian peripheral nerve. Melatonin may actually be secreted from the pineal gland into the blood; if this is true, the pineal gland is indeed a neuroendocrine organ. Recent evidence suggests that melatonin acts through the hypothalamus to regulate the content of MSH in the adenohypophysis. Melatonin also appears to affect the ovary (p. 354), but the mechanism is unknown.

In addition to melatonin, the pineal gland is rich in histamine, acetylcholine, and a melatonin derivative, 1-methyl-6-methoxy-1,2,3,4-tetrahydro-2-carboline, which was thought to be involved in regulating the secretion of aldosterone. Subsequent studies have failed to support a role of the pineal gland in control of aldosterone secretion.

Another derivative of the cells lining the third ventricle is the subcommissural organ. It constitutes a collection of columnar cells lining the roof of the caudal end of the third ventricle. The secretory granules which can be seen in these cells stain like those found in the cells of the neurohypophysis which secrete vasopressin, and it has been suggested that they may be involved in water regulation. Proof for this hypothesis is still lacking, however.

We know almost nothing about the fetal pineal gland. Indeed, the role of the pineal in the adult is still unclear. Nevertheless, a considerable amount of interest in the role of the pineal, particularly in regulating the menstrual cycle, will undoubtedly provide some answers to the question of pineal-hypothalamic-pituitary interactions.

HYPOTHALAMUS

The lateral walls and the floor of the diencephalon are divided by a longitudinal groove into a dorsal *thalamus* and a ventral *hypothalamus*

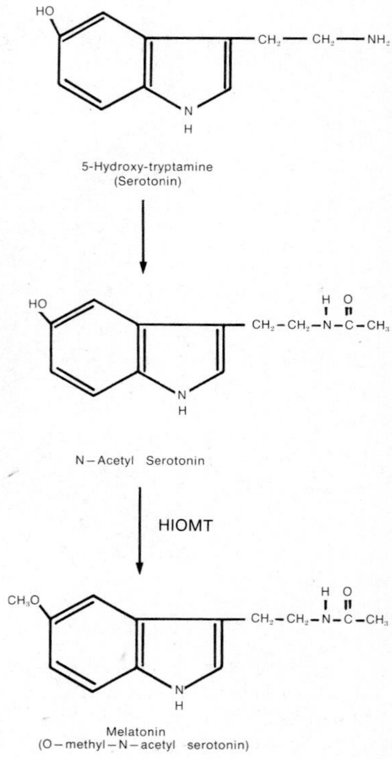

FIGURE 3–5. The synthesis of melatonin from serotonin. (Adapted from Villee, C. and Dethier, V. *Biological Principles and Processes.* Philadelphia: W. B. Saunders Company, 1971, p. 664.)

(Figure 3–6). The latter differentiates into a number of separate nuclei which are the sources of releasing and inhibiting factors. These control the synthesis and release of hormones of the adenohypophysis. The hypothalamus also contains nuclei (supraoptic and paraventricular) from which fibers pass to the *neurohypophysis* (see following discussion).

The hypothalamus is readily outlined by the optic chiasm anteriorly, the mammillary bodies posteriorly, and the temporal lobes laterally. The smooth rounded base of the hypothalamus is termed the *tuber cinereum.* To the central region of the latter, the *median eminence,* is attached the pituitary stalk. The median eminence plus the posterior pituitary are known as the *neurohypophysis.*

NEUROHYPOPHYSIS

The neurosecretory neurons which produce the octapeptide hormones *vasopressin* and *oxytocin* are located in the supraoptic and paraventricular nuclei of the hypothalamus (Figure 3–7). Fibers from these nuclei terminate primarily in the posterior pituitary (pars nervosa). In contrast, fibers from the basal hypothalamic nuclei, which produce the releasing factors, terminate largely in the median eminence.

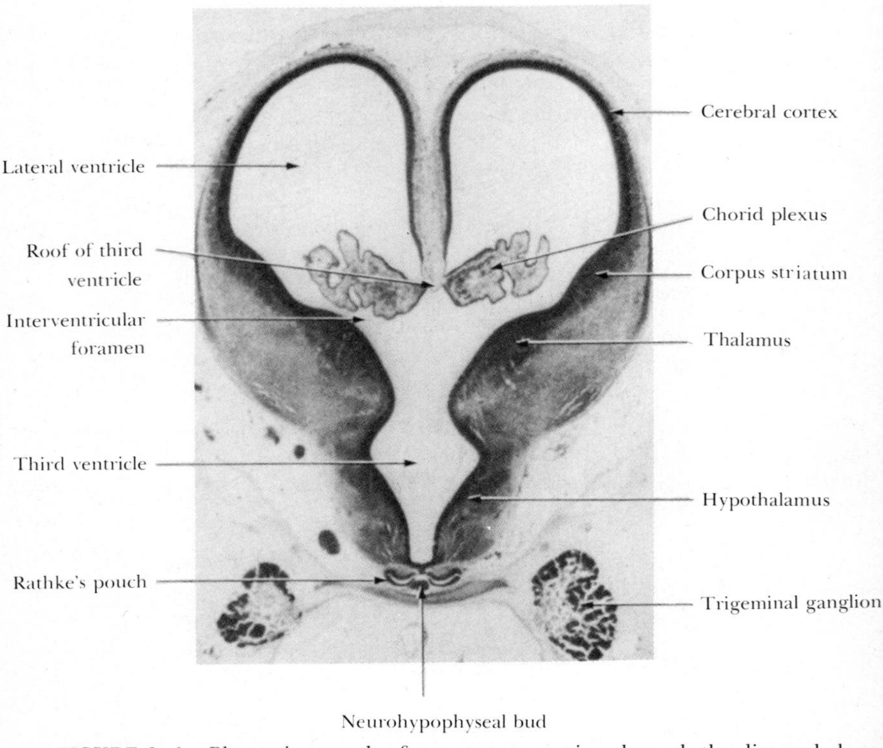

FIGURE 3–6. Photomicrograph of a transverse section through the diencephalon and the cerebral vesicles of a 20 mm human embryo of about 40 days at the level of the interventricular foramina (× 20). (From Moore, K. *The Developing Human.* Philadelphia: W. B. Saunders Company, 1973, p. 321.)

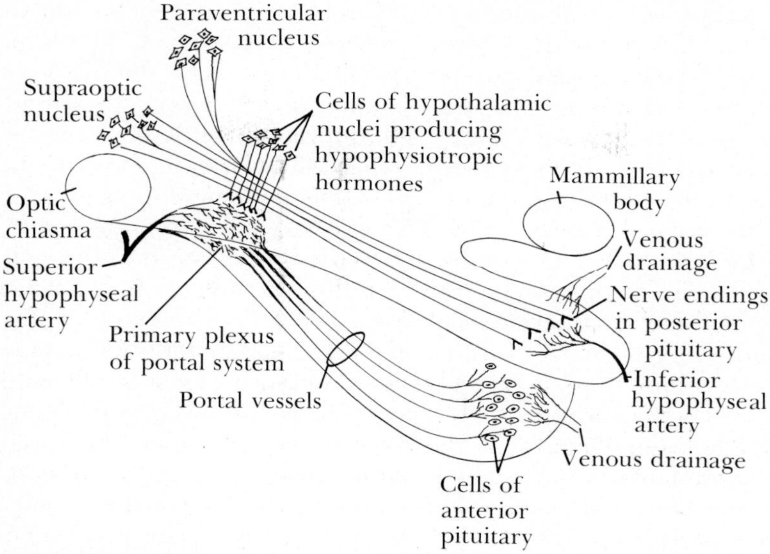

FIGURE 3–7. Diagram of hypothalamus and pituitary gland showing the portal system of the vasculature.

Phylogenetically, the median eminence appears to be the oldest part of the neurohypophysis. It represents the region where hypothalamic nerve terminals come into contact with the primary capillaries of the portal vessels, where nerve impulses become converted into biochemical messages. The rate of secretion of both releasing factors and hormones of the posterior pituitary is immediately and directly due to action potentials arriving at the nerve terminals. The transmission of signals across synapses in the neuroendocrine system involves monoamines such as acetylcholine, 3,4-dihydroxyphenyl-ethylamine (dopamine), norepinephrine, and serotonin. These neurotransmitter substances that are released by monoaminergic nerve endings diffuse a short distance to neuroendocrine cells, which are stimulated to secrete their releasing factors. Since humoral transmitter agents seem generally to be concentrated at the nerve terminal, as compared with the rest of the nerve fiber, the highest concentration of releasing factors per weight of tissue is obtained by extraction of tissue from the median eminence rather than from the hypothalamus. By analogy with other neurosecretory neurons, the releasing factors are probably synthesized in the cell bodies and transported down the axons to the median eminence.

The major blood supply of the anterior pituitary is derived from the portal vessels arising as capillaries in the median eminence (Figure 3–7). The activity of the anterior pituitary is controlled by impulses originating in the hypothalamic nuclei. The impulses pass to the median eminence, where the releasing factors are secreted and taken up in the capillaries of the portal vessels, passing through the portal system to the anterior pituitary.

A downward extension of the floor of the diencephalon, the *infundibulum,* gives rise to the posterior lobe of the pituitary. The hormones oxytocin and vasopressin are released from nerve fibers in the posterior pituitary. These fibers originate in the paraventricular (oxytocin) and supraoptic (vasopressin) nuclei. The supraoptic nucleus can be seen in the 6½-week-old fetus (29 mm), whereas the paraventricular nucleus is not seen until the eighth week. The median eminence is distinguishable by about 8½ weeks. The primary plexus of the portal system can first be seen at age 3 months. Capillaries penetrate into the nervous tissue of the median eminence in the fourth month. It is not known when the monoaminergic mechanism needed for the secretion of the hypothalamic hormones is functional in the human fetus. One approach to determining this has been through the measurement of monoamines in the hypothalamus of the human fetus. Concentrations of dopamine are significantly higher in the hypothalamus than in the forebrain of the human fetus. As the human organism grows to adulthood, the concentration of dopamine in the hypothalamus decreases, while that of norepinephrine increases to about double the fetal value. Fluorescence due to monoamines increases slowly in intensity in the median eminence of the human fetus from the thirteenth week on. Fluorescence can also be seen in many of the hypothalamic nuclei and nerve fibers by this time, but no fluorescent material can be found in the cerebral cortex.

Both vasopressin and oxytocin (Figure 3–8) have been isolated from fetal pituitaries. Although the term vasopressin denotes an action on blood pressure, it is clear that the major action of this hormone relates to its potent antidiuretic activity. In fact, it is frequently called antidiuretic hormone (ADH). Dehydration provides the usual physiologic stimulus for release of the hormone, and it is generally accepted that osmoreceptors are localized in the supraoptic nucleus. Vasopressin acts (probably via stimulation of adenyl cyclase) to increase the permeability of kidney tubules to water (p. 203).

Oxytocin exerts its major action by causing contraction of uterine

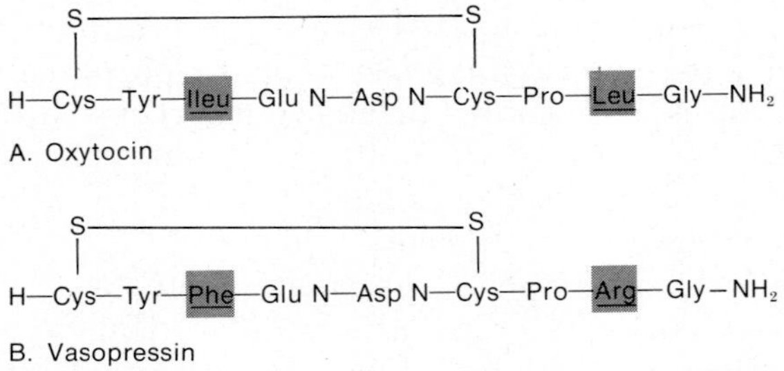

B. Vasopressin

FIGURE 3–8. The structure of oxytocin and vasopressin (antidiuretic hormone). Note that the two hormones have amino acid sequences which differ only in two amino acids. These two hormones are termed "octapeptides" by some investigators who regard the two cysteines as one cystine. (From Villee, C. and Dethier, V. *Biological Principles and Processes.* Philadelphia: W. B. Saunders Company, 1971, p. 655.)

musculature. Its amino acid sequence was reported in 1953 by du Vigneaud and his colleagues (Figure 3–8). Apparently, oxytocin is synthesized initially in the form of a large precursor molecule, from which the active hormone is split at some stage before its release from the posterior pituitary. The active peptides in the posterior pituitary are bound to a protein, neurophysin. It is possible that neurophysin may represent the inactive part of the precursor molecule.

During pregnancy a circulating enzyme, oxytocinase (an aminopeptidase), can destroy the biological activity of oxytocin. This is accomplished by cleaving the link between the N-terminal hemicystine residue and the adjacent tyrosine residue (Figure 3–8). Thereafter, it breaks successive bonds up to the proline residue of the side chain. There is no evidence that the concentration of oxytocinase changes before labor.

Both vasopressin and oxytocin share physiological actions with one another. Thus pure synthetic oxytocin has definite antidiuretic activity, and vasopressin has some of the activities of oxytocin. This is not surprising in view of their similar structures (Figure 3–8). Both vasopressin and oxytocin are released from the fetal posterior pituitary during labor (p. 110); however, the importance of these hormones in parturition is not clearly established.

Hypothalamic Hypophysiotropic Hormones

At the base of the hypothalamus are the tuberal, ventromedial, infundibular, and arcuate nuclei. The evidence presently available suggests that these nuclei produce the tropic hormone releasing factors and constitute the hypophysiotropic area (Figure 3–7). The area, confined mainly to the region around the base of the third ventricle, and lying close the midline, extends dorsally into the anterior hypothalamus.

Corticotropin Releasing Hormone (CRH). CRH was the first of the hypothalamic hypophysiotropic substances to be identified as a distinct entity. (The identification was arrived at independently in 1955 by the team of Saffran, Schally, and Benfey and the team of Guillemin and Rosenberg.) For a long time vasopressin and CRH were thought to be identical. Intraneurohypophyseal injection of vasopressin evokes a significant release of ACTH. More recent experiments suggest that vasopressin mobilizes neurohypophyseal CRH, which in turn causes the release of ACTH. Epinephrine, in large doses, can also stimulate ACTH release directly, and it has been postulated that both epinephrine and CRH may lead to the release of ACTH by processes involving the stimulation of the adenyl cyclase of pituitary cells. Exogenous cyclic AMP or derivatives of cyclic AMP have been shown to stimulate the release of ACTH. It has been suggested that the enhanced ACTH secretion may involve glycogenolysis. Stress has been shown to deplete the glycogen content of the anterior pituitary and median eminence. In vitro studies by Goodner and Freinkel have shown clearly that glycogen of the anterior pituitary can undergo extensive turnover. An increase in cyclic AMP (via increased activity of adenyl cyclase) could activate pituitary phosphorylase and increase glycogen breakdown. The energy thus provided could be used for the production and secretion of ACTH.

Unfortunately, CRH is present in very small amounts in the median eminence and therefore, though highly purified preparations have been obtained, the chemical structure is still unknown. Until pure CRH is available, its action on the anterior pituitary must remain uncertain.

By using bioassay techniques it has been possible to show that glucocorticoids inhibit and adrenalectomy increases CRH release. A circadian rhythm apparently exists for several of the hypophysiotropic hormones, including CRH, TRH, and GHRH.

Thyrotropin Releasing Hormone (TRH). The long search in several laboratories for an understanding of the chemical nature of releasing hormones achieved its first success in 1970 with the determination of the chemical structure of TRH by Bowers et al. This tripeptide, composed of pyroglutamate, histidine, and proline residues, has been synthesized and shown to be biologically active in the release of thyrotropin from the anterior pituitary.

Bound by a receptor to thyrotrophs of the anterior pituitary, TRH stimulates the release of TSH. Both adenyl cyclase and the receptor for TRH are localized almost exclusively in the plasma membrane. Since TRH stimulates adenyl cyclase in pituitary cells, it is reasonable to assume that its stimulation of TSH release is mediated via cyclic AMP. Exogenous cyclic AMP or derivatives of cyclic AMP have been shown to stimulate the release of TSH. Indeed, as data accumulate it seems reasonable to suppose that ACTH, GH, TSH, LH, and FSH are released from distinct cells, each of which possesses an adenyl cyclase sensitive to a specific hypothalamic hormone. The level of cyclic AMP is increased in the appropriate pituitary cells in response to the appropriate releasing hormone, and this in turn leads to release of the corresponding pituitary hormone. This general hypothesis is not likely to be put to the test until methods become available for studying the various pituitary cells in isolation. In addition, there is some evidence that prostaglandins may play an essential role at a step between the interaction of TRH with its plasma membrane receptor and the activation of adenyl cyclase (p. 84).

It is of interest that administration of pyroGlu-His-ProNH_2 to humans or to monkeys causes a release of both prolactin and TSH. Thus TRH may be a physiologic regulator of the release of prolactin as well as of TSH in primates, or it may be very similar chemically to the prolactin releasing hormone.

Gonadotropin Releasing Hormone (GRH). The possibility that gonadotropin secretion from the anterior pituitary may be influenced by the function of the central nervous system has been suggested for a long time. There is now no doubt that there are substances in extracts of the median eminence which can raise plasma concentrations of gonadotropins, induce release of FSH and LH from pituitary tissue in vitro, and rapidly lower the content of these hormones in the pituitary gland. It is quite possible that a single factor (GRH) regulates the output of both gonadotropins.

Porcine and ovine LH releasing hormone (LRH) have been shown to have the sequence pyroGlu-His-Trp-Ser-Tyr-Gly-Leu-Arg-Pro-GlyNH_2. Synthetic preparations of LRH and the peptide isolated from extracts of the median eminence show identical dose-response curves in regard to release and synthesis of LH and FSH by pituitary tissue (p. 356). As determined by assays both in vivo and in vitro, LRH is localized in the basal hypothalamus in a rather broad zone which extends from the suprachiasmatic region to include the median eminence and pituitary stalk. It seems likely that the secretory neurons which elaborate LRH have their cell bodies in the suprachiasmatic region and axons which project to the median eminence and pituitary stalk, terminating there in juxtaposition with the hypophyseal portal vessels. Other neurons elaborating LRH have cell bodies in the arcuate nucleus, immediately overlying the median eminence. At present, evidence supports the concept that the arcuate neurons regulate the tonic discharge of LH, while the suprachiasmatic neurons regulate the burst of LH which triggers ovulation (p. 352).

It is still uncertain whether there is a separate FSH releasing hormone (FRH) or not. There is some evidence that FRH can be separated from LRH and the other releasing hormones. FRH activity tends to be located more caudally to LRH activity, again suggesting separate entities. Nevertheless, many investigators believe that LRH regulates the release of both FSH and LH, and they refer to this hypothalamic hormone as GRH.

Growth Hormone Releasing Hormone (GHRH). It is well established that hypothalamic lesions can produce impairment of growth and a decreased content of GH in the pituitaries of rats, cats, and dogs. The first convincing experimental evidence of the existence of a hypothalamic neurohormone which affects GH secretion was made in 1964 by Deuben and Meites. They showed that rat hypothalamic extracts release GH in tissue cultures of rat pituitaries. It seems clearly established now that GHRH is present in hypothalamic extracts of several species, including man. Schally and his colleagues have shown that bilateral lesions of the paraventricular nuclei result in growth retardation and a reduction of GHRH in the median eminence. Analyses of porcine GHRH indicate that it is an acidic polypeptide with a molecular weight of about 1600. Some evidence points to the existence of a GH inhibitory hormone (GHIH). This substance, called somatostatin, has been reported to have the following amino acid sequence: Ala-Gly-Cys-Lys-Asn-Phe-Phe-Trp-Lys-Thr-Phe-Thr-Ser-Cys.

Prolactin Inhibitor and Releasing Factors (PIF and PRF). In sharp contrast to its stimulatory effects on other pituitary hormones, the hypothalamus exerts an inhibitory influence on the secretion of prolactin in both males and females. A prolactin inhibiting factor (PIF) is present in extracts of hypothalamus. Stimuli which induce a release of prolactin (suckling, for example) ultimately produce their effect by reducing the hypothalamic secretion of PIF. This hypothalamic hormone has been purified and separated from most other releasing factors.

In birds there appears to be a hypothalamic stimulatory influence on prolactin secretion. This is mediated by a prolactin releasing factor (PRF). The existence of PRF in mammals is uncertain, and the chemical identities of both PRF and PIF are unknown.

MSH Releasing and Inhibitory Factors (MRF and MIF). The secretion of MSH in the adenohypophysis is regulated by hypothalamic factors. The factor involved in the release of MSH is produced in the paraventricular area, and the factor which inhibits MSH secretion is produced in the supraoptic area. Celis has shown that an exopeptidase exists in the stalk median eminence regions which cleaves a tripeptide, prolylleucylglycinamide, from oxytocin; this tripeptide is considered to be MIF on the basis of its biological activity.

Other Hypothalamic Factors

Much more study of the neuroendocrine system needs to be done before we can put together the morphologic, histochemical, and biochemical data of the developing hypothalamus and neurohypophysis. Though we now have evidence for the existence of neurohypophyseal hormones and hypophysiotropic hormones, there is undoubtedly other biologically active material in the hypothalamus. Recent studies showing the isolation of hypothalamic factors which induce salivation and raise the blood glucose in rats suggest that there may well exist a whole host of regulatory factors which function not via the adenohypophysis, but rather, directly on target tissues elsewhere in the body. The role(s) of these factors and the hypophysiotropic factors in the developing fetus is yet to be determined.

THE ULTIMOBRANCHIAL BODY

Branchiogenic tissue from a diverticulum of the fifth branchial pouch (sometimes considered part of the fourth pouch) joins the thyroid anlage in mammals during the early embryonic period. This tissue, sometimes referred to in the plural as the lateral thyroids, becomes part of the thyroid and ultimately is the site of formation of calcitonin. In other species this tissue forms a discrete calcitonin-secreting gland called the ultimobranchial body. The cells in these tissues which store and secrete calcitonin are called *C-cells.*

Le Dourain and her associates (1970) demonstrated that these calcitonin-secreting cells arise from the neural crest. She transplanted segments of neural crest from embryonic Japanese quail into embryonic chicks (the cells are readily identifiable in quail because of their characteristic nuclear chromatin). The quail neural crest cells were observed to migrate to the ultimobranchial bodies of chicks. Pearse and Polak (1971) also showed the neural crest origin of calcitonin-secreting cells in mice. Thus, although the ultimobranchial tissue is derived from the last pharyngeal pouch, the calcitonin-secreting cells are of neuroectodermal origin.

The ultimobranchial body can be demonstrated outside the thyroid anlage only in embryos less than 1.9 cm long (39 days). At about the sixth week of gestation the ultimobranchial body joins the thyroid anlage. In embryos over 3 cm in length, the development of primitive follicles can be observed in this bilateral anlage. Cysts of varying size occur in fetuses after the twelfth week of gestation and it is in the walls and vicinity of the ultimobranchial cysts that immature C-cells are found. (Only after the twelfth week of gestation can C-cells be identified in the thyroid.) The C-cells are immature throughout the embryonic period, and remain immature up to the seventeenth week of gestation. Contact of C-cells with the colloid of thyroid follicles has never been demonstrated conclusively. C-cells are usually larger than follicular cells, and may possess long finger-like projections extending between the follicular cells or along the basement membrane. The large pale nucleus is situated in the center of the C-cell.

Human calcitonin is a polypeptide with 32 amino acid residues. There is an amide group in place of a free carboxyl group at the C-terminus and a disulfide bond linking residues one and seven. It exists as a monomer of molecular weight 3600 (Calcitonin M), or as a dimer (by intermolecular rearrangement of the disulfide bonds in two monomers to give an antiparallel arrangement) of 7200 (Calcitonin D). The hormone is released in response to increased concentration of calcium in the serum. The hypocalcemic effect of calcitonin lowers the raised plasma calcium, and this in turn limits further secretion of the hormone. Thus calcitonin secretion is controlled by a negative feedback mechanism. The plasma calcium is lowered by suppressing the resorption of bone. Because calcitonin is effective in parathyroidectomized animals, the inhibition of bone resorption is probably not due to competition of calcitonin with PTH at a single site of action.

The hormone is most effective in lowering calcium in young, rapidly growing animals. It is not known, however, what role calcitonin may have in the human fetus. Although the fetal skeleton takes on form by the eighth to tenth week of intra-uterine life, it is only in the last trimester that appreciable amounts of calcium are required for osteogenesis. Well over half the total calcium content of the fetus, amounting to 10 to 12 g, is stored during the last 8 weeks of pregnancy. If calcitonin suppresses the resorption of bone in the fetus, the reportedly high values for serum calcitonin in the human fetus may be of some importance.

THE ADRENAL MEDULLA

Cells derived from the neural crest migrate from the primitive spinal ganglia to form the sympathetic primordium, which lies posterior to the dorsal aorta and is a recognizable structure in the 5 mm embryo (4 weeks). From the cells of the sympathetic primordium, called *sympathogones,* are derived both the neuroblasts which form the sympathetic ganglion cells and the chromaffin cells (pheochromoblasts and pheochromocytes), which are involved in the synthesis of catecholamines.

Starting at about the 14 mm stage (6 weeks), primitive cells migrate from the sympathetic primordium, moving along the central vein, into the fetal adrenal cortex. This migration continues until the fetus is 270 mm in length. Other chromaffin cells migrate along the aorta and form the paraganglia.

The early fetal medulla is composed of both sympathogones and pheochromoblasts. Maturation of the latter into pheochromocytes commences at the 27 to 47 mm stage (9 to 10 weeks). Initially, the cells form whorl- or rosette-like structures in which pheochromoblasts occupy a central position. When the predominant cell becomes a pheochromocyte, the cellular arrangement is replaced by anastomosing cords. Granules, with a positive chromaffin reaction, are not seen in the cells under the light microscope until the fetus is 55 mm in length (12 weeks).

Sympathetic nerve endings, chromaffin cells, and the brain are capable of synthesizing the catecholamines. Epinephrine is released from secretory cells of the adrenal medulla and appears to function primarily as a circulating hormone (p. 251). Norepinephrine may also function in this capacity to some extent, but this catecholamine plays a more important role as the principal neurotransmitter of the sympathetic nervous system. Dopamine appears to be a particularly important substance within the central nervous system.

The catecholamines interact with specific receptors (adrenergic receptors). Originally, the effects of the catecholamines were classified according to their mode of mediation (α or β adrenergic receptors). More recently, catecholamine effects have been classified as: (1) those producing a rise in intracellular cyclic AMP (p. 275), (2) those producing a fall in cyclic AMP, and (3) those producing no effect on cyclic AMP. Many of the effects classified as β-adrenergic are the same as those mediated by increases in the intracellular concentration of cyclic AMP. Those classified as α-adrenergic effects overlap with those associated with a fall in cyclic AMP. Thus the two classifications may be related.

The pathway of synthesis for the catecholamines is shown in Figure 3–9. Both liver and adrenal medulla can convert phenylalanine to tyrosine (the first stage shown in Figure 3–9); however, dietary tyrosine can serve equally well for the synthesis of norepinephrine. Tyrosine hydroxylase is the rate-limiting enzyme for catecholamine formation. Once DOPA is formed, it is readily converted to dopamine.

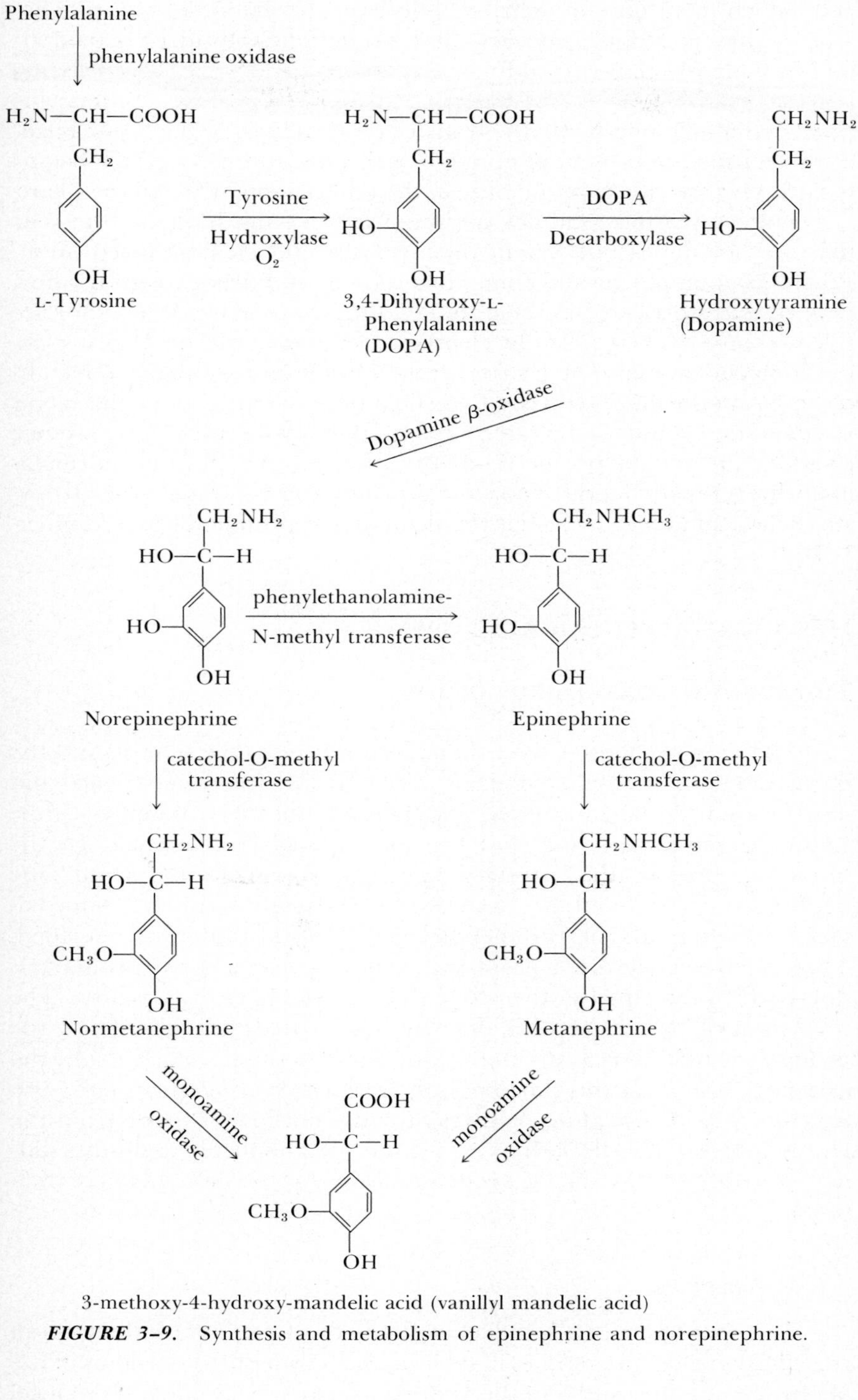

3-methoxy-4-hydroxy-mandelic acid (vanillyl mandelic acid)

FIGURE 3–9. Synthesis and metabolism of epinephrine and norepinephrine.

Large amounts of DOPA decarboxylase are found in the cytoplasm of cells which form norepinephrine. The actual formation of norepinephrine occurs in cytoplasmic granules present in the adrenal medulla and in sympathetic nerve endings. Norepinephrine is the principal catecholamine of the adrenal medulla in fetal and neonatal life. The enzyme phenylethanolamine-N-methyl transferase develops largely after birth, at which time the content of epinephrine in the adrenal medulla begins to rise. This enzyme is found only in the adrenal medulla and the heart.

The cytoplasmic granules are important not only in the synthesis of the catecholamines but also in their storage and biologic inactivation. When norepinephrine and epinephrine are bound to adenosine triphosphatase and stored within the granules, they are inactive. When they are released into the cytoplasm by chemical or nervous stimuli, they are active. Catecholamines that are free in the cytoplasm are subject to metabolism by monoamine oxidase. Catecholamines circulating in the blood are degraded primarily by catechol-O-methyltransferase. The excretory products are metanephrine (O-methylation of epinephrine), normetanephrine (O-methylation of norepinephrine), and 3-methoxy-4-hydroxymandelic acid (VMA), which is the deaminated product of both (Figure 3–9).

MESODERMAL ENDOCRINE TISSUE

THE ADRENAL CORTEX AND GONADS

The development of the urinary and reproductive systems and the development of the adrenal gland occur in close interdependence and must, therefore, be considered together. Of the three "kidneys" to be found in vertebrates, the *pronephros* is vestigial in mammals. In the human embryo, the vestigial pronephros develops from the nephrogenic cord and lies anterior to the eighth somite. Approximately seven pairs of rudimentary pronephric tubules are formed. These soon degenerate, but not before they give rise to the pronephric ducts, which remain after the pronephric tubules have disappeared. The formation of the pronephric duct by fusion of the distal ends of the pronephric tubules is a very important phase in the development of the excretory system, as this duct not only serves the pronephros but is also instrumental in providing pathways for the outflow of urine from the mesonephros ("middle kidney") and the metanephros (definitive kidney). In addition, the duct is needed in males for the passage of spermatozoa.

Mesonephros

The *mesonephros,* or Wolffian body, is the functional kidney of all vertebrates below the reptiles. The human mesonephros develops in the nephrogenic cord caudal to the pronephric area, beginning at the level of the eighth or ninth somite. The mesonephric or *Wolffian duct* arises from the dorsal surface of the nephrogenic cord, forming a linear *nephrogenic ridge* which later canalizes to form the duct. The duct parts company with the nephrogenic cord at about the level of the thirteenth somite and grows freely in close apposition to the ectoderm. The duct opens into the cloaca at about the twenty-eighth day in embryos of about 5 mm length (Chapter Four, Figure 4–8).

The mesonephric tubules, some 35 to 40 on each side, form in a strictly craniocaudal sequence. The anterior tubules begin to degenerate while the caudal tubules are still differentiating from the nephrogenic cord. The tubules from about the seventh to the eleventh somites are modified as the efferent ductules of the testis. The mesonephric tubules are S-shaped and consist of a glomerular segment, a postglomerular or proximal segment, and a distal segment which opens into the Wolffian duct. The mesonephros of embryos about 25 mm long is supplied by 8 or 10 mesonephric arteries arising from the abdominal aorta. From these the afferent glomerular arteries arise.

As the tubules and their glomeruli increase in bulk and complexity, the mesonephros bulges into the dorsal wall of the abdominal cavity, forming a linear swelling or *urogenital ridge.* At the same time, the coelomic cavity expands into the base of the urogenital ridge, cutting off all but a narrow urogenital mesentery from the dorsal wall. The mesonephros, adrenal cortex, and gonad develop in close proximity to one another. Experiments with amphibians indicate that the cells of the intermediate mesoderm are pluripotential: they may differentiate into nephrons, adrenal cortex, or gonadal medulla, depending on environmental influences. For example, the addition of one or two milligrams of estradiol per liter of aquarium water causes a more than tenfold increase in the size of the adrenals of exposed tadpoles, and a more than proportional reduction of the kidneys. On the other hand, early hypophysectomy is followed by a reduction of adrenal size. We do not know what factors may control the early differentiation of the nephrogenic blastema in the human, but there seems little doubt that the cells from the mesonephric blastema contribute to the development of both the adrenals and gonads.

Development of the Adrenal Cortex

Several days before there is any indication of a gonadal primordium, cells from the coelomic epithelium on the medial surface of the urogenital ridge, in the dorsomedial angle of the body cavity, begin to proliferate and gradually condense into a discrete mass—the primordium of the adrenal cortex. The tendency of the adrenal cortical cells to form strands with cylindric arrangement of the cell nuclei is reminiscent of tubule formation in the urinary mesonephros and, as we shall see, in the gonadal medulla. The proliferation of the cortical cells begins in embryos about 6 mm long (28 days), a time when the mesonephros is

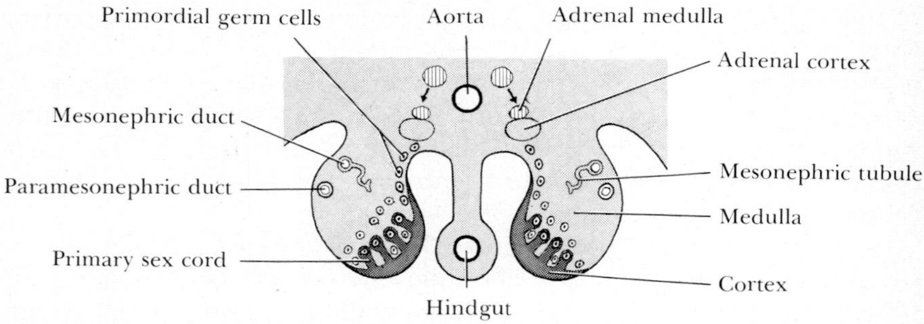

FIGURE 3–10. The developing adrenals and gonads. (From Moore, K. *The Developing Human.* Philadelphia: W. B. Saunders Company, 1973, p. 209.)

well-developed, the thyroid diverticulum is elongated and bilobed at its extremity, the ultimobranchial body is well defined and epithelial proliferations of thymus and parathyroids are evident, the pancreatic primordia are formed, the liver is conspicuous, and Rathke's pouch has come in contact with the infundibular process of the diencephalon. In other words, all the endocrine primordia except the gonads are visible. By 34 days (10 mm), the cortical anlage is seen as a discrete mass of cells medial to the mesonephros and ventral to the aorta (Figure 3–10). It is about this time that primitive cells from the sympathetic primordium begin to invade the adrenal cortex. Slightly later, cells from Bowman's capsule of the mesonephros migrate to the adrenal cortex and the developing gonad.

At 5 to 6 weeks gestation the adrenal gland is composed of rather immature cells surrounded by a thin fibrotic capsule. The gland is highly vascularized, and the cells are dividing rapidly, but as yet there is no division of the cortex into an outer and inner zone. This division, so characteristic of the human fetal adrenal cortex, occurs sometime after 6 weeks and is associated with the appearance of more mature cells in the inner or *fetal zone.* These cells possess well-developed endoplasmic reticulum, Golgi apparatus, and mitochondria. Johannisson, in her electron microscopic studies of the human fetal adrenal, concluded that the outer zone of the adrenal cortex, at least early in gestation, appeared to have mainly a proliferative activity, whereas the inner zone revealed intracellular changes indicating steroidogenic activity. After midgestation, Johannisson found changes in the outer zone suggesting a beginning of functional activity of these cells.

Many studies, utilizing in vitro incubations of adrenal glands or perfusions of human fetuses, have helped to answer the question of the possible steroidogenic properties of the fetal zone. Namely, if the fetal zone of the fetal adrenal cortex is steroidogenic, what steroids does it make? Since the fetal zone comprises about 80 percent of the volume of the fetal adrenal, any incubations of the entire gland probably reflect the activity of the fetal zone. Such incubations revealed that although the fetal adrenal could synthesize cholesterol from acetate and could convert cholesterol to pregnenolone, the latter steroid was not converted to progesterone to any appreciable extent (Figure 3–11). Rather, the pregnenolone was hydroxylated in position 17 to form 17-hydroxypregnenolone, the latter then losing its side chain (desmolase enzyme) to form dehydroepiandrosterone. Some of the pregnenolone and some of the dehydroepiandrosterone were hydroxylated in the 16α position to form 16α-hydroxypregnenolone and 16α-hydroxydehydroepiandrosterone (Figure 3–11). Even with dehydroepiandrosterone as a substrate, only a small conversion to androstenedione could be observed. In essence, then, the fetal adrenal appears to have a relative lack of the enzyme 3β-hydroxysteroid dehydrogenase. Thus the conversion of Δ5-3β-hydroxysteroids such as pregnenolone or dehydroepiandrosterone to their respective Δ4-3-ketosteroids (progesterone or androstenedione) is severely limited.

The enzyme 3β-hydroxysteroid dehydrogenase uses NAD as a cofactor and can be detected histochemically by coupling the hydrogen transfer to a formazan dye. Such histochemical studies were performed

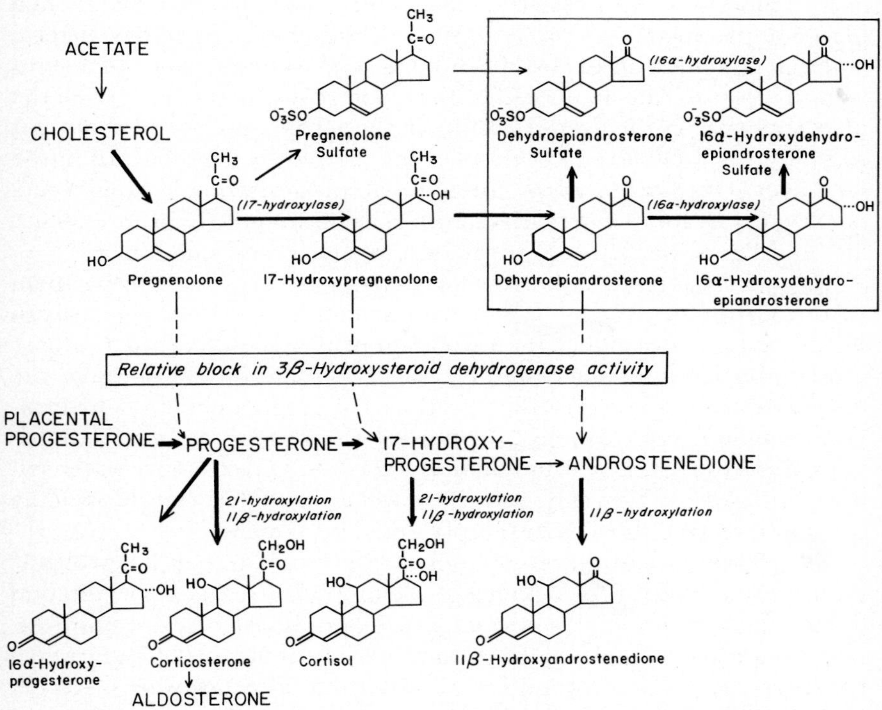

FIGURE 3–11. Pathways of steroid metabolism in the human fetal adrenals. The relative block in 3β-hydroxysteroid dehydrogenase activity is indicated by the dotted lines connecting the Δ5, 3β-hydroxysteroids and the Δ4, 3-ketosteroids. (From Page, E., Villee, C., and Villee, D. *Human Reproduction.* Philadelphia: W. B. Saunders Company, 1972, p. 234.)

by Goldman, and they demonstrated that although this enzyme was present in placenta, in fetal testis, and even in the outer or *definitive zone* of the fetal adrenal, little or none could be shown to be present in the fetal zone of the fetal adrenal. Other studies, in which the fetal and definitive zones were incubated separately and examined, corroborated the histochemical work.

Does this mean that the fetal adrenal cannot form cortisol? Not at all. If the adrenal gland is incubated with labeled progesterone as substrate (bypassing the 3β-hydroxysteroid dehydrogenase block), a variety of labeled products can be isolated from the incubation medium (Figure 3–11). If the adrenals come from a fetus of less than 8 weeks gestation, the principal products of progesterone in vitro are 16α-hydroxyprogesterone, 17α-hydroxyprogesterone, and androstenedione. (The enzymes 16α-hydroxylase, 17α-hydroxylase, and desmolase are present very early in development.) After about 8 weeks gestation, when the enzymes 21-hydroxylase and 11β-hydroxylase are active, progesterone can be converted to 11-deoxycorticosterone, corticosterone, and cortisol. The fetal adrenal can also form aldosterone from progesterone.

What is the source of the progesterone in vivo? The placenta forms large amounts of progesterone (Chapter Two); it is estimated that placental production of progesterone reaches 250 mg per day at term and that roughly half of this reaches the fetus. The presence of a sinus venosus ensures that about half of the blood reaching the fetus from the placenta bypasses the liver. Thus the progesterone has a good chance of reaching the fetal adrenal without being altered by the enzymes in the fetal liver. Once taken up by the adrenal, progesterone is rapidly metabolized. The complementarity of the placenta and the fetal adrenal has inspired Egon Diczfalusy to speak of a "fetoplacental unit" (p. 85).

The fetal adrenal can conjugate steroids as well as synthesize them from appropriate precursors. The conjugation is restricted primarily to sulfurylation and includes the formation of the 21-sulfates of 11-deoxycorticosterone and corticosterone, the 17-sulfate of testosterone, the 3α-sulfate of pregnanediol, the 3β-sulfates of pregnenolone, 17-hydroxypregnenolone, dehydroepiandrosterone (Figure 3–11), and the 3-sulfates of the estrogens. Sulfurylation renders the steroids more water soluble and less biologically active; however, sulfates can be readily converted to free steroids in the placenta and "reused."

The growth and differentiation of the fetal adrenal are probably under tropic influence. In anencephalic monsters of 20 weeks gestation or less, the fetal adrenal is normal in size and differentiation; however, after 20 weeks the fetal zone of the adrenal cortex atrophies. Benirschke has interpreted these findings as showing that after 20 weeks, ACTH from the fetal pituitary (atrophic in anencephalics) is necessary for normal growth of the adrenal. Prior to 20 weeks, hCG may play some role in adrenal development. Experimental work in rats indicates that the adrenal X-zone (perhaps analogous to the human fetal zone?) is maintained by a pituitary gonadotropin, LH. Since hCG is similar to LH in biological activity and is formed in large amounts by the placenta, enough of this placental hormone may reach the human fetal adrenal to maintain its fetal zone until fetal pituitary LH can take over this role. We do not know whether ACTH or LH is involved in the growth and development of the fetal zone. If the fetal zone cells are under the control of LH (or hCG), they may share a common origin with the interstitial cells of the gonads, namely the mesonephric blastema. ACTH may act solely on the definitive zone of the adrenal gland.

Why does the fetal zone involute after birth? Does the newborn pituitary cease to form tropic hormone in sufficient amounts to maintain this zone? Many questions remain to be answered about the function and control of the fetal zone of the human fetal adrenal.

Development of the Gonads

INDIFFERENT GONAD. The gonad develops as a linear thickening of the coelomic epithelium on the medial side of the urogenital ridge. At first this linear thickening, or *gonadal ridge,* extends almost the full length of the urogenital ridge. Later it is restricted to about its middle third.

In the early stages of gonadal development the testis and ovary are indistinguishable and the gonads are said to be in the *indifferent stage.* The genetic sex of the embryo, however, is determined from the time of fertilization. Thus the cells comprising the indifferent gonad are either male (46XY) or female (46XX). This genetic constitution determines the phenotypic expression of the embryonic gonad.

It is probable that, as in many lower forms, the mammalian germ cell line is set apart from the somatic cell line early in development. The germ cells have been found in many animals in the yolk sac. Witschi described human primordial germ cells as large, pale cells containing glycogen and possessing alkaline phosphatase activity. The latter can be used to trace these cells in their journey from the yolk sac lining to the gonad. The germ cells move independently, apparently by ameboid motion, each cell choosing its own path. Although individually following no set route, the primordial germ cells in the normal embryo show no tendency to settle anywhere but in the genital ridge (Figure 3–10).

At the same period in embryonic development, the blood cell precursors are also migrating from the yolk sac, but these cells end in the liver. What controls the sites to which these two populations of cells migrate? One theory states that the cells of the developing genital ridge are producing a substance that chemotactically attracts primordial germ cells.

During their migration the primordial germ cells undergo repeated division, and even after they reach the gonad mitosis continues. The germ cells pass through the mesenchyme of the urogenital ridge and lodge in the coelomic epithelium. Although retaining their alkaline phosphatase activity, these cells lose their glycogen and become smaller, thus seeming to blend in with the surrounding epithelial cells. The cells of the genital ridge now proliferate rapidly. Growth is more rapid in the central portion of the ridge than in the peripheral regions, and consequently the gonad develops an elliptical shape.

The gonad starts this period of rapid growth composed of an underlying layer of densely cellular mesenchyme containing many small blood vessels and a dense cap of epithelioid cells derived from the coelomic epithelium. Whether the cells derived from the coelomic epithelium "invade" the underlying mesenchyme or the mesenchyme pushes upward to break up the proliferating epithelium into cords is not known. By the end of this period the cell populations are organized into a set of epithelial cell cords *(sex cords)* lying in a vascularized mesenchymal bed. These cells are continuous from the outer coelomic epithelium to the clumps of small cells deep in the gonad that will form the rete systems.

Sex cords begin to develop in embryos between 6.7 and 8.7 mm in length. Once the sex cords appear, development of the gonad is rapid. The mesenchymal primordium forms the supporting tissue of the sex cords. It receives an accession of cells from the medial aspect of the Bowman's capsules of the mesonephric tubules. Other mesonephric cells migrate to the primordium of the adrenal cortex. Thus both the indifferent gonad and the adrenal cortex receive mesonephric cells in this early stage of development. What the role of these cells might be in the later function of these endocrine tissues is unknown; however, it is tempting to speculate that they might serve as the precursors of the steroid producing cells of these organs.

Testis

The differentiation of the indifferent gonad into a testis occurs much earlier than ovarian differentiation. In male embryos of 14 to 16 mm length, the sex cords (seminiferous tubules) become more prominent and are widely separated by mesenchymal tissue. The number and size of the cells of the germinal epithelium decrease; later this outer layer of cells forms the tunica albuginea. Germ cells seem to disappear or become so modified that they are difficult to identify.

The cells between the seminiferous tubules undergo a remarkable metamorphosis during development. From small spindle-shaped cells lying between the tubules of the recently differentiated testis, they increase rapidly in size and number to occupy a large volume of the gonad. Individual cells may be enormous. These interstitial cells *(Leydig cells)* arising from the mesenchymal part of the indifferent gonad continue to develop and comprise a maximum proportion of the fetal testis. At 130 mm length, one half to two thirds of the testis (by volume) consists of Leydig cells.

Differentiation and growth of the interstitial cells of the testis occur during a phase of development in the male when, in the female, the ovary is increasing in size with little evidence of morphological differentiation. It is also a period in gestation when the production of hCG by the placenta is maximal. hCG has been found in physiological amounts in fetal tissues, suggesting that this gonadotropin may play a role in the differentiation of the Leydig cells of the fetal testis. At this point the fetal pituitary has not begun to form gonadotropins and could not be responsible for stimulating the Leydig cells.

When fetal testes are incubated with labeled steroid precursors such as acetate, cholesterol, pregnenolone, or progesterone, labeled testosterone can be isolated from the incubation mixture. The amount of testosterone formed tends to increase as the number of Leydig cells in the testis increases. The studies by Bloch have shown that from about 9 to 15 weeks gestation, the fetal testis is capable of forming testosterone in vitro.

The differentiation of the Leydig cells and their ability to form testosterone just precede the male differentiation of the gonaducts and the external genitalia. Without a fetal testis, female differentiation of these structures occurs (p. 185). Abnormalities in androgen synthesis, or in end organ sensitivity, can result in abnormal sexual differentiation (p. 175).

Ovary

The young ovary is identified chiefly by the fact that it is not a testis. The developing ovary undergoes steady growth, while there is a reduction in the size of the primitive germ cells (now called oogonia). The cord-like arrangement of the indifferent gonad is no longer present, but rather a more uniform appearance is evident. As development proceeds the oogonia become encapsulated by cells derived from the coelomic epithelium *(follicular* or *granulosa cells).* The germ cell surrounded by follicular cells is called a *follicle.* After the oogonia are encapsulated by follicular cells the fetal stroma (derived from mesenchyme) invades the ovary from the area of the rete system. Apparently, the fetal stroma has a lethal effect on "naked" oogonia, and to counter this effect follicular formation precedes stromal invasion. The stroma has permeated the whole ovary in embryos of 280 to 300 mm. In contrast to the interstitial cells of the testis (also derived from mesenchyme), the ovarian stroma differentiates late, being first seen in fetuses between 100 and 130 mm. Since the fetal ovary is relatively inactive in steroid synthesis, it must be presumed that none of the stromal cells or their derivatives (such as the theca cells which surround the follicles) are capable of synthesizing progesterone or estrogens. The cells lining the follicles (granulosa cells) would also appear to lack one or more of the enzymes necessary for steroid synthesis.

The early follicles of the fetal ovary eventually develop into *Graafian follicles,* which contain fluid. Many of the follicles undergo atresia, an event which, along with follicular growth, occurs only in the second half of fetal life. The underdeveloped character of the human ovary in the first half of gestation, and its poor capacity for steroid synthesis, suggest an inability to respond to gonadotropic hormones. The fetal pituitary is capable of producing FSH and LH by 12 to 14 weeks gestation, yet the ovary remains relatively undifferentiated. Perhaps the fetal ovarian cells lack the receptors for FSH and LH.

ENDODERMAL ENDOCRINE TISSUE

THE BRANCHIAL REGION

Three endocrine tissues—thyroid, parathyroid, and ultimobranchial tissue—develop as derivatives of the pharynx. If the thymus is included among the endocrine tissues, a fourth endocrine derivative of the pharynx exists. The endodermal cavity in the branchial region bulges laterally, producing a series of pockets or *branchial pouches.* As the endodermal branchial pouches reach the epidermis, pushing aside the intervening mesoderm, the epidermis becomes folded inward. Thus a series of *branchial grooves* between the pouches (or arches) forms on the surface of the embryo (Figure 3–4). The outer wall of the branchial pouch fuses with the inner wall of the epidermal groove. A variety of structures having nothing to do with respiratory function develop from these branchial pouches, though in lower animals they form the gills. The first pair of branchial pouches, for instance, becomes the eustachian tubes. The tips of the third and fourth branchial pouches give rise to the parathyroid glands, while the ultimobranchial tissue develops from the fifth pouches (rudimentary in the human embryo). The thyroid, of course, forms as a diverticulum from the floor of the pharynx at the base of the tongue, during the 3 to 4 mm stage.

Thyroid Gland

The thyroid is made up of *follicles,* each consisting of epithelial cells arranged in a hollow sphere; the cavity of the follicle is filled with *colloid,* a pink-staining material composed largely of the protein *thyroglobulin.*

Early in development the endodermal cells comprising the thyroid diverticulum multiply rapidly. Masses of cells form and in time are broken up by the ingrowth of mesenchyme carrying blood vessels. The endodermal masses become arranged in follicles, whereas the mesenchyme forms the capsule and stroma of the gland.

By the seventh week, the thyroid has reached its definitive location, and the thyroglossal duct has atrophied.* Thyroid follicles begin to form

*Abnormal embryonic migration may leave the thyroid anlage in the tongue (lingual thyroid), in the upper neck, or in the mediastinum. Vestiges of the thyroglossal duct may persist as benign chronic cysts.

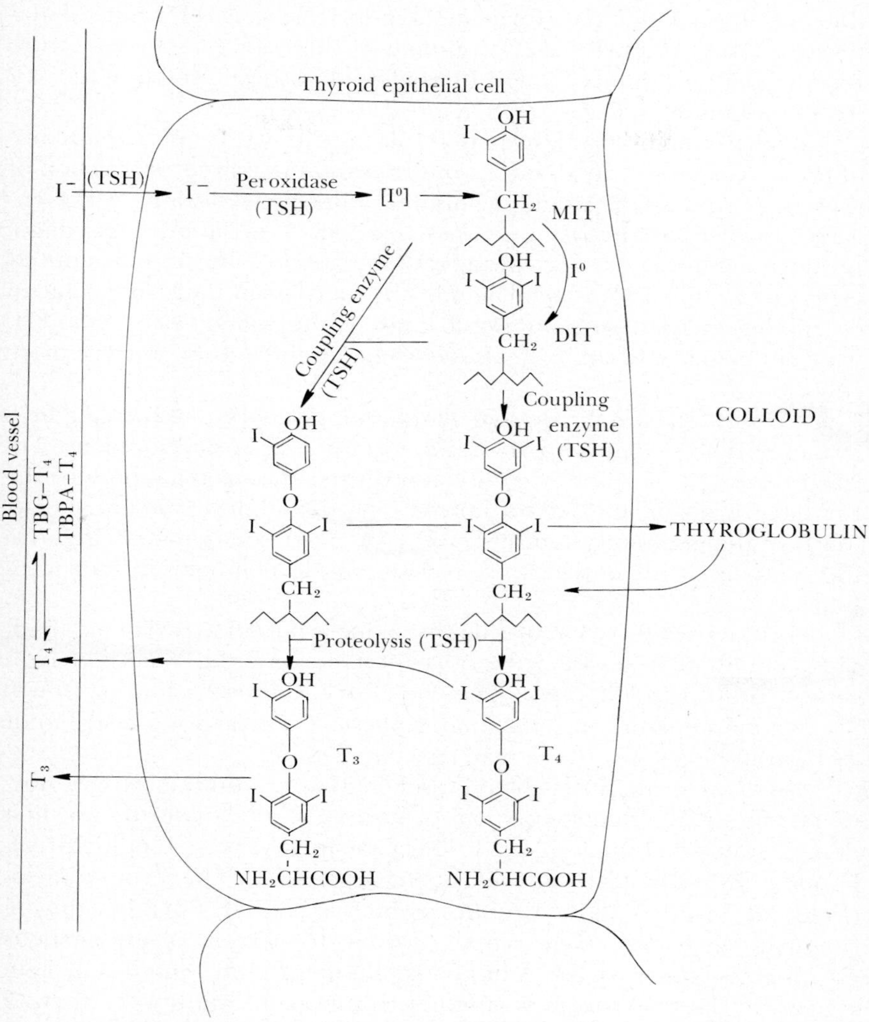

FIGURE 3–12. The iodination of tyrosine (attached to thyroglobulin) in the formation of triiodo thyronine (T_3) and thyroxine (T_4) in the thyroid cell.

at about 8 weeks of age. The epithelial cells lining the follicles secrete thyroglobulin into the central cavity of the follicle. Fetal thyroid cells gradually assume a columnar shape and show morphologic evidence of secreting thyroglobulin.

By 10 weeks gestation the fetal thyroid can accumulate iodide. This involves the uptake of iodide ion and its subsequent oxidation by the thyroid peroxidase system (Figure 3–12). In the process of oxidation I^- is organified; one or two atoms of iodine are added to the tyrosine residues of thyroglobulin to form monoiodotyrosine (MIT) and diiodotyrosine (DIT) (Figure 3–12). Coupling of these iodinated tyrosines to form triiodothyronine (T_3) and thyroxine (T_4) is well established by 12 weeks gestation.

Defective embryogenesis may result in complete or partial absence of the thyroid. Such an absence would result in impaired production of thyroid hormones, as would a hereditary deficiency in any of the enzymes involved in thyroxine synthesis (p. 288). The latter defect might produce a goiter in the fetus owing to stimulation of the thyroid gland by elevated levels of TSH in fetal blood. Any state which can lead to a fall in circulating thyroid hormone would cause an increased release of TSH, which in turn would stimulate the follicular epithelium to produce more colloid.

Early in fetal life the thyroid gland, though capable of forming hormone, probably does not play an important role in development. Toward the end of intra-uterine life and during the neonatal period, the thyroid is probably needed for normal growth and development, particularly of the nervous system and bones. (p. 106). Though not doing so in the fetus, athyrosis nearly stops growth and development in immature persons.

A large fraction of circulating thyroxine is bound to thyroxine-binding globulin (TBG), an acidic glycoprotein with the relatively high carbohydrate content of 32 percent. TBG is present in very much smaller amounts in the fetus than in the mother, favoring distribution of thyroid hormones to the maternal circulation.

Other proteins in the blood bind thyroxine. Binding of this hormone to a prealbumin component of normal plasma or serum was first demonstrated by Ingbar in 1958. This protein, thyroxine-binding prealbumin (TBPA), has been purified and characterized. The serum concentration of TBPA is about 10 times as high as that of TBG, but during pregnancy it is depressed. Approximately 15 percent of endogenous thyroxine is bound to TBPA in normal human serum. Another protein which can bind thyroxine is albumin; however, its affinity for thyroid hormone is much lower than that of either TBG or TBPA.

Because of contributions of thyroid hormone from the mother, abnormalities of fetal thyroid function may not be clearly evident at birth. As we shall see (in Chapter Five), however, the importance of thyroid hormone in the maturation of the central nervous system suggests that critical assessment of the function of the thyroid in the newborn is a necessity.

Pharyngeal Pouches

PARATHYROID GLANDS. The human embryo has five pairs of endodermally lined pharyngeal pouches located along the lateral walls of the pharyngeal gut and approaching each other ventrally toward the midline. The last of these pouches is rudimentary and is often considered as part of the fourth. In the fifth week of development the epithelium of the dorsal parts of the third and fourth pouches differentiates into parathyroid tissue. The differentiating cells in each pouch multiply rapidly to form a solid nodule. By the sixth week the gland primordia lose their connection with the pharynegal wall. The parathyroid tissue of the third pouch migrates with the thymus (derived from the ventral portion of the third pouches) and comes to rest finally on the dorsal surface of the lower part of the thyroid gland and, in the adult, forms the *inferior parathyroid glands.* The parathyroid tissue of the fourth pouches attaches itself to the caudally migrating thyroid and finally is found on the dorsal surface of the mid or upper portion of the thyroid gland *(superior parathyroid glands).*

Each parathyroid gland is surrounded by a connective tissue capsule from which septa extend into the substance of the gland, dividing it into lobules. The substance of the gland consists of densely packed masses and cords of epithelial cells between which are interspersed numerous small blood vessels. The cells of the developing parathyroid gland appear to be variants of the *chief cell,* the cell which synthesizes and secretes PTH. The large acidophilic cells that will represent the "oxyphilic" cells of the parathyroid gland do not appear until late childhood.

Parathyroid hormone has been isolated from bovine and porcine glands and is a straight-chain polypeptide consisting of 84 amino acid residues. The hormone increases serum calcium and decreases serum phosphate concentrations by a direct action on bone, kidney, and probably the intestinal mucosa (Chapter Twelve). The secretion of PTH is regulated directly by the fluctuating levels of plasma calcium, and indirectly by the levels of plasma phosphate.

According to current concepts PTH acts principally on bone and kidney (p. 336). The normal concentration gradient continuously moves calcium from the fluid compartments of the body into surface bone, and PTH is required to replace this loss from the plasma. The replacement is accomplished by the breakdown of bone collagen and apatite crystals, releasing both calcium and phosphate into the circulation. PTH acts upon the kidney tubules to increase the reabsorption of calcium and to decrease the reabsorption of phosphate (p. 336). The net result of this renal action is to return calcium to the plasma and thus minimize the amounts of calcium that would otherwise have to be supplied by bone.

It is not known at what point in fetal life parathyroid hormone is first secreted. Glands from a fetus of 12 weeks gestation demonstrated PTH activity when grown in culture with bone. There is a striking increase in the rate of growth of parathyroid tissue from the fourteenth to the twentieth week of gestation. At about the same time vesicular cells appear in the gland. Such cells are thought to be associated with increased parathyroid function because vesicular cells often predominate in hyperfunctioning glands. Thus the morphologic features of the fetal parathyroids and their biologic activity in culture suggest that the fetal parathyroid is a functional gland.

In considering the control of mineral metabolism in the fetus it would be well to remember that in addition to parathyroid hormone, vitamin D and calcitonin may play important roles. Vitamin D, or more correctly its metabolites, plays a more or less permissive role and enables PTH to exert its normal action upon bone resorption. There are also strong indications that vitamin D has important effects upon all types of bone cells and upon the cells of the intestinal mucosa (p. 329). These effects involve the synthesis of a calcium-activated ATPase, which is required for the bulk transport of calcium across intestinal mucosal cells and across osteoclasts (see Chapter Twelve). However, the exact mechanism of action of vitamin D remains obscure.

THE THYMUS GLAND. The ventral portions of the third pharyngeal pouches, with contributions from ectodermal cells of the branchial grooves, give rise to the primordia of the thymus gland. Although this gland is not usually considered an endocrine gland, its very large size in the fetus and some recent evidence of a diffusible substance from the gland suggests it should be considered in this survey of developmental endocrinology.

The primordia of the thymus gland begin to migrate early in development in a caudal and medial direction, pulling the parathyroid primordia with them. The main portions of the primordia move rapidly to a final position in the thorax where they fuse. The thymus gland is the first organ to develop as a true lymphoid tissue: by the third gestational month the human thymus has a well-developed lymphocyte population, and even though other embryonal tissues, such as liver, may show immunocompetence at this stage, this property depends on the presence of the thymus.

It is known that the thymus gland is essential for the establishment and maintenance of immunologic competence in neonatal rodents; however, its role in the human fetus is unknown. Several types of experiments indicate that, in rodents at least, the thymus is the source of a blood-borne factor which induces the differentiation of lymphoid precursor or stem cells, rendering them capable of participating in immune reactions. Thus the thymus itself does not produce antibodies; rather, it confers on the stem cells of the bone marrow the potentiality of reacting to antigens.

Goldstein and White have isolated and purified a material from calf thymus which they call *thymosin.* This partially purified fraction prevents wasting disease (Chapter Fourteen) and restores cell-mediated host immunity of neonatally thymectomized mice. It is still not known whether the thymus secretes a single hormone or a multiplicity of factors that act to modulate lymphoid tissue structure and function.

The thymus is extremely responsive to endocrine stimuli throughout life. Thymic weight is particularly sensitive to endocrine regulation, being reduced by gonadal and adrenocortical hormones and increased by growth and thyroid hormones.

THE LIVER

The liver, strictly speaking, is not an endocrine gland; however, its role in steroid metabolism in the fetus and its contribution to estriol synthesis in pregnancy deserve consideration. Just as the thyroid rudiment first appears in the third week of gestation, so the liver primordium appears at that time as a thickening of the endodermal epithelium at the distal end of the foregut (Figure 1–8). This thickened area, known as the *hepatic diverticulum,* consists of rapidly proliferating cells which penetrate the mesodermal layer (septum transversum) between the pericardial cavity and the stalk of the yolk sac. The connective tissue of the liver is formed by the mesodermal cells of the septum transversum. The hepatic diverticulum splits into two components; one forms the liver and biliary duct system, the other forms the gall bladder.

The liver grows continuously and rapidly, and by the tenth week of development, it accounts for about 10 percent of the total body weight. Part of the large size of the liver early in development is due to its important hematopoietic constituents. Large nests of proliferating cells, which produce red and white blood cells, are found between the hepatic cells and the walls of the vessels. This hematopoietic activity gradually subsides in the latter part of gestation.

The liver is also of prime importance in the metabolism of steroids. Hepatic steroid metabolism usually involves an hydroxylation or a reduction which yields a steroid product with little or no biological activity. For instance, the hydroxylation of progesterone at either the 15α or 16α position yields 15α-hydroxyprogesterone and 16α-hydroxyprogesterone respectively, both very weak progestins. The fetal liver has very active 15α- and 16α-hydroxylases and thus provides a means of "inactivating" some of the large amounts of progesterone secreted to the fetus from the placenta. Any of the androgens (dehydroepiandrosterone, androstenedione, testosterone) can be hydroxylated at carbon 15 or 16 in the fetal liver. Consequently, androgens synthesized in the gonads or adrenals can reach the liver via the blood and can be metabolized to less active androgens. The androgens which are 16α-hydroxylated in the fetal liver can be transported to the placenta and serve as precursors of estriol. Estrone and estradiol, made in the placenta, can be 16α-hydroxylated in the fetal liver to a 16α-hydroxyestrone and estriol respectively.

The fetal liver also possesses highly active sulfokinases. Indeed, many fetal tissues appear to be capable of sulfurylating steroids, and as a result it is largely as the sulfates that one isolates steroids from fetal fluids. In contrast, the activity of the fetal liver enzymes uridine diphosphate glucose dehydrogenase (UDPG dehydrogenase) and glucuronyl transferase is rather low (p. 136). The former catalyzes the conversion of uridine diphosphate glucose (UDPG) to uridine diphosphate glucuronic acid (UDPGA), and the latter catalyzes the transfer of glucuronic acid from UDPGA to either steroid hormones or to bilirubin. Thus only small quantities of steroid glucosiduronates are found in the fetus. By the same token, conjugation of bilirubin to the water soluble diglucuronide is limited. Even at birth these enzymes are poorly developed in the liver, and the handling of a bilirubin load, which may be large because of accelerated breakdown of red cells, is seriously impaired. This abnormality is primarily responsible for the "physiologic" jaundice of the newborn.

The pancreas

The fetal pancreas arises as two outgrowths of the foregut. The dorsal bud, originating opposite to and slightly above the hepatic diverticulum, eventually forms the body and tail of the pancreas. A smaller ventral bud grows in the angle between the duodenum and the hepatic diverticulum and forms the common bile duct and the head of the pancreas. Dorsal and ventral outgrowths fuse at about 7 weeks in the human embryo.

The pancreas is both an exocrine and an endocrine gland. The cells having endocrine function originate from the duct epithelium, budding off to form the *islets of Langerhans.* The exocrine or acinar cells of the pancreas differentiate at about the third month of gestation, at a time when distinct islets of Langerhans are present.

By 12 weeks gestation, not only are islets of Langerhans detectable in the fetal pancreas, but insulin can be isolated from either pancreatic tissue or fetal blood. The insulin can be measured by either its immunoreactivity or its biological activity.

Steiner showed in 1969 that when isolated islets from rat pancreas or human pancreatic tumors were incubated with labeled amino acids, radioactivity appeared first in association with proteins of molecular weight 9000 rather than those corresponding with the molecular weight of insulin (6000). It was later demonstrated that this high molecular weight material, called *proinsulin,* consists of a single polypeptide chain 84 amino acids long and is composed of a C peptide which connects the N-terminal amino acid of the A chain of insulin to the C-terminal amino acid of the B chain of insulin. Since proinsulin contains the intact amino acid sequence of the insulin molecule it is not surprising that it cross-reacts with antibodies against insulin.

Extracts of human fetal pancreases contain proinsulin. It comprises 0.26 to 1.6 percent of the total immunoreactive insulin in the pancreas, irrespective of the age of the fetus. After partial tryptic digestion of this fetal proinsulin, the insulin immunoreactivity was enhanced by 40 percent, and the biological activity by over 800 percent. Thus it seems likely that different portions of the insulin molecule are responsible for the immunoreactivity and the biological activity.

The concentration of insulin in umbilical cord plasma ranges from 10 to 36 μU/ml, and it does not appear to vary with fetal age. Since there is little or no transfer of insulin across the placenta the insulin measured in fetal blood probably reflects secretion of the hormone by the fetal pancreas.

Though the pancreas develops early in fetal life, and apparently secretes insulin, it is still unknown how this secretion is controlled and how important insulin may be for normal growth and development in utero. In the adult a slight increase in blood glucose is a powerful stimulant for insulin secretion. The administration of glucose to pregnant women led to a fourfold increase in insulin in maternal plasma, but the insulin content of fetal plasma remained unchanged. The glucose had reached the fetuses and produced hyperglycemia (122 mg percent), but the β (insulin synthesizing) cells of the islets were unable to respond by secreting more insulin. No correlation was found between the concentration of insulin and that of glucose in fetal plasma. Thus in the fetal period the secretion of insulin appears to be controlled by different mechanisms from those operative in adult life. Some recent studies by Milner and colleagues suggest that the manner in which the pancreas responds to stimuli varies with age. The first stimuli to become effective are those operating via cyclic AMP, such as glucagon (p. 122). This is seen at 14 weeks, and a little later leucine is effective; later still the pancreas responds to arginine. Glucose becomes effective only at birth. If this is so, the means of insulin release may be dissociated into two mechanisms: a glucoreceptor mechanism developing late in gestation, and a much more primitive cyclic AMP-dependent mechanism present early in gestation.

The fetal pancreatic islets contain α cells as well as β cells. Indeed, the preponderance of α cells over β cells in the fetal pancreas suggests that glucagon may be an important regulator of glucose concentration in fetal blood.

Recent experiments have shown that a variety of human fetal tissues, including skin, muscle, brain, adrenal, and kidney tissues, respond in vitro to insulin by increased incorporation of labeled amino acids into protein. Insulin could be either increasing the transport of the labeled amino acids across the cell membrane, or directly increasing protein synthesis, or both. In many species (e.g., the chicken and the rat) insulin does not increase uptake of glucose in the fetus until relatively late in gestation. It is quite possible that the insulin-dependent transport systems for glucose and amino acids do not develop in fetal tissues until the end of gestation. However, protein synthesis may be stimulated by insulin in the fetus by a separate mechanism, provided amino acids can cross the cell membrane at a rapid enough rate.

The role of insulin as a "growth hormone" in the human fetus will be discussed further in Chapter Four. Just what factors control the synthesis and release of insulin in the fetus are not yet clear. Apparently the usual stimuli—glucose and amino acids—are not effective during the first half of gestation. Even at birth the response of the pancreas to these agents may be sluggish. There is no indication at present that insulin is necessary for normal fetal growth; however, human fetal tissues can respond to insulin in vitro.

SUMMARY

We have traced the development of each of the endocrine tissues from the original primordium in one of the three germ layers. Organogenesis is essentially complete after 3 months of gestation, and the fetal tissues have the potential to synthesize and secrete hormones. The controls of endocrine secretion in fetal life are poorly understood; however, there is some evidence that the controls are different from those operating in adult life. The failure of the fetal pancreas to respond to hyperglycemia is an example in point. Once organogenesis is complete we can begin to appreciate the role these endocrine tissues may play in the overall metabolism of the developing fetus.

SUGGESTED READINGS

Hormones of the adenohypophysis. C. H. Li, Proceedings of the American Philosophical Society, *Vol. 116*, p. 365, 1972.

An excellent summary of the present state of isolation and identification of the adenohypophyseal hormones. For the student who is interested in structure of hormones, this paper, by a renowned expert in the field, is very helpful.

Hypothalamic control of adenohypophyseal secretions. R. E. Blackwell and R. Guillemin, Annual Rev. of Physiology, *Vol. 35*, p. 357, 1973.

An up-to-date review of this rapidly changing area of endocrinology. The references provide the reader with original experimental details as well as pertinent review articles.

Development of steroidogenesis. D. B. Villee, American Journal of Medicine, *Vol. 53*, p. 533, 1972.

This review article is designed for the student who wants more detailed information on steroidogenesis in the fetus and placenta.

Developmental Physiology and Aging, P. S. Timiras, The Macmillan Company, New York, 1972.

The approach in Part I of this book is developmental and considers fertilization, embryogenesis, and neonatal and childhood changes in various organ systems. Endocrine aspects are covered in those sections where appropriate. Part II is devoted to the physiology of aging. An excellent reference book.

CHAPTER FOUR

Endocrine Control of Fetal Metabolism and Differentiation

In order to achieve the growth and differentiation necessary for extra-uterine survival, the human embryo and fetus must have adequate sources of energy. Ultimately these energy sources must come from the mother, whether it be in the form of carbohydrate, lipid, or protein. The modulation of the flow of energy-yielding compounds is achieved by the placenta, and the fate of these compounds is determined by the fetus. Undoubtedly, as in the adult, many of these metabolic processes are under endocrine regulation. Growth is much more rapid in the early part of gestation than it is in the latter part. The metabolic processes associated with growth and with the concomitant differentiation of cells involve the whole gamut of biochemical reactions. Let us consider them in some detail.

CARBOHYDRATE METABOLISM

Glycolysis

In the breakdown of carbohydrate to carbon dioxide and water, the initial changes occur equally well in the absence or presence of oxygen. The reactions of anaerobic glycolysis are mediated by the enzymes of the Embden-Meyerhof system of phosphorylating glycolysis, and the end result of the breakdown of glycogen or glucose is pyruvic acid (Figure 4–1). In the absence of oxygen, pyruvic acid is reduced to lactic acid by

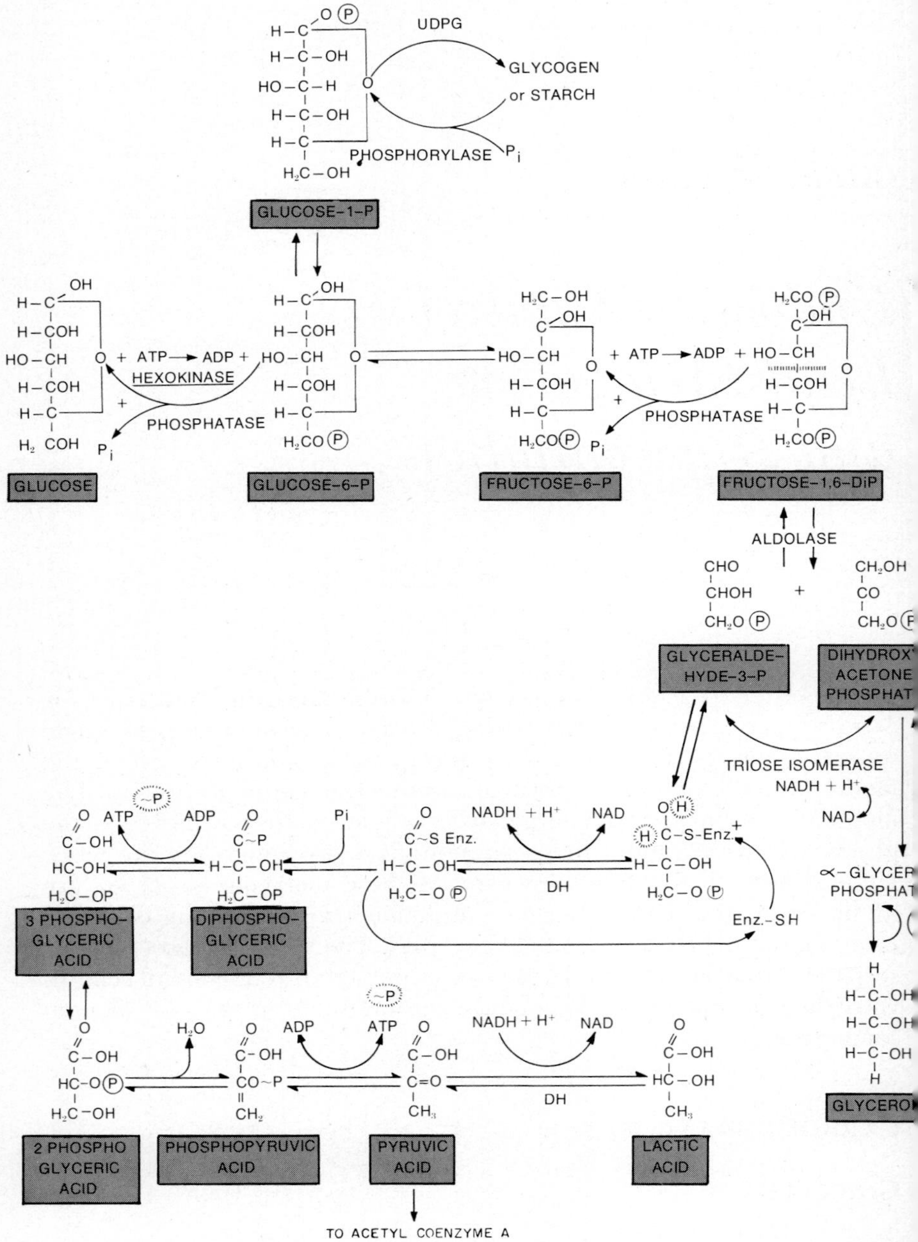

FIGURE 4–1. Glycolysis, the series of reactions by which glucose and other sugars are metabolized to pyruvic acid. The reversible steps are indicated by double arrows. Other steps are essentially irreversible; two different enzymes catalyze the reaction in the two different directions. For example, glucose-6-phosphate is converted to glucose by glucose-6-phosphatase but hexokinase catalyzes the conversion of glucose to glucose-6-phosphate. (From Villee, C. and Dethier, V. *Biological Principles and Processes.* Philadelphia: W. B. Saunders Company, 1971, p. 138.)

hydrogen transferred from reduced nicotinamide adenine dinucleotide (NADH). During the anaerobic reactions, some energy is conserved and stored in energy-rich phosphate bonds such as those in adenosine triphosphate (ATP). The important features of this pathway are that it consumes no oxygen and that it produces H^+.

The *phosphogluconate shunt* (or *hexose monophosphate shunt*) is an alternate path for the conversion of glucose to pyruvate. In this path, glucose-6-phosphate is oxidized to 6-phosphogluconic acid, and then through several intermediate steps to glyceraldehyde-3-phosphate (Figure 4–1). The initial reaction of the phosphogluconate shunt is catalyzed by a specific enzyme, glucose-6-phosphate dehydrogenase, and NADP is an obligatory cofactor. The NADPH generated by this oxidation must be converted back to NADP (oxidized) in order to accept another hydrogen from another molecule of glucose-6-phosphate. The NADPH is reoxidized by reactions in which the hydrogen is used in reductive biosynthetic processes, such as the synthesis of fatty acids (p. 81) and steroids (p. 159). Glyceraldehyde-3-phosphate is an intermediate in the Embden-Meyerhof pathway, and thus the phosphogluconate shunt can feed into the latter and yield pyruvate.

CITRIC ACID CYCLE

Though avian and mammalian embryos can derive energy through anaerobic processes, oxygen seems to be indispensable for normal development. The pathway for the further metabolism of pyruvate to carbon dioxide and water is called the *tricarboxylic acid* or *citric acid cycle* and has a much higher yield of ATP than does the glycolytic pathway. The first step in this pathway, the decarboxylation of pyruvate, is catalyzed by a very complex group of enzymes called the pyruvate dehydrogenase system. It requires coenzyme A, NAD^+, lipoic acid, and thiamine pyrophosphate and takes place in the mitochondria of the cell. Three molecules of ATP are generated during this reaction.

The two-carbon fragment that is generated, acetyl coenzyme A, combines with oxaloacetate to enter the cycle as citrate (Figure 4–2). In the steps involved in the conversion of citrate to oxaloacetate, electrons and hydrogen are removed and are transferred to nicotinamide adenine dinucleotide (NAD) and thence to oxygen via the system of cytochromes and cytochrome oxidase *(electron transmitter system)*. During the operation of the citric acid cycle (acetate to carbon dioxide and water), 12 high energy phosphate bonds are generated, as contrasted with the net gain of two ATP molecules in the conversion of glucose to pyruvate. Thus the citric acid cycle is an important, and probably *the* most important source of cell energy; however, oxygen must be present to accept the electrons released in the cycle.

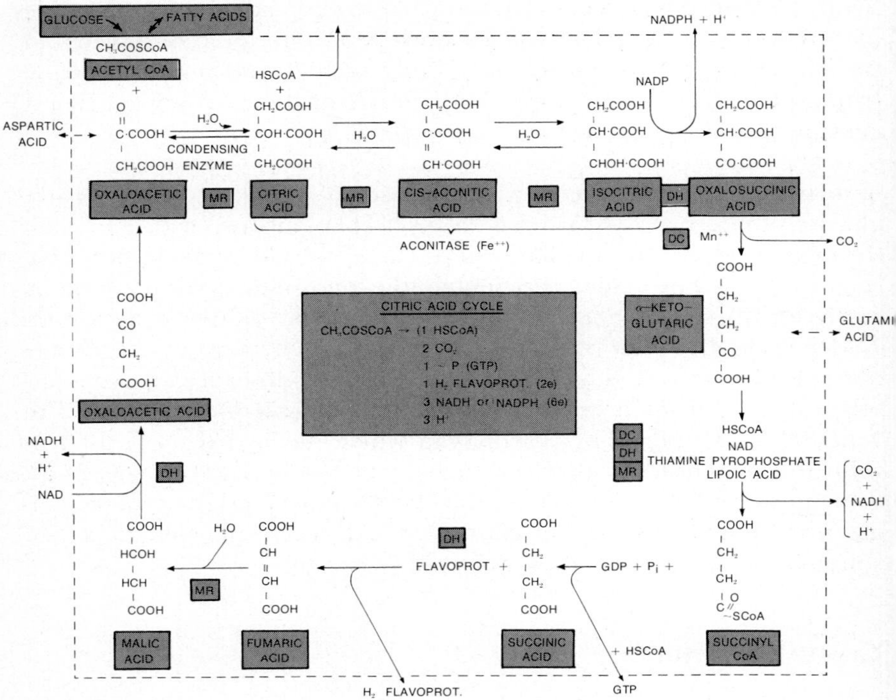

FIGURE 4–2. The cyclic series of reactions, termed the Krebs citric acid cycle, by which the carbon chains of sugars, fatty acids and amino acids are metabolized to yield carbon dioxide. The reactions are of three types, designated *DH*, dehydrogenations; *DC*, decarboxylations; and *MR*, make-ready reactions. The overall reaction effected by one "turn" of the cycle is summarized in the center. (From Villee, C. and Dethier, V. *Biological Principles and Processes.* Philadelphia: W. B. Saunders Company, 1971, p. 132.)

Glucose transport and storage

Undoubtedly all the enzymes involved in the conversion of glucose to carbon dioxide and water are present in all embryonic cells. The pathways of carbohydrate metabolism are essential for the production of biologically useful energy. Regulation of these pathways is equally vital in order to conserve energy not needed immediately. Glucose is supplied to the fetus from the maternal blood and all present evidence suggests that is the major source of energy for the human fetus. Glucose enters the cell by means of a "carrier protein" located on the cell membrane. This transport of glucose across the cell membrane is stimulated in the adult by insulin. Studies of glucose transport in chick embryos and rat fetuses indicate that uptake of glucose by fetal cells may not respond to insulin until relatively late in gestation. It is possible that the carrier protein in the cell membrane develops late in gestation and that early in development the membrane structure is such that glucose can cross freely.

Once within the cell, glucose is phosphorylated. In adult liver a specific enzyme (glucokinase) catalyzes the phosphorylation of glucose; however, this enzyme is active only when the concentration of blood glucose is high (p. 228). At low concentrations the less specific hexokinase is active. In the rat fetal liver no specific glucokinase can be observed. Since the concentration of glucose in fetal blood is rather low (56 mg/100

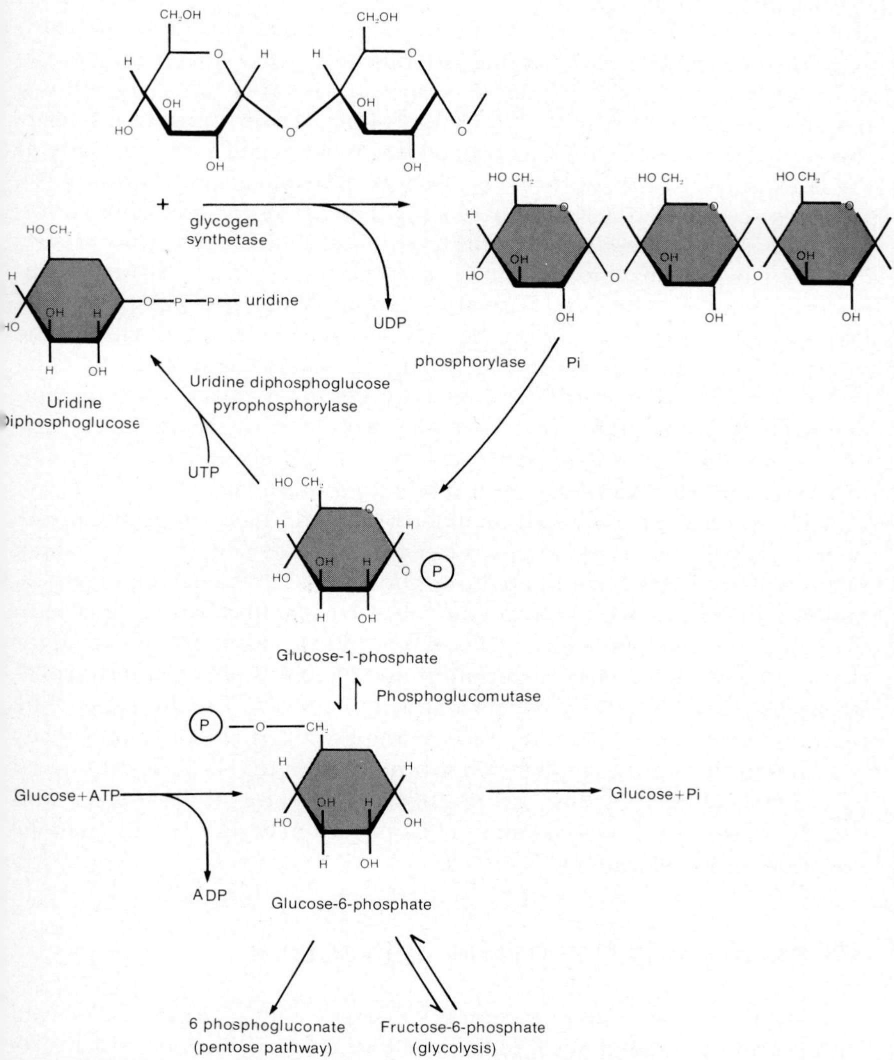

FIGURE 4–3. The synthesis and cleavage of glycogen occur by different pathways. Glycogen is synthesized by reactions involving uridine triphosphate (UTP) and the formation of uridine diphosphoglucose (UDPG). Glycogen is broken down by the action of phosphorylase, which strips off individual glucose units as glucose-1-phosphate. (From Villee, C. and Dethier, V. *Biological Principles and Processes.* Philadelphia: W. B. Saunders Company, 1971, p. 157.)

ml in the human fetus), it is quite likely that hexokinase is the more active enzyme in the fetus.

Once phosphorylated, glucose can be metabolized for energy or stored for future use. Carbohydrate is stored in the form of glycogen by a series of steps involving the enzymes phosphoglucomutase, uridine diphospho-glucose pyrophosphorylase, and glycogen synthetase (Figure 4–3). In the human fetus a variety of tissues are capable of forming and storing glycogen, including liver, heart, skeletal muscle, placenta, lung, and skin. Liver, heart, and skeletal muscle in particular serve as reservoirs of glycogen. Under normal circumstances the fetus begins to lay down glycogen at about 10 weeks gestation. At birth this glycogen is a major source of energy in the first hours of life. To be utilized for energy this complex molecule must be broken down by specific enzymes. One of the key enzymes in this process is glycogen phosphorylase (Figure 4–3), which exists in active and inactive forms. The active form of phosphorylase is phosphorylated; the phosphorylation of inactive phosphorylase is catalyzed by an enzyme—a kinase, the activity of which is under endocrine control. Hormones such as epinephrine and glucagon act through adenyl cyclase and cyclic AMP to increase the activity of the phosphorylase kinase. At birth, when the blood sugar falls (causing release of glucagon) and the body temperature falls (releasing epinephrine), glycogen is broken down to glucose to provide via the glycolytic pathway and the citric acid cycle the energy needed for metabolic processes and the maintenance of body temperature.

The fetus is primarily an anabolic organism. Early in gestation the fetal liver lacks the enzyme glucose-6-phosphatase (Figure 4–1), which releases free glucose from glucose-6-phosphate. This enzyme is important in adult life, since the liver controls the concentration of glucose in the blood and must be able to release free glucose when the blood sugar is low. The placenta early in gestation possesses this enzyme and probably helps maintain steady concentrations of glucose for the fetus. The placenta is capable of forming and storing glycogen, and one of the key enzymes in this pathway, glycogen synthetase (Figure 4–3), is stimulated by insulin. Quite possibly the glycogen synthetase of fetal liver and muscle is also sensitive to insulin. Thus insulin may serve as an anabolic hormone of development.

AMINO ACID AND PROTEIN METABOLISM

Peptide bond synthesis requires energy, energy which is derived largely from the metabolism of glucose in the fetus. The amino acids required as substrates for protein synthesis are supplied by the maternal blood. The concentration of free amino acids in fetal plasma is higher than that in maternal plasma as a result of the transport of amino acids across the placenta against a chemical gradient by an active process requiring energy.

Little is known directly about the energetics of protein synthesis in the embryo; however, in vitro cultures of human fetal skin, muscle, brain, kidney, and adrenal have been shown to incorporate labeled amino acids into protein rapidly. The specific activity of the protein from these tissues was increased 50 to 150 percent when insulin was added to the culture medium (0.1 to 1.6 I.U. ml). Here again, insulin may be functioning as an anabolic hormone in the human fetus.

Studies of human fetal pituitaries show that labeled GH, TSH, FSH, and LH can be formed from labeled amino acids by these tissues in vitro. The release of insulin by the fetal pancreas has been well documented.

The amino acid tyrosine serves as a precursor in the synthesis of epinephrine and thyroxine, and several amino acids are used in the synthesis of the releasing factors of the hypothalamus. There is evidence for the formation of thyroxine in the fetal thyroid, and epinephrine is present in fetal blood; as yet, however, we have no information as to when the synthesis of hypothalamic releasing factors begins. Human fetal pituitaries do respond to exogenous releasing factors in vitro by secreting more of the appropriate tropic hormone (Chapter Three).

LIPID METABOLISM

Fatty Acids and Triglycerides

In the adult organism a large portion of energy is derived from fat. This fat, in the form of triglyceride, is formed in adipose tissue cells and in certain other cells of the body. During the first half of gestation the human fetus contains about 0.5 percent fat, but by the twenty-eighth week of gestation the fat content may reach 3.5 percent. The deposition of fat in the last two months of pregnancy is rapid; indeed, fat makes up about 16 percent of the 3.5 kg weight of the normal full term baby.

Acetyl coenzyme A is the building block for the de novo biosynthesis of fatty acids. Its carboxylation to malonyl coenzyme A is catalyzed by the enzyme acetyl coenzyme A carboxylase. Malonyl coenzyme A is coupled to a molecule of acetyl coenzyme A to form acetoacetyl coenzyme A. By a process of alternate reductions (using hydrogen from NADPH), dehydrations, and repetitive additions of two-carbon units, fatty acids are formed (Figure 4–4). By a series of enzymatic reactions, glycerol (via glycerol phosphate) can be esterified with fatty acids, and triglycerides are formed (Figure 4–4). In liver and adipose tissue, the major sites of triglyceride biosynthesis, fat is stored for future use.

When energy is needed, triglyceride in adipose tissue can be split to glycerol and free fatty acids. The latter are transported in the blood and are used by many tissues as a source of energy. The breakdown of triglyceride is under hormonal control. The cleavage is very much like that of the phosphorylase involved in the breakdown of glycogen. A key enzyme in the breakdown of triglyceride, lipase, exists

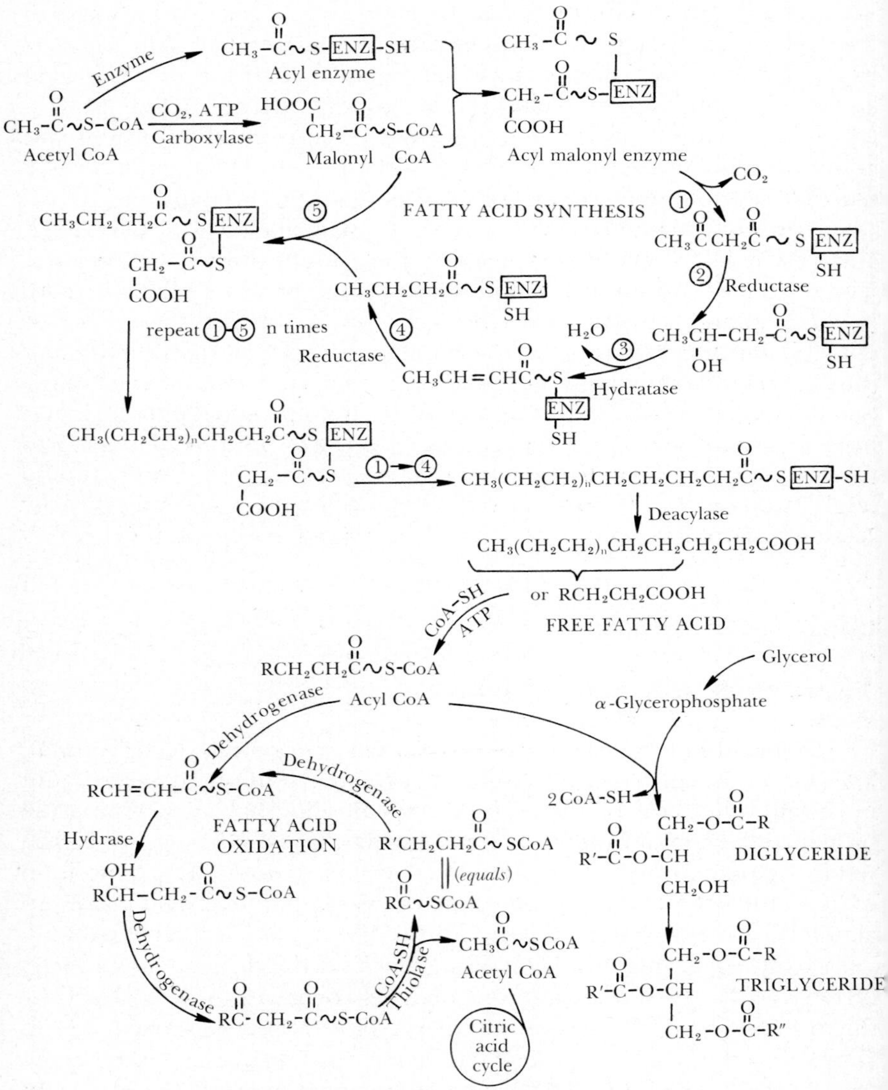

FIGURE 4–4. Pathways of fatty acid metabolism.

in an active phosphorylated form and in an inactive unphosphorylated form. A kinase catalyzes the phosphorylation of the inactive lipase. The activity of the kinase is increased by cyclic AMP, which is increased in the cell when the enzyme adenyl cyclase is stimulated. A variety of *lipolytic* hormones can stimulate the adenyl cyclase of adipose tissue and bring about the rapid breakdown of fat. Amongst the most powerful of lipolytic hormones are epinephrine and ACTH.

Fatty acids are oxidized by a process called β-oxidation, with the removal of two-carbon fragments (Figure 4–4). These two-carbon fragments are in the form of acetyl coenzyme A and can enter the citric acid cycle to be further metabolized. Ultimately, then, the energy of fat or fatty acids is made available via the citric acid cycle.

PROSTAGLANDINS

Within the last two decades a group of lipid derivatives of prostanoic acid have been characterized. These derivatives were called prostaglandins because they were isolated in large quantities from semen and were thought to be formed in the prostate gland. We know now that it is the seminal vesicle rather than the prostate gland which is responsible for most of the prostaglandins in human semen, where the concentration approaches one millimolar. These substances, however, are not formed solely by the seminal vesicle—almost every tissue in the body is capable of synthesizing prostaglandins. Their effects on uterine motility and the number of their other influences on reproductive organs suggest that one of the principal roles of the prostaglandins is concerned with reproduction.

The prostaglandins are oxygenated and cyclized twenty-carbon fatty acids formed from arachidonic acid. The carbon atoms 8, 9, 10, 11, and 12 form a cyclopentane ring. One group of prostaglandins (E) has an oxygen at carbon 9 and a hydroxyl at carbon 11, whereas another group (F) has hydroxyls at both carbons (Figure 4–5). In general, the E compounds cause inhibition of uterine motility, whereas the F compounds cause contraction. In human seminal fluid the ratio of E:F is about 7:1; therefore, it is not surprising that the overall effect of seminal fluid on human myometrium in vitro was found to be inhibition of uterine motility. Human menstrual fluid contains at least two prosta-

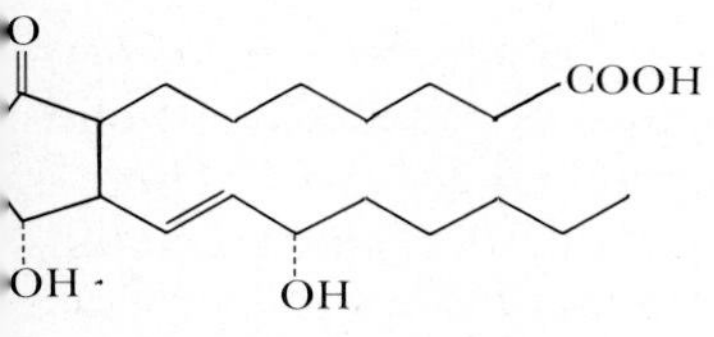

Prostaglandin E_1

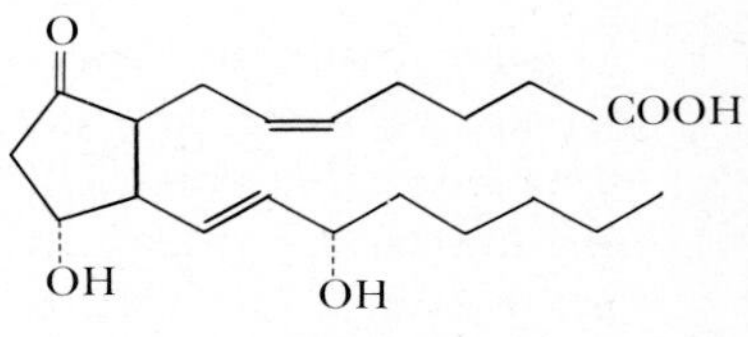

Prostaglandin E_2

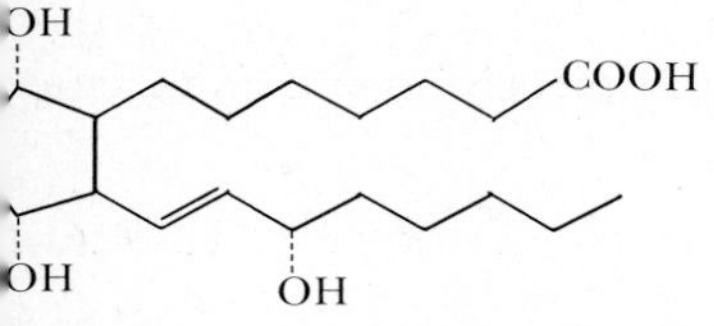

Prostaglandin F_{1a}

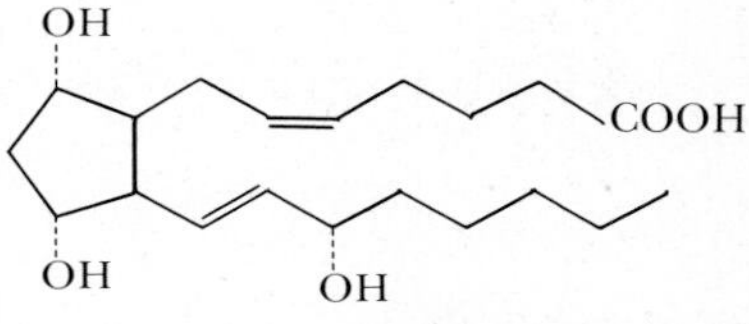

Prostaglandin F_{2a}

FIGURE 4–5. Structural formulas of biologically important prostaglandins.

glandins, and it has been suggested that these substances are liberated into the blood stream from the endometrium during menstruation and are transported to the muscular part of the uterus where they induce rhythmical contractions which assist in the expulsion of the menstrual fluid.

Many tissues have the capacity for synthesizing prostaglandins from essential fatty acids; accordingly, it seems unlikely that the prostaglandins are part of a classical endocrine-target organ system. However, it is possible that they serve as local regulators of cell function. Aside from their effects on uterine motility, prostaglandins are capable of stimulating adenyl cyclase in a variety of tissues, including the ovary. (Indeed, Marsh has recently shown that prostaglandin E can stimulate adenyl cyclase of corpus luteal cells in broken cell preparations.) The ability of prostaglandins to increase the concentration of cyclic AMP (by stimulating adenyl cyclase) has been shown to exist in adipose tissue, platelets, thyroid, lung, spleen, diaphragm, fetal bone, adenohypophysis, heart, and kidney medulla also. Interestingly enough, prostaglandin E_1 in small quantities can also *lower* the concentration of cyclic AMP in fat cells. Thus it can inhibit the activation of adenyl cyclase in the fat cell by several hormones, including the catecholamines and ACTH. Concentrations of prostaglandin E_1 as low as four nanomolar prevent the effects of epinephrine on fat cells.

The ubiquitous distribution of these compounds and their profound effects on the ovary, uterus, and other tissues of the body justify the enormous amount of interest in and research on prostaglandins at present. The whole area of fetal synthesis of and response to prostaglandins is virtually untouched. The effects of these compounds on uterine motility has prompted trials of various prostaglandins as abortifacients or as inducers of labor. Do they play a role in sperm migration? What is their role in luteinization? The recent work of Channing suggests that prostaglandins are capable of inducing luteinization of granulosa cells in vitro.

Aside from their effects on the reproductive system, the prostaglandins may very well produce profound alterations in metabolism secondary to their effects on cyclic AMP in fat cells and in the thryoid. There is some indication, at least in fat cells, that the synthesis of prostaglandins may be under hormonal control. If so, the fat cell may be able to form these compounds under the appropriate stimulus and self-regulate its rate of lipolysis. The roles of prostaglandins in reproduction and metabolic homeostasis remain at the frontier of our knowledge; future studies may enable us to fit the prostaglandin piece into the endocrine puzzle.

STEROIDS

By virtue of their solubility properties, the steroids are classified in the lipid family. The synthesis of steroid hormones by the fetus and

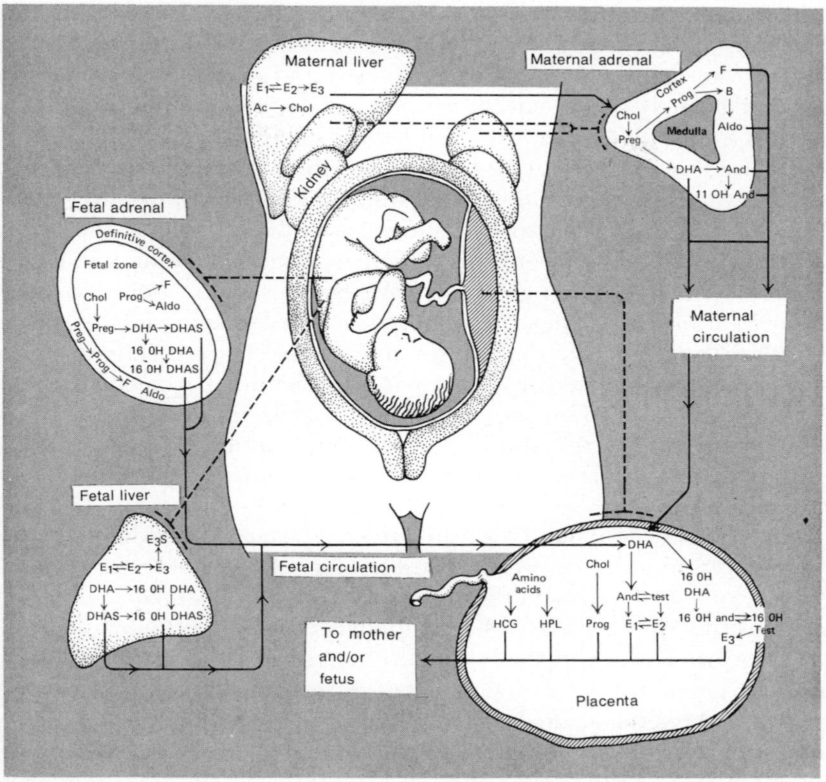

FIGURE 4–6. Steroid metabolism in the materno-feto-placental unit. *Abbreviations*: Chol, Cholesterol; Preg, Pregnenolone; Prog, Progesterone; DHA, Dehydroepiandrosterone; 16OH DHA, 16α-hydroxydehydroepiandrosterone; B, Corticosterone; F, Cortisol; Aldo, Aldosterone; And, Androstenedione; 11OH And, 11-hydroxyandrostenedione; 16OH And, 16α-hydroxyandrostenedione; Test, Testosterone; 16OH Test, 16α-hydroxytestosterone; E_1, Estrone; E_2, Estradiol; E_3, Estriol. (From Page, E., Villee, C., and Villee, D. *Human Reproduction.* Philadelphia: W. B. Saunders Company, 1972, p. 242.)

placenta has been studied extensively. The fetal adrenal cortex and testes develop during embryonic life and are capable of forming steroid hormones. These steroids, plus those formed by the placenta, contribute to the overall steroid metabolism of the *feto-placental unit.* As we saw in Chapter Three, the major steroid product of the fetal adrenal cortex is dehydroepiandrosterone. This nineteen-carbon androgen can serve as a precursor for the synthesis of estrone or estradiol in the placenta. If dehydroepiandrosterone is 16α-hydroxylated by either the fetal adrenal cortex or the fetal liver, the product, 16α-hydroxydehydroepiandrosterone, can serve as a precursor of placental estriol. Thus a close association exists between the fetal adrenal cortex, the fetal liver, and the placenta, in that they share in the overall biosynthesis of estrogens (Figure 4–6).

Estrogens are not formed exclusively from fetal nineteen-carbon precursors. Dehydroepiandrosterone formed in the maternal adrenal cortex can reach the placenta and can be used there as a substrate for estrogen synthesis. Since the maternal liver has an active 16α-hydroxylase, 16α-hydroxydehydroepiandrosterone may also come from the mother. Though the maternal contribution to estrogen precursors is undoubtedly much less than the fetal contribution, it is probably better to think in terms of a *materno-feto-placental* unit for estrogen synthesis (Figure 4–6).

Steroids with the Δ5-3β-hydroxy configuration are rapidly conjugated in the fetus, and they are found in the blood primarily as sulfates. The placenta, however, has little or no sulfokinase, and the steroid sulfates reaching the placenta are rapidly hydrolyzed by placental sulfatases. Accordingly, when any dehydroepiandrosterone sulfate circulating in fetal blood reaches the placenta, the active sulfatases there will hydrolyze the steroids to their free compounds. The free dehydroepiandrosterone can then be converted to androstenedione, which in turn can be converted to testosterone (Figure 4–6). Both androstenedione and testosterone can be aromatized to estrone and estradiol respectively. By a similar pathway, free 16α-hydroxydehydroepiandrosterone can be converted to estriol.

Fetal blood contains large quantities of 16α-hydroxylated Δ5-3β-hydroxysteroid sulfates. Most of these steroids originate in the fetal adrenal cortex, though modification may occur in the fetal liver. The relative lack of a Δ5-3β-hydroxysteroid dehydrogenase in the fetal adrenal cortex prevents the conversion of Δ5-3β-hydroxysteroids to Δ4-3-ketosteroids. Thus, at least in the first half of gestation, the biosynthesis of cortisol by the fetal adrenal cortex is probably dependent on a supply of progesterone from the placenta. The latter produces about 260 mg of progesterone per day at term and it has been estimated that roughly half of this goes to the fetus. The progesterone content of the whole placenta rises steadily during gestation; thus a source of this steroid is available even in early pregnancy. It is possible, then, that placental progesterone could serve as a precursor for adrenal corticosterone or cortisol. It is equally possible that the cortisol circulating in the fetus comes from the mother. If the maternal adrenal can synthesize enough cortisol for the fetus and the mother, there may be no need for glucocorticoid synthesis in the fetus.

Similarly, though the fetal adrenal cortex can synthesize aldosterone in vitro from progesterone, the maternal adrenal may supply the fetus with this important mineralocorticoid. Or, since electrolyte homeostasis is maintained in all probability by the mother, mineralocorticoids may not be needed at all in the fetus.

Within recent years, clinicians have found the measurement of estriol in maternal urine or amniotic fluid helpful in assessing the condition of the fetus. The concept that neither the fetal adrenal cortex nor the placenta are of themselves complete endocrine organs, but that their combined activity is required for estriol synthesis, leads naturally to the theory that the amount of estriol formed is a reflection of the activity of the fetal adrenal and liver, and indirectly of fetal viability. The amniotic fluid contains a high concentration of estriol, and sampling of this fluid in high risk pregnancies has become almost routine. Many authors are agreed that estriol output is reduced when intra-uterine fetal growth is retarded. Some authors have gone further and claimed that the weight of a normal fetus at birth and the preceding maternal estriol output are related. However, fetal growth is the outcome of many factors, and it seems unlikely that there is a single factor simultaneously operative on growth and estriol production.

There are many occasions in obstetrical practice when it becomes of great concern to ascertain the possibility of intra-uterine fetal death. If indeed one could predict when fetal death is imminent, immediate efforts to remove the fetus could be instituted. Estriol assays may be helpful in this regard. In the common causes of intra-uterine death, such as toxemia, retarded intrauterine growth, or fetal abnormality, the impending disaster is frequently foreshadowed by a fall in estriol excretion. There is no doubt that once the fetus is dead, the estriol output drops rapidly to very low levels, whatever the state of the placenta. In late pregnancy, values of less than 1 mg of estriol in the urine passed in 24 hours are an indication of fetal death, and values below 3 mg give a strong indication of possible intra-uterine death.

Steroid Hormones and Development

Aside from their possible diagnostic value, do steroid hormones subserve any special roles in fetal growth and development? There is some evidence that steroid hormones, in particular cortisol, may induce certain enzymes and thus play an important role in the maturation of certain tissues. Cortisol may also be involved in the onset of parturition. There seems no doubt that testosterone is critical for normal sexual differentiation.

MATURATION OF FETAL TISSUES. It has been known for some time that premature babies run a greater risk of hyaline membrane disease than do full term babies. It has also been shown that infants dying of hyaline membrane disease are deficient in surfactant, a lipid material composed largely of dipalmityl phosphatidylcholine (dipalmityl lecithin) that is capable of reducing surface tension (p. 136). The work of several investigators using fetal lambs and rabbits has shown clearly that the enzymes involved in lecithin synthesis in the alveolar cells of the lungs of these fetuses develop in the latter weeks of gestation. Administration of cortisol to the fetus in utero accelerates the appearance of these enzymes both in lambs and in rabbits. If a similar condition obtains in the human, cortisol therapy prior to delivery of premature infants may be valuable. The ability of the fetus to form surfactant can be assessed by sampling the amniotic fluid and measuring the concentrations of lecithin and sphingomyelin. If the ratio of these substances (the L/S ratio) is less than two, the chances of the infant developing hyaline membrane disease after birth are high, according to Gluck (p. 136).

Both Jost's work with fetal rats and Greengard's work with newborn rats have shown the importance of hormonal induction of enzymes in the liver, particularly those enzymes involved in glycogen synthesis (p. 233) and gluconeogenesis (p. 235). Just how much of this work is applicable to the human is uncertain; however, undoubtedly the synthesis of many liver enzymes is under some sort of hormonal control in primates as well as in rodents.

ONSET OF PARTURITION. Anencephalic babies with hypoplastic adrenals often have prolonged gestation periods. This fact, coupled with the extensive studies by Liggins linking adrenal function and cortisol with the onset of parturition in sheep, has suggested to many investigators that cortisol may somehow trigger labor (possibly via prostaglandins p. 109). In the human fetus, during the first half of gestation (8 to 18 weeks), the concentrations of serum cortisol and cortisone are 7.3 ng/ml and 32.5 ng/ml, respectively, but late in pregnancy, the concentrations are tripled. There is an an abrupt rise in serum cortisol in association with labor. Whether the rise in cortisol in the human fetus is secondary to the stress of labor or is the instigator of labor still remains somewhat unclear. It has been shown, however, that weights of adrenals from infants born prematurely without apparent cause were greater than the weights of adrenals from premature babies of preeclamptic or hemorrhaging mothers. Also, hypophysectomy of fetal rhesus monkeys at the beginning of the third trimester was associated with significant prolongation of gestation. The birth weights of these hypophysectomized fetuses were normal, suggesting that growth hormone is not necessary for normal fetal growth. Adrenals, gonads, and thyroid glands were hypoplastic in these animals.

Undoubtedly, the factors controlling the onset of parturition will continue to receive attention as more evidence points to hormonal (in particular adrenal) factors in the process.

SEXUAL DIFFERENTIATION

The role of androgens in sexual differentiation is worthy of detailed consideration. Studies by Jost, using fetal rabbits, have contributed immensely to our knowledge and understanding of the process whereby an essentially bisexual system differentiates as female and male.

The cells of the gonads in males and females are derived from three different sources: the primordial germ cells, the coelomic epithelium on the medial wall of the mesonephros, and the mesonephric blastema. In Chapter Three we discussed the contribution of the mesonephric blastema to the development of the adrenals and gonads. The cells from the mesonephric blastema and the coelomic epithelium differentiate in situ. The primordial germ cells must migrate into the developing gonad (Chapter Three).

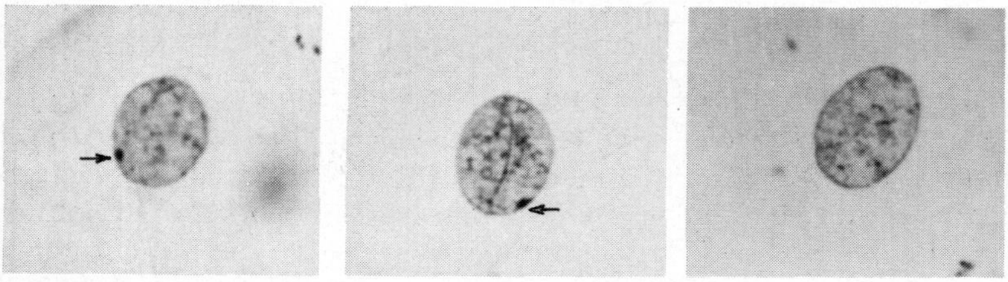

FIGURE 4–7. Sex chromatin in the epithelial cells of the human buccal mucosa. Arrows point to the sex chromatin at the nuclear membrane. The male cell (right) shows no sex chromatin. These photographs appeared in the original paper describing the buccal mucosa technique for observation of the sex chromatin. (From Moore and Barr 1955. *Lancet 2*: pp. 57–58.)

SEX CHROMATIN

Though the gonads are identical early in development, male and female human embryos can be distinguished by nuclear chromatin well before the primitive gonad stage. The X chromosomes in the female are necessary for normal ovarian development as well as for a large variety of somatic functions. The major portion of the second X in female cells is in a highly condensed (heteropyknotic) state during interphase. Barr and his associates were the first to describe the sexual dimorphism in nuclear structure. They found that the highly condensed chromatin appeared as a focal mass against the inner surface of the nuclear membrane in 25 percent or more of female cells (Figure 4–7). This chromatin mass is now known as the sex chromatin. It completes DNA synthesis later than any other chromosome in the complement, and the action of genes located on these condensed segments is suppressed. The other X chromosome, the single X chromosome in male somatic cells, is in a highly extended (isopyknotic) state during interphase. It completes DNA replication with most of the complement of chromosomes and is genetically active. Thus, in the female, the "inactivation" of one of the two homologous X chromosomes serves as a mechanism of dosage compensation. Though the second X in the female is probably genetically inactive, it is apparently necessary for normal human ovarian development, since XO individuals have rudimentary gonads (p. 189). In some animals, such as mice, normal female development occurs even in the absence of the second X chromosome.

After the sixteenth day of intra-uterine life, a high proportion of female somatic cells in interphase show condensed chromatin at the periphery of the nucleus. According to Lyon, this sex chromatin is alternately either the maternal or paternal X in a specific proportion of cells fixed by chance in embryonic life. Thus, with respect to maternal and paternal X chromosomes, each female would be a mosaic (again, according to Lyon). The germ cell line is a very important exception to this rule. Sex chromatin is never seen in the primitive germ cell, the oogonium, or, of course, the oocyte.

Gonadal differentiation

The Y chromosome has potent male determiners and induces testicular differentiation of the primordial bipotential gonad. After the primitive gonad stage, the gonads begin to develop their characteristic structures, and the courses of testicular and ovarian development diverge. The embryonic ovary continues to grow—in the human, for several weeks—before developing structures similar to the adult's. The characteristic testicular structure, under genetic control of the Y chromosome, becomes recognizable immediately.

In the male the epithelial cells of the sex cords (Chapter Three) continue to proliferate. As the testis develops, these cords become arranged into compact tubes of cells, the seminiferous tubules. Meanwhile, the free ends of the original sex cords, deep within the mesenchymal core of the gonad, form the rete of the testis. In the final organization, each coiled tubule is connected via a straight tubule to the rete complex. Within the primitive gonad, the germ cells are scattered throughout the sex cords, the mesenchyme, and the coelomic epithelium. In the male these germ cells become incorporated into the developing seminiferous tubules. The Leydig cells, the major steroid hormone-producing cells, develop from the mesenchyme between the sex cords (p. 64). They rapidly increase in size and number, filling the spaces between the seminiferous tubules.

Even after the testis has developed an adult cell organization, the ovary continues to show no sexual differentiation. Embryonic gonads during this period are distinguishable as male and not-male, rather than as male and female. The coelomic epithelium and its daughter cells continue to divide, soon forming a solid epithelioid cell parenchyma around the mesenchyme and the epithelial cell cords of the primitive gonad. This outer parenchymal cap is termed the gland's cortex, and the inner region is called the medulla.

The germ cells in the female, as in the male, are scattered throughout the primitive gonad. They become concentrated within the cortex of the developing ovary. These germ cells, or "oogonia," enlarge and proliferate. Later they cease mitosis and enter meiosis. Meiotic prophase from leptotene to diplotene takes several days for individual cells (now called oocytes). The oocytes become arrested in diplotene until ovulation in the mature individual.

Gonaduct differentiation

There is little or no evidence that steroid hormones play any role in controlling gonadal differentiation; however, steroids produced by the fetal testis are critical in male differentiation of the external genitalia. In addition the fetal testis probably produces a substance which acts locally to induce development of the Wolffian duct structures (Wolf-

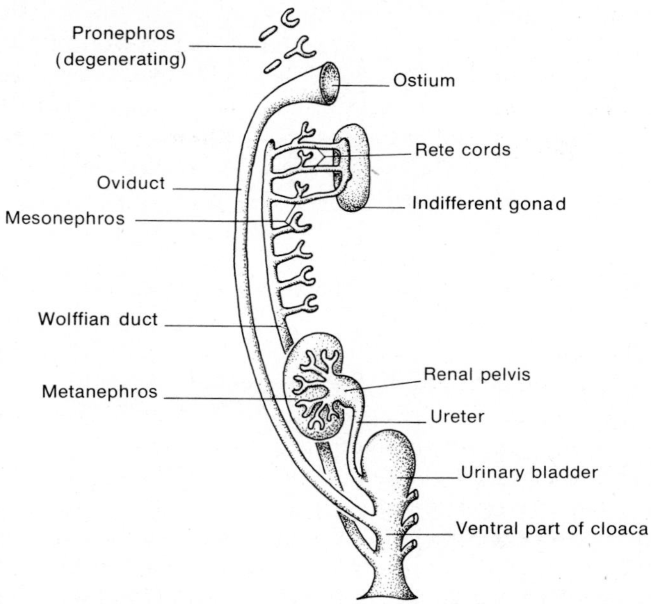

FIGURE 4–8. A ventral view of the urogenital organs of the sexually indifferent stage of an embryo. (From Villee, C. and Dethier, V. *Biological Principles and Processes.* Philadelphia: W. B. Saunders Company, 1971, p. 824.)

fian inducer). Human fetal testes have the capacity to produce significant amounts of androgens, including testosterone, from 9 to 15 weeks gestation (Chapter Three). This is the period of gonaduct differentiation, and androgens plus the Wolffian inducer stabilize the Wolffian duct system and induce its differentiation into epididymis, vas deferens, and seminal vesicles. The Wolffian duct derivatives and the prostate glands develop only the presence of these testicular products. Androgens prevent the invagination of the vagina and the development of the breast rudiments. Androgens also produce masculine development of the external genitalia. In the absence of the testis during the period of sexual differentiation, all of these systems develop in the female pattern.

The Mullerian ducts (oviducts) form as a second pair of ducts that are anterior and external to the mesonephros (Figure 4–8). Cranially, they appear as a funnel of the coelomic epithelium, the funnel which becomes the ostium of the Fallopian tube. The blind end of this funnel proliferates posteriorly and pushes a cord of cells lateral to the Wolffian duct. The Mullerian ducts reach the urogenital sinus (cloaca) at about 32 mm (10 weeks). At this stage the fetus may be considered to be provided with both Mullerian and Wolffian structures and is sexually undifferentiated and bisexual with regard to the gonaducts (Figure 4–8). Near the cloaca the two Mullerian ducts join in the midline and fuse. It is evident that some product of the fetal testis is responsible for the inhibition of fetal Mullerian ducts. The Mullerian duct repressor may also be involved in stimulating differentiation of the Wolffian ducts. The repressor is generally considered to be a protein but there is no real proof of this hypothesis. No steroid tested has been effective. It has been noted that the Mullerian repressor acts only locally and is probably diffusion limited. In cases of mixed testicular dysfunction, with one essentially normal and one grossly abnormal testis, the Mullerian duct regresses only on the side by the normal testis.

DIFFERENTIATION OF THE EXTERNAL GENITALIA

Like the other portions of the genital tract, the external genitalia pass through a bisexual period. The urogenital sinus and the anlage of the external genitalia are neutral primordia which give rise to the homologous structures in the male and female (see Chapter Eight). At early stages the external genitalia consist of: (1) a genital tubercle or phallus, (2) the urethral groove which is limited laterally by the two urethral folds, and (3) the genital swellings (scrotolabial swellings) which appear on either side of the phallus. Testosterone and other androgenic hormones play the decisive role in the differentiation of external genitalia. Like the genital ducts, in the absence of the testis the external genitalia develop in the feminine pattern; this requires no hormonal stimulant. Differentiation of the external genitalia along male lines will occur only if androgenic stimulation is received during early fetal life. Androgenic hormones stimulate growth of the genital tubercle and induce fusion of the urethral folds and labioscrotal swellings. They also inhibit growth of the vesicovaginal septum, thereby preventing the separation of a vagina from the urogenital sinus. After the twelfth fetal week, when the vagina has already separated from the urogenital sinus, fusion of the labioscrotal folds will not occur, even under an intense androgenic stimulus. Androgen stimulation will cause clitoral hypertrophy, however, at any time during intra-uterine existence, as well as after birth.

SUMMARY

So much of fetal development and relationship to the mother is unknown. We can discuss in a fairly sophisticated manner steroid metabolism in the materno-feto-placental unit. After all, enormous numbers of experiments from many different laboratories have contributed to this fund of knowledge. However, we know almost nothing about the effects of steroid hormones on fetal metabolism. Does cortisol produce the same changes in metabolism in the fetus as it does in the adult? We don't know. Does aldosterone regulate sodium excretion in the fetus? Again, we don't know.

The single exception to this bleak picture of ignorance lies in the area of our knowledge of the role of androgens in sexual differentiation.

Once again, many investigators have been interested in sexual differentiation, and countless experiments in lower animals have paved the way for interpretation of mammalian differentiation. The beautiful experiments by Jost, in which he demonstrated the necessity of a fetal testis for normal male differentiation, and the organ culture experiments by Price, serve as examples of painstaking research in this filed. As physicians we are confronted all too often with "experiments of nature" which require interpretation in the light of our knowledge of normal sexual differentiation.

The information we have gained about steroids in the developing human fetus has come from several studies over the past years. Comparable studies should be performed in other areas of fetal endocrinology. The fetal thyroid has been of considerable interest to investigators, as has the fetal pancreas and pituitary. Much less is known about the fetal parathyroid or the parafollicular cells of the thyroid, thymus, and hypothalamus. The prostaglandins, too, may be of some importance in the fetus, but we know very little indeed about their synthesis, concentration, or effects in the human fetus. The study of the human fetal endocrine system and its metabolism is coming into its own now, and in the near future this discipline may help in the interpretation of and therapy for many of the clinical problems which confront the obstetrician and pediatrician in the perinatal period.

SUGGESTED READINGS

Mammalian conception, sex differentiation and hermaphroditism as viewed in historical perspective. Dorothy Price, American Zoologist, *12*:179, 1972.

An excellent review of concepts of sexual differentiation from earliest times to the present.

Fetal Growth and Development, H. A. Waisman and G. Kerr, McGraw-Hill Book Company, New York, 1970.

The papers reported at a symposium on Fetal Growth and Development (San Diego, 1968) are reported in this book. Pertinent chapters are (a) Energy Metabolism and Fetal Development, by John Sinclair, and (b) Fetal and Postnatal Development of Lipid and Carbohydrate Metabolism, by Pater Hahn. Factors affecting fetal growth, such as malnutrition, are discussed in some detail.

PART TWO

THE NEWBORN

CHAPTER FIVE

Endocrine and Metabolic Changes in the Perinatal Period

Our discussions so far have concerned possible endocrine control of growth and differentiation in utero. Fetal growth is such that although the human fetus develops a variety of organ systems, many of these are used very little or not at all prior to birth. The mother has been supplying the fetus with oxygen and nutrients. She has also maintained the proper pH, temperature, and electrolyte balance of the fetus, and she has removed fetal metabolic wastes as well. Suddenly, when newborn, the infant must perform all of these functions independently. The perinatal period, defined as extending from 20 weeks gestation through 28 postnatal days, is fraught with problems for the fetus-newborn. Fortunately, a variety of prepartum preparations and postpartum adjustments reduce the peril of the change from intra- to extra-uterine existence.

ENDOCRINE CHANGES IN THE MOTHER

Throughout pregnancy the mother must undergo adaptations to meet the needs of her offspring. These adaptations include alterations in circulatory and respiratory functions and profound shifts in metabolism to maintain the nutrient and oxygen supplies to the fetus. The metabolic alterations of pregnancy are in large part under hormonal control and thus it is not surprising that changes in the maternal endocrine system are observed.

Estrogens and Progestins

Some of the early maternal endocrine changes were discussed in the section on the fetus. The maternal ovary and subsequently the placenta secrete large amounts of progesterone and estrogens. The concentrations in the maternal blood and urine of progesterone and of all three estrogens—estrone, estradiol, and estriol—rise progressively throughout pregnancy. The much greater increase in estriol is the result of contributions of 16α-hydroxylated precursors from the fetus. In contrast to the synthesis of estrogens, the synthesis of progesterone by the placenta can occur without the intervention of fetal enzymes.

Certainly at no time in the normal life span is one exposed to greater quantities of estrogens and progestins than in pregnancy. These hormones are obviously important in the maintenance of pregnancy and have marked effects on uterine structure and function. Under the influence of estrogen, the endometrium grows and becomes thicker and relatively dense (p. 379). In addition, the spiral arterioles elongate. Under the influence of progesterone, the previously estrogen-primed endometrium becomes secretory. Other target tissues respond to these hormones. Cornification of the vaginal cells and the initial stimulation of growth of the mammary glands are produced by estrogens. Progesterone also plays a role in regulating breast development, particularly the budding of the alveolar system.

Aside from the effects of these hormones on the breasts and the reproductive tract, there is abundant evidence that estrogens and progesterone can produce alterations in other tissues of the body. During pregnancy, estrogens increase the concentration of a variety of plasma proteins such as renin substrate, thyroxine binding globulin (TBG), and corticosteroid binding globulin (CBG). The latter two specific hormone binding plasma proteins have been studied extensively as models of hormonal transport. Many steroid hormones are transported in the blood stream, bound to protein. For example, estradiol is bound to albumin and to a β-globulin (sex hormone binding globulin, or SBG) which will also bind testosterone. This β-globulin is present in higher concentrations during pregnancy and may represent another plasma protein which is increased by estrogens.

The steroid-protein complex is in equilibrium with the free steroid. Only the latter is actually taken up by tissues. The interaction between SBG and estradiol can be represented by the equation:

$$\text{Estradiol} + \text{SBG} \underset{k_2}{\overset{k_1}{\rightleftarrows}} \text{Estradiol-SBG}$$

At equilibrium: $k_1\,[\text{Estradiol}]\,[\text{SBG}] = k_2\,[\text{Estradiol-SBG}]$

The binding shows high affinity and specifity. These high affinity binding proteins have been widely used in recent years for assaying steroids. In these assays, the hormone to be measured competes with radioactively labeled steroid for sites on the binding protein. The binding of the radioactive hormone with the protein is similar to that of the nonradioactive hormone.

Estradiol-^{14}C + SBG $\rightleftharpoons$ Estradiol-^{14}C-SBG + Add sample of Estradiol $\rightarrow$

{Estradiol-^{14}C-SBG, Estradiol-SBG} + {Estradiol-^{14}C, Estradiol}

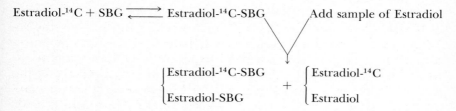

The amount of displaced radioactive estradiol is therefore a measure of the amount of nonlabeled estradiol in the sample. Such competitive protein binding assays are highly sensitive and are now being used to measure estradiol, testosterone, progesterone, and cortisol.

Just how the various effects of estrogens and progestins are produced has occupied the attention of numerous investigators. It seems clear that target tissues possess specific protein receptors that bind steroid hormones such as estradiol or progesterone (Figure 5–1). Jensen

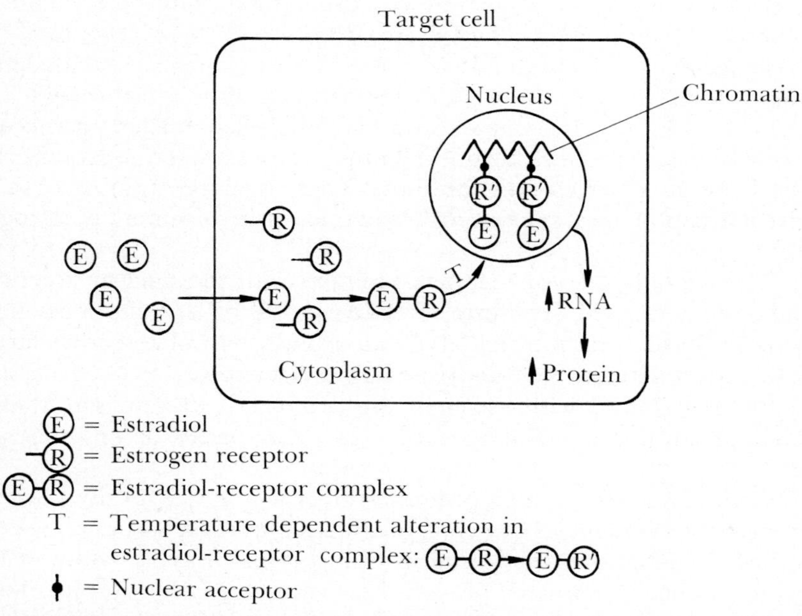

FIGURE 5–1. Model of mechanism of action of estradiol. Comparable models exist for other steroid hormones and their respective cytoplasmic receptors and nuclear acceptors.

proposed that estradiol is taken up and bound to a receptor present in the cytoplasm of the uterine cells (uterine cytosol). The estrogen cytosol receptor complex sediments as a discrete band on ultracentrifugation in a sucrose gradient. The sedimentation coefficient is about 8S. In the presence of sodium or potassium chloride (0.2M or higher), the 8S complex is reversibly transformed into a smaller, more slowly sedimenting entity (4S).

Estrogen receptor proteins can be isolated from the uterine cytosol of hormone-deprived animals. When combined with estradiol, the resulting estradiol-receptor complex is transformed by a temperature-dependent process to a 5S complex. Exposure of uterine nuclei to estrogen and the cytosol receptor at 2°C results in a small uptake of the complex by the nuclei and conversion to a 4S complex. If the same mixture is heated to 25 to 37°C, a much greater uptake of estrogen-receptor complex occurs, and the transformation yields a 5S complex. Simply warming a cytosol-estradiol mixture in the absence of nuclei yields a 5S complex. Jensen concludes that the estradiol-4S protein of the cytosol complex is first converted to a 5S form which then associates with an "acceptor" site in the uterine nucleus.

More recently Puca and his colleagues have reported the purification of a receptor-transforming factor. This factor is apparently a Ca^{++}-dependent protease which transforms the 5S-estrogen complex to a 4S complex. On the basis of the molecular weights of the 5S (5.3S molecule = 118,000) and 4S (4.5S molecule = 61,000) material, Puca suggests that the parent protein (5S) is cleaved into two equimolecular fragments by the receptor-transforming factor. According to these investigators, the 5S complex is converted to a 4S complex in the cytoplasm, and the latter penetrates the nucleus, where it forms a strong, although reversible, interaction with the chromatin. Puca has identified nuclear acceptors, which are basic proteins (histones) binding only estrogen-receptor complexes, not the estrogen-free receptors. There is a large number of these nuclear acceptor sites, suggesting broad nuclear involvement in estrogen action.

The steroid-receptor complex interacts with the nuclear acceptor, producing increased synthesis of RNA, including specific messenger RNA. This estrogen-induced RNA can actually be isolated from target tissues, and when estrogen-deprived tissues are exposed to it, effects similar to those found with estrogen are produced. Protein synthesis is increased, and as a result the activities of a variety of enzymes are increased.

O'Malley has found that progesterone is bound specifically to a protein receptor present in the chick oviduct. The receptor increases the synthesis of RNA and the synthesis of a specific protein, avidin, if the oviduct has been stimulated previously by estrogen. Other studies of this nature in mammalian systems indicate that probably all steroid hormones interact with specific receptors in their target tissues and are thus concentrated in these tissues (Figure 5–1). We may take this theory a step further. All available evidence suggests that protein hormones also interact with specific receptors in their target cells (p. 274). Since many protein hormones (ACTH, vasopressin, LH, glucagon) are known to increase the intracellular concentration of cyclic AMP by altering the adenyl cyclase system, and since the adenyl cyclase system resides on the inner surface of the cell membrane, once the hormone is bound to the cell surface, it may act directly on adenyl cyclase. In contrast to steroid hormones, there is little evidence as yet that protein hormones are transported to the nucleus of the cell, or that they even enter the cell.

Pituitary hormones

Although changes in the production of estrogens and progesterone during pregnancy are of pre-eminent interest to many researchers, other endocrine changes are worth noting. It is well established that the pituitary, primarily the anterior pituitary, enlarges in pregnancy. Specific, transitional "pregnancy" cells appear. The function of these these cells is uncertain, but they may be concerned with an increased secretion of prolactin.

Spellacy and Buhi have shown that the output of GH in late pregnancy is markedly decreased. At the same time, the concentration of human placental lactogen (hPL) in maternal blood is high. There may be some reciprocal relationship between these two "somatotropic" hormones; however, the hyposecretion of GH persists into the early postpartum period, despite the disappearance of hPL from the blood. By 6 weeks postpartum, GH is released from the pituitary gland in normal amounts.

Adrenal hormones

Cortisol and similar adrenocortical steroids exist in plasma in two forms; a protein-bound form and a free form. The estrogen-induced rise in CBG during pregnancy is paralleled by an increased concentration of cortisol; however, classic signs of adrenal hyperfunction are not often seen. Only free cortisol is metabolically active, and it is this concentration in maternal blood which is important. The studies by Doe suggest that the concentration of free cortisol is increased in pregnancy. Pregnant women may have purplish striae, diabetic glucose tolerance curves, easily bruised skin, hypertension, and fluid retention—all compatible with hypercortisolism.

Although there is still some question about free cortisol in pregnancy, there is no doubt that the secretion of aldosterone by the mother is increased significantly, especially during the last months of pregnancy. Undoubtedly, some of the rise in aldosterone secretion is due to the estrogen-induced increase in plasma renin activity.

Thyroid hormones

The thyroid gland is moderately enlarged in pregnancy owing to hyperplasia of the gland and increased vascularity. The basal metabolic rate (BMR) progressively increases from the fourth month of pregnancy to term by as much as 15 to 20 percent. The rise in oxygen consumption which occurs can be ascribed largely to the products of conception and is not due to hyperthyroidism.

Both the glomerular filtration rate (GFR) and renal plasma flow increase early in pregnancy, and the mean renal clearance of iodine is high. The increased renal clearance of iodine continues throughout pregnancy and is associated with a persistent loss of maternal iodide and a decreased concentration of plasma inorganic iodine. Thus in pregnancy there is a state of relative iodide insufficiency. The thyroid gland must increase its clearance of iodine to maintain the absolute iodine uptake within the euthyroid range. Hence the hyperplasia of the gland is a compensatory phenomenon and is not due to increased TSH in the circulating blood (Table 5–1).

The serum protein-bound iodine (PBI) value gradually rises during the first 12 weeks of pregnancy until it reaches a plateau. The values for butanol extractable iodine (BEI) also rise to a plateau during pregnancy. Tests of these values to determine levels of iodine are non-specific, for they measure iodides from other sources, such as medications (KI, iodinated drugs), organic dyes (cholecystogram, intravenous pyelography, angiography, myelography), or abnormal iodinated proteins (p. 289). Both the PBI and BEI tests have been replaced by measuring the serum thyroxine. Since thyroxine is 65 percent iodine by weight, the PBI will be equal to two thirds of the concentration of thyroxine.

There are three proteins in serum that bind thyroid hormone: thyroxine-binding globulin (TBG), thyroxine-binding prealbumin (TBPA), and albumin. TBG migrates electrophoretically in a zone intermediate between α_1 and α_2 globulin. The concentration of TBG in serum may be expressed as thyroxine-binding capacity, and for a normal

TABLE 5–1. Representative Values in Serum for Some Clinically Useful Thyroid Function Tests*

	Nonpregnant Euthyroid	Pregnant or on Estrogen Therapy
Thyroxine (μg/100 ml)	4.0 to 10.0	5.1 to 13.9
Free thyroxine (ng/100 ml)	2.5 ± 0.4	2.7 ± 0.6
Immunoreactive TSH (μU/ml)	3.9 ± 2.0	3.9 ± 2.0
Resin T_3 (%)	25 to 35	Less than 25

*Summarized from Selenkow, H. A., Birnbaum, M. D., Hollander, C. S.: Thyroid function and dysfunction during pregnancy, pp. 66–108, in *Obstetrical Endocrinology*, ed. K. J. Ryan, Clin. Obst. and Gyn., *Vol. 16*, No. 3 (New York: Harper and Row, 1973).

human this value would equal 16 to 25 $\mu g/100$ ml serum. Assuming one thyroxine-binding site per TBG molecule, the concentration of TBG in normal human serum is about 2.5×10^{-7} M. This value rises in pregnancy about 2.5 times over and apparently results from the high levels of estrogen, since the administration of estrogens to nonpregnant women causes a similar rise in TBG.

TBPA is a binding protein of relatively low affinity, as compared to the high affinity of TBG. Each molecule of TBPA has a single binding site for either T_4 or T_3. The serum concentration of TBPA is normally about 10 times greater than that of TBG, but during pregnancy it is depressed. Approximately 15 percent of endogenous thyroxine is bound to TBPA in normal human serum. Another protein which can bind T_4 or T_3 is albumin; however, its affinity for thyroid hormone is much lower than that of either TBG or TBPA. Roughly 75 percent of thyroxine is bound to TBG, and another 10 percent is bound to albumin. Approximately 99.97 percent of thyroxine is protein-bound, while about 99.7 percent of triiodothyronine is protein-bound, predominantly to TBG.

It is often helpful in assessing thyroid function to measure the TBG capacity. An indirect measurement is afforded by the red cell or resin uptake test. In this test, $^{131}I\text{-}T_3$ plus either red blood cells or resin are incubated with the patient's serum. If the TBG in the serum is fully saturated with thyroid hormone, no $^{131}I\text{-}T_3$ can bind to it, and all the labeled hormone will remain bound to the resin. The serum and resin are separated and the latter counted. The amount of radioactivity present is inversely proportional to the number of unsaturated binding sites. In pregnancy, with the large increase in TBG, there is a marked increase in the number of binding sites, and though there is more thyroid hormone formed, only about half of these sites are occupied. Thus less of the $^{131}I\text{-}T_3$ remains bound to the resin in the resin uptake test (Table 5–1). Estrogen therapy also decreases the resin (or red blood cell) uptake of $^{131}I\text{-}T_3$. It should be remembered that measuring resin T_3 uptake is an in vitro test which has nothing to do with the concentration of either T_3 or T_4 in the serum. It is a test which measures the available binding sites for thyroid hormones on serum proteins.

Certain conditions cause a decrease in the amount of TBG in the blood. In the nephrotic syndrome and in patients on androgen therapy, TBG is diminished, as is the concentration of T_4 in the serum. Certain compounds, such as diphenylhydantoin, can displace T_4 from TBG.

The concentration of thyroxine in serum is essentially the concentration of bound thyroxine. The method of Murphy and Pattee is the technique of choice in measuring serum thyroxine. It utilizes the techniques of competitive protein binding: just as labeled and unlabeled estradiol compete for binding sites on SBG, so labeled and unlabeled T_4 compete for binding sites on TBG. A standard curve is prepared by incubating known amounts of thyroxine with TBG saturated with radioactive T_4. Depending upon the amount of T_4 in the patient's serum, a certain amount of radioactive T_4 will be displaced, and this displaced T_4 can be counted. By reference to the standard curve, the amount of T_4 in the serum can be determined. In pregnancy there is an increase in serum thyroxine, and as a consequence the amount of displaced radioactive T_4 is elevated (Table 5–1).

It is possible to measure the concentration of free thyroxine by equilibrium dialysis. The values for the pregnant woman are similar to those of the nonpregnant woman (Table 5–1). What the values indicate is that although total thyroxine concentration of the serum in pregnancy is elevated, the increase over the nonpregnant state is due to increased thyroxine bound to TBG.

Although the amount of triiodothyronine in the circulation is miniscule in comparison with the amount of thyroxine, the much greater biological potency of this hormone and its much more rapid turnover render its measurement of some significance. During normal pregnancy, there is a steady but slight rise in serum T_3 (as measured by radioimmunoassay). The peak of this rise is reached by the end of the first trimester. The concentration of free T_3 in maternal serum, however, falls below normal values and remains in the low range to term.

OTHER HORMONES

There seems to be a definite rise in the amount of serum parathyroid hormone (PTH) during the latter half of pregnancy. This is the period when the fetal demands on maternal calcium are maximal, and hyperparathyroidism in late gestation is probably explainable on this basis.

The concentration of insulin in pregnancy serum is also elevated; however, unlike other hormones, it is rapidly degraded by a placental insulinase. In late pregnancy, glucose utilization by maternal tissues is impaired. The contradictory co-existence of decreased glucose uptake with higher blood insulin values has been attributed to anti-insulin factors such as the high circulating hPL. This hormone is diabetogenic in man and counteracts the effects of insulin. Grumbach believes that hPL has a specific role in pregnancy: to increase lipolysis in order to provide non-carbohydrate calories for the mother and thereby conserve carbohydrate and amino acids for the fetus.

ENDOCRINE CHANGES IN THE FETUS

The developing fetus needs a constant supply of glucose and amino acids. It may well be that maternal metabolic adjustments ensure that ample amounts of these materials are provided via the placenta. If the functions of supplying the fetus are such that amounts of each material are indeed adjusted on the maternal side, then perhaps there is no need for endocrine regulation of these functions in the fetus. Moreover, if fetal growth is dependent simply on the supply of nutrients alone, and if differentiation is programmed and independent of hormonal control, there may be no need for fetal hormones. We know that various fetal endocrine tissues differentiate morphologically and biochemically (Chapter Three), but whether they actually function in vivo remains somewhat uncertain. It is clear, however, that testosterone must be produced in the fetus to provide for male sexual differentiation.

THYROID HORMONES

Let us consider the thyroid first. Studies of aborted human fetuses have shown that during fetal life, there is a gradual increase in plasma proteins, with the early appearance of TBPA and, later, TBG. The concentrations of these binding proteins in fetal blood increase up to term. Associated with this rise in plasma binding proteins is a progressive increase in fetal serum T_4 and T_3; however, T_3 values are low and in the adult hypothyroid range, whereas T_4 values are comparable to, or even exceed, maternal values. The concentration of free T_4 in cord blood at birth is slightly higher than the comparable value in maternal blood. Free T_3 values, in contrast, are significantly lower than maternal free T_3 values.

Thus in the fetus the ratio of circulating T_4 to T_3 is higher than that in the normal adult. This high ratio is not reflected in the fetal thyroid gland. The mean T_4/T_3 content of fetal thyroid glands is similar to that of euthyroid adult glands. In the adult, a significant fraction of circulating T_3 is derived from peripheral conversion of T_4 to T_3, and it has been suggested that in the fetus, the rate of this conversion may be decreased.

Despite the low concentrations of both total T_3 and free T_3 in fetal blood, the normal newborn is not hypothyroid. Throughout pregnancy, the concentrations of free T_4 in maternal and fetal sera remain within normal limits, which may explain the euthyroid state of the normal newborn. It is of some interest to consider the source and function of these thyroid hormones circulating in fetal blood.

The human fetal thyroid is capable of synthesizing thyroglobulin and thyroid hormones by 10 weeks gestation, but does it need to? Is thyroid hormone necessary for growth and development in utero? The experiments by Kerr, using rhesus monkeys, indicate that the primate fetus *does* require thyroid hormone. Can the maternal thyroid supply all of the hormone required? The gross appearance of athyrotic babies born of euthyroid mothers is normal at birth; however, the development of bones and teeth is usually retarded. Dental anlagen seem to develop normally without fetal thyroid hormone, but enamel and dentine formation, tooth eruption, and development of the jaw bones are dependent on thyroid hormone. Thus not enough maternal thyroid hormone reaches the athyrotic fetus to permit normal maturation of all bones. Is this true also for maturation of the brain?

Thyroid hormones in the fetus and neonate can pass the blood-brain barrier. The development of the central nervous system, particularly the cerebellum, is influenced by thyroid function. Lack of thyroid hormones during growth and maturation of the brain may result in irreparable mental deficiency. Most of the experiments in this area have been performed using neonatal rats. Solokoff noted that thyroxine increased cerebral oxygen consumption and caused a more rapid rise of the cerebral metabolic rate. These effects, however, could be produced in rats only during the period of growth and development. Once the brain was mature, thyroid hormone was without effect. (Thyroid hormones cannot pass the blood-brain barrier in later life.) Solokoff's experiments with cell-free systems indicate that the action of thyroid hormone in the target cell is dependent on the presence of mitochondria and results in enhanced protein synthesis. Of even greater interest is Solokoff's discovery that the source of the mitochondria determines whether thyroxine can stimulate protein synthesis. The hormone stimulates protein synthesis in the presence of mitochondria from immature brain, but it fails to stimulate in the presence of adult mitochondria, regardless of the source of the microsomes and cell sap. It appears, then, that the mitochondria of immature brain, like those of liver and other thyroxine sensitive tissues, contain functional sites which are a locus of action of thyroxine.

If all the data on developing rats apply to the human, a similar thyroid-dependent change in brain cells may occur with maturation. The proliferation as well as the character of brain cells at a critical stage of development may depend on thyroid hormone, and in its absence, the growth and maturation of these cells could be arrested. The dependence of brain growth and development on thyroid hormone would be expected to involve the perinatal period, for maturation is occurring most rapidly then.

If the development of the nervous system in late gestation is dependent on thyroid hormone, can the thyroid hormone reach the fetus from the mother? Moreover, *does* the hormone reach the fetus from the mother? Thyroxine crosses the placenta very slowly, and many investigators believe that the rate is too slow to maintain an athyrotic fetus. They would argue that athyrotic newborns of euthyroid mothers only *appear* normal and that the evidence of hypothyroidism is too subtle to be picked up readily at this time. This may be particularly true of changes in the central nervous system.

Though TSH does not cross the placenta, and thyroxine crosses very slowly, there is abundant evidence that the long acting thyroid stimulator (LATS) crosses the placenta and is probably the cause of neonatal hyperthyroidism in some babies born of mothers with Grave's disease. The disorder in the newborn is self-limited and lasts until LATS disappears from the blood.

Iodides and antithyroid drugs also cross the placenta and can produce goiters in the fetus. Accordingly, the treatment of hyperthyroidism in the pregnant woman must be conducted with great care, and the use of KI in asthmatic pregnant women should be restricted. The minimum dose of antithyroid drug should be used. Selenkow recommends the addition of thyroxine to the therapeutic regimen to guard against maternal hypothyroidism.

ADRENAL HORMONES

Both the natural and synthetic glucocorticoids (prednisolone and prednisone) can cross the placenta and in so doing can pose a potential threat to the fetus. This is particularly true in mothers treated for a variety of diseases requiring large daily doses of glucocorticoids. There have been occasional reports of adrenal insufficiency in babies born of steroid-treated mothers; however, actual measurements of cortisol production rates in babies of prednisone-treated mothers show no difference from normal values. Warrell and Taylor have reported a rather high incidence of stillbirths to mothers treated with prednisolone throughout pregnancy. They are of the opinion that babies of prednisolone-treated mothers are at high risk and that glucocorticoid administration during pregnancy is not without danger. Often, however, there is no choice but to use steroids in treating some patients.

It is generally believed that protein hormones do not cross the placenta in significant amounts. Thus if insulin, PTH, or GH are necessary for development in utero, the fetal endocrine tissues must supply the hormones. Growth hormone is present in high concentrations in fetal blood, but its role is unknown. Insulin is present in fetal blood, but the response of the fetal pancreas to hyperglycemia is sluggish. The preponderance of α cells in the fetal islets of Langerhans suggests that glucagon may be quantitatively significant in the fetus.

Catecholamines may play a special role in utero. The large amount of extra-adrenal chromaffin tissue in the fetus contains impressive amounts of norepinephrine. These tissues are responsive to anoxia in vitro, with a marked decline in the amount of fluorescent material (catecholamines) they contain. Such responses, if they exist in vivo, may be important in maintaining circulatory function. It has been suggested that the release of norepinephrine under the stimulus of hypoxia at birth may be involved in the constriction of the ductus venosus and ductus arteriosus.

PARTURITION

The mean duration of human pregnancy is 266 days from conception to birth, with a standard deviation of 12 days. Labor is triggered by

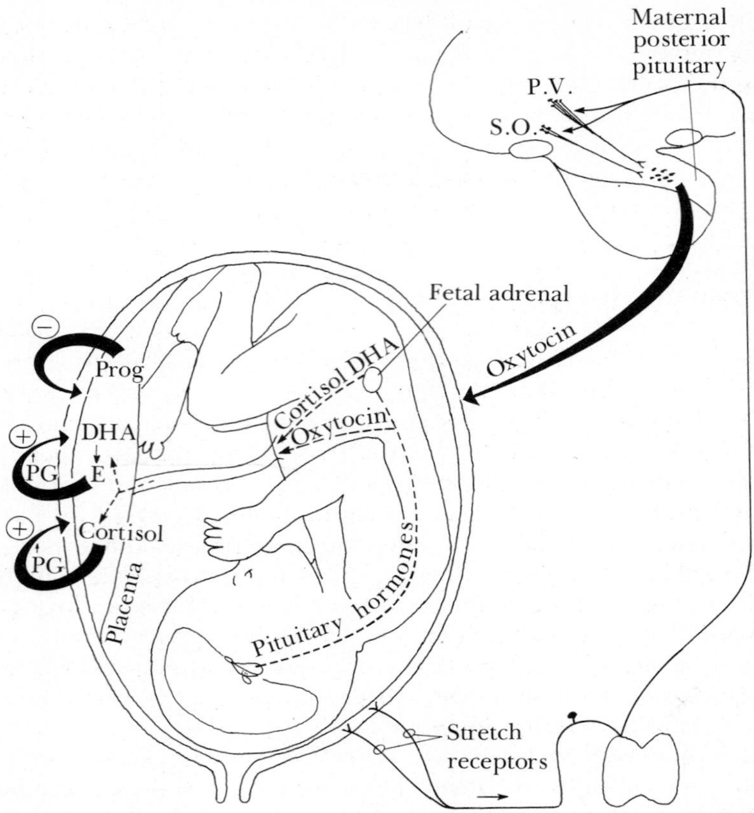

FIGURE 5–2. A hypothetical scheme for the control of parturition. Either estrogen (E) formed from fetal dehydroepiandrosterone (DHA) or glucocorticoids may act by increasing prostaglandin (PG) synthesis in the uterus or placenta. The latter increases (+) the sensitivity of the uterus to oxytocin from either maternal or fetal supraoptic (S.O.) or paraventricular (P.V.) nuclei. Progesterone decreases (−) the sensitivity of uterine musculature.

different factors in different species. For example, in the rabbit, labor follows a decrease in plasma progesterone secondary to the decline of the corpus luteum; however, in the human, there is no such decrease in maternal plasma progesterone concentration before labor. The possibility remains, however, that changes in local concentration or in uterine metabolism of progesterone in the human near term could influence the sensitivity of the myometrium to hormonal stimuli or to changes in uterine volume (Figure 5–2). Increased uterine volume can stimulate mechanical activity of the myometrium (Figure 5–2). Hydramnios usually precipitates premature delivery, and on the average twins are born 22 days earlier than term.

Recently, opinion has shifted toward assigning a greater role to the fetus in the onset of parturition. One of the clearest examples of the influence of the fetus on the duration of pregnancy is seen in hybrids of the horse and donkey. The mean duration of pregnancy for a mare carrying a horse fetus is 340 days, but the mean for a mare carrying a mule fetus is 355 days.

Ingenious experiments by Liggins have implicated the fetal pituitary-adrenal axis in the initiation of labor in sheep. Hypophysectomy of fetal lambs results in prolongation of gestation, whereas administration of glucocorticoids to the fetuses can induce premature labor. In the human, too, the fetal pituitary and adrenal cortex may influence the onset of parturition. Fetuses with hypoplastic adrenals (as in anencephaly) are frequently subjected to prolonged gestational periods, whereas spontaneous premature terminations of human pregnancy are often associated with unusually high fetal adrenal weights. It is not certain what product of the human fetal adrenal may be involved in the onset of parturition. Both cortisol and estrogen precursors have been suggested (Figure 5–2).

The onset of labor in the human is apparently much more gradual than the sudden changes which occur in other species, such as the sheep. The increase in uterine contractility develops gradually over a period of 8 weeks or more. Concomitant with this altered uterine contractility, plasma and urinary estrogens rise more steeply, and plasma progesterone and urinary pregnanediol concentrations reach a plateau. In essence, the ratio of estrogen to progesterone increases in the last weeks of pregnancy, and these hormonal changes may be important in preparing the uterine musculature for labor. In the absence of estrogen, the resting electrical potential of the myometrial cell is extremely low. Under the influence of estrogen, this potential rises. Such an alteration in potential would help "prime" the uterus and make it more receptive to the effects of other stimuli such as oxytocin and prostaglandins.

The increase in estrogens noted in late pregnancy may be secondary to increased activity of the fetal adrenal, which provides precursors for estrogen synthesis (Figure 5–2). The fetal adrenals grow rapidly after 32 weeks gestation, perhaps in response to tropic influences of the fetal pituitary. The concentration of cortisol in fetal blood rises in late pregnancy, and it has been suggested that fetal corticosteroids may regulate placental synthesis of prostaglandins.

Liggins has shown that, in sheep, relatively high concentrations of cortisol in fetal blood act on the placenta by unknown mechanisms to reduce the secretion of progesterone and to increase the secretion of estrogen. Associated with the rising concentration of unconjugated estrogen, and possibly induced by it, is an equally sharp increase in the concentration of prostaglandin $F_2\alpha$ in uterine venous blood. According to the work done by Liggins, progesterone inhibits the release of prostaglandin $F_2\alpha$. Thus the decrease in progesterone produced by cortisol would increase the release of prostaglandin $F_2\alpha$. Estrogen itself promotes the synthesis of prostaglandin $F_2\alpha$. The myometrium of sheep responds to prostaglandin $F_2\alpha$ with heightened sensitivity to oxytocin.

If human parturition is controlled in a similar manner, one would expect a rise in prostaglandin $F_2\alpha$ with the onset of labor. This prostaglandin has been identified in the peripheral venous blood of women in labor, whereas no prostaglandins were found before the onset of labor. The decidua or the placenta are likely sources of these prostaglandins. There are indications, however, that when one subjects the human fetus to pharmacological concentrations of corticosteroids, estrogen production falls, a finding which suggests that species variation in control of parturition is quite likely. The final common pathway for all the hormonal effects on parturition may very well relate to prostaglandin alterations in the intracellular concentration of cyclic AMP. It is known that increased concentrations of cyclic AMP in myometrial cells inhibit uterine contraction, whereas diminished cyclic AMP enhances contraction.

The fetus may also be involved in the release of oxytocin and thus influence its own delivery (Figure 5–2). Near the end of pregnancy, the concentration of oxytocin in fetal blood increases and is higher than that in maternal blood. Concomitantly, the uterine muscle becomes progressively more sensitive to the hormone (an estrogen effect?). Once labor has started, stimuli from the cervix and vagina cause reflex secretion of oxytocin from the maternal posterior pituitary. This "fetus ejection reflex" is readily inhibited by stress or by ethanol. The latter has been used successfully in the treatment of threatened premature labor in women. Although the uterus can be sensitized to oxytocin, it is still uncertain whether maternal oxytocin is necessary for normal labor. Women with diabetes insipidus, who lack both vasopressin and oxytocin, as well as women from whom the pituitary has been surgically removed, have given birth without incident.

During the progress of labor, changes occur in the fetus. A progressive fall in P_{O_2} and oxygen content of fetal blood (measured from the blood vessels of the scalp), with a concomitant rise in P_{CO_2} and fall in pH, have been observed during labor. Failure of cardiorespiratory adjustments is the most frequent cause of death in the perinatal period. During uterine contraction there is fetal bradycardia. This bradycardia is usually of brief duration but may become prolonged in fetal hypoxemia.

ADAPTATION TO EXTRA-UTERINE LIFE

The fetus must adapt rapidly to extra-uterine life and for this many hormonal factors play a role. Once cardiorespiratory function is established, maintenance of body temperature represents one of the main physiologic challenges to the newborn.

THERMAL BALANCE

The smaller size and greater ratio of surface to body weight of infants (compared to that of adults), together with their scanty layer of insulating subcutaneous fat, renders them far less capable than adults of keeping body temperature constant. The human newborn exposed to cold responds with an increase in both metabolic rate and oxygen consumption. By this device, heat production is increased. How is this effect mediated at birth? Immediately at birth glycogen in various fetal tissues is probably used as a source of energy. The breakdown of glycogen is under hormonal control, and a release of either epinephrine or glucagon would activate glycogen phosphorylase. Studies of newborns in distress reveal that the infant is capable of autonomous glucagon secretion at delivery.

Another and more important source of energy for thermogenesis is triglyceride in adipose tissue. In human newborns, distinct masses of brown adipose tissue are found in the abdomen, around the kidney and adrenal, and around the neck and in the interscapular and axillary regions as well. This tissue represents the main site of thermogenesis in the newborn. Brown adipose tissue has undergone a curious adaptation in which electron transport is not coupled to phosphorylation in the cytochrome system. Therefore the rate of oxidation is no longer governed by the concentration of ATP and ADP in the mitochondria, and energy is released as heat instead of being stored as ATP. Under the influence of catecholamines, brown adipose tissue is activated to break down stores of triglyceride to glycerol and fatty acids and to oxidize them with the local production of heat. This is a form of chemical thermogenesis. The effect of catecholamines, though rapid, is transient.

A more prolonged increase in heat production depends upon thyroid hormone. Fisher and Odell have shown that during delivery and the early postpartum period, the concentration of TSH in fetal blood rises rapidly, reaching a maximum of 86 μU/ml at 30 minutes of age. Between 30 minutes and 4 hours, serum TSH decreases and thereafter gradually levels off at a value of 13 μU/ml by 48 hours. The half-time of disappearance of TSH in the newborn is similar to that of administered radioactive TSH in the adult. Thus the rapid rise and fall in serum TSH concentration in the newborn may represent release of stored pituitary TSH.

This acute discharge of TSH in the newborn provokes a marked thyroid hyperfunction, as reflected in the high total and free thyroxine concentrations found in blood during the hours following birth. At 12 hours they are still elevated but begin to decline after 2 days. In the premature infant, the acute release of TSH is more marked and prolonged than in the term fetus. Many investigators believe that cold exposure at birth triggers the release of TSH from the fetal pituitary; however, Fisher and Odell found a similar release of TSH in infants kept warm during the first 3 hours of life.

Water balance

Inasmuch as most cell membranes are completely permeable to water, water exchange between extracellular and intracellular compartments is governed largely by changes in osmotic pressure in the two compartments. With age, there is an increase in the intracellular water compartment, which probably reflects an intracellular increase in non-diffusible proteins. The extracellular water compartment decreases with maturation, a decrease which is undoubtedly responsible for the decline in total water content. At birth, total body water is 700 to 800 ml/kg body weight, whereas in the older child the value decreases to 600 ml/kg.

The kidney and gastrointestinal tract act as regulators of water volume and salt composition of the body; however, the newborn kidney is limited in function. Following its relative inactivity in utero, the kidney undergoes a transition period with marked limitation of most activities. The newborn is less able to handle a water load and less able to conserve water than the older child. The immaturity of the newborn kidney is reflected in its decreased glomerular filtration rate and even greater decrease in tubular function. As maturation proceeds, water excretion gradually increases.

The ability to concentrate urine is dependent upon the activity of the antidiuretic hormone vasopressin. The relative inability of the newborn kidney to concentrate urine suggested to several investigators either that an insufficient amount of vasopressin is released from the newborn pituitary or that the target cells in the collecting tubules are unresponsive to the hormone. The pores of the collecting tubules are normally sensitive to vasopressin, and in the presence of the hormone they permit free passage of water into the cells, providing there is an osmotic gradient. In the presence of an excess of water, the hypothalamic osmoreceptors are not stimulated and vasopressin is not released from the neurohypophysis.

Recent studies seem to indicate that the inability of the neonatal kidney to concentrate urine is not due to an insufficiency of vasopressin. Osmoreceptor activity in the newborn stimulates the secretion of vasopressin, but some studies have raised the question of just how responsive to vasopressin the newborn kidney is. The response to vasopressin differs in the newborn and the adult. Urine is slightly more concentrated in infants 2 hours after intramuscular administration of vasopressin, but the osmolarity of the urine returns to preinjection levels thereafter. In contrast, in adults, urinary osmolar concentrations rise sharply and continue to rise after vasopressin injection. It is possible that the target site receptors are not fully functional in the immature kidney, or that the countercurrent system in the medulla is relatively immature. The loop of Henle is short in the fetus and infant and may thus be unable to produce the necessary gradient for water transport into the cells of the collecting tubules.

Electrolyte balance

Though a wide range of electrolyte intakes is tolerated by the newborn, there is some evidence to suggest that the kidney of the newborn continues to reabsorb sodium chloride in situations in which the adult kidney would excrete it. For instance, infants on high sodium diets develop larger extracellular compartments than do infants on normal sodium diets. We know little or nothing about the effects of aldosterone on the newborn kidney, but it is possible that the mechanism for the control of aldosterone release is faulty in early neonatal life and predisposes the newborn to salt retention on high salt diets. Extracellular volume *is* regulated, however, for if the high salt diet is discontinued and a normal diet instituted, the extracellular compartment returns to normal size.

Mineral balance

It is not unusual to encounter a jittery, hyperactive newborn in the nursery. Increased neuromuscular irritability and convulsions are the most common and characteristic symptoms of neonatal hypocalcemia; therefore, a consideration of calcium homeostasis in these children is in order. Ordinarily, the concentration of calcium in serum is maintained within narrow limits, very close to a value of 10 mg/100 ml. Of this, about 6.6 mg per 100 ml is diffusible calcium, the majority of which (5.2 mg) is ionized. It is the concentration of ionized calcium which determines the onset of clinical tetany.

If hypocalcemia (serum calcium less than 8 mg/100 ml) develops in the first day or two of life (before oral feedings), the infant is most likely to be the product of an abnormal pregnancy or labor (as in births complicated by maternal diabetes mellitus, premature delivery, prolonged or difficult labor, or caesarean section). The cause of the hypocalcemia in these conditions is unknown.

Hypocalcemia occurring after the first few days of life (classical neonatal tetany) is most frequently related to diet. When feedings are started, changes in the concentrations of calcium and phosphorus in the serum are influenced by the kind of food given the newborn. Gardner (1950) showed that babies fed evaporated milk formulas had higher concentrations of inorganic phosphate in the serum than did breast-fed babies. Babies may have a relatively low serum calcium if their kidneys are unable to excrete the large amounts of phosphate associated with the formulas. Because of renal immaturity the newborn infant excretes phosphate less efficiently than the older child or the adult. Thus serum phosphate concentrations tend to rise, and this would predispose the infant to a reciprocal fall in calcium and to possible tetany.

Since breast-fed babies may develop hypocalcemia also, other factors must be considered as well. The high concentrations of parathyroid hormone in maternal blood in late pregnancy may influence indirectly the activity of the fetal parathyroid gland. In one study, measurements of serum PTH at the time of delivery showed that maternal PTH (6.6 ng/ml) was significantly higher than umbilical cord PTH (1.8 ng/ml), whereas the concentration of calcitonin in all the patients studied was greater in umbilical cord blood (2.2 ng/ml) than in maternal blood (0.76 ng/ml). In this study serum calcium was higher in cord blood (10.29 mg/100 ml) than in maternal blood (8.82 mg/100 ml). A functional insufficiency of the newborn parathyroid gland due to suppression by high calcium levels in utero may predispose to hypocalcemia. Babies born of mothers with parathyroid adenomas have developed hypocalcemia, supporting this theory.

Another possibility which could account for hypocalcemia would be unresponsiveness to PTH, a theory which is supported by other recent studies. The response of the newborn kidney to exogenous PTH in the first day of life, as measured by an increase in the tubular rejection of phosphate relative to the filtered load, was minimal, with a rise in serum phosphate. In contrast, the response on the third day of life showed a phosphaturia of sufficient magnitude to lower the serum phosphate concentration. One effect of PTH on the kidney is to increase the concentration of cyclic AMP in the urine. Linarelli found the cyclic AMP excretion in newborns to be 2.37 nmoles/mg creatinine, and by three days of age, this value had risen to 6.93 nmoles/mg creatinine. Thus an impaired sensitivity to PTH or diminished secretion of PTH could account for the hypocalcemia often seen in the newborn.

Neonatal tetany is treated by the administration of calcium salts. A 10 percent solution of calcium gluconate (1 ml/min or less) may be given intravenously. Calcium chloride has acidic properties and should not be given intravenously. After the acute symptoms are controlled, calcium therapy should be continued orally for about one week (3 to 4 g of calcium gluconate divided in three or more doses daily, or 1 to 1.5 g of calcium chloride in divided doses daily). A low phosphorus milk, similar to breast milk, would be indicated also.

LACTATION

During pregnancy, the breast is subject to the effects of elevated amounts of estrogen and progesterone. Both types of hormones are necessary for complete mammogenesis. Estrogens are primarily responsible for proliferation of the mammary ducts, progesterone for the development of lobules and alveoli. In addition, estrogens and progesterone inhibit (via prolactin inhibiting factor) prolactin release, and as a result prolactin accumulates in the pituitary gland during gestation. Other hormones also appear to influence mammary gland development. Several hormones have been found to regulate the proliferation of mammary epithelial cells in organ culture. Insulin, GH, and epithelial growth factor (EGF) can induce DNA synthesis and subsequent division of the cells in vitro (the protein EGF has been derived from mouse submaxillary gland). In addition, there is some evidence that estrogens may increase proliferation of mammary epithelial cells, but only if insulin is present to initiate DNA synthesis. Thyroid hormone may also be involved in mammary development.

Undifferentiated mammary epithelial cells can divide. Differentiation of these cells to secretory alveolar cells requires the action of cortisol. It is the differentiated alveolar cell which is capable of responding to prolactin (or to hPL) and forming milk proteins. During pregnancy, all these hormones bring about full mammary development. After delivery, with the decline in estrogen and progesterone concentrations in maternal blood, release of prolactin from the pituitary gland occurs, bringing about copious milk secretion and, in the presence of oxytocin, ejection of milk ("milk ejection reflex").

There are two phases to lactation. The first consists of the secretion of milk from the cytoplasm of the alveolar cells into the milk ducts. This phase is under the influence of prolactin. The second phase consists of the ejection of the milk through the nipples and is dependent upon oxytocin. The relation of prolactin to the secretion of milk has been worked out by Turkington and his colleagues. A specific receptor in the plasma membrane of the secretory alveolar cell binds prolactin. The effect of the prolactin-receptor complex is to induce the transcription in the nucleus of RNAs necessary to synthesize more protein kinase enzyme molecules. This protein kinase can subsequently phosphorylate specific proteins in the plasma membrane, ribosomes, and nucleus. The net result is the synthesis of characteristic milk proteins such as casein and the secretion of milk components into the ductal system of the gland. Turkington finds no evidence to support an effect of prolactin on adenyl cyclase activity.

Prolactin bound to mammary particles is displaced not only by prolactin, but also by GH and hPL. Thus the receptor recognizes all lactogenic hormones; however, the greatest competitive displacement is found using prolactin. Prolactin receptors have also been found in seminal vesicles and in liver, kidney, brain, ovary, testis, and adrenal tissue. In each of these tissues, the binding showed high affinity and specificity and was saturable. Such data suggest that prolactin may have many target tissues.

Milk ejection represents a neuroendocrine reflex activated by the tactile stimulation of the nipple with sucking (Figure 5–3). Impulses are relayed to the hypothalamus, where the neurosecretory cells of the paraventricular nuclei are stimulated. Discharge of the paraventricular neurons causes liberation of oxytocin from the posterior pituitary. Oxytocin stimulates the contraction of the myoepithelial cells that line the ducts of the mammary gland and forces the milk out of the alveoli into the large ducts and thence out of the nipple (Figure 5–3). Suckling not only affects oxytocin secretion but also acts on the median eminence to inhibit the release of PIF. As a result, prolactin release is enhanced.

Lactation has specific effects on the endocrine system and the reproductive cycle. During lactation the pituitary undergoes characteristic changes. The acidophilic cells increase in number, while the "preg-

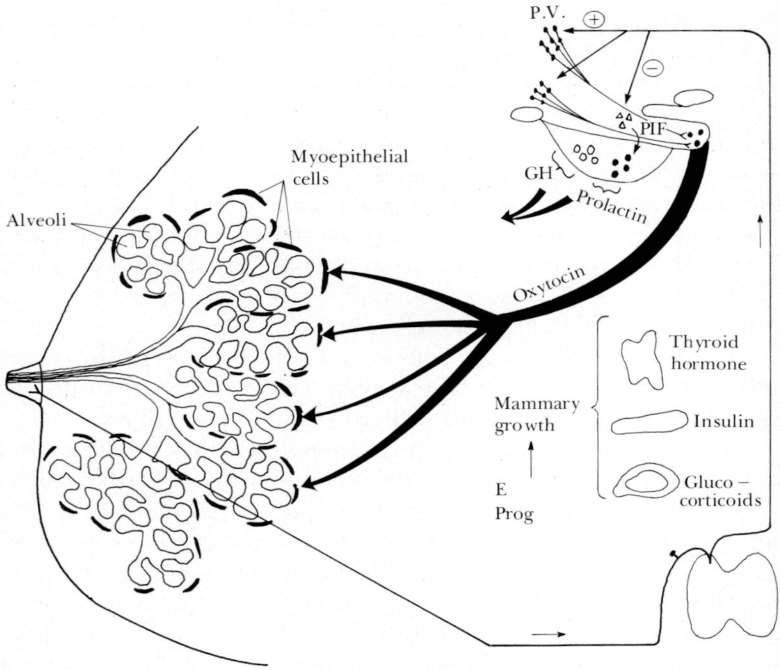

FIGURE 5–3. Endocrine regulation of lactation. See text for details of the mechanisms involved.

nancy cells" decrease. At the same time, gonadotropin release is suppressed. Ovulation does not occur, and amenorrhea or irregular periods are usual.

If lactation persists (galactorrhea) after the period of nursing and the patient continues to be amenorrheic, the possibility of a pituitary lesion should be considered. Galactorrhea is frequently encountered in patients with pituitary neoplasms, and for this reason radiologic examination of the sella turcica should be performed.

SUMMARY

By an intermingling of hormonal effects, the maternal and fetal organisms prepare for separate existences. Labor is triggered, probably in part by the fetus, and the maternal uterus undergoes rhythmic contractions to expel the fetus. During labor the fetus may be subjected to hypoxia, to which extra-adrenal chromaffin tissue can respond, via catecholamines, to maintain vascular tone. Once released from the uterus, the fetus undergoes immediate cardiorespiratory changes compatible with pulmonary oxygenation of blood. Hormonal changes help maintain body temperature and water and electrolyte homeostasis.

The changes in the breast during gestation and the onset of lactation at parturition are under hormonal control. Once released from the suppressive effects of the sex hormones, at parturition, the anterior pituitary releases prolactin. This hormone stimulates the synthesis and secretion of milk proteins into the ductal system of the breast. By way of a neuroendocrine reflex, oxytocin is released, bringing about the ejection of milk through the nipples. This same reflex inhibits PIF in the median eminence, permitting continued release of prolactin. During lactation (or at least in the initial phases), gonadotropins are not released, ovulation is suppressed, and amenorrhea is usual.

The newborn has now adapted to extra-uterine existence and has established alimentation. Not all, however, have such a smooth transition. Some of the endocrine problems peculiar to the neonatal period will be discussed in the next chapters.

SUGGESTED READING

The Thyroid Gland in Pregnancy, Gerard N. Burrow, W. B. Saunders Co., Philadelphia, 1972.
A lucid discussion of thyroid physiology and its alterations in pregnancy. Various thyroid function tests are described and interpreted. Conditions of maternal and neonatal hyper- and hypothyroidism are also covered.

The mechanism of initiation of parturition in the ewe. G. C. Liggins, R. J. Fairclough, S. A. Grieves, J. Z. Kendall, and B. S. Knox, in *Recent Progress in Hormone Research, Vol. 29*, edited by Roy O. Greep, Academic Press, New York, 1973.
A beautifully presented discussion of the initiation of labor in the sheep by an outstanding authority on the subject. The roles of estrogens, progestins, prostaglandins, glucocorticoids, and oxytocin are discussed. At the end of the paper is a very stimulating discussion by various experts in the field with some references to data in the human.

Hormonal regulation of gene expression in mammary cells. R. W. Turkington, G. C. Majumder, N. Kadohama, J. H. MacIndae, and W. L. Frantz, in *Recent Progress in Hormone Research, Vol. 29*, edited by Roy O. Greep, Academic Press, New York, 1973.
A detailed discussion of the endocrine regulation of mammary cell function. Evidence for a prolactin receptor and the induction of protein kinase is presented.

Thyroid function in the premature and the full term newborn. Th. Lemarchaud-Beraud, A. R. Genazzani, F. Bagnoli, and M. Casoli, Acta Endocrinologica, *70*:445, 1972.
A discussion of the physiologic hyperthyroidism of the premature and full term newborn. Values for total and free serum thyroxine and plasma TSH for the two groups are compared.

The metabolic clearance rate, blood production, interconversion, and transplacental passage of cortisol and cortisone in pregnancy near term. I. Z. Beitins et al., Pediatric Research, 7:509, 1973.
An attempt to resolve some of the questions regarding fetal and maternal glucocorticoid synthesis and metabolism. Calculations of maternal and fetal contributions to circulating cortisol and cortisone suggest that the fetus at term secretes most of its circulating cortisol, but that cortisone is mainly of maternal origin.

Obstetrical Endocrinology. Edited by K. J. Ryan, Clin. Obst. and Gyn. *Vol. 16*, No 3, 1973.
A series of papers on endocrine function in pregnancy. Particularly appropriate to this chapter are: Thyroid function and dysfunction during pregnancy, by H. A. Selenkow, M. D. Birnbaum, and C. S. Hollander; and Endocrine regulation of metabolic homeostasis during pregnancy, by S. S. C. Yen.

CHAPTER SIX

Endocrine Disorders of Carbohydrate Metabolism in the Newborn: The Infant of the Diabetic Mother

The products of every endocrine gland can influence carbohydrate metabolism. Glucose homeostasis is regulated very closely by an interplay of several hormones, especially insulin, glucagon, GH, epinephrine, and the glucocorticoids. A change in the rate of secretion or degradation or in the action of any of these hormones can upset the delicate balance between hyperglycemia and hypoglycemia. The latter occurs frequently in the newborn infant and deserves detailed consideration. Cornblath's definition of neonatal hypoglycemia is generally accepted; it states that a blood glucose concentration of less than 30 mg per 100 ml in the first 72 hours of life, or of less than 40 mg per 100 ml after the third day in full term, full-sized infants constitutes hypoglycemia. In infants of low birth weight, the lower limit of normal concentration is set at 20 mg per 100 ml.

THE MAINTENANCE OF NORMAL BLOOD GLUCOSE

There are two readily available sources of glucose in the normal individual: carbohydrate in the diet and liver glycogen. In addition, glucose can be formed from amino acids. Most of the polysaccharides ingested in food are rapidly converted to glucose by enzymes secreted by cells lining the intestinal tract. The conversion is accomplished by a combination of nervous and hormonal controls of enzyme secretion and applies not only to carbohydrate but to protein and fat as well.

Gastrointestinal hormones

Gastric secretion is initiated by nervous or reflex mechanisms (parasympathetic system) which in turn stimulate the release of the hormone *gastrin.* This heptadecapeptide hormone is produced primarily by pyloric glands in the antral part of the stomach, and to a lesser extent in the duodenum and apparently also in the delta cells of the pancreatic islets. Gastrin is absorbed into the blood, which carries it back to the stomach. There gastrin acts to stimulate gastric secretion. In particular, gastrin is a strong stimulator of acid secretion and has been implicated in the etiology of peptic ulcer. Many of its effects can be mimicked by cyclic AMP. Gastrin, histamine, and the parasympathetic nervous system seem to interact in a highly complex manner in regulating gastric secretion. In addition, glucagon (which decreases gastrointestinal motility and the volume of gastric secretion) and prostaglandin E_1 (which inhibits gastric secretion in mammals in vivo) may be involved. Of some interest is the fact that gastrin, some of which is probably secreted by the delta cells of the islets, stimulates insulin release. The chief digestive function of the stomach is the partial digestion of protein by means of the enzyme pepsin, produced by the gastric chief cells.

Like the stomach, the pancreas secretes its digestive juice almost entirely by means of hormonal stimulation. The hormones are secreted in the duodenum and upper-jejunum under the stimulation of HCl and partially digested foodstuffs. There are several hormonal factors in the duodenum. *Secretin,* a polypeptide containing 27 amino acids, stimulates the production by the pancreas of a thin, watery fluid, high in bicarbonate but low in enzyme content. Secretin was the first substance to be called a hormone (Bayliss and Starling, 1902); however, to this day, we know little about its mechanism of action. The response to secretin is enhanced by theophylline and can be mimicked by exogenous cyclic AMP. Secretin has been shown to stimulate adenyl cyclase in rat adipose tissue. The chemical resemblance between secretin and glucagon might suggest similar effects on cyclic AMP; however, all the present evidence indicates that separate receptors (often in different tissues) exist for the two hormones. Secretin does not stimulate liver adenyl cyclase; however, like glucagon, it stimulates the release of insulin from pancreatic islets. A separate "gut" glucagon, distinguishable from secretin and pancreatic glucagon, has also been reported.

Another hormonal factor, *pancreozymin,* stimulates the production by the pancreas of a viscous fluid low in bicarbonate but high in enzyme content. The enzymes in pancreatic juice include trypsin and chymotrypsin (secreted as the inactive zymogens trypsinogen and chymotrypsinogen), the carboxypeptidases, amylase, lipase, cholesterol esterase, ribonuclease, deoxyribonuclease, and collagenase. The effects of pancreozymin may be mediated via cyclic AMP. Like other gastrointestinal hormones, it stimulates the release of insulin. Cholecystokinin (which induces contraction and emptying of the gall bladder), originally thought to be a separate hormone is identical to pancreozymin. Thus this single polypeptide chain of 33 amino acids (cholecystokinin-pancreozymin) has effects on both gall bladder contraction and on pancreatic enzyme secretion.

Other hormones secreted by the duodenum include *hepatocrinin* (which causes the liver to secrete a thin, salt-poor type of bile), and *enterocrinin* (which induces the flow of intestinal juice). It is in this intestinal juice that we find, in addition to the proteolytic enzymes already described, specific disaccharidases (sucrase, maltase, and lactase). The products of carbohydrate digestion are absorbed from the intestine into the blood of the portal venous system in the form of monosaccharides (glucose, fructose, mannose, and galactose). The disaccharide lactose (galactose plus glucose) forms about 40 percent of the caloric intake of the breast-fed infant. The activity of the enzyme which hydrolyzes lactose, *lactase* (β-glycosidase), reaches maximal values at term or within a few days of birth.

The other source of glucose, glycogen, is found in many fetal tissues, especially liver, heart, and muscle. Thus the newborn has a reserve of glycogen to provide glucose during the first hours of life before alimentation is begun. If the store of glycogen is inadequate (owing to prematurity, intra-uterine growth retardation, or injury due to exposure to cold, or if the child lacks one of the enzymes involved in glycogen synthesis (glycogen synthetase), or if glycogen breakdown is impaired (as in glycogen storage diseases), hypoglycemia will ensue.

Insulin Release

Without insulin, the concentration of glucose in blood after a meal would continue to rise until the renal threshold was exceeded. The glucose concentration is maintained within certain limits by a variety of factors which trigger insulin release from the pancreatic islets (Figure 6–1). We may divide these factors into those directly altering the concentration of cyclic AMP in the β cell and those mediating their effects by acting as metabolic substrates.

Cyclic AMP-Mediated Insulin Release

A large number of hormones have been shown to act by stimulating or inhibiting the adenyl cyclases of certain tissues. Stimulation increases

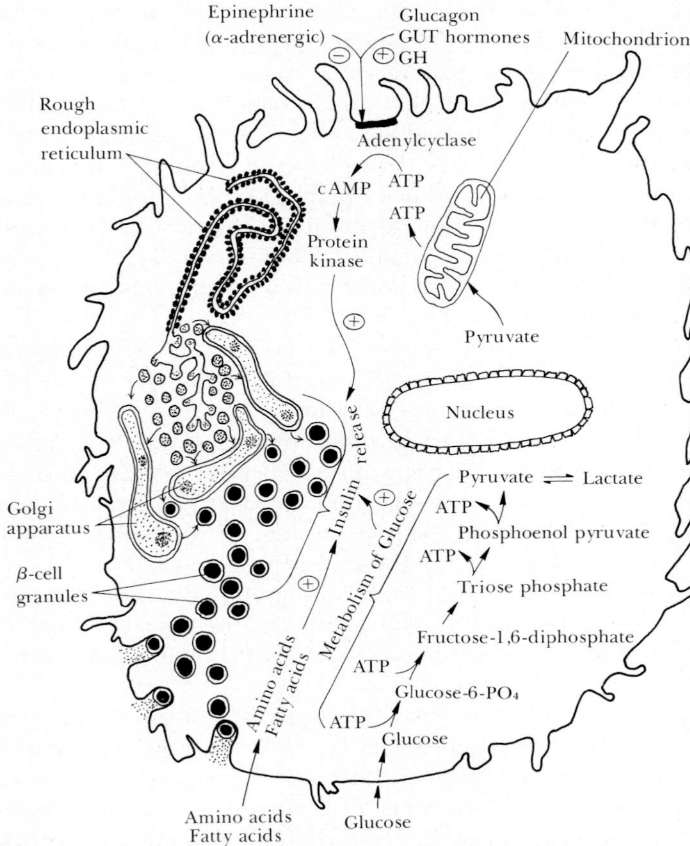

FIGURE 6–1. Schematic drawing of insulin release from pancreatic β cell. Factors which increase (⊕) and decrease (⊖) insulin release are depicted.

the rate of formation of cyclic AMP within the cell, whereas inhibition decreases the rate. Sutherland has suggested a scheme of hormonal activity wherein the hormone acts as the *first messenger* (carrying information), and cyclic AMP acts as a *second messenger.* This second messenger concept has proved fruitful and lends itself to consideration of alternate second messengers, such as Ca^{++} (p. 327), or even to *third* or *fourth messengers* within the cell. Glucagon is known to stimulate adenyl cyclase in liver and adipose tissue and to be a potent stimulator of insulin release from the pancreatic β cell. The latter stimulation is a direct effect on the pancreas, and all available evidence is compatible with its being mediated by cyclic AMP. In experiments using organ cultures of fetal rat pancreas, glucagon stimulated the release of insulin even in the absence of added glucose. The release of insulin is an exocytotic process that requires calcium. Similar processes have been shown to be regulated by cyclic AMP, but the mechanism is unknown. It has been postulated that phosphorylation of one or more membrane proteins (via cyclic AMP) may be a prerequisite for fusion of insulin granules with the inner plasma membrane of the β cell. Rupture of the membrane at the site of fusion would follow, discharging the contents of the granules into the extracellular space.

The effect of glucagon on insulin release presents the intriguing possibility that the α cells of the islets may help regulate β cell function. We think of glucagon as the hormone of "glucose need," and certainly its effects on liver support this view; however, insulin has a quite opposite effect, so much so that it decreases levels of cyclic AMP in target tissues. It is becoming clear that the β and α cells possess the capability of controlling the balance of glucose, fatty acids, and amino acids within target tissues by varying the relative concentrations of insulin and glucagon. An increase in the insulin/glucagon ratio would promote storage of nutrients and favor protein synthesis, whereas a decrease in the insulin/glucagon ratio would favor mobilization of glucose and fatty acids and the utilization of protein for energy. There does seem to be a relationship between the insulin/glucagon ratio and diet, for the ratio increases with higher carbohydrate diets.

Does the newborn maintain a careful balance between these two hormones? Glucagon has been found in the portal plasma of both normal infants and infants of diabetic mothers. The administration of glucose intravenously to either group of children did not suppress plasma glucagon, as it does in adults. Milner and his coworkers measured glucagon, insulin, and glucose in maternal and umbilical cord blood and found that the values for glucagon were very similar in maternal blood (177 pg/ml) and fetal blood (162 and 174 pg/ml for umbilical arterial and venous blood, respectively). Glucose concentrations, on the other hand, were higher in maternal vein (99 mg/100 ml) than in either umbilical vein (80 mg/100 ml) or umbilical artery (72 mg/100 ml). Insulin values were also higher in maternal vein (30 μU/ml) than in umbilical blood (20 μU/ml). Neither protein hormone crosses the placenta to any significant extent, therefore, the values in umbilical blood probably represent fetal hormone synthesis. The concentrations of glucagon are low in comparison to those found in normal fasting adults. Perhaps they represent a basal plasma concentration for the fed state. After birth, the concentration of glucagon in plasma rises slowly, and the newborn liver responds to rising glucagon by increasing glucose output. It is not known at what stage in development the α cell becomes sensitive to changes in glucose concentration, but present evidence suggests that, like the β cell, the α cell of the newborn is relatively unresponsive to glucose infusions. The rise in glucagon after birth may indicate that the α cell can respond to hypoglycemia.

Insulin secretion can be enhanced by hormones which increase the amount of intracellular cyclic AMP (glucagon and, to a lesser extent, ACTH and TSH), by cyclic AMP itself, or by agents which increase the amount of cyclic AMP (theophylline). The sulfonylureas, such as tolbutamide, bring about the release of insulin from β cells, and their activity is largely independent of glucose concentration. It has been suggested that the sulfonylureas inhibit the phosphodiesterase which breaks down cyclic AMP, and the resulting rise in intracellular cyclic AMP then triggers insulin release.

When the same degree of hyperglycemia is produced by intravenous or intraduodenal glucose, the resulting rise in blood insulin is greater during the latter infusion. This suggests that gastrointestinal hormones released during intestinal glucose infusion have a physiologic role in insulin release, apparently via cyclic AMP.

Epinephrine is a potent inhibitor of insulin release. This effect can be reversed by ergotamine, suggesting the participation of α-adrenergic receptors. It has been known for some time that the catecholamines can interact with at least two different types of receptors—α-adrenergic and β-adrenergic. These two types of receptors can be distinguished on the basis of the type of blocking agent which can prevent the response in question. Derivatives of *isoproterenol,* which are closely related chemically to the catecholamines, are β-adrenergic blocking agents. The α-adrenergic blocking agents constitute an assortment of compounds including some ergot alkaloids, imidazole derivatives such as *phentolamine,* and the long-lasting β-haloalkylamine derivatives such as *phenoxybenzamine.* In general, the stimulation of adenyl cyclase is a β-adrenergic receptor effect, whereas a fall in cyclic AMP is associated with α-adrenergic effects.

Stimulation of insulin release by β-adrenergic receptors has also been demonstrated. Turtle and his colleagues suggest that α-adrenergic receptors and β-adrenergic receptors in the β-cells of the pancreas mediate divergent effects of epinephrine on cyclic AMP, α-adrenergic receptors decreasing and β-adrenergic receptors increasing the concentration of cyclic AMP. The β-adrenergic effect of catecholamines is of doubtful physiologic significance. Under normal conditions, the β-effect is obscured by the more powerful α-adrenergic effect. That this latter effect may involve a metabolite of cyclic AMP has been suggested recently.

Vagal stimulation in the dog and the baboon leads to an increased release of insulin into the portal veins. Pancreatic islets of various species are richly innervated, and activation of the parasympathetic nervous system or inhibition of the sympathetic nervous system may play a role in the control of insulin release. The effect of vagal stimulation on insulin release in the dog is magnified if the blood glucose concentration is raised. This synergism between cyclic AMP-mediated stimulation and substrate-mediated stimulation may be important in providing optimal conditions for insulin release.

SUBSTRATE-MEDIATED INSULIN RELEASE. Glucose itself directly stimulates the release of insulin within 30 to 60 seconds both in vivo and in vitro. Several theories have been proposed to account for the effect of glucose on the release of insulin from the β cell of the pancreatic islets. One theory, proposed by Matchinsky and others, suggests that glucose interacts with a membrane receptor on the surface of the β cell. It is not clear how this initial binding to a receptor is linked to insulin release. There is no evidence of a rise in cyclic AMP in islets when insulin release is stimulated by glucose.

Another possibility is that the transport of glucose across the β cell membrane might initiate secretion of insulin, or, once inside the cell, glucose might be metabolized to a substance which acts directly as a trigger for insulin release (Figure 6–1). Other sugars such as mannose and the pentoses also appear to induce insulin release. Sugars that do not undergo metabolism are not effective. Experiments by Gabbay suggest that the conversion of glucose to sorbitol (p. 245) may be involved in the mechanism of insulin release.

The response of the β cell to prolonged glucose stimulation (one hour) is biphasic. There is an initial, rapid phase of insulin release lasting for 15 minutes or so, then a slight decline in rate of release to about two to three times the non-stimulated rate, followed by a second increase. This pattern of release has suggested the concept of two insulin storage pools. Most likely the initial rapid rise represents the release of preformed insulin. The later rise may depend in part on newly synthesized insulin.

Amino acids, particularly leucine and arginine, can bring about the release of insulin; in fact, one of the causes of hypoglycemia in children is an unusual reactivity to the amino acid leucine. The diagnosis of intolerance to leucine can be established in children by administering the amino acid (150 mg/kg orally or 75 mg/kg intravenously) and measuring the change in glucose concentration in the blood; however, steps must be taken to cope with hypoglycemia should it occur. Within a relatively short period (15 to 45 minutes) following the administration of leucine, the blood sugar of leucine-sensitive children falls to at least 50 percent of the fasting level, with a concomitant rise in plasma insulin. The hypoglycemia associated with *maple syrup urine disease* (an inherited metabolic error in the metabolism of valine, leucine, and isoleucine) may be due to hyperinsulinism secondary to high leucine values in the blood. The *idiopathic hypoglycemia* of childhood may represent another example of altered β cell response to some as yet unknown stimulus.

Amino acids can also stimulate the release of glucagon from α cells in the pancreas. Glucose appears to modulate the effects of amino acids. For example, the stimulation of insulin release from isolated perfused rat pancreas by amino acids occurred only when glucose was present in the medium. In contrast, the release of glucagon in response to amino acids was inhibited by glucose. The possibility of a reciprocal control of insulin and glucagon release by glucose makes for an attractive hypothesis.

Although there is clear evidence for an action of fatty acids and ketone bodies on insulin release in certain species (e.g., the dog and the rat), the significance of these substances as inducers of insulin release in man is unknown. *Ketotic hypoglycemia,* seen in young children, develops after a long fast and is associated with acetonuria.

It is possible that substrate-mediated effects on insulin release simply provide the chemical energy needed for discharge of the insulin from the cell. The ATP generated by the metabolism of the substrates (glucose, amino acids, fatty acids) could also serve as substrate for production of cyclic AMP (Figure 6–1). Thus, cyclic AMP may be a common denominator in insulin release. Another common denominator is the absolute requirement for Ca^{++} ions in order for the β cell to respond to *any* stimulus, regardless of the concentration of glucose. Calcium ions may constitute *second messengers* for a variety of physiologic phenomena (p. 327). In contrast, Mg^{++} is inhibitory to insulin release. Changes in Na^+ and K^+ concentrations can also effect secretion of insulin.

Insulin Action

Once released from the β cell, insulin enhances the transport of glucose and related monosaccharides, amino acids, K^+, nucleosides, and inorganic phosphate across certain cell membranes. Insulin thus decreases the concentration of glucose in the blood—by increasing its peripheral uptake. These effects are not secondary to glucose metabolism, for increased uptake can be demonstrated in in vitro systems when nonmetabolizable sugars are tested. Insulin is firmly bound to a highly specific receptor site in the membrane fractions of muscle and adipose tissue (these are the two most important tissues in regard to insulin's effects on transport). The amount of membrane-bound insulin quantitatively parallels its biological activity in the tissue, which suggests that binding is a requisite of hormone activity. There is some evidence that the membrane receptor is a glycoprotein.

In addition to its effects on transport in muscle and adipose tissue, insulin has been shown to counteract the lipolytic activities of epinephrine and glucagon, to enhance protein synthesis, and to increase the activities of certain enzymes (hexokinase, glycogen synthetase).

The effects of insulin on the liver are complex and will be discussed in detail in Chapter Ten. Of particular interest is the role of insulin in inducing or activating certain glycolytic enzymes.

Insulin Synthesis

In the β cells of the pancreas, insulin is synthesized, as is any other protein, on ribosomes. The molecule that is synthesized is actually *proinsulin,* consisting of insulin plus a connecting peptide (C-peptide). Proinsulin can be measured by specific radioimmunoassay or after separation from insulin by chromatography. The conversion of proinsulin to insulin occurs in the granules of the β cells (Figure 6–1).

Insulin, proinsulin, and C-peptide are all secreted by the β cells and circulate in the blood. In order to measure the insulin in the blood of patients who are receiving exogenous bovine or porcine insulin, one must find a means of eliminating the effects of circulating insulin antibodies.

The measurement of immunoreactive C-peptide instead of immunoreactive insulin circumvents this difficulty and can serve as an index of pancreatic function.

The role of other hormones

Glycogen synthesis and breakdown are controlled by an intricate enzymatic and hormonal mechanism. Several hormones are capable of accelerating the breakdown of glycogen, but only insulin and glucocorticoids stimulate glycogen synthesis. Thus in addition to its effects on the transport of glucose and amino acids, insulin directly enhances the activity of glycogen synthetase. This contributes to the action of insulin in decreasing the blood glucose; also, when glucose is in excess, it can be stored as glycogen.

Glucagon activates phosphorylase and in so doing causes the breakdown of glycogen. When glucose is needed, glycogen can be broken down to glucose-1-phosphate and then to glucose-6-phosphate; the latter, via phosphatase, yields free glucose. Epinephrine also activates phosphorylase and can raise blood glucose concentrations.

The glucocorticoids induce the synthesis of (1) enzymes involved in the transamination of amino acids to intermediates in the citric acid cycle and (2) enzymes involved in the reversal of the glycolytic cycle. The glucocorticoids increase the supply of glucose by gluconeogenesis at the expense of amino acids (protein).

THE DIABETIC MOTHER

The interplay of the hormones involved in glucose homeostasis ensures a steady supply of carbohydrate for cellular metabolism. The newborn usually adjusts quickly to extra-uterine existence and, unless subjected to overwhelming insults, can maintain a normal blood glucose. One of the most frequently encountered exceptions to this rule is the infant of the diabetic mother. Even under the best of control, the diabetic mother must have periods of hyperglycemia. The elevated glucose, when transmitted to the fetus, undoubtedly requires the fetal pancreas to function much earlier and to a greater extent than in the normal pregnancy. Somehow the fetal hyperglycemia and fetal pancreatic hyperplasia seem to be related to a variety of perinatal problems which result in increased morbidity and mortality for the infant of the diabetic mother.

Potential, latent, and gestational diabetics

White (1965) has estimated that in the United States, one delivery in a thousand is by a diabetic mother. Though this represents a rather low incidence, the need for close medical supervision of pregnant diabetic patients in order to ensure a successful delivery requires that the obstetrician devote special attention to diagnosing possible abnormalities of carbohydrate metabolism.

Women who have a strong family history of diabetes, or who have given birth previously to a baby weighing more than 4.5 kg, have a greater than normal chance of developing diabetes. Even if these women manifest normal results on the glucose tolerance test, they remain in the category of *potential diabetic* and should be tested periodically for evidence of reduced ability to utilize glucose.

Pregnancy itself represents an altered metabolic state, and consequently even nondiabetic women show changes in carbohydrate and lipid metabolism. As pregnancy progresses, the plasma glucose tends to decrease, and plasma free fatty acids tend to increase during fasting. Ketonuria may occur and glycosuria is common. In addition, in the last trimester of pregnancy, the insulin response to either glucose or tolbutamide is augmented. However, under normal circumstances, the glucose tolerance test is normal.

Pregnancy may reveal the *latent diabetic*. Such individuals have a normal glucose tolerance test ordinarily, but under stress (such as pregnancy) the test results become abnormal. Some women have an abnormal glucose tolerance test during pregnancy which reverts to normal after delivery. These women are called *gestational diabetics*, and like most latent diabetics, they are more likely to develop overt diabetes in later life than is the general population.

The Glucose Tolerance Test

The diabetic—or the potential diabetic—cannot utilize glucose as rapidly as the normal individual can. One can measure the ability to utilize glucose by presenting the patient orally or intravenously with glucose. The oral glucose tolerance test measures the balance of (1) intestinal absorption, (2) uptake by tissues, and (3) excretion in urine. The intravenous test bypasses the first variable. In general, the oral glucose tolerance test is more satisfactory for the detection of diabetes.

Ideally, the patient is placed on a high (300 g) carbohydrate diet for three days before the test is given. This is important, for a low carbohydrate intake can produce a "diabetic" curve similar to that seen in starvation. After an overnight fast (at least 10 hours), glucose in the form of a flavored 25 percent solution (1.75 g glucose per kg of "ideal" body weight) is administered by mouth. Venous blood specimens are taken at 0, 0.5, 1, 1.5, 2, and 3 hours after the glucose ingestion. Urine specimens are obtained at the same time intervals.

In a study of 10 normal mothers and 9 gestational diabetic mothers, Kalkhoff (1964) found that the concentration of glucose in the blood of the gestational diabetic exceeded that of the normal mother (Figure 6–

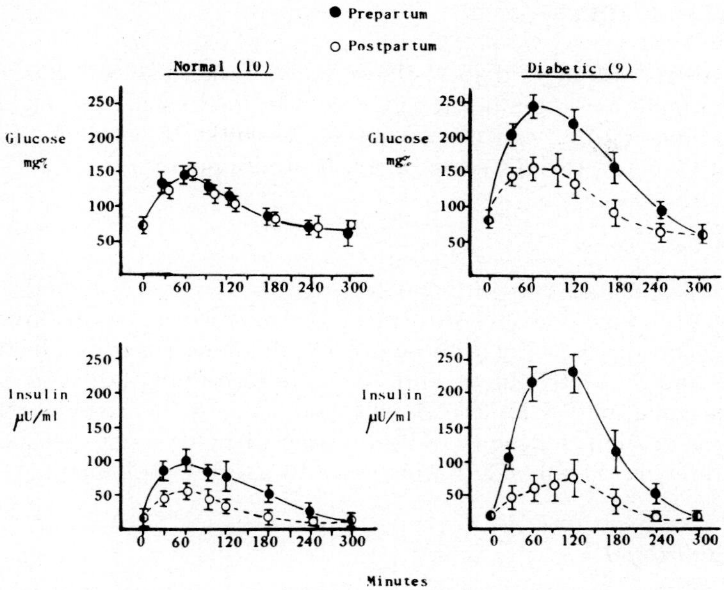

FIGURE 6–2. Effect of pregnancy on oral glucose tolerance and plasma insulin response. (From Kalkhoff, R. et al. Diabetogenic factors associated with pregnancy. Trans. Assoc. Am. Phys., 1964, 77:p. 271.)

2). Measurements of insulin in the same blood specimens revealed that the gestational diabetic attained a much higher peak (250 μU/ml) than did the normal patient (100 μU/ml), and the increased insulin persisted for a longer time.

Intravenous glucose (25 g) elicits a similar difference between the diabetic mother and the normal mother. What both types of test establish is that even though a supernormal concentration of insulin appears in the blood after glucose administration, the ability of the diabetic to utilize glucose rapidly is impaired.

CHEMICAL DIABETES

A stage of diabetes more advanced than gestational (or latent) diabetes is the condition in which the patient manifests an abnormal glucose tolerance test (even without stress) but has no clinical symptoms of diabetes. The fasting blood glucose may or may not be elevated. In the gestational or latent diabetic, the fasting blood glucose is usually normal. In any case, long before there is evidence of hyperglycemia or glucosuria, the asymptomatic diabetic manifests his inability to cope with the glucose administered in a glucose tolerance test.

Clinical diabetes

Patients with overt diabetes have many of the classical symptoms of diabetes mellitus. Not only is the glucose tolerance test abnormal, but the fasting blood glucose concentration is usually high. Depending upon the type of diabetes, various symptoms will predominate.

Juvenile-Onset

Clinical diabetes beginning before age 15 is usually classified as *juvenile diabetes.* This is a severe form of diabetes with a rapid onset and progression (p. 244). Early in the disease, the pancreas is usually hyperplastic and hypertrophied, and the concentration of insulin in the plasma is elevated; later the β cells atrophy and the juvenile diabetic manifests insulin deficiency. The juvenile diabetic, when pregnant, is more difficult to control and thus presents greater problems.

Adult-Onset

Diabetes which develops later in life tends to be of a milder nature and more readily controlled. The adult-onset diabetic tends to be relatively resistant to insulin. In contrast to the underweight juvenile diabetic, the adult diabetic is usually overweight. Though the two types of diabetes may represent distinct entities, undoubtedly considerable overlap exists, particularly when diabetes becomes clinically manifest between ages 15 and 40. Vascular complications of diabetes occur more gradually in the adult-onset diabetic than in the juvenile-onset diabetic.

Complications in the diabetic mother

Obstetric complications tend to increase with impaired control of maternal diabetes. Especially tight control of diabetes must be maintained during pregnancy because of the detrimental effect of periodic hyperglycemia on the fetus.

Hydramnios

Severe hydramnios (the accumulation of excessive amounts of amniotic fluid) is usually associated with poor control of maternal diabetes, and often with preeclampsia. The amniotic fluid itself does not differ qualitatively from that found in the non-diabetic, except that it has a higher glucose content. There is no direct relationship between the concentration of glucose in the amniotic fluid and the volume of the fluid; therefore, fetal osmotic diuresis is probably not the explanation for the hydramnios. Most investigators believe that the amount of hydramnios can be reduced by strict control of maternal diabetes.

Hydramnios with diabetes mellitus is a bad prognostic sign and calls for immediate hospitalization of the mother and maintenance of her blood glucose below 160 mg/100 ml.

Preeclampsia

This syndrome is arbitrarily defined as a rise in blood pressure (of at least 30 mm Hg systolic and 15 mm Hg diastolic), accompanied by proteinuria. Symptoms (in some cases) include generalized edema occurring after the twenty-fourth week of pregnancy. The old term, toxemia of pregnancy, includes all cases of hypertension in pregnancy, with or without proteinuria or edema. About 25 percent of diabetic women develop preeclampsia during pregnancy, an incidence about five times greater than that in the non-diabetic. The preeclampsia is frequently associated with hydramnios. These complications are more likely to occur in those diabetic mothers with vascular disease, particularly if there is renal damage.

Dystocia

Because of the large size of the babies of diabetic mothers, mechanical dystocia may occur following induction of labor. Many obstetricians deliver their patients by caesarean section.

Ketoacidosis

In the diabetic state there are biochemical changes in the target tissues which cause the accumulation of metabolites ordinarily present in small amounts. Among these metabolites are the *ketone bodies:* acetoacetic acid, β-hydroxybutyric acid, and acetone. High concentrations of ketone bodies in the blood can produce a metabolic acidosis, or ketoacidosis. The two major tissues implicated in the development of diabetic ketoacidosis are the liver and adipose tissue.

One of the major actions of insulin is its stimulation of triglyceride synthesis in adipose tissue. The stimulation is accomplished by (a) enhanced transport of glucose into the cell, thereby providing more glucose for conversion to fatty acids and to glycerol within the cell and (b) inhibition of lipolysis, thereby reducing the amount of free fatty acids released into the circulation. In the absence of the antilipolytic influence of insulin, the effects of lipolytic hormones are unopposed. This is particularly pertinent in the pregnant state because the large amounts of hPL secreted by the placenta exert a powerful lipolytic action. The result of lipolysis is an increased concentration of free fatty acids and glycerol in the plasma.

In the diabetic, free fatty acids reach the liver in increased amounts. What then occurs is the β-oxidation of the fatty acids, with a resulting accumulation of acetyl coenzyme A. Two molecules of acetyl coenzyme A can condense to form acetoacetyl coenzyme A, and cleavage of the coenzyme A yields free acetoacetic acid. The latter may be reduced to β-hydroxybutyric acid by the mitochondrial enzyme β-hydroxybutyric dehydrogenase and to acetone by decarboxylation. More ketone bodies are formed in the liver than can be utilized peripherally, producing a metabolic acidosis.

Vascular Disease

Pregnancy intensifies the manifestations of diabetes. The ultimate prognosis for diabetic women who are pregnant may be worse than that for diabetic women who are not pregnant, especially if the diabetes is complicated by renal, retinal, or vascular disease.

THE INFANT OF THE DIABETIC MOTHER

It was Pedersen (1954) who proposed originally that prolonged exposure of the fetus in a diabetic pregnancy to hyperglycemia stimulated the pancreas to produce excessive insulin. This may indeed explain the hyperplastic β cells of the fetal pancreas, but the increased morbidity and mortality of these infants require further explanation.

PERINATAL MORTALITY

It seems clear that the perinatal mortality of infants of diabetic mothers is related both to the severity of the maternal diabetes and to the gestational age of the infant at the time of delivery. If we use the White classification of diabetic pregnancies (Table 6–1), the least perinatal mortality (4.8 percent) is associated with Class A diabetics and the

TABLE 6–1. White Classification of Diabetes Mellitus in Pregnancy

Grouping	Characteristics of the Disease
Class A	Diagnosis based upon abnormal glucose tolerance test only (chemical diabetes).
Class B	Onset of clinical diabetes after age 20, duration less than 10 years, no demonstrable vascular disease.
Class C	Onset between ages 10 and 20, duration 10 to 19 years, no x-ray evidence of vascular disease.
Class D	Onset before age of 10 or duration over 20 years, x-ray diagnosis of vascular disease in legs, retinal changes on funduscopy.
Class E	Same as D, with addition of calcification of pelvic arteries (determined by x-ray examination).
Class F	Diabetic nephropathy (Kimmelstiel-Wilson syndrome).

highest (47.8 percent) with Class F. Because of the high incidence of stillbirths in the last 3 or 4 weeks of pregnancy, babies of diabetic mothers are usually delivered prematurely. Stillbirth is unusual before 36 weeks gestation; however, the problems of immaturity greatly increase the risk of early delivery. A compromise must be reached between the risks of immaturity and the risk of stillbirth, and most obstetricians aim for delivery of the infant of the diabetic mother by the end of the thirty-seventh week. Obviously each case requires an individual decision; many patients can wait until 38 weeks, while others are best delivered at 36 weeks.

In order to make this decision the obstetrician must obtain as much information as possible about the status of the fetus and the diabetic control of the mother. By using L/S ratios, estriol determinations, ultrasound, and fetal heart recording, a judgment can be made as to the optimal time for delivery.

Appearance and Clinical Findings

The characteristic feature of babies born to diabetic mothers is their large size. This excessive size is apparently due to an increased accumulation of body fat and an increase in the size of the viscera. Visceromegaly is particularly striking in the heart and liver. The babies are not usually edematous; in fact, they have less extracellular and total body water than do normal infants. The islets of Langerhans are prominent in the newborn pancreas; the β cells are hyperplastic. Steinke and Driscoll (1965) extracted insulin from fetal pancreases close to term and found that the pancreas from infants of diabetic mothers contained almost twice as much insulin (21.1 ± 5.2 units/g pancreas) as did the pancreas from normal babies (12.7 ± 3.2 units/g pancreas).

The infant of the diabetic mother is usually a fat, almost puffy baby. He is frequently limp, with legs flexed and abducted. The prominent fat pad over the upper back suggests a "cushingoid" condition. The umbilical cord is large. Those babies delivered vaginally may be subject to birth trauma owing to their excessive size and the resulting cephalopelvic dystocia.

Neonatal Complications

Hypoglycemia

Immediately after birth, the blood glucose concentration of the newborn falls. This decline is more rapid in infants of diabetic mothers than in normal babies (Figure 6–3). A true blood glucose below 30 mg per 100 ml was noted in the first 6 hours of life in 54 percent of babies born to diabetic mothers and in only 14 percent of babies born to nondiabetic mothers. The disappearance of glucose from peripheral blood

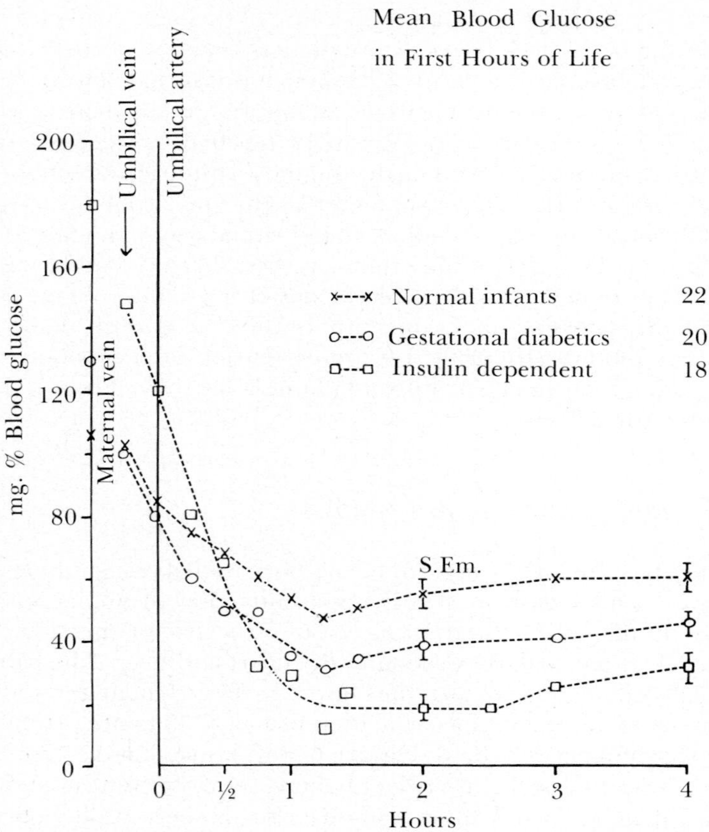

FIGURE 6–3. Serial changes in the concentration of glucose in the blood of infants immediately following delivery. The group from mothers with gestational diabetes had abnormal intravenous glucose tolerance tests during pregnancy but received no insulin therapy. (From Cornblath, M. and Schwartz, R. *Disorders of Carbohydrate Metabolism in Infancy.* Philadelphia: W. B. Saunders Company, 1966, p. 65. The figure is adapted from McCann et al. Proc. Soc. Ped. Res., May, 1965.)

is a reflection of uptake of glucose by the tissues of the newborn when the maternal supply of glucose has been cut off. The blood glucose continues to fall until the newborn can begin either to mobilize endogenous stores of carbohydrate or to convert amino acids, lactate, and pyruvate into glucose. The latter process is called *gluconeogenesis.* The breakdown of glycogen depends upon the activity of glycogenolytic enzymes, whereas gluconeogenesis requires transaminases and the enzymes involved in the reversal of glycolysis. The hepatic glycogen concentration declines to values below those in fasting adults after 24 to 48 hours of extra-uterine life. We infer that the newborn liver secretes glucose during the first few days of life. Indeed, the blood glucose, after reaching a nadir at around 2 hours of life, starts to rise and eventually reaches equilibrium at a concentration of about 70 mg/100 ml by the third postnatal day.

The infant of the diabetic mother (on insulin therapy) starts at birth with a much higher blood glucose concentration than that of the infant of the non-diabetic mother (Figure 6–3); however, within the first 2 hours of life, the glucose level has fallen to about 20 mg/100 ml in the former, while that of the latter falls to about 50 mg/100 ml. Thus the infant of the diabetic mother removes glucose from the plasma more rapidly than does the normal infant. This is clearly seen when the babies are given an intravenous glucose load. Babies of diabetic mothers show an immediate rise in their blood glucose, as do the control babies, but the former exhibit a far more rapid decline in glucose than the latter over a two-hour period.

The usual explanation for the rapidly developing hypoglycemia of the infant of the diabetic is hyperinsulinism. Presumably, after repeated hyperglycemic episodes in utero, the pancreas of these fetuses is stimulated to secrete more and more insulin. The assay for insulin in the blood of these babies is complicated by the presence of insulin antibodies (if the mother has been taking insulin). The insulin values may be excessive, since a part of the ^{131}I-insulin (used for radioimmunoassay of insulin) may be bound to human insulin antibodies which are not precipitated quantitatively by the antiserum. Nevertheless, there is good evidence that the concentration of insulin is indeed higher in plasma from infants of diabetic mothers than in normal babies. High concentrations of insulin have been measured in cord blood of infants of diabetic mothers who have not received insulin therapy. In these infants no insulin antibodies could be found, indicating that the elevated insulin value represents a real phenomenon.

As a group, infants of diabetic mothers are characterized by responding to glucose injection with a very rapid increase in insulin. In contrast, infants of non-diabetic mothers show a rather sluggish insulin response to administered glucose. You will remember that the fetal pancreas is relatively unresponsive to a glucose stimulus. One must conclude that during intra-uterine exposure to hyperglycemia, the pancreas of the fetus develops a system which responds to glucose with the release of insulin. From our present knowledge of the role of glucose in triggering insulin release, we must conclude that, although ordinarily this system does not develop fully until after birth, the fetus of the diabetic mother becomes sensitized to glucose much earlier, and thus in the early hours and days of life is more prone to hypoglycemia than is the normal newborn.

Immaturity

Because babies of diabetic mothers must be delivered prematurely, they suffer all the hazards of the immature infant. Many enzymes (glucuronyl transferase, N-methyl transferase, certain enzymes in the pathway for lecithin synthesis) develop late in gestation and are important in the survival of the newborn. Of all the most life-threatening complications, none ranks so high as the *respiratory distress syndrome* (hyaline membrane disease) engendered by the immaturity of the newborn lung. This syndrome has become the most common cause of death in the first week after delivery in babies born to diabetic mothers.

As the fetus matures, the synthesis of phosphatidylcholine (lecithin) increases in the fetal lung. Two pathways are available to the alveolar cells: one route involves the direct incorporation of choline into phosphatidylcholine, and the other route is via phosphatidylethanolamine, which is methylated three times to form phosphatidylcholine (Figure 6–4). The methylation pathway develops earlier in gestation (22 weeks); however, it is very sensitive to anoxia, and the phosphatidylcholine that is formed has unsaturated fatty acids in it, reducing the surface activity of the lecithin. The choline pathway yields largely dipalmityl phosphatidylcholine (a very good surface-acting lecithin) but develops late in gestation (35 weeks). Another lipid, sphingomyelin, is also synthesized, and the maturity of the fetal lung can be assessed by measuring the relative amounts of lecithin and sphingomyelin in amniotic fluid (L/S ratio). If this ratio is less than two, according to Gluck, the probability of the infant developing respiratory distress syndrome is high. Using lecithin values alone, Bhagwanami, Fahmy, and Turnbull found that a concentration of 3.5 mg/100 ml of amniotic fluid was almost invariably associated with normal respiratory function. Below this value, there was a high incidence of respiratory distress. Liggins has recently suggested that cortisol may be able to induce certain key enzymes in the choline pathway, thereby triggering the formation of pulmonary surfactant (the surface-active material secreted by the lung), which protects the premature baby. Liggins studied sheep, but Farrell has achieved much the same results with rabbits. In addition, initial clinical trials by Howie and Liggins suggest that antepartum cortisol therapy may be effective in the human.

Glucuronyl transferase activity rises sharply after birth; consequently, premature babies must develop this enzyme several weeks before the full term baby. Because the liver enzymes required for conjugation of bilirubin (and steroids) have not developed fully as yet, hyperbilirubinemia is more of a problem in the premature infant in general, and in the infant of the diabetic mother in particular. The peak of the jaundice in premature babies usually occurs between the fifth and seventh days postpartum, somewhat later than in term infants.

Still another enzyme which develops late in gestation is the N-methyl transferase of the adrenal medulla. This enzyme methylates norepinephrine to form epinephrine. Infants of diabetic mothers have much lower excretion rates of both epinephrine and norepinephrine than do normal infants. In addition, there is no increase in catecholamine excretion as accompanies hypoglycemia in otherwise normal infants. The N-methyl transferase is another enzyme which is presumably induced by cortisol.

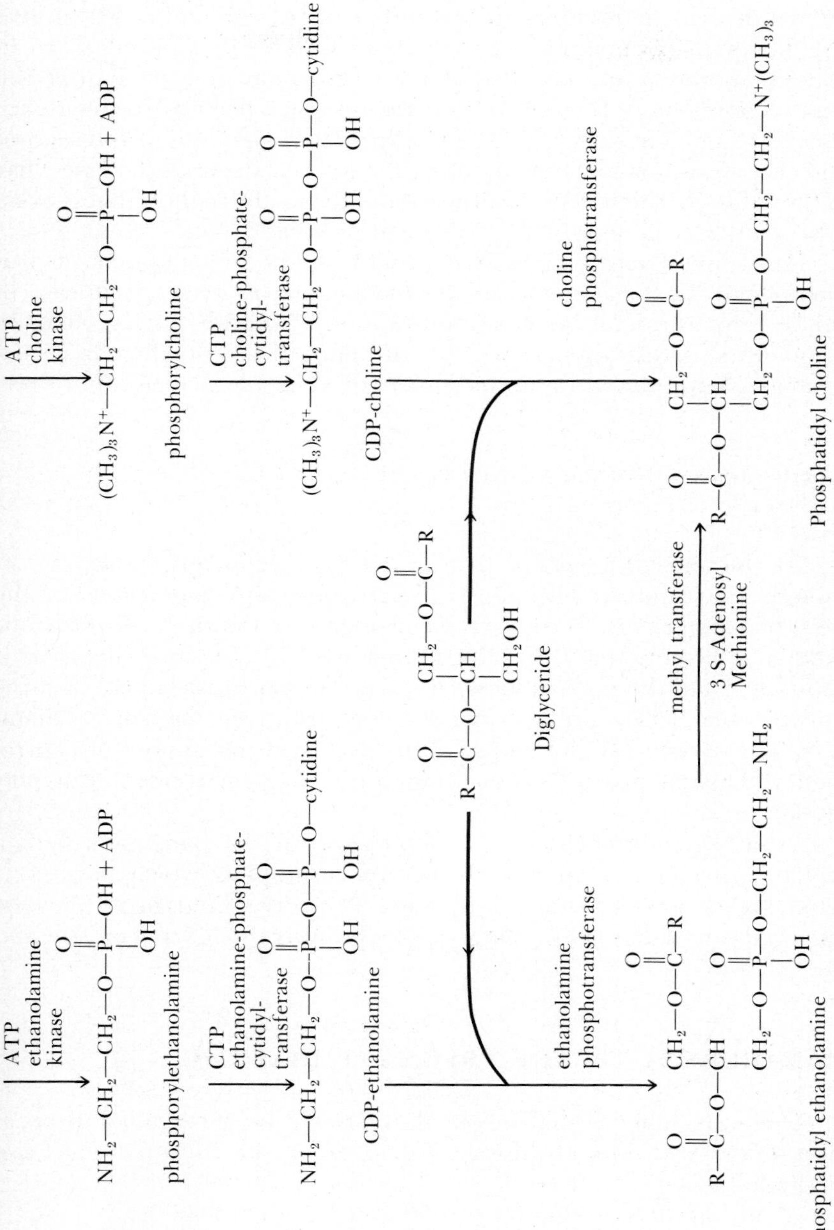

R = fatty acid

FIGURE 6–4. Biosynthesis of phosphoglycerides. (From Page, E., Villee, C., and Villee, D. *Human Reproduction.* Philadelphia: W. B. Saunders Company, 1972, p. 339.)

Congenital malformations

Malformations involving any organ system occur more frequently in infants of diabetic mothers than in other infants of similar gestational age. Major malformations occur in about 5 percent of infants born to diabetic mothers, an incidence about seven times greater than in the general population. If maternal vascular disease is present, the incidence rises to 10 percent. Among these malformations agenesis of the sacrum and coccyx and/or malformations of the lower extremities are peculiar to the infant of the diabetic mother. Another malformation that is over-represented in these infants is ventricular septal defect.

Most investigators agree that insulin (or the hypoglycemia it produces) can be teratogenic. Abnormalities have been produced in chickens by intra-embryonic administration of insulin. There seems to be no clear correlation between the incidence of severe congenital malformations and the duration or control of maternal diabetes, however.

Pathologic findings in infants of diabetic mothers

In the fetus of a diabetic mother the most characteristic finding, although not an invariable one, is hypertrophy and hyperplasia of the islets of Langerhans. A comparable change is noted in erythroblastotic infants, indicating that the change is not specific. The total islet mass is about 20 times the normal mass, and the number of islets may be three times normal. The average diameter of an islet is twice the normal diameter. The severity of the maternal diabetes and the degree of control seem to have no bearing on the magnitude of hypertrophy and hyperplasia.

Another common finding is infiltration of the pancreatic stroma and, to a lesser extent, the islets by mature eosinophils, which may represent a response to insulin antibodies. Both liver and heart may be enlarged and laden with glycogen. The brain is small for fetal size and age.

MANAGEMENT OF THE PREGNANT DIABETIC

The possibility of diabetes mellitus should be entertained in pregnant women with a family history of diabetes or with a history of any two of the following:

1. an infant weighing over 4000 g or less than 2400 g
2. fetal death in utero or neonatal death
3. preeclampsia
4. congenital abnormality
5. monilial vulvovaginitis

6. excess weight gain and/or excessive exogenous obesity
7. hydramnios
8. significant and repeated glycosuria

Such women should have a glucose tolerance test, repeated, if negative, each trimester. The classification of diabetes should be established as early in pregnancy as possible.

Insulin

The control of diabetes with insulin is discussed in detail in Chapters Ten and Fourteen. There are differences, however, in the control of diabetes in the pregnant and nonpregnant woman. Because of the increased elaboration of insulin antagonists (such as hPL) and the increased degradation of insulin (by the placenta), the patient's insulin requirement usually increases during pregnancy. Often patients who do not require insulin in the nonpregnant state require the hormone during pregnancy. Oral antidiabetic agents cross the placenta and can influence the fetal pancreas. Therefore, they are contraindicated in pregnancy.

Diet and care

An intake of 30 calories/kg body weight is recommended, with a daily intake of at least 150 g carbohydrate and 100 g protein. In order to control fluid balance to prevent edema and to limit hydramnios, salt intake is usually restricted.

Weekly prenatal visits to the physician and antepartum hospitalization (for a minimum of one week) are the usual procedures. One of the most difficult decisions for the obstetrician is the time and mode of delivery of the diabetic mother's infant. No diabetic of any classification should be allowed to go beyond the expected date of confinement. In most cases, it is a question of how soon before term the baby should be delivered. Several variables must be considered. If the baby is not too large, the pelvis is adequate, the diabetes has been present less than fifteen years, and there is no toxemia, the obstetrician might consider letting the pregnancy go to term. However, if unexplained fetal loss has occurred in previous pregnancies, earlier delivery is indicated. If the cervix is favorable, labor can be induced and the child delivered vaginally. Such inductions require careful management, with constant monitoring of the fetal heart rate and the progress of labor. If the cervix is not favorable, the infant should be delivered by caesarean section. With a very large baby or a Class C to F diabetic, early delivery is advisable. The baby of the Class C diabetic is usually delivered at 36 to 37 weeks, while babies of Class D to F diabetics should be delivered no later than 36 weeks.

MANAGEMENT OF THE INFANT OF THE DIABETIC MOTHER

In spite of the large size of offspring of diabetic mothers, these babies are fragile physiologically and metabolically. They are prone to hypoglycemia, hypocalcemia, respiratory distress, hyperbilirubinemia, and venous thrombosis. Not all of these infants have neonatal complications. Indeed, it has been estimated that about one half have an uneventful neonatal course.

Babies of diabetic mothers belong in the "high risk" category and should be handled by specially trained personnel. The classification and control of the maternal diabetes enter into the assessment of neonatal care. At birth, a sample of umbilical cord blood can provide baseline values of glucose and calcium. If needed, resuscitation can be provided at birth or in the special care nursery after birth. These babies are often jittery, even with normal calcium concentrations in the blood. Calcium and glucose concentrations should be measured regularly during the neonatal period, and calcium therapy is indicated when the blood calcium is less than 7 mg/100 ml and there are manifest signs of hypocalcemia—e.g., irritability or convulsions. The concentration of bilirubin in the blood should be monitored if there is any evidence of hyperbilirubinemia. Any signs of respiratory distress call for immediate assessment of blood P_{O_2}, P_{CO_2}, and HCO_3.

There is some disagreement as to the need to treat asymptomatic infants with a blood glucose of less than 30 mg/100 ml. In view of the possible damage to the central nervous system by prolonged hypoglycemia, it would seem advisable to administer glucose to these babies. Symptomatic hypoglycemia is always treated, and it must be remembered that the prognosis is worse for the baby with symptomatic hypoglycemia than for the infant who shows no symptoms. Avery recommends that symptomatic babies be given 50 percent glucose (1 to 2 ml/kg) intravenously followed by 10 or 15 percent glucose (75 ml/kg/24 hours). Others have reported that although blood glucose concentrations can be raised immediately by administration of intravenous 25 percent or 50 percent glucose, there is often a reactive hypoglycemia. In such cases an infusion of 10 percent glucose for the first 24 hours is preferred. Oral feedings should be instituted as soon as possible.

McCann has recently suggested that long-acting epinephrine (Susphrine 1:200, 0.01 ml/kg intramuscularly every 6 hours for the first 24 hours) might be beneficial in the management of the infant of the diabetic mother. The rationale is based on the known effects of epinephrine: (1) hyperglycemia, (2) inhibition of insulin release, and (3) mobilization of fat (which would correct the low circulating free fatty acids in these bab.es). It has been postulated that there is a deficiency of catecholamines at birth and thus the administration of epinephrine would help repair this deficiency. There is, however, disagreement regarding the efficacy of epinephrine, and its use in the infant of the diabetic mother remains controversial.

The use of glucagon has been suggested for the alleviation of hypoglycemia, but its effectiveness is disputed. Cornblath found that injection of 300 μg/kg raised the blood glucose concentration in nine infants of insulin-dependent diabetic mothers. McCann showed that rapidly injected fructose (0.5 to 2 g/kg) raised the blood glucose concentration in six of seven infants of insulin-dependent diabetic mothers.

Children of diabetic mothers show no difference in growth and development from those of non-diabetic mothers. The probability that these children will develop diabetes, although small, is real. White estimates that 7 percent of them will have diabetes by the age of 20 years. Farquhar estimates their risk of diabetes to be about 20 times that of infants of non-diabetic mothers.

DIFFERENTIAL DIAGNOSIS OF NEONATAL HYPOGLYCEMIA

Aside from the infant of the diabetic mother, two other conditions of the newborn are frequently associated with hypoglycemia: (1) the "small-for-dates" infant, and (2) the erythroblastotic baby.

THE LOW BIRTH WEIGHT INFANT (SMALL-FOR-DATES)

The birth of an infant whose weight is below the normal range for gestational age may be associated with a higher risk of neonatal hypoglycemia. Low weight infants tend to have low hepatic carbohydrate stores; however, a causal relationship has not been established between the inadequate liver glycogen and the hypoglycemia. Some of these infants also have a reduced catecholamine secretion rate postnatally.

Carbohydrate metabolism in the infant who is small for his gestational age is typically unstable, and both hypoglycemia and hyperglycemia may occur (the latter is discussed further on in relation to transient neonatal diabetes mellitus). The rate of glucose disappearance from the blood is increased in hypoglycemic small-for-dates babies whether they have normal or increased insulin secretion rates. Therefore, one cannot attribute the hypoglycemia solely to hyperinsulinism.

If the low birth weight is associated with signs of placental dysfunction, the infant is often called "dysmature." The infant's failure to grow adequately in utero is attributed to inadequate materno-fetal transfer of nutrients, which is caused by reduced placental function. In essence, these factors represent intra-uterine growth retardation.

The hypoglycemia is treated by continuous infusion of glucose, and if glucose homeostatis is difficult to maintain, treatment may be supplemented with cortisone (5 mg/kg/day) or ACTH (5 U/kg/day). The hypoglycemia, though transient, may persist for several weeks; therefore, oral feedings should be instituted as rapidly as possible.

THE ERYTHROBLASTOTIC INFANT

The newborn infant with erythroblastosis fetalis resembles the infant of the diabetic mother in many ways. There is β cell hyperplasia and increased insulin-like activity in the pancreas. The plasma concentration of insulin is also elevated; however, the insulin molecule is inactivated more rapidly in these babies. The mechanism for the hyperinsulinism is unknown but seems to be related to the severity of the disease in utero.

NEONATAL DIABETES MELLITUS

A rare disorder of metabolism in the neonatal period is transient diabetes mellitus. At the onset of the illness, the infant fails to gain weight and has hyperglycemia with glycosuria but no ketonuria. Most of these infants are "small-for-dates" and in utero experienced poor placental function. In the few cases in which insulin concentrations have been measured in these children, the amounts have been found to be low.

The cause of neonatal diabetes mellitus is unknown in the great majority of cases, but most of the evidence is compatible with an immaturity of the β cells of the neonatal pancreas. Such immaturity is in marked contrast to the presumed early maturation and function of the β cells of the infant of the diabetic mother. Can we learn anything about the controls of β cell maturation from a comparison of these two clinical entities? In the small-for-dates baby we have undernutrition in utero; in the infant of the diabetic mother we have overnutrition in utero. There is good evidence that extra-uterine malnutrition, especially in infants, produces serious impairment of insulin release. Is this just a reflection of diminished concentrations of compounds such as glucose and amino acids that trigger insulin release?

The situation is probably not as simple as that. Evidence is accumulating that hormonal factors (particularly glucocorticoids) are important in β cell maturation. Differentiation of the β cells of fetal rat pancreas grown in organ culture occurred only if the tissue was incubated in the presence of fetal adrenal cortex. In other cultures of fetal rat pancreas, with cortisol added to the medium, the β cells developed granules and contained more insulin than the β cells of those pancreases which had developed in utero. Precocious development of rabbit fetal exocrine and endocrine pancreas was noted when cortisone or ACTH was administered to pregnant rabbits. These studies, coupled with the evidence of the importance of cortisol in the development of mammary gland, fetal lung, fetal liver, and fetal adrenal medulla, suggest that the availability of glucocorticoids may be critical for maturation of many tissues.

The small-for-dates baby often manifests intra-uterine growth retardation, and one of the organs which is usually smaller for age in this condition is the adrenal gland. If the usually small adrenals in intra-uterine growth retardation are functioning at a reduced level, fetal glucocorticoids may be reduced in concentration in fetal blood. In addition, maternal glucocorticoids may be less available in the presence of placental insufficiency.

Recently, Ferguson and Milner (1970) reported transient neonatal diabetes mellitus in two siblings; the mother of these two children had persistently low blood glucose levels. If fluctuations of blood glucose are necessary for normal functional development, maternal hypoglycemia might be an etiologic factor in the lack of development of functional β cells.

Presumably, after birth the β cells of the small-for-dates baby mature, since spontaneous regression of the diabetes usually occurs. However, in some cases, the diabetes mellitus is permanent.

SUMMARY

In the pre-insulin era few diabetic pregnancies were reported. Most juvenile diabetics died in adolescence and, in general, early adult diabetics were infertile. With insulin therapy the picture has changed. Diabetes mellitus has now become one of the commonest medical causes of problems to the fetus and newborn. The occurrence of diabetic pregnancies varies widely from hospital to hospital; nevertheless, the trend is upward.

The infant of the diabetic mother must sustain the effects of a possible diabetic genotype as well as an unfavorable hormonal environment engendered by the maternal diabetes. Ketoacidosis of the mother is only one of many hazards in utero. The perinatal mortality is increased in these infants. The hyperinsulinism, presumably secondary to hyperglycemia in utero, paves the way for hypoglycemia in the neonatal period. Of even greater hazard to the infant is the respiratory distress syndrome, undoubtedly due to the morphologic and enzymatic immaturity of the lung of the prematurely delivered baby.

Other causes of hyperinsulinism or hypoglycemia, or both, exist, and in the neonatal period the dysmature (small-for-dates) baby and erythroblastotic infant must be considered at risk. In addition, in cases of the birth of twins, the smaller of the twins is frequently hypoglycemic.

Less frequently encountered, but equally interesting, is hyperglycemia in the neonatal period. Examples of hyperglycemia are usually seen in small-for-dates babies; the presumed etiology is immaturity of the pancreatic β cells. It is possible that the β cells, like the alveolar cells of the lung, the chromaffin cells of the adrenal medulla, and the hepatocytes of the liver, may require glucocorticoids for full maturation.

We are discovering that symptomatic neonatal hypoglycemia is far commoner than had been previously thought. We are also learning that the maturation of the system(s) controlling glucose concentration in the blood is more complex than heretofore suspected. The interplay of hormones in the perinatal period is undoubtedly dependent upon genotype and environmental factors. The infant of the diabetic mother serves as an example of survival in an abnormal endocrine environment, possibly coupled with a diabetic genotype.

SUGGESTED READING

Diabetes in pregnancy, M. Brudenell and R. Beard, Clinics in Endocrinology and Metabolism, November, 1972, W. B. Saunders Co., Philadelphia.

An overview of the subject with discussions of maternal and fetal complications. The section on management is offered in some detail.

Control of glucose metabolism in the fetus and newborn infant, Peter A. J. Adam, Adv. Metab. Disorders 5:183, 1971.

An exhaustive review of the metabolism of mother and conceptus. The biochemical and hormonal controls of glucose metabolism are covered in great detail. There is a section on the infant of the diabetic mother as well as discussions of small-for-dates babies and erythroblastotic infants. The bibliography is complete and should serve the student who wishes to explore certain aspects in depth.

Respiratory Distress Syndrome, edited by C. A. Villee, D. B. Villee, and J. Zuckerman, New York, Academic Press, 1973.

An up-to-date book in this rapidly advancing area of research. Particularly pertinent are the discussions relating to the control of enzyme activity in the fetal lung. Hormonal and environmental factors are considered. For the student interested in the molecular events of differentiation, there are several papers dealing with the chemistry of phospholipids and the phenomenon of surface tension.

CHAPTER SEVEN

The Adrenal Gland of the Newborn: Congenital Adrenocortical Hyperplasia

The fetal zone of the adrenal cortex of the newborn infant undergoes rapid involution and loses about half its total mass by about 2 weeks of age. Usually, degeneration is not evident to any great extent prior to 3 or 4 days after birth. The most active period of involution occurs during the second week of life. At the end of the first week of life, a growth of cells of the definitive cortex down into the degenerating area is discernible. Gradually, these "definitive" cells assume the typical arrangement of the adult adrenal cortex, with a peripheral zona glomerulosa, a prominent zona fasciculata, and an ill-defined zona reticularis adjacent to the adrenal medulla. During the first month of life, concomitant with the degeneration of the fetal zone, the definitive or adult adrenal cortex may double or triple in size.

As one might expect, the pattern of steroids found in blood and urine also changes as the products of the fetal zone disappear and the definitive cortex becomes more active. Moreover, changes in steroid production produce physiological alterations. For instance, inborn errors in the synthesis of adrenal hormones can produce changes in the external genitalia resulting in a form of pseudohermaphroditism in the female (p. 154). These changes are brought about by the excessive production of androgens in adrenal glands stimulated by elevated levels of ACTH caused in turn by impaired production of cortisol.

THE PATTERN OF STEROID METABOLISM IN THE NEONATAL PERIOD

The adrenal gland is actively producing steroid hormones in the newborn. The gonads are relatively inactive at birth, although the fetal testis had been active in the synthesis of testosterone in utero, particularly in the first half of gestation. The adrenal cortical hormones are classified as (1) *glucocorticoids* (21-carbon steroids which control the activities of certain enzymes involved in the intermediary metabolism of carbohydrates, amino acids, and lipids and also suppress certain inflammatory processes), (2) *mineralocorticoids* (21-carbon steroids which regulate electrolyte transport), and (3) *androgens* (19-carbon steroids which possess varying degrees of virilizing activity). One might add estrogens and progestins as fourth and fifth categories of steroid hormones; however, under normal circumstances, these hormones are not synthesized in biologically significant amounts in the human adrenal cortex.

Steroids are transformed by various tissues of the body. These transformations in the adult may involve hydroxylation, dehydrogenation, oxidation of the side chain, reduction of the 4,5 double bond, or conjugation. Enzymes involved in steroid catabolism are confined in large part to the liver. For example, the liver can reduce the 4,5 double bond of steroid hormones, rendering them biologically inactive. In the reduction of the double bond between carbon 4 and carbon 5 in cortisol, two hydrogens are incorporated in the A ring, forming the biologically inactive dihydrocortisol (Figure 7–1). The ketone group at carbon 3 can be reduced (producing tetrahydrocortisol, or THF), and subsequently the 3α-hydroxyl group can be coupled with uridine diphosphoglucuronic acid (UDPGA) to give the glucosiduronate (THF-3α-glucosiduronate) or with $3'$-phosphoadenosyl-$5'$-phosphosulfate (PAPS) to form the sulfate (THF-3α-sulfate). Cortisol can also be inactivated in the liver by reversible conversion to cortisone (11β-hydroxysteroid dehydrogenase). Cortisone can undergo similar transformations in the liver to yield dihydrocortisone and tetrahydrocortisone (THE). Both cortisol and cortisone can be reduced at carbon 20 also, to form cortol and cortolone respectively. These two steroids can be reduced to their respective dihydro- and tetrahydro derivatives in the liver (Figure 7–1).

Other tissues can also metabolize steroids, although to a much lesser degree. Kidney tissue can (1) convert cortisol to cortisone, (2) reduce the ketone at carbon 20 (progesterone $\rightarrow$ 20α-dihydroprogesterone), and (3) oxidize or reduce estrogens and androgens by means of a 17β-hydroxysteroid dehydrogenase. The skin has 17β- and 3β-hydroxysteroid dehydrogenases as well as a 5α-reductase, and skeletal muscle contains 3β-, 17β-, and 20α-hydroxysteroid dehydrogenases. These chemical transformations are very important in eliminating the biological activity of steroid hormones. Both biologically active and inactive steroids are excreted in the urine, but, by far, most steroid hormones have been converted to inactive products before being excreted.

Glucocorticoids in urine

The major glucocorticoid in the human is cortisol (originally termed compound F). In contrast to corticosterone (found in about one third the quantity of cortisol), cortisol has a 17-hydroxyl group. The 21-carbon metabolites of cortisol as well as its immediate precursor, 11-deoxycortisol (compound S), are classified with cortisol as 17-hydroxycorticosteroids (17OHCS). In these corticosteroids, carbons 17, 20, and 21 constitute a dihydroxyacetone side chain (Figure 7–1). In plasma, the principal 17-hydroxycorticosteroid is cortisol itself, whereas in the urine of the adult, reduced derivatives of cortisol and cortisone are found. A measurement of the 17OHCS in the urine passed in 24 hours does not, however, measure all the cortisol produced over that period, since about 10 percent of cortisol and cortisone are oxidized in the liver to 17-ketosteroids by removal of the side chain at carbon 17 (Figure 7–1). Measurement of the 17-ketosteroids (17KS) in urine would include both androgens with a 17-keto group (such as androstenedione, androsterone, and etiocholanolone) and 17OHCS which have been oxidized to 17KS.

The dihydroxyacetone side chain of the 17OHCS can react with phenylhydrazine and sulfuric acid to give a characteristic yellow color. This reaction was first described by Porter and Silber; fittingly, the reaction is used to measure material referred to as "Porter-Silber chromogens." Use of the Porter-Silber reaction is one method for assaying 17OHCS and measures approximately one third of the total cortisol produced. By this Porter-Silber method, normal infants were found to excrete in the urine about 500 μg of 17OHCS per 24 hours. Premature infants excrete about half as much 17OHCS as do term infants.

This value for 17OHCS in the newborn's urine is rather low, and it led some investigators to propose a state of adrenal insufficiency in the newborn infant. A glance at the Porter-Silber method may help explain these low values. In the method, methylene dichloride is used for extracting the Porter-Silber chromogens. Cortisol is metabolized differently in the newborn than in the adult, and the very polar metabolites of the newborn are not so readily extracted by methylene dichloride. These compounds, however, can be extracted by ethyl acetate, and methods using this solvent yield much higher values. Thus the relatively low 17OHCS of the newborn measured by the standard Porter-Silber method may represent, in part, an artifact of the extraction procedure.

Another method of measuring 17-hydroxycorticosteroids, the "17-ketogenic method" of Norymberski, has the advantage of including the group of 17OHCS excretory products in which the 20-keto group has been reduced to a hydroxyl group (namely, the cortols and cortolones shown in Figure 7–1). In the Norymberski method, the side chains of these compounds and of their 17-hydroxycorticosteroid precursors are split off by reacting with sodium bismuthate. The resulting 17KS can be measured colorimetrically by the Zimmermann method, which couples the reactive 17-keto group with metadinitrobenzene, producing a blue-

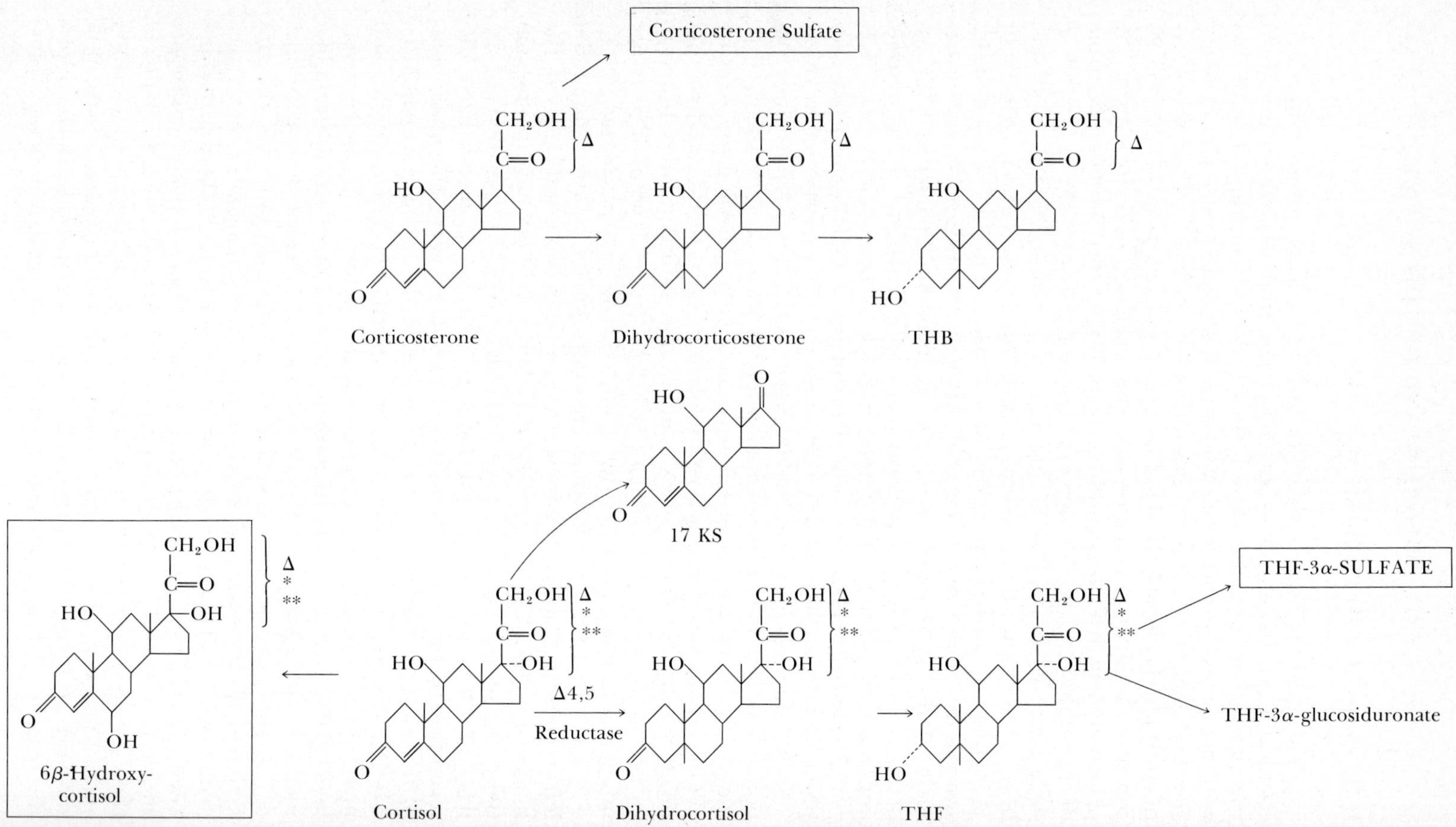
Corticosterone Sulfate
Corticosterone
Dihydrocorticosterone
THB
17 KS
6β-Hydroxy-cortisol
Cortisol
Δ4,5 Reductase
Dihydrocortisol
THF
THF-3α-SULFATE
THF-3α-glucosiduronate

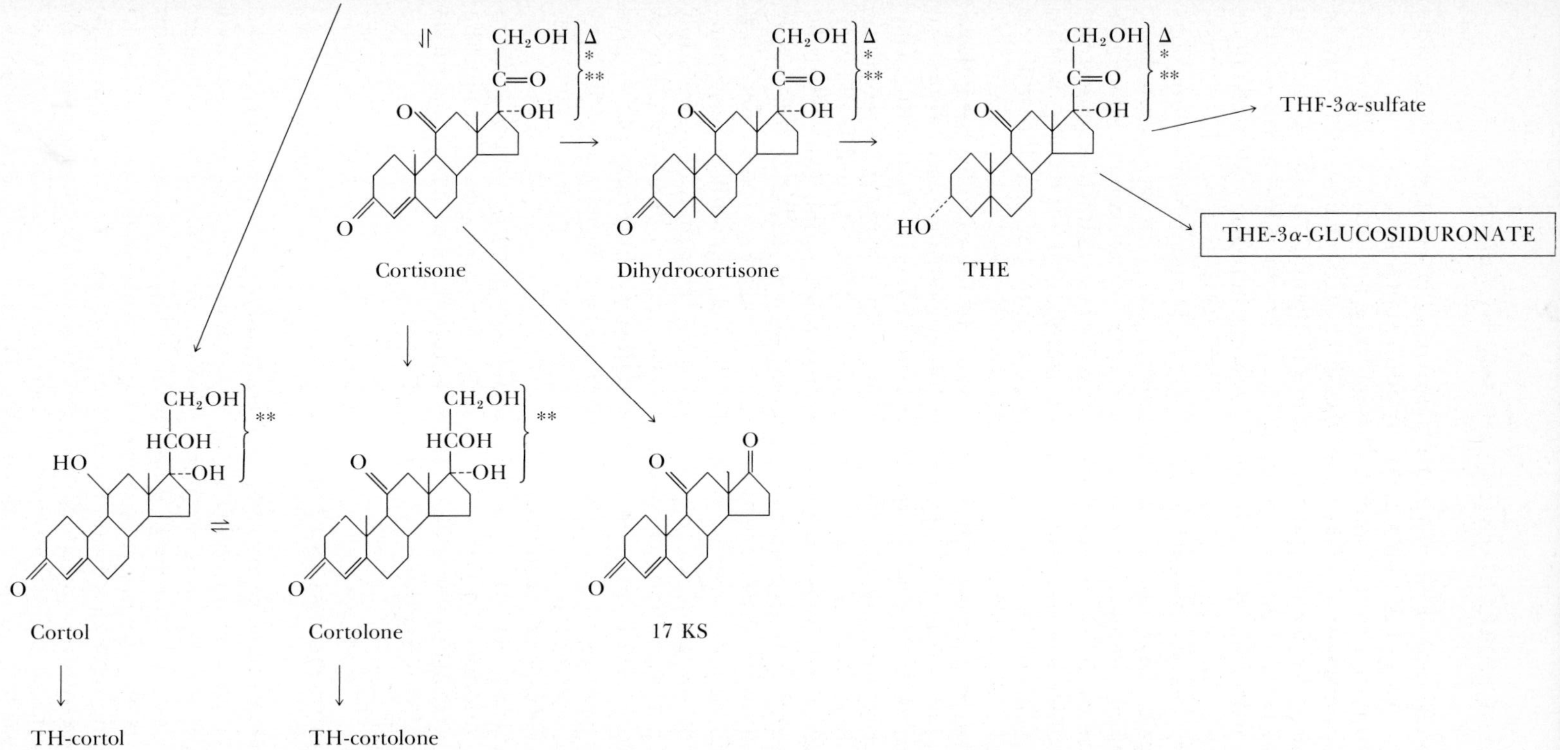

*Dihydroxyacetone side chain → P-S chromogens
**17-Ketogenic steroids → 17 KS
Δ α-ketol

FIGURE 7–1. Metabolism of glucocorticoids. Major metabolites in the urine of the newborn are set off as boxed labels.

colored compound. This method of assaying the urine of young children also yields values that are low by adult standards.

Corticosterone and its metabolites are not measured by either the Porter-Silber or Norymberski methods. Since this steroid is of relatively more importance in the perinatal period than in adulthood, other methods of assay should be utilized. Methods which are based on the sugar-like sidechain (α-ketol) of the corticosteroids, although non-specific, have the advantage of measuring 17OHCS as well as corticosterone and its metabolites (Figure 7–1). Triphenyltetrazolium has proved particularly useful as an oxidizing agent in these reactions. These methods do not, of course, measure the cortols and cortolones. A comparision of the excretion of 17-deoxycorticosteroids (corticosterone and its metabolites principally) with the excretion of 17OHCS— that is, 17-deoxyCS/17OHCS— yields, in infants, a ratio of 3:1, and in adults, a ratio of 1:3.

The specific glucocorticoids excreted by the infant differ from those found in adult urine. Tetrahydrocortisol and tetrahydrocortisone are the most abundant reducing steroids in adult urine, but not in the urine of infants (Figure 7–1). Only 10 percent of the cortisol-4-^{14}C administered to infants was recovered in the urine as THE, THF, and alloTHF (5α hydrogen), whereas comparable values in the adult were 25 to 30 percent. The newborn apparently carries out less reduction of ring A and instead utilizes hydroxylation at various positions (particularly 6β) in the catabolism of corticosteroids (Figure 7–1). In addition, the newborn excretes far less 17OHCS as glucosiduronates than does the adult (10 to 20 percent versus 60 percent, respectively). These data are in keeping with several observations that indicate a lower activity of glucuronyl transferase in the newborn. Most of the glucocorticoids in newborn urine are present as sulfates; however, cortisone is excreted primarily as THE-3α-glucosiduronate.

There is no evidence that the normal newborn is unable to form cortisol in amounts equal to or exceeding adult values. In addition, the newborn adrenal appears to be normally responsive to ACTH, as far as enhanced cortisol synthesis is concerned.

Mineralocorticoids in urine

The term *mineralocorticoid* is applied to such steroids as aldosterone and deoxycorticosterone which act upon renal tubules and the sweat and salivary glands to produce sodium retention and potassium exchange. Estimation of the very small quantity of aldosterone excreted in the urine is difficult. The procedure involves the acidification of the urine to pH 1, freeing the aldosterone from its association with glucuronic acid, and then extracting and purifying the free aldosterone. Accuracy of measuring the purified aldosterone is increased by the addition of radioactive aldosterone to the urine samples, which helps to provide an estimation of losses incurred in the measuring process. The double isotope derivative technique of Kliman and Peterson has greater precision than the single isotope method. The Kliman and Peterson method involves the use of two different isotopic forms (usually tritium and ^{14}C) of the steroid. One form is injected into the patient; the second is added to the sample taken for analysis. The steroid (aldosterone) is rigorously purified through a series of chromatographic procedures, and the final recovery is calculated from the recovery of the isotopic form added to the sample. The specific activity of the recovered injected steroid can be used to calculate the secretion rate of the steroid.

Weldon and colleagues reported low aldosterone secretion rates in normal infants during the first week of life, but older infants had mean aldosterone secretion rates equivalent to those of normal adults. In most patients there is a good correlation between aldosterone secretion rate and urinary excretion of aldosterone. When the excretion of aldosterone was correlated with surface area, New found that normal subjects of any age excrete 3 to 13 $\mu g/m^2/24$ hours.

No measurement of aldosterone has significance unless the dietary intake of sodium and potassium is known. In fact, one method for assessing aldosterone production is to deprive the patient of salt by placing him on a diet containing 10 mEq Na/24 hours or less for five days. The secretion of aldosterone under these conditions should increase. Obviously, such tests must be conducted with great care in the infant because of his greater susceptibility to electrolyte imbalance.

Androgens in Urine

Most androgens have a ketone group at carbon 17 in the steroid nucleus and are called 17-ketosteroids (17KS). The classical Zimmermann method for assaying these steroids is not entirely specific for 17KS, and a correction formula must be applied to compensate for interfering non-specific chromogens. In neonatal and infant urines, these non-specific chromogens are present in large amounts. Extracts of infant urine, when examined by paper chromatography, reveal several very polar materials which react with the Zimmermann reagent. These polar compounds are present in the urine of the premature infant in even greater quantities—about twice as much as the amount in the urine of term infants. Probably a large portion of this polar material can be accounted for by 16α-hydroxydehydroepiandrosterone and 16-ketodehydroepiandrosterone. In contrast, urine of the newborn contains only small amounts of dehydroepiandrosterone, androsterone, or etiocholanolone. By the end of the first week of life, the polar compounds which react with Zimmermann reagent are almost undetectable.

The ease of the Zimmermann assay makes it useful in the investigation of virilizing states; however, it must be remembered that the most powerful androgens—testosterone and dihydrotestosterone (p.

368)—are not 17KS. Thus it is possible to have normal 17KS values and still have increased biologically active androgens.

Most workers agree that in the first week of life the excretion of 17KS is elevated (2 to 5 mg/24 hours); thereafter, however, in normal children up to 8 years old, the value rarely exceeds 2 mg/24 hours. During the first few days of life, the total urinary excretion of Δ5-3β-hydroxysteroids actually increases. Of these steroids the major components of neonatal urine are: 16α-hydroxydehydroepiandrosterone, 16-ketodehydroepiandrosterone, androstenetriol (3β,16α,17β-trihydroxyandrost-5-ene), 16α'hydroxypregnenolone, and 21-hydroxypregnenolone. These steroids are excreted primarily as 3β-sulfo conjugates. When expressed as μg steroid/m²/24 hours, the concentration of Δ5-3β-hydroxysteroids in infant urine is about 10 times that in adult urine.

Another difference between adult and infant urine is the predominance of the 17α epimer of androstenediol in the latter and the 17β epimer in the former. Both 17α- and 17β-androstenediol are excreted as disulfates (3β,17α, or 17β).

When the change in concentration of 17KS (especially dehydroepiandrosterone) in the urine is used as a criterion of ACTH effect, it is found that the newborn does not respond as well as the adult to the administration of ACTH. The usual increase in cortisol secretion after the administration of ACTH *does* occur in the newborn.

STEROIDS IN PLASMA

Many of the group-specific methods used for urinary steroids can be used to measure hormones in plasma. Because of the diurnal variation in the concentration of hormones in plasma it is important to carry out analyses on samples drawn at standard times. This diurnal variation may be absent in early infancy. In general, the concentration of Porter-Silber chromogens in cord blood of babies delivered vaginally is about 20 μg/100 ml plasma. Babies delivered by caesarean section tend to have less Porter-Silber chromogens in cord blood (less than 10 μg/100 plasma). By one month after birth, the concentration of Porter-Silber chromogens in plasma of both caesarean and vaginally delivered babies reaches normal adult values (14± 1.36 μg/100 ml plasma).

A more specific method for measuring cortisol and other 11-hydroxylated corticosteroids, reported by Mattingly in 1962, is based upon the fact that 11-hydroxylated steroids react with sulfuric acid to give an intense blue fluorescence during exposure to ultraviolet light. In this assay, corticosterone fluoresces with two and a half times the intensity of cortisol. Unfortunately, the relatively high concentration of corticosterone in neonatal fluids interposes difficulties in interpreting concentrations of cortisol (this is not a drawback in analyzing plasma from adults). The contribution of corticosterone to total plasma corticosteroids is maximal during the first week of life. Cortisone does not give sulfuric acid fluorescence, nor do the synthetic compounds prednisolone (Δ1-cortisol), dexamethasone (9α-fluoro-16α-methyl prednisolone), and betamethasone (9α-fluoro-16β-methyl prednisolone).

More recently, methods for assaying steroid hormones by competitive protein binding have come into vogue. These techniques and the techniques of radioimmunoassay offer greater sensitivity as well as specificity. In time, these techniques will undoubtedly supplant the group-specific methods.

Using such specific assays it is possible to get a better idea of the relative amounts of the various glucocorticoids in umbilical cord and infant plasma. For instance, it appears that at birth there are about equal quantities of cortisol and cortisone in the plasma. The concentration of cortisol in cord blood is about one third that in maternal blood, whereas the concentration of cortisone is three times that in maternal blood. The relatively low cortisol concentration in cord blood may in part result from the decreased cortisol-binding capacity of fetal and neonatal blood. The low plasma cortisol-binding capacity in the neonate may in turn result from the high concentration of progesterone in fetal plasma. Progesterone has a threefold greater affinity for CBG than does cortisol, and consequently it could occupy a large percentage of the binding sites. After about 1 week of age, the concentration of cortisol in plasma approaches adult values, and the concentration of cortisone falls. Because the rate of metabolism of cortisol in the newborn is two to four times less than that of the adult, administered cortisol disappears slowly from the plasma.

The 17KS in neonatal plasma are largely Δ5-3β-hydroxysteroids. The very high values at birth fall to low levels during the first weeks of life. There is, however, a postnatal rise in plasma testosterone concentration in male infants (p. 359). Such a rise is not detected by the 17KS assay.

CONGENITAL ADRENOCORTICAL HYPERPLASIA

Several hereditary defects in the synthesis of cortisol have been described. An understanding of the clinical manifestations of each of these enzyme deficiencies requires a thorough knowledge of the biosynthesis of cortisol and its controls. Under normal conditions, the concentration of cortisol in the blood perfusing the hypothalamus regulates the secretion of CRH from the median eminence. This in turn regulates the secretion of ACTH by the anterior pituitary. Thus the final endocrine product, cortisol, exerts feedback control at the hypothalamic level. In addition glucocorticoids can act directly on the anterior pituitary to suppress the response of the corticotropin cell to CRH.

A reduced concentration of cortisol in the blood signals the hypothalamic receptors to release CRH, which in turn triggers the release of ACTH. The increased production and secretion of ACTH results in hyperplasia of the adrenal cortex. In congenital adrenocortical hyperplasia, the hyperplastic gland may be able to synthesize normal amounts of cortisol, provided the enzyme defect is not too severe. If the cortisol output can be increased by ACTH to values adequate to support life, the enzyme defect is said to be compensated. The cost, however, is high. In order to produce enough cortisol, excessive amounts of other adrenal products are formed. Among these are the adrenal androgens, which are responsible for the virilization found in patients with certain forms of adrenocortical hyperplasia.

The *adrenogenital syndrome* is that condition of hyperfunction of the adrenal cortex associated with sexual changes. The manifestation of the sexual changes depends upon when the onset of the disorder begins. Adrenal hyperplasia developing in the female fetus usually results in *pseudohermaphroditism.* Pseudohermaphroditism is characterized by the presence of gonads of only one sex (in contrast to true hermaphroditism, in which the gonads of both sexes are present), but associated with this are abnormalities of the external genitalia which cast some doubt on the sex of the patient.

The female pseudohermaphrodite usually has an enlarged clitoris, fused labioscrotal folds, and a urogenital sinus (Figure 7–2). The external appearance of the female genitalia (Figure 7–3) resembles that of the bilaterally cryptorchid male with hypospadias (p. 186). Occasionally, fusion of the labioscrotal folds is so complete that the urethra traverses the penis. Subjects with a penile urethra are often reared as boys. Prostatic tissue may be noted; ovaries, uterus, and tubes, though usually normal, may remain rudimentary. Hirsutism and a tendency to a male body configuration usually develop if treatment is not instituted early.

Adrenocortical hyperplasia may not be recognized in the male at

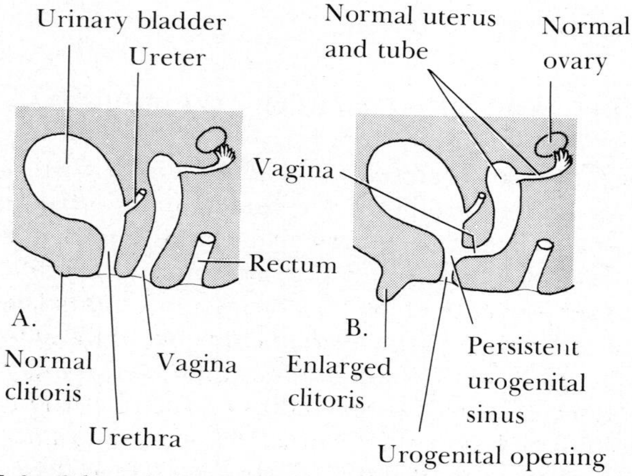

FIGURE 7–2. Schematic lateral views of the female urogenital system. *A*, normal; *B*, female pseudohermaphrodite caused by congenital virilizing adrenal hyperplasia. Note the enlarged clitoris and the persistent urogenital sinus. (From Moore, K. *The Developing Human.* Philadelphia: W. B. Saunders Company, 1973, p. 230.)

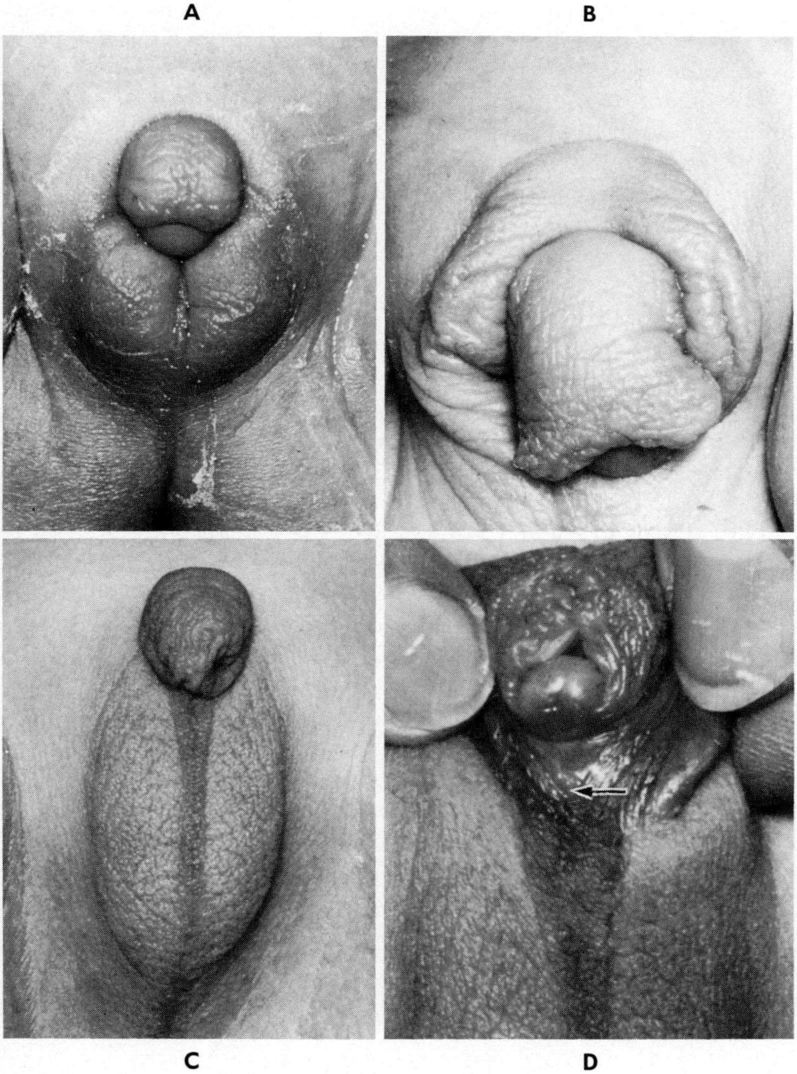

FIGURE 7–3. Photographs of the external genitalia of female pseudohermaphrodites resulting from congenital virilizing adrenal hyperplasia. *A*, external genitalia of a newborn female, exhibiting enlargement of the clitoris and fusion of the labia majora. *B*, external genitalia of a female infant, showing considerable enlargement of the clitoris. The labia majora are rugose as in a scrotum. *C* and *D*, external genitalia of a 6-year-old girl showing an enlarged clitoris and fusion of the rugose labia majora to form a scrotum-like structure. In *D*, note the glans clitoridis and the opening of the urogenital sinus (arrow). (From Moore, K. *The Developing Human.* Philadelphia: W. B. Saunders Company, 1973, p. 229.)

birth unless there are associated symptoms of salt loss. Starting shortly after birth, rapid somatic and osseous development occurs, along with the appearance of secondary sexual characteristics (acne, deepening of voice, penile enlargement, erections, excessive muscular development). This condition has been termed *macrogenitosomia praecox.*

The extent of anomalous sexual development and the presence of other clinical symptoms such as hypertension and salt loss depend upon the kind and extent of enzyme deficiency. The enzyme deficiencies described so far range from defects early in the biosynthetic path (congenital lipoid hyperplasia) to flaws in the final steps of cortisol synthesis (11β-hydroxylase deficiency).

Congenital lipoid adrenal hyperplasia

In 1955, Prader and Gurtner described a defect in the enzymatic conversion of cholesterol to pregnenolone. This defect blocks the synthesis of all steroid hormones (Figure 7–4) and results in large lipid-filled adrenals; cholesterol and its esters accumulate in the adrenal cortex. The enzyme deficiency also involves the gonads, and affected male infants lack male differentiation of the external genitalia and have an apparently normal female phenotype *(male pseudohermaphroditism).* The severe electrolyte disturbances resulting from the lack of aldosterone allow few of these patients to survive. The normal architecture of the adrenal cortex is destroyed. There is an increase in the size and number of foam-filled cortical cells which show a positive Schultz reaction for cholesterol.

The impaired conversion of cholesterol to pregnenolone could result from a deficiency of the 20,22-desmolase or from a defect in the hydroxylation of either carbon 20 or 22 of cholesterol (Figure 7–4). Both carbons must be hydroxylated before the six-carbon side chain of cholesterol can be removed. In vitro studies using postmortem adrenal tissue from a patient with lipoid adrenal hyperplasia suggest that the defect resides in the 20α-hydroxylase.

Δ5-3βHydroxysteroid dehydrogenase deficiency

In 1951, Samuels and his coworkers first described the enzyme Δ5-3β-hydroxysteroid dehydrogenase in testicular tissue. This enzyme catalyzes the oxidation of the hydroxyl group at the 3β carbon. A second enzyme, isomerase, converts the double bond from Δ5 to Δ4. A variety of substrate-specific Δ5-3β-hydroxysteroid dehydrogenases probably exist in many tissues, including the ovary, testis, adrenal, and placenta. Enzyme activity, which has been localized to the microsomal fraction of the cell, requires NAD as a cofactor. In the process of oxidation of preg-

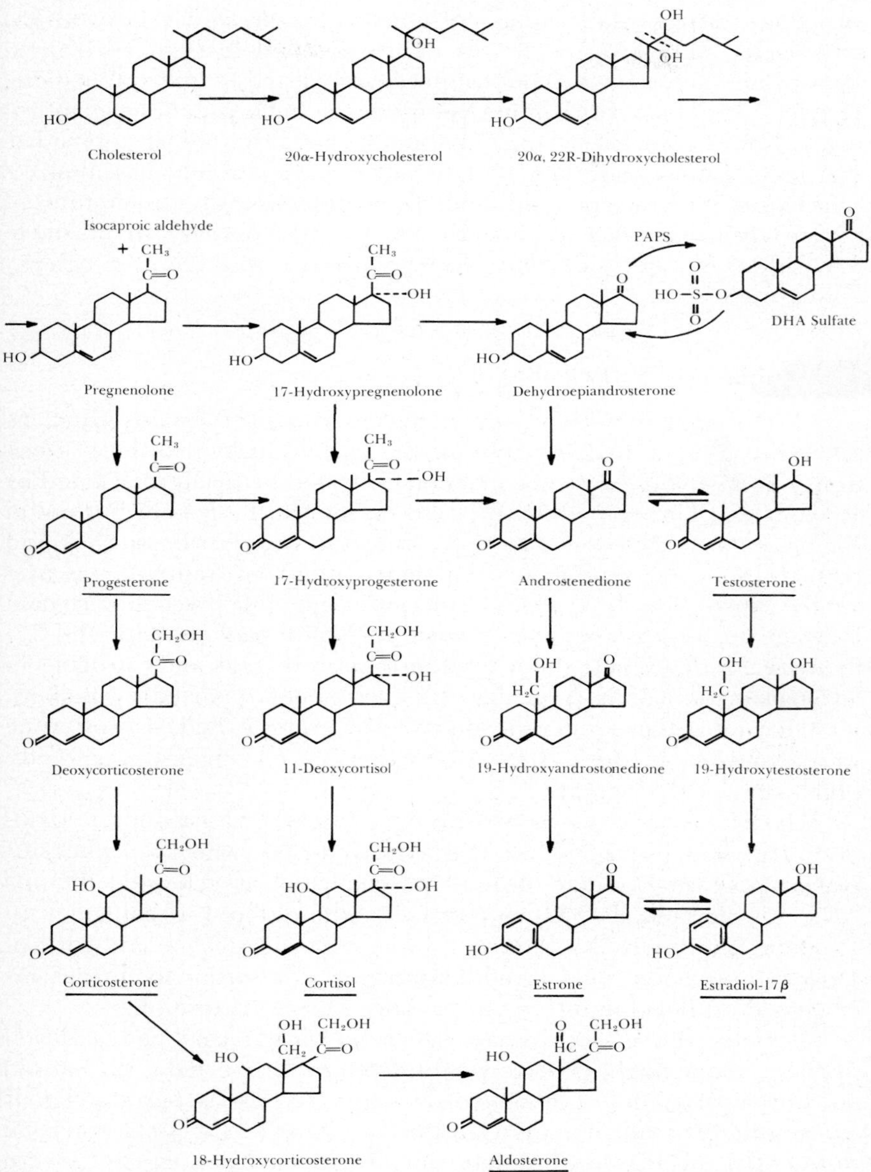

FIGURE 7–4. The synthesis from cholesterol of progestins, corticoids, androgens, and estrogens. (From Page, E., Villee, C., and Villee, D. *Human Reproduction.* Philadelphia: W. B. Saunders Company, 1972, p. 53.)

nenolone to progesterone, NADH is generated (the hydrogen of the OH group of pregnenolone being transferred to NAD).

As might be expected, a deficiency of $\Delta5$-3β-hydroxysteroid dehydrogenase impairs the synthesis of glucocorticoids, mineralocorticoids, androgens, and estrogens. By the nature of the defect, dehydroepiandrosterone can be formed but cannot be converted to androstenedione (Figure 7–4). Males with this hereditary defect (male pseudohermaphrodites) show incomplete masculinization, because dehydroepiandrosterone is a weak androgen. The female may be partially masculinized. The lack of mineralocorticoids and glucocorticoids leads to symptoms of severe adrenal insufficiency in early infancy. Most of these infants die in early life. The infants excrete urinary steroids with the $\Delta5$-3β-hydroxy configuration.

17-Hydroxylase deficiency

A more recently described defect in cortisol synthesis (Biglieri, 1966) involves the hydroxylation of the steroid nucleus in the 17 position. The 17-hydroxylase was first demonstrated in the adrenal gland by Hechter and Pincus in 1954. It is also present in the gonads but not in the placenta. With a defect in 17-hydroxylase, deoxycorticosterone and corticosterone are synthesized, but the synthesis of androgens is prevented, since 17-hydroxylation of progesterone must precede side chain cleavage to androstenedione (Figure 7–4). In patients with the 17-hydroxylase deficiency, the biosynthesis of androgens and estrogens in adrenals or gonads is negligible. (In the patient reported by Biglieri, secretory rates of progesterone, deoxycorticosterone, and corticosterone were elevated, but aldosterone production was nil, suggesting an additional enzyme deficiency.)

Hypertension is associated with the 17-hydroxylase disorder. Urinary 17KS and estrogens are markedly reduced, whereas values for plasma progesterone and urinary pregnanediol are elevated. Plasma ACTH is elevated also. When cortisol is administered to patients with the deficiency, there is a reduction in deoxycorticosterone and corticosterone production, with a gradual return of aldosterone to normal. Estrogens must be administered to produce sexual maturation.

Females with 17-hydroxylase deficiency have normal genital development, as one might expect. New and Peterson reported a 12-year-old boy with a partial defect in 17-hydroxylation. In this case, production of aldosterone was not impaired and classic signs of excess aldosterone were noted. In this boy, the defect in 17-hydroxylation was not severe enough to alter androgen production in the testis, and consequently sexual differentiation and postnatal development were normal. New also reported the case of a 24-year-old male (46/XY) with a small penis, a vagina, and gynecomastia. He had a deficiency in 17-hydroxylation. It is interesting that genetic females with this condition have little or no breast development.

21-Hydroxylase deficiency

By far the most commonly encountered hereditary defect in cortisol synthesis involves hydroxylation at carbon 21. Like other steroid hydroxylases, 21-hydroxylase requires both molecular oxygen and NADPH and belongs in the general category of mixed function oxidases. These enzymes catalyze the incorporation of only *one* atom of the oxygen molecule into the substrate. The other oxygen atom is reduced to water; therefore, reducing equivalents are needed. The true *oxygenases* incorporate *both* atoms of oxygen into the substrate.

Studies by several investigators have brought us to our present concept of just how one atom of oxygen is introduced into the steroid molecule (Figure 7–5). The overall equation is:

$$\text{Steroid-H} + O_2 + \text{NADPH} + H^+ \longrightarrow \text{Steroid-OH} + H_2O + \text{NADP}^+$$

NADPH provides reducing equivalents via a chain of intermediates including a flavoprotein and, in mitochondria, a non-heme iron protein called *adrenodoxin.* The latter interacts with a special cytochrome, cytochrome P_{450}, which in its reduced form yields with oxygen an activated complex the chemical structure of which has not yet been established. The active oxygen-P_{450} complex then interacts with the steroid substrate to produce a hydroxylated steroid and a molecule of water, regenerating the ferric form of P_{450}. The NADPH can be generated by the first step of the pentose pathway that is catalyzed by glucose-6-phosphate dehydrogenase. Indeed, one theory of the mode of action of ACTH is that the hormone stimulates a specific adrenal glucose-6-phosphate dehydrogenase, thus producing more NADPH to provide reducing equivalents for the hydroxylation of steroids.

It must be remembered that in all the forms of adrenocortical hyperplasia the enzyme deficiency has not been directly proved. Rather, it has been inferred on the basis of the steroid precursors that accumulate in body fluids and in tissue incubated in vitro. Such "proof" does not rule out the possibility of a defect in the generation or synthesis of any of the intermediates required for steroid hydroxylation. The term hydroxylase refers to the whole complex involved in the hydroxylation reaction. The high concentration of ascorbic acid in the adrenal cortex suggests that this substance serves as a reservoir of electrons for the mixed function oxidases.

The enzyme 21-hydroxylase is located in the microsomes, and a specific alteration of an intermediate in the P_{450} path could prevent the hydroxylation reaction from occurring. A similar defect in the mitochondria might prevent the action of 11β-hydroxylase. At present, evidence suggests that congenital adrenocortical hyperplasia is due to a genetic failure to produce specific proteins needed for the catalysis of steroid hydroxylation involved in hormone synthesis.

About 30 percent of patients with a defect in 21-hydroxylase show

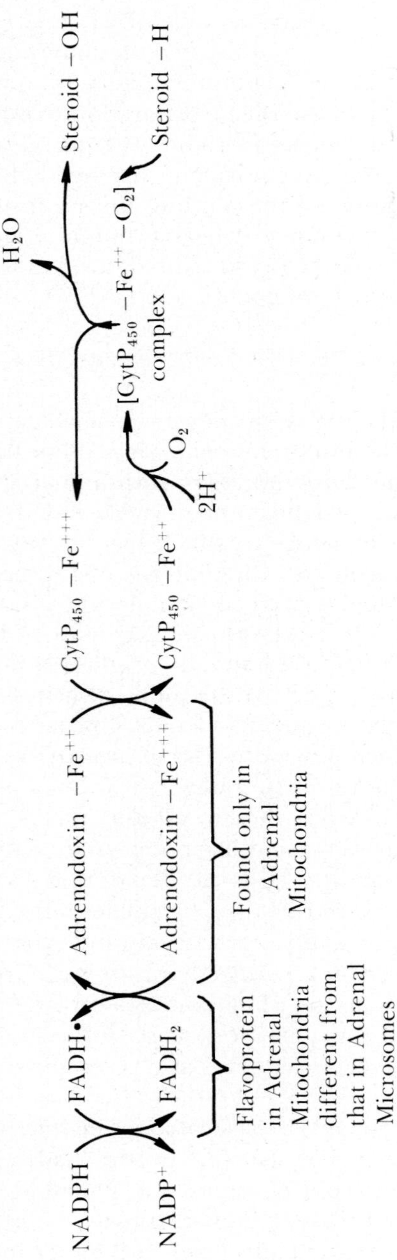

FIGURE 7–5. Steroid hydroxylation in the adrenal gland.

evidence of a salt-losing syndrome with hyperkalemia, hyponatremia, and metabolic acidosis. When the loss of salt and water is severe, the infant may show symptoms of adrenal crisis shortly after birth. Such infants are in grave danger, and without immediate treatment mortality is high.

Females with 21-hydroxylase deficiency usually show evidence of virilization at birth, and the virilization progresses further after birth if treatment is not instituted. Phallic enlargement occurs in both sexes. Pubic hair usually appears before the age of 3 years. Other signs of virilization (axillary hair, voice changes, acne) occur early. In untreated patients, normal pubertal development does not occur at the time of adolescence, and the female patient fails to menstruate.

Adrenal androgens normally accelerate growth at puberty, but in patients with virilizing adrenogenital syndrome this accelerated growth occurs much earlier. The possibility exists that GH may also be involved in this acceleration of growth. Finkelstein and coworkers found that GH secretion in two patients with congenital adrenocortical hyperplasia was increased for chronological age. This increased secretion of GH was not suppressed by glucocorticoid therapy. The increase in height in adrenocortical hyperplasia occurs earlier than normal; however, because fusion of the epiphyses occurs even earlier, untreated children are dwarfed. By the sixth year of life, the height age may reach that of 12 or 13 years while the bone age may exceed 15 or more years. Rapid muscular development in early life and evolution of a masculine habitus occur. Because many of these alterations are irreversible, the importance of early therapy is obvious, especially in the female.

If the defect in hydroxylation at carbon 21 is mild, the onset of virilization may not occur until later in life. Stress, such as puberty, may trigger the onset of clinical manifestations of the disease. In such cases the development of the genitalia is normal, but clitoral hypertrophy and hirsutism in females occur.

There is still disagreement about the biochemical defect in the salt-losing form of the 21-hydroxylase deficiency. Bongiovanni and Eberlein postulate that both forms of the 21-hydroxylase defect are due to a single enzyme deficiency. The patient who is a salt loser, however, has an almost complete lack of the enzyme, precluding synthesis of mineralocorticoids. According to the Bongiovanni and Eberlein hypothesis, patients without salt loss have a milder defect which permits the synthesis of mineralocorticoids in sufficient amounts.

Bryan and his colleagues (1965) proposed that there are substrate-specific 21-hydroxylases, analogous with the situation for the $\Delta 5$-3β-hydroxysteroid dehydrogenases. A deficiency in both the progesterone and 17-hydroxyprogesterone 21-hydroxylases would block both mineralocorticoid and glucocorticoid synthesis and produce the salt-losing variety of adrenocortical hyperplasia. A deficiency in only the 17-hydroxyprogesterone 21-hydroxylase would permit the synthesis of mineralocorticoids, thus preventing salt loss. The possibility that such specificity exists is strenghened by Kowarski's report (1965) that patients without the salt-losing form of adrenocortical hyperplasia have aldosterone secretion rates above normal and that further increase occurred on a low sodium intake. Treatment with glucocorticoids brought the aldosterone secretion rate to normal. Until in vitro studies can show clearly whether several substrate-specific 21-hydroxylases or one nonspecific 21-hydroxylase is involved in the synthesis of glucocorticoids and mineralocorticoids, the disagreement will remain unresolved.

11-Hydroxylase deficiency

Eberlein and Bongiovanni (1955) described an additional rare enzyme deficiency, an 11β-hydroxylase defect. This enzyme completes the synthesis of cortisol by inserting the final and most characteristic hydroxyl group of the adrenal hormones. Approximately 5 percent of patients with virilizing adrenocortical hyperplasia have a deficiency of this enzyme. In these patients, 17- and 21-hydroxylation occur in such a manner that 11-deoxycorticosterone (DOC) and 11-deoxycortisol (compound S) are formed in excessive amounts. The latter has a dihydroxyacetone sidechain and can form Porter-Silber chromogens. Initial studies of blood and urine in patients with 11-hydroxylase deficiency showed the Porter-Silber chromogens to be abnormally high, and the material was thought to be cortisol. Eberlein and Bongiovanni showed that the chromogen in blood was 11-deoxycortisol and that in urine a metabolite of 11-deoxycortisol.

The sodium-retaining properties of DOC are probably responsible for the hypertension characteristic of the 11-hydroxylase disorder. Both urinary deoxycorticosterone and the secretion rate of deoxycorticosterone are elevated. The secretion rates of cortisol, corticosterone, and aldosterone, on the other hand, are diminished.

The site of 11β-hydroxylation of steroids is in the mitochondria of the cell. One obvious difficulty in mitochondrial hydroxylations is the availability of the NADPH necessary to provide reducing equivalents. The membranes of mitochondria are impermeable to pyridine nucleotides, and therefore the NADPH generated by the pentose pathway in the cytoplasm of the cell is not available to the mitochondria. In 1969 Simpson and Estabrook suggested an attractive hypothesis to resolve this problem. They found that adrenal cortical cells contain an intramitochondrial *malic enzyme* as well as the usual cytoplasmic malic enzyme. The malic enzyme catalyzes CO_2 fixation to pyruvic acid to form L-malic acid. The mitochondrial and cytoplasmic enzymes are distinctly different. The reaction malate + $NADP^+ \rightarrow$ pyruvate + CO_2 + NADPH + H^+ is favored in the mitochondria, whereas the reverse (normal) direction is favored in cytoplasm. Thus NADPH and pyruvate produced in the cytoplasm (via the pentose pathway and glycolysis respectively) give rise to malate. The mitochondrion is freely permeable to malate, which within the mitochondrion can give rise to NADPH for steroid hydroxylation.

18-Hydroxylase deficiency

In contrast to the other enzyme defects described, a deficiency of 18-hydroxylase does not impair the synthesis of cortisol; therefore, the concentration of ACTH in the blood should not be elevated. Nevertheless, in one case of this deficiency, the patient's adrenals were enlarged, with hypertrophy of the zona reticularis. The outstanding clinical feature of this defect is salt loss. The external genitalia of both males and females are normal.

THE DIAGNOSIS OF CONGENITAL ADRENOCORTICAL HYPERPLASIA

Antenatal Diagnosis

Infants suffering from salt-losing syndromes due to adrenocortical hyperplasia should have steroid treatment as soon as possible after birth. When a pregnancy occurs in a mother who has already given birth to a child with congenital adrenocortical hyperplasia, there is one chance in four that her child will have this disorder. If the previous child had the salt-losing variety of hyperplasia, it may be of some importance to have advance information about the fetus in utero. Amniotic fluid can be examined for the presence of specific steroids. Several investigators have diagnosed congenital adrenocortical hyperplasia antenatally by this technique.

Any enzyme defect in the fetus would exist in the trophoblast (fetal tissue). Thus a defect in the conversion of cholesterol to pregnenolone or a defect in $\Delta 5$-3β-hydroxysteroid dehydrogenase would be present in the trophoblast, and in vitro incubation of trophoblastic tissue at birth might be of interest. However, since the placenta normally lacks 17, 21, 11β, and 18 hydroxylases, defects in these enzymes would not be detected in this manner.

Neonatal diagnosis

A family history of abnormal genitalia in a sibling should alert the attending physician to the possibility of an hereditary defect in cortisol synthesis. Virilization in the newborn infant is most likely to be due to congenital adrenocortical hyperplasia. Other causes of neonatal sexual anomalies are described in Chapter Eight and will not be discussed further here.

Of most immediate concern to the physician is the possibility of adrenal crisis. Salt loss should be detected early so that an adrenal crisis can be prevented. Characteristic symptoms can occur immediately after birth but more usually begin sometime between the sixth and fourteenth day of life.

The birth is usually normal as are the length and weight of the newborn. During the first few days of life, weight loss (over 10 percent) occurs, and despite adequate caloric intake, no weight gain occurs. If the correction of salt loss is delayed, the serum sodium falls, the potassium and urea rise, and a metabolic acidosis ensues, accompanied by vomiting, diarrhea, and dehydration. Peripheral circulatory failure and possible cardiac arrest (due to hyperkalemia) may follow.

Prevention of irreversible deterioration—an endocrine emergency—is essential. The treatment should include intravenous fluids and electrolytes as well as glucocorticoids (up to 10 mg cortisol hemisuccinate per kg body weight intravenously several times a day) and mineralocorticoids (2 to 5 mg DOC acetate per day intramuscularly). In adrenocortical insufficiency, the deficit is largely one of extracellular water, and therefore the volumes of replacement fluid are not as large as those for other types of dehydration. It is advisable to plan on a fluid replacement of about 120 ml/kg body weight in early infancy. The electrolyte concentrations of the serum are measured at frequent intervals. The loss of sodium exceeds that of chloride; hence, additional sodium may be given as sodium citrate.

Hyperkalemia may be troublesome. Rehydration and mineralocorticoid therapy will usually correct the condition. Only rarely are additional agents required. Calcium infusion is a rapidly effective, although transient, measure if cardiac toxicity is severe. The calcium does not change the concentration of potassium in the serum but acts directly on the heart. Elimination of potassium may be achieved by oral or rectal cation exchange resins.

Biochemical diagnosis of hereditary defect

If possible, a 24 hour urine specimen should be collected before cortisol therapy is instituted. In both 21- and 11β-hydroxylase deficiencies, 17-ketosteroids are excreted in increased amounts (3 to 40 mg per 24 hours) (Table 7–1). Both 11-oxy and 11-deoxy 17KS are elevated in the 21-hydroxylase defect, whereas only the 11-deoxy 17KS are elevated in the 11-hydroxylase defect. In addition, 11-oxy 17KS are depressed or absent in the 11-hydroxylase defect. It is important to remember that the excretion of 17KS in the normal newborn is elevated and does not usually fall below 1 mg/24 hours until after 1 week of age.

Specific steroids may be diagnostic of certain defects. In the 21-hydroxylase deficiency, the conversion of 17-hydroxyprogesterone to 11-deoxycortisol (Figure 7–4) is impaired. Large amounts of 17-hydrox-

TABLE 7–1. Biochemical Characteristics in Various Forms of Congenital Adrenal Hyperplasia

Enzyme Defect	Viril-ization	Salt Loss	17KS	DHA	17 OHCS	Pregnan-etriol	Aldo-sterone
Lipoid adrenal hyperplasia	0	yes	low	low	low	low	low
3β-hydroxy-steroid dehydrogenase	+	yes	high	high	low	normal or low	low
17α-hydroxylase	0	no	low	low	low	low	high
21-hydroxylase	+++	often	high		low	high	low in salt losers
11β-hydroxylase	+++	no	high		high	slightly high	low
18-hydroxylase	0	yes	normal		normal	normal	low

yprogesterone accumulate and are metabolized by the liver to pregnanetriol (3α,17α,20-trihydroxypregnane), pregnanetriolone (3α,16α,17α-trihydroxypregnane-20-one), and pregnanetetrol (3α,16α,17α,20-tetrahydroxypregnane). Normally, only a trace—or none—of these steroids is demonstrable in the urine of young infants. Pregnanetriol excretion is most often measured for diagnostic purposes. The metabolites that characterize the 21-hydroxylase deficiency may also be slightly elevated in the 11-hydroxylase deficiency. Characteristic metabolites in 3β-hydroxysteroid dehydrogenase deficiency are pregnenetriol (3β,17α,20-trihydroxy-Δ5-pregnene) and dehydroepiandrosterone.

If the defect in cortisol synthesis is compensated, the 17OHCS in the urine and plasma will be normal. However, this level of production allows for little if any adrenal reserve. As a result, stimulation of the adrenal with exogenous ACTH yields little or no rise in 17OHCS. It must be remembered, however, that 17OHCS measured by the Porter-Silber technique include 11-deoxycortisol (compound S) or its metabolites. Consequently, unexpectedly high values for Porter-Silber chromogens are found in infants with the 11-hydroxylase defect because of the accumulation of 11-deoxycortisol and its metabolites.

The 17-ketogenic steroids are usually a good measure of cortisol production, but again, anomalous results are obtained in the 21-hydroxylase deficiency. Pregnanetriol, which appears in excessive amounts, has a 17 and a 20 hydroxyl group and can be oxidized to a 17KS. Therefore the value for 17-ketogenic steroids is high in the presence of this steroid.

If available, techniques to measure individual steroids are always preferable to group analysis. For example, though patients with certain defects have high values of 17KS and evidence of virilization, it is not possible to say which, if any, of the steroids measured in the group assay is responsible for the virilization. Incidentally, it now appears that none of the 17KS is responsible for masculinization, except in so far as it is converted to testosterone. Significantly increased excretion and production rates for testosterone have been demonstrated. Much of this testosterone is derived from the peripheral conversion of androstenedione formed in the adrenal to testosterone. Estrogens are also produced in significantly increased amounts in congenital adrenal hyperplasia.

Specific assays for pregnanetriol are now used in many laboratories (instead of determining total 17KS) in testing for possible congenital adrenocortical hyperplasia due to a deficiency of 21-hydroxylase. This steroid theoretically should reflect the enzyme deficiency more exactly than the 17KS determination; however, in the first 2 weeks of life, pregnanetriol values may be normal in patients with 21-hydroxylase deficiency. In such patients, measurement of plasma 17-hydroxyprogesterone is helpful, since the concentration of this steroid is elevated even in early life.

An important aspect of the laboratory diagnosis is that therapy with glucocorticoids should decrease the ACTH secretion from the pituitary and return the pregnanetriol or 17KS values to normal. (Determining the effect of glucocorticoids on these values is in essence an ACTH suppression test.) If the excess steroids are produced by a tumor, administration of cortisone would not be so likely to influence the steroid level. Thus in a child with ambiguous genitalia—with or without signs of adrenal insufficiency—a 24 hour urine sample and/or a blood sample should be procured for the analysis of the 17KS, 17OHCS, and pregnanetriol. A buccal smear or karyotype should also be obtained to determine the genetic sex of the patient. If the 17KS and pregnanetriol values are elevated, and the 17OHCS values are normal or low, a tentative diagnosis of congenital adrenocortical hyperplasia should be made. If the patient is a boy with signs of adrenal insufficiency, the diagnosis is made more readily than if no adrenal insufficiency (salt loss) is present. Suppressive therapy with glucocorticoids should produce a fall in both 17KS and pregnanetriol.

If hypertension is present, 11-deoxycortisol should be measured in blood or urine. If this steroid is elevated, therapy with suppressive glucocorticoids should be started. Appropriate doses of glucocorticoids will return the steroid pattern in the blood or the urine of the patient to normal and reduce the blood pressure.

Experimental adrenogenital syndrome

Unfortunately, there are no spontaneous animal models of the adrenogenital syndrome; however, by the use of enzyme inhibitors, it has been possible to produce analogous situations in experimental animals. A synthetic inhibitor of 3β-hydroxysteroid dehydrogenase, 2α-cyano-4,4,17α-trimethyl-17β-hydroxyandrost-5-en-3-one (cyanoketone), has been used in rats to produce a counterpart to the adrenogenital syndrome found in humans. The adrenals are very large, and the clinical features of the adrenogenital syndrome are seen in newborn rats of mothers given the cyanoketone on either day fifteen or sixteen of gestation.

Another specific enzyme inhibitor, metyrapone, has been used to reproduce the 11β-hydroxylase deficiency of certain forms of adrenogenital syndrome. Pregnant rats given the drug on day fifteen or sixteen of gestation gave birth to pups displaying the clinical features of this syndrome.

THERAPY FOR CONGENITAL ADRENOCORTICAL HYPERPLASIA

GLUCOCORTICOIDS

In 1950, Wilkins demonstrated that the administration of cortisone to patients with congenital adrenal hyperplasia markedly reduced the urinary output of 17KS. Since that momentous discovery, the use of glucocorticoids to substitute for the relative enzyme deficiency of the adrenal has become standard practice. The choice of glucocorticoid is dictated by certain considerations. The steroid chosen for therapy should be an active glucocorticoid, ideally with a long half life and of such a nature as to cause little or no interference in the urinary assays for 17KS, 17OHCS, and pregnanetriol.

The corticosteroids have numerous and diversified physiological functions, including effects on (1) carbohydrate, fat, protein and purine metabolism, (2) electrolyte and water balance, and (3) functional capacities of the cardiovascular system, the kidney, lymphoid tissue, skeletal muscle, and the nervous system. Certain of these multiple biological actions of the corticosteroids lend themselves to quantitative measurement. Estimates of potencies of natural and synthetic corticosteroids usually fall into one of three categories: (1) sodium retention (reduction of sodium excretion by the kidney of the adrenalectomized animal), (2) deposition of liver glycogen, and (3) anti-inflammatory effect (inhibition of the action of an agent that induces inflammation). Calculations of potencies that are based on the ability of the steroids to maintain an adrenalectomized animal in a state of well-being closely parallel calculations of potencies that are based on the ability of the steroids to induce sodium retention. Evaluations of corticoid activity based on liver glycogen deposition, anti-inflammatory effect, work capacity of skeletal muscle, and involution of lymphoid tissue closely parallel one another. However, clear-cut dissociations exist between the sodium retentive activities (mineralocorticoids) and the liver glycogen deposition (glucocorticoids). For example, deoxycorticosterone is highly potent in sodium retention but practically without effect on liver glycogen deposition. Cortisol is powerful in stimulating liver glycogen deposition, but only a weak stimulus to sodium retention. Corticosterone has activities in both categories.

Changes in the molecular structure of the steroid nucleus may cause changes in biological activity. Such changes may be the result of altered absorption, protein binding, rate of metabolic transformation, rate of excretion, or effectiveness at the target site. Certain structural features such as the 4,5 double bond and the 3-ketone are absolutely necessary for glucocorticoid activity. The reduction of the 3-ketone of cortisol and the saturation of the 4,5 double bond produce tetrahydrocortisol, which lacks glucocorticoid activity. Introduction of a 1,2 double bond, as in prednisone (Δ1-cortisone) or prednisolone (Δ1-cortisol), results in a fourfold enhancement (approximately) of glucocorticoid activity over that of cortisol. Prednisolone has the added advantage of a longer biological half life (200 min) than that of cortisol (80 minutes).

A further modification of prednisolone, 6α-methylation, causes slightly greater biological potency than that of the parent compound. Another maneuver which enhances glucocorticoid anti-inflammatory activity is fluorination in the 9α position, producing 9α-fluorocortisol. As a result of 9α fluorination, there is a tenfold enhancement of glucocorticoid activity over that of cortisol, and mineralocorticoid activity becomes 125 times greater than that of cortisol. Thus for all intents and purposes 9α-fluorocortisol is a powerful mineralocorticoid.

An oxygen function at carbon 11 is indispensable for glucocorticoid activity. Compound S, 11-deoxycortisol, has essentially no activity. Oxidation of 11β-hydroxy compounds to 11-keto compounds results in significant loss of activity. Indeed, it has been suggested that any activity that exists in 11-keto compounds is dependent upon metabolic transformation to the 11-hydroxy compound. Thus cortisone is a weaker glucocorticoid than is cortisol; however, it is readily convertible to the more powerful steroid.

Methylation or hydroxylation at carbon 16 reduces the mineralocorticoid activity while maintaining or enhancing glucocorticoid activity. Examples of compounds with such activities are triamcinolone (9α-fluoro-16α-hydroxyprednisolone), betamethasone (9α-fluoro-16β-methylprednisolone), and dexamethasone (9α-fluoro-16α-methyl-prednisolone). These compounds or their metabolites do not react with dinitrobenzene (Zimmermann reaction) and thus do not alter the value for 17KS. In contrast, the metabolites of cortisol, cortisone, prednisolone, and prednisone do increase the estimated urinary 17KS.

We know very little about the specific actions of the synthetic glucocorticoids in the target cells. Presumably, their actions are similar to those of cortisol. Perhaps it is appropriate at this point to review our present knowledge of the mechanism of action of cortisol. As seems to be the case with all hormones, specific receptors exist either on or just within the target cell (see Figure 5–1). The cortisol receptor binds the hormone and concentrates it within the nucleus of the cell. Here cortisol acts to alter the genetic material in such a way that specific RNA is formed. This RNA (including messenger RNA) enhances the synthesis of specific proteins.

The overall effects of cortisol are almost the opposite of those of insulin. In response to cortisol, amino acids are mobilized from peripheral tissues and utilized in the accelerated gluconeogenesis of the liver. Peripheral utilization of glucose is suppressed. Indeed, it has been claimed that uptake of glucose by thymus cells is suppressed within about 20 minutes of cortisol administration. In addition, nucleic acid synthesis in thymus cells is decreased. We don't know how these effects of cortisol on thymus cells relate to the known anti-inflammatory influence of this steroid. Glucose utilization in muscle and adipose tissue is also decreased following cortisol treatment.

The liver exhibits a variety of effects after cortisol administration. In order of occurrence in vivo, there are increases in uptake of amino acids, synthesis of RNA (2 to 4 hours), glucose production (2 to 6 hours), urea production (4 to 8 hours), and protein synthesis (8 to 20 hours). The synthesis of specific enzymes (glucose-6-phosphatase, fructose-1,6-diphosphatase) which are rate-limiting for gluconeogenesis is enhanced by cortisol.

The stimulation of hepatic deposition of glycogen by glucocorticosteroids has been extensively studied. When adrenalectomized rats are deprived of food, a rapid depletion of liver glycogen occurs. Treatment of adrenalectomized rats with glucocorticoids leads to rapid and extensive deposition of glycogen in the liver. It was not until the discovery of hepatic glycogen synthetase that the regulation of glycogen synthesis could be studied in detail. This enzyme catalyzes the transfer of glucosyl units from UDPG to glycogen. The enzyme exists in glucose-6-phosphate dependent (D) and independent (I) forms. In adrenalectomized rats, the enzyme is almost entirely in the D form. In starved intact rats given cortisol, the enzyme is almost entirely in the I form. The interconversion of the I and D forms is critical for control of glycogen synthesis and it is at this site that several hormones act. Glucocorticoids apparently activate a phosphorylase phosphatase which dephosphorylates glycogen synthetase to yield the I (active) form. Glucagon, epinephrine, or cyclic AMP can reverse this glucocorticoid effect.

In spite of the enhanced protein synthesis produced by cortisol in the liver, this hormone in general has a catabolic effect in most tissues. In Cushing's syndrome, in which excessive quantities of cortisol are synthesized by the adrenal and circulate in the blood, muscle wasting occurs along with a loss of protein from skin and bones, leading to osteoporosis and thinning of the skin.

From the preceding discussion it is clear that excessive corticoid therapy in adrenocortical hyperplasia may produce catabolic effects. Such effects in the immature individual would impair normal growth. Thus the use of glucocorticoid therapy for this disorder must be accompanied by close supervision of urinary steroid excretion, linear growth, and bone maturation.

MINERALOCORTICOIDS

Only two mineralocorticoids are now used for therapy of salt-losing adrenocortical hyperplasia. Deoxycorticosterone acetate is devoid of glucocorticoid activity. Its major disadvantage is that it is not absorbed well by the gastrointestinal tract and must therefore be given as an injection or be implanted subcutaneously. The most potent synthetic mineralocorticoid, 9α-fluorocortisol acetate, also has high glucocorticoid activity. It can be administered orally and is usually given in a dose of 0.05 to 0.1 mg per day.

The natural mineralocorticoid in the normal individual is aldosterone, and it exerts profound effects on sodium transport. The mechanism of action of this hormone has been studied in the toad bladder, a tissue which is exquisitely sensitive to aldosterone. Tritium-labeled aldosterone is preferentially localized in the nuclear and perinuclear areas of the cells of the toad bladder. Once taken up by the target cell, the hormone is bound to a nuclear aldosterone-binding protein. The activated complex (aldosterone-nuclear receptor complex) acts upon the genetic machinery of the cell to bring about the synthesis of aldosterone-specific messenger RNA. This messenger RNA codes for the synthesis of specific proteins (aldosterone-induced proteins) which are located on the plasma membrane and act to increase the rate of transepithelial sodium transport. The one- or two-hour latent period in the renal and extrarenal effects on sodium transport represents the time required to synthesize the aldosterone-induced proteins. At the same time that renal reabsorption of sodium is enhanced, the excretion of potassium, magnesium, and hydrogen ion in the distal convoluted tubule is increased by aldosterone. As early as 1927, Baumann and Kurland noted that adrenalectomy in the cat lowered the concentrations of sodium and chloride and increased the concentrations of potassium and magnesium in the plasma. In turn, the lowered concentration of sodium in the plasma acts to increase the secretion of aldosterone by the adrenal cortex. Other factors involved in the control of aldosterone synthesis are discussed in Chapter Nine.

The prompt use of mineralocorticoids is particularly critical in the infant manifesting signs of salt loss. Immediate measures, such as addition of salt to the formula, or intravenous saline if the infant is vomiting, should be instituted, while a 24 hour urine sample is collected for analysis of steroid metabolites. The elevation of certain steroids and the state of the external genitalia permit the diagnosis of a specific enzyme defect. If adrenal steroids in general are low, and the external genitalia are normal, adrenal hypoplasia (or insufficiency) should be considered. In any case, therapy with salt and mineralocorticoids is mandatory. Glucocorticoid therapy is necessary if there is a defect in cortisol synthesis. During the acute phase of salt loss, one or two milligrams of deoxycorticosterone acetate can be given intramuscularly each day. After the electrolytes have returned to normal, the child can be maintained on oral sodium chloride, one to four grams daily in four to six divided doses. Oral 9α-

fluorocortisol acetate (0.025mg two or three times daily) can be used in place of intramuscular deoxycorticosterone acetate when vomiting is controlled. By the time some patients are 6 to 9 months of age, therapy with salt and cortisol is sufficient to control the disease. Implanting one or two pellets (75 mg) of deoxycorticosterone acetate subcutaneously in the young infant will provide salt retaining activity for four to six months. A second pellet may be inserted at that time if needed. Those children requiring mineralocorticoid therapy after the first or second year of life can be given 9α-fluorocortisol acetate orally (0.1 mg per day).

It has become increasingly clear in recent years that proper treatment of congenital adrenocortical hyperplasia must take into consideration the diurinal variation in secretion of ACTH from the anterior pituitary. Studies of the concentration of 17-hydroxyprogesterone in plasma from patients with congenital adrenal hyperplasia indicate that the main suppressive dose of steroids is required to cover the period from 3:00 a.m. to 3:00 p.m. Hamilton and Moodie (1970) have suggested that these patients should be given steroids in the late evening to suppress the early morning secretion of ACTH. Indeed, late night therapy in these patients may permit the use of smaller doses of steroid. The usual procedure is to give one half the daily dose in the late evening (waking the child when the parent retires); the remainder of the steroid is divided between a morning and afternoon dose. A rough guide is to administer 10 to 30 mg cortisone acetate daily for age 0 to 5 years, 25 to 50 mg for age 5 to 10 years, and about 50 mg for children over 10 years of age. During the growing years, the dose of glucocorticoids must be carefully titrated to produce normal linear growth with no advancement of virilization or bone age. The maintenance of normal serum electrolyte values is the best guide to the adequacy of mineralocorticoid replacement. Continued absence of hypertension in the 11-hydroxylase deficient state is a favorable sign. It must be remembered, however, that continuing hypertension and high serum sodium concentrations indicate inadequacy of *glucocorticoid* replacement in the 17α-hydroxylase and 11β-hydroxylase deficiency states.

Surgical correction of the female perineum

By a combination of intravenous pyelography and retrograde instillation of radiopaque material into the vagina it should be possible to ascertain the presence or absence of a lower vagina and the relationship of the urethral meatus to the urogenital sinus. The aim of surgery is to establish an adequate communication between the exterior and the uterine cervix via the vagina. If the lower segment of the vagina is absent, the creation of an artificial vagina should be considered.

The degree of clitoral enlargement varies considerably. With very minor degrees of enlargement, no surgical correction is necessary. Adequate glucocorticoid therapy will prevent further enlargement, and with continued body growth the enlargement will become less and less conspicuous. In most cases, however, clitoral reduction is necessary.

ENZYME-BLOCKING DRUGS IN TREATMENT

The virilization and rapidity of bone maturation which can occur under the influence of inadequately suppressed androgens has suggested to some investigators the possibility of using antiandrogens as therapy. One such antiandrogen, cyproterone acetate (6-chloro-6-dehydro-17α-acetoxy-1,2α-methylene progesterone), is also a potent progestational agent (1000 times as active as progesterone). Given to the pregnant rat (1 to 10 mg daily), this steroid led to feminization of the male fetuses. In these fetuses the penis was underdeveloped and resembled a clitoris, the prostate was missing, and the testes were small and undescended. This steroid is the most active antiandrogen so far encountered; however, trials of cyproterone acetate in the treatment of congenital adrenal hyperplasia have not been particularly successful.

Another drug of possible use in congenital adrenocortical hyperplasia is aminoglutethimide. Its structure is very similar to the hypnotic drug glutethimide. The decreased urinary 17OHCS brought about by the use of aminoglutethimide suggested to Hamilton that although the drug was originally used as an anticonvulsant, it might be used in congenital adrenocortical hyperplasia. In animal experiments, aminoglutethimide has been shown to block the conversion of cholesterol to pregnenolone. Studies using beef adrenal slices and monolayer cultures of functional adrenal tumor cells suggest that this drug inhibits the 20α-hydroxylation of cholesterol. In higher concentrations, it is a competitive inhibitor of 11β-hydroxylation.

In the human, the drug would essentially destroy the ability of the adrenal cortex to form hormones, and by the appropriate use of substitution therapy, the dangers of excessive androgens could be avoided in children with congenital adrenocortical hyperplasia. The initial results of a regimen of aminoglutethimide (30 mg/kg/day in three divided doses) plus one to two mg prednisolone daily were favorable. It must be emphasized, however, that the use of aminoglutethimide for this disorder is still very much in the experimental stage. It has been reported that long term treatment (six years) may cause ovarian dysfunction and virilization in young women.

THE INHERITANCE OF ADRENOCORTICAL HYPERPLASIA

The exact genetic basis for these inherited defects of cortisol synthesis is unknown; however, the nature of the inheritance of the defects suggests that each is due to an autosomal recessive. The gene frequency of the disorder varies in different parts of the world, being relatively high in Alaska (the figure for natives is 0.026) and in Switzerland (0.014) and low in the United States (0.004). The sex incidence is equal. Apparently, the same gene controls the synthesis of the enzyme in both gonad and adrenal.

PSYCHOLOGICAL ASPECTS OF CONGENITAL ADRENOCORTICAL HYPERPLASIA

Male sexual differentiation of the brain in mammals is dependent upon the presence of androgens. The critical period for this differentiation seems to vary from species to species. Studies in rodents suggest that the absence of androgens at certain crucial periods of neural differentiation may lead to behavioral and physiological feminization. Male rats castrated at birth, when several structures of the central nervous system are still immature, display feminine mating behavior as adults. Small doses of androgens given to such animals during the critical first week after birth have been found to be capable of partially restoring some degree of masculine type of behavior.

Apparently, prenatal androgenization in the human, as would occur in certain forms of congenital adrenocortical hyperplasia, has limited effects on the child. Money has found that certain predominantly masculine types of behavior may occur more often in patients with adrenocortical hyperplasia than in normal individuals; however, the difficulties of eliminating environmental influences in such studies are obvious. This area of investigation—sexual maturation of the brain—has proved fruitful in rodents and may provide a better understanding of behaviorial aberrations in man.

SUMMARY

Inborn errors of metabolism frequently manifest themselves in the early neonatal period. Those encountered most often in the field of hormone metabolism are disorders in the synthesis of thyroid hormone (Chapters Five and Eleven) and steroid hormones. The first clue to an inborn error in cortisol synthesis is usually the presence of abnormal external genitalia at birth. Other causes of anomalies in sexual differentiation (Chapter Eight) must be considered; however, congenital adrenocortical hyperplasia is one of the most frequently encountered. All individuals with congenital adrenocortical hyperplasia should be considered potential salt losers until proved otherwise. With present laboratory techniques, it should be possible to make an accurate diagnosis so that appropriate therapy can be instituted. Avoidance of salt-losing crises and the suppression of pituitary ACTH secretion are the immediate goals. If ACTH is suppressed, linear growth and bone maturation can be maintained within the normal range. If ACTH is secreted in excessive amounts, the adrenal produces proportionally more androgens, which can cause further virilization and more rapid bone maturation. Excessive glucocorticoid therapy causes a depression in the rate of linear growth. Thus the suppression of ACTH must be carefully maintained at all times within the appropriate limits.

Long range goals of therapy include surgical repair of the external genitalia where indicated. As the need for more glucocorticoids occurs (under conditions of stress), the patient should be aware of changes in the dose of steroids which will be required. As a general rule, patients with the salt-losing form of adrenocortical hyperplasia who are febrile and have an infection should double the dose of glucocorticoid. Preparations of cortisone acetate and deoxycorticosterone for intramuscular injection with sterile syringes should be available in the home. The patient should wear an identification bracelet with information regarding his disease. A cautious, continuous surveillance by the physician can permit children with congenital adrenocortical hyperplasia to grow normally, mature, and lead normal reproductive lives.

SUGGESTED READING

Congenital adrenal hyperplasia, Rolf P. Zurbrugg, in *Endocrine and Genetic Diseases of Childhood,* edited by Lytt E. Gardner, Philadelphia, W. B. Saunders Co., 1969.

A comprehensive review of the pathophysiology, diagnosis, and therapy of the inborn errors of cortisol synthesis. A preceding chapter by Lytt Gardner discusses the normal fetal and neonatal adrenal.

Diseases of the Adrenal Cortex, edited by A. Stuart Mason, Clinics in Endocrinology and Metabolism, Philadelphia, W. B. Saunders, July, 1972.

Chapters on the chemistry of steroids and the morphology of the adrenal cortex precede discussions of various disease states. Included is an excellent chapter by William Hamilton on congenital adrenal hyperplasia.

CHAPTER EIGHT

Ambiguous Genitalia in the Newborn: Abnormalities of Sexual Differentiation

One of the first questions asked of the physician attending a delivery is in regard to the sex of the infant. Our concepts of "boy" and "girl" are established early in life and depend primarily upon psychosocial aspects of sex. The reversal of sex later in life is a highly traumatic procedure in almost all cases. Once an infant has been called "male" or "female," it adopts that psychosocial sex, irrespective of his or her genetic or endocrinologic sex. Specific attitudes of society come into play, and the child learns from these attitudes what he or she "is." Before 18 to 24 months of age, the psychosexual assignment is not absolutely fixed and a change in sex assignment, when indicated, can be accomplished with less trauma than later in life.

Upon what do we base this assignment of sex? Although the phenotypic expression of sex (in large measure the appearance of the external genitalia) determines the subsequent sexual role of the individual, this criterion is not completely infallible. For example, the female with congenital adrenocortical hyperplasia may be born with an enlarged clitoris that has the appearance of a hypospadiac penis. A casual glance might suggest that the patient is a boy with cryptorchidism. It is important to remember that the phenotypic expression of sex depends upon a variety of factors, including karyotype (genetic sex), gonadal development (gonadal sex), and endocrine function of the gonads (endocrinologic sex).

If development proceeds normally during intra-uterine life, the newborn infant will possess external genitalia characteristic of his or her genotype. In general, this means that an individual with a 46/XY karyotype (chromosomal complement) will have external genitalia consisting of penis and scrotal sacs containing testes. This male differentiation of the genitalia, as we have learned, is dependent upon the presence of biologically active androgens during fetal life. In the absence of androgens, the individual develops as a phenotypic female, irrespective of the karyotype. In the presence of androgens, the genetic female (46/XX) undergoes virilization; the extent of the virilization depends upon the time of elaboration and the biological activity of the androgen. These androgens may be produced by the fetal adrenals or the fetal gonads, or they may originate in the mother.

The definitive sex of rearing must be determined as rapidly as possible. This is accomplished by a careful history, physical examination, and laboratory studies. The latter should include analysis of urinary excretion of 17KS and/or pregnanetriol, analysis of the sex chromatin pattern, and determination of karyotype.

PHYSICAL EXAMINATION OF THE NEWBORN GENITALIA

The examination of the external genitalia of the newborn should be systematic and complete. The penis of the normal male newborn varies in size; however, there should be no real confusion with the virilized clitoris. The phallus of the masculinized female tends to be smaller than the male penis and in addition may be bound ventrally by fibrous bands in a condition known as *chordee.* In this condition, the phallus is contracted ventrally and bowed.

Depending on the extent of masculinization in utero, the urethral meatus may be at the tip of the penile shaft (as in the normal male) or at any point down the shaft to the perineum (as in the virilized female or incompletely masculinized male). The position of the urethral opening at birth can perhaps be best understood by considering the embryologic sequences involved. The genital tubercle elongates and is called a *phallus.* A *urethral groove* forms on the ventral surface of the phallus and is continuous with the urogenital opening. Under the influence of androgens, the phallus elongates to form a penis, pulling the urogenital folds forward. These folds form the lateral walls of the urethral groove, and as they fuse progressively from the perineum to the tip of the glans, the outlet of the urethra is moved along the shaft of the penis to the tip of the glans. If the urethra of the glans penis fails to become canalized, or if the urethral folds fail to fuse, *hypospadias* will result. In essence, hypospadias represents an arrested state of embryonic development. Cessation of production of androgens by the fetal testis or an inadequate supply of androgens during the progressive fusion of the urethral folds could result in hypospadias in the male. In turn, exposure of the female to androgens in utero at the time of development of the penile urethra could produce an apparent hypospadias.

During the third month of gestation a fold of skin at the base of the glans penis begins to grow toward the tip of the glans. This tubular prepuce, or *foreskin*, surrounds the glans by 5 months. For some time, the foreskin is fused to the glans and is usually not retractable at birth. The fused surfaces normally separate during infancy. The corpora cavernosa penis and the corpus cavernosum urethrae (corpus spongiosum) arise from the mesenchymal tissue in the phallus.

Like the fusion of the urogenital folds, the midline approximation of the genital swellings to form the scrotal sacs is a continuous process and may proceed normally (as in the fully virilized male) or be arrested at various stages of fusion. The degree of fusion usually parallels the closure of the urethral folds. Thus the virilized female may display a complete spectrum, from fused labia and an apparent hypospadias to partial fusion with a single opening into the urogenital sinus to minimal fusion and separate urethral and vaginal orifices.

Descent of the testis into the scrotum is abnormal in most intersexes; however, apparent bilateral cryptorchidism in intersexes may reflect bilaterally deficient testes or the absence of any testicular tissue. The presence of a palpable gonad in the scrotum is extremely helpful in diagnosis, since an ovary is almost never found there.

After careful examination of the external genitalia, a rectal examination should be performed. The uterus at birth is larger than it will be in subsequent weeks and may be palpable. In the presence of bilateral cryptorchidism, a determined effort should be made to ascertain whether or not a uterus is present.

CYTOGENETICS

In preparation for the process of cell division, each chromosome makes an exact copy of itself. During the relatively short period of division, the chromosomes contract and become thicker and shorter. They are dense enough to be seen in the light microscope. In order to observe the chromosomes "in action," cells are grown in culture. The most commonly used cells are white blood cells. After separation from the red cells by centrifugation, the white cells are placed in an antibiotic-enriched medium and are incubated for three days. After about 60 hours at 37°C, there is a burst of mitotic activity. Mitosis can be arrested in metaphase by treating the cells with colchicine. This drug apparently acts by interfering with the formation of the mitotic spindle. The cells thus arrested are exposed briefly to a hypotonic solution which causes

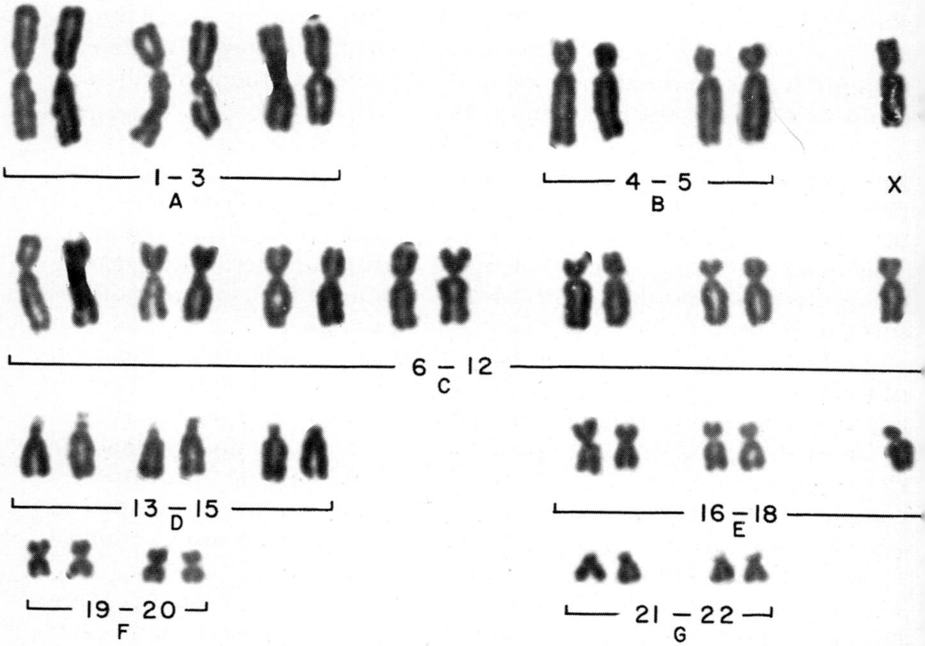

FIGURE 8–1. The karyotype of a normal male. The numbers represent the Denver classification; the letters show the terminology of Patau. The main characteristics of the groups are:

A (1–3): The largest chromosomes, distinct from each other as well as from the other groups; 1 and 3 have median centromeres, and 2 has a submedian centromere.

B (4–5): Large chromosomes with submedian centromeres.

C (6–12 plus X): Medium-sized chromosomes with submedian centromeres; 6 is often distinctly larger than 7–12, and some cytogeneticists therefore group 6 and X separately.

D (13–15): Medium-sized chromosomes with subterminal centromeres. Often called the large acrocentric chromosomes to contrast with 21–22, the short acrocentrics. All members of this group may bear satellites, well seen in the first pair here.

E (16–18): Medium-short chromosomes with median (16 or submedian (17–18) centromeres.

F (19–20): Short chromosomes with median centromeres.

G (21–22): Short, acrocentric chromosomes. All may bear satellites.

X: A medium-sized chromosome with submedian centromere.

Y: A short acrocentric chromosome. The Y is distinguished from 21–22 by several features: it never has satellites; its long arms are close to parallel; it often stains either more or less deeply than the other short acrocentrics. Its length also varies in different persons. (From Federman, D. *Abnormal Sexual Development.* Philadelphia: W. B. Saunders Company, 1967, p. 9.)

them to swell. The individual chromosomes are spread out. The cells can now be fixed and stained for microscopic analysis. A photograph is taken of a typical metaphase plate, the photograph is enlarged, and the individual chromosomes are cut out and placed in sequence according to a standard classification (the Denver system, shown in Figure 8–1). A careful study of the chromosomal complement of the cells from various tissues of the body helps assess the genetic sex of the patient.

Sex chromatin

The analysis of sex chromatin is particularly important in diagnosing intersexes, for it provides a rapid means of classification of patients by genetic sex (Figure 8–2). The chromatin positive intersex patient may be either a *true hermaphrodite* (an individual with both an ovary and a testis, or with one or two ovotestes) or a *female pseudohermaphrodite* (an individual with ovaries plus variable degree of ambisexual development). The latter is almost always a patient with congenital adrenocortical hyperplasia (see Chapter Seven).

The chromatin negative intersex patient may be either a true hermaphrodite, a *male pseudohermaphrodite* (an individual with testes plus ambiguous genitalia), or a patient with *gonadal dysgenesis* (failure of the gonads to function normally).

Intermediate sex chromatin counts may suggest a mixture of male and female cells or a mixture of XO and female cells. If an individual is derived from a single fertilized egg, and if genetic changes during somatic cell division establish two or more distinct lines of cells within the body, the individual is said to be a *mosaic.* Among the types of mosaics possible are those with a mixture of male and female cells. The kinds of genetic alterations which can occur to produce mosaics include nondisjunction, anaphase lag, or both.

In the process of mitosis, chromosomes which had replicated during interphase form a spindle *(prophase),* line up on the equatorial plate *(metaphase),* and then separate *(anaphase).* If one of the X chromosomes of an XX individual moves too slowly (anaphase lag) and fails to be incorporated in the chromosome complement of one of the daughter nuclei, that chromosome is lost. Subsequent divisions of that cell line (hypoploid, 45) will have only one X, whereas the other, euploid (46) cell line

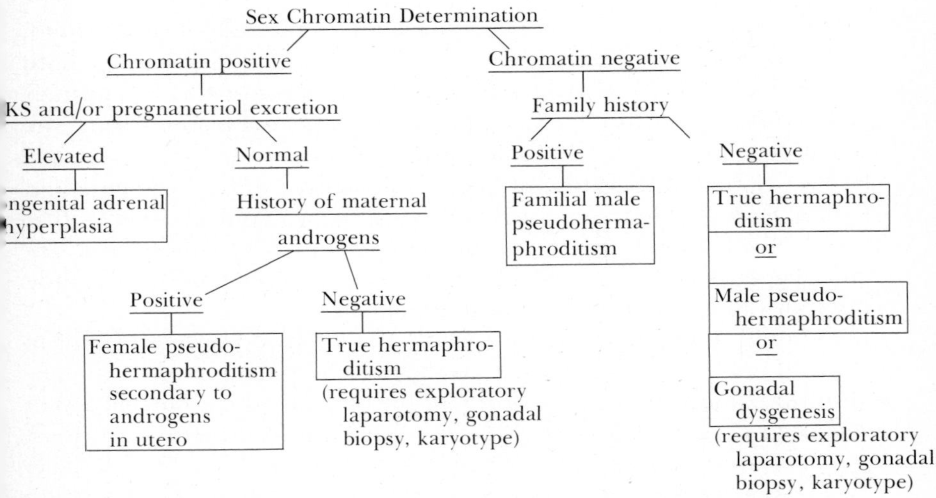

FIGURE 8–2. Differential diagnosis of infants with ambiguous external genitalia.

will have two X's. Such abnormal mitosis can occur at any time, and the individual is an XO/XX mosaic.

If one pair of X chromosomes fails to separate at anaphase (nondisjunction), both X's will be incorporated into one daughter nucleus, whereas the other will receive neither X. If the other pair of X chromosomes separates normally, one cell line will have a 47/XXX chromosomal complement, the other 45/X. Combinations of nondisjunction and anaphase lag may occur and yield a variety of mosaics.

If anaphase lag or nondisjunction occurs during meiosis, the germ cell may be hypoploid (22), or, with nondisjunction, hyperploid (24/XX, 24/YY) (Figure 8–3). Assuming that such gametes are viable and are fertilized by normal gametes with 23 chromosomes, zygotes with 45 or 47 chromosomes will be formed. For example, Klinefelter's syndrome (47/XXY) probably results from the fertilization of an egg with 24 chromosomes (24/XX) by a sperm with 23 chromosomes (23/Y) or from the union of a 23/X egg with a 24/XY sperm. Mosaics also can occur in Klinefelter's syndrome as a result of anaphase lag or nondisjunction during mitosis (Figure 8–3).

Since the sex chromatin seen in squash preparations of cells represents supernumerary X chromosomes, the mosaics just described will have some chromatin positive cells (XX, XXX) and some chromatin negative cells (XO). Chimeras produced by double fertilization of a binucleate egg—that is, XX/XY individuals—would also show a mixture of chromatin positive and chromatin negative cells. A definitive analysis of the chromosomal complement (karyotype) should always be made in those patients with ambiguous genitalia who are clearly diagnosed as not having congenital adrenocortical hyperplasia.

TRUE HERMAPHRODITISM

One might expect, from a consideration of the role of sex chromosomes in gonadal differentiation, that individuals possessing both ovarian and testicular tissues would have both XX and XY cells in their gonads. Such mosaicism has been described in several patients with true hermaphroditism and it has been postulated that this may occur as a result of double fertilization of either a binucleate egg or an ovum and its polar body. By definition, such an individual would be a *chimera*—that is, an individual with more than one cell line, each of which has a different genetic origin. Often the term mosaicism is used loosely to include conditions more accurately termed chimerism.

Though there have been cases of XX/XY true hermaphroditism, about 80 percent of true hermaphrodites are chromatin positive on buccal smear examination; the majority of the patients whose chromosomes have been studied had a 46/XX karyotype. Thus the karyotype of most true hermaphrodites is indistinguishable from that of a normal female. Does this mean that a Y chromosome is not necessary for the formation

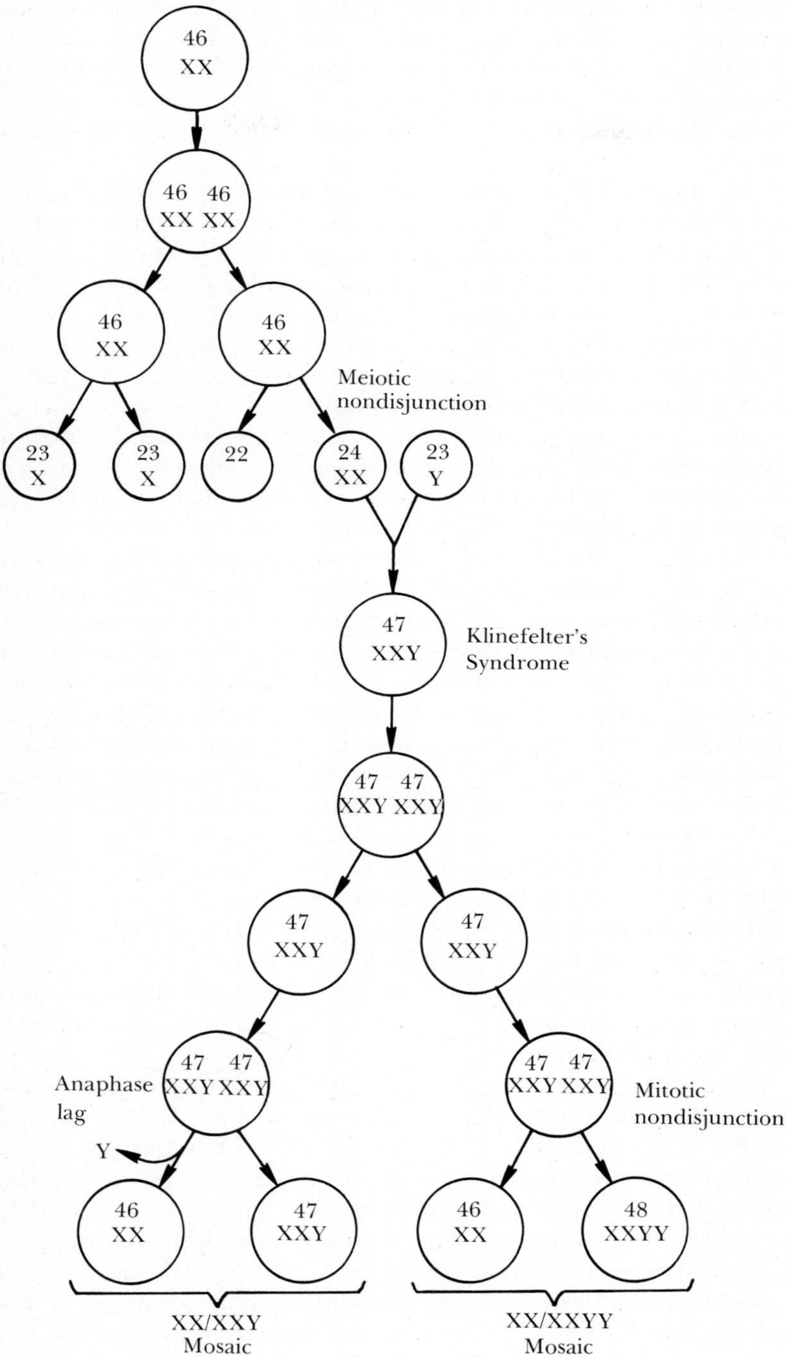

FIGURE 8–3. Normal and abnormal meiosis and mitosis.

of a testis? One can always suggest that these individuals are mosaics and that culturing of many tissues might reveal XY cells. Another possibility is that the portion of the Y chromosome needed to induce testicular development could have undergone translocation to an X chromosome. Such an X chromosome would be designated X^Y and the karyotype $46/XX^Y$.

The internal and external sexual differentiation in the true hermaphrodite varies widely from almost normal female to male with some degree of hypospadias. Most true hermaphrodites (some 76 percent) are reared as males after surgical correction of the hypospadias. Such individuals frequently show breast development at puberty and many menstruate or show evidence of cyclic hematuria. The structure of the internal ducts reflects the type of gonad present. The side with a testis will usually show a vas deferens and epididymis, whereas the ovarian side will show a uterus and a fallopian tube. Most patients with an ovotestis have predominantly female development of the genital ducts. In all cases of true hermaphroditism, the ovarian tissue contains large numbers of primordial germ cells or developing oocytes. Ovulation has been demonstrated in over 25 percent, but spermatogenesis in testicular tissue is extremely rare. None of these patients has ever begotten a child.

Unfortunately, most hermaphrodites are not diagnosed at birth. The typical case history is that of an infant born with perineal hypospadias, a bifid scrotum, and unilateral cryptorchidism. The hypospadias is surgically corrected and the child, reared as a boy, is not seen until puberty, when breast development occurs in 80 percent of patients. The growth of axillary and pubic hair is normal, with a female escutcheon. Facial hair is usually absent. Urinary estrogens and androgens are within the normal range; gonadotropins are not increased. The sex chromatin is usually positive, and surgical exploration reveals that the "undescended testicle" is an ovary or ovotestis. A uterus is present in virtually all patients and the vagina varies from very small to normal in size. Only a few of the true hermaphrodites are reared as girls. The external genitalia may show hypertrophy of the clitoris and slight labioscrotal fusion. A gonad may be palpable in one of the labial folds, and inguinal hernia is not uncommon.

A variety of sex chromosome mosaicisms associated with true hermaphroditism have been described. Among these are XX/XY, XX/XXY, XX/XXYY, XX/XXY/XXYY, XO/XY, and XX/XY/XXY. The XX/XXY mosaicism may arise by loss of a Y chromosome at an early cleavage division of an XXY zygote, whereas the XX/XXYY and XX/XXY/XXYY patterns could be a consequence of mitotic nondisjunction in an XXY zygote (Figure 8–3). A more likely cause of XX/XY mosaicism is chimerism. How does one prove chimerism? A readily available method is to test for specific blood group antigens among the population of red cells from a single individual. An XX/XY true hermaphrodite tested at 2½ years of age was found to have two populations of red cells with multiple differences in blood group antigens. The father was heterozygous at two loci, MNS_S and Rh, and contributed both alleles to the patient.

The mother was homozygous at these loci and of course contributed the same alleles to both populations of red cells in the patient. These facts suggest that the patient was the result of the fertilization of a binucleate egg by two sperm, one Y-bearing and one X-bearing. Segregation of the haptoglobin phenotype in an XX/XY true hermaphrodite has been studied by Josso, and a similar interpretation of the results was reached.

The chromosomal pattern has little bearing on the definitive sex of rearing in this disorder. The earlier a sex role can be assigned, the better. In this regard, careful consideration of the extent of masculinization of the external genitalia is important. It is comparatively simple to remove a hypertrophied clitoris and to separate the labioscrotal folds. If the hypospadias can be successfully corrected surgically, then a male role is possible. At puberty those patients reared as boys should have breasts, uterus, and ovarian tissue removed. The hermaphrodites reared as females should receive estrogen therapy at puberty and all testicular tissue should be removed.

FEMALE PSEUDOHERMAPHRODITISM

Congenital adrenocortical hyperplasia

Any female fetus exposed to androgens may undergo virilization in utero and be born with ambiguous genitalia. The masculinization involves only the external genitalia; internal duct structure is that of a normal female. By far the most frequently encountered form of female pseudohermaphroditism is that due to congenital adrenocortical hyperplasia secondary to an inherited lack of the 21-hydroxylase (p. 159). Patients with this form of female pseudohermaphroditism are genetically female and chromatin positive. The virilization results from the excessive production of androgens in the hyperplastic adrenals. Ordinarily, the enzymes involved in cortisol synthesis develop in the human fetal adrenal at about 8 to 10 weeks gestation. At this time the sexual differentiation of the genital ducts is under way. Differentiation of the external genitalia occurs later. The genital tubercle begins to elongate in the eleventh week under the influence of androgens. If the female fetus fails to develop one of the enzymes necessary for the synthesis of cortisol, there will be less glucocorticoid to suppress ACTH secretion by the fetal pituitary, and the fetal adrenal cortex will be subjected to stimulation by high levels of ACTH.* Precursors of the glucocorticoids, among which are adrenal androgens, will then be released from the adrenal. At this time the internal ducts have already developed normally in these females; however, the external genitalia undergo varying degrees of masculinization. Once normally developed, the internal ducts are no longer altered by androgens.

*Glucocorticoid will not be entirely absent, because some comes from the mother.

Patients with adrenocortical hyperplasia can be treated with cortisol, preventing further masculinization. Any surgical alterations of the external genitalia that are required should be performed at as early an age as possible (after age 4 months).

Maternal androgens

Virilization of the female fetus may also result from exposure to androgens of maternal origin. Tumors of the maternal ovary have caused virilization in the fetus in two documented cases. More commonly, virilization of the fetus may result from the administration of androgenic steroid hormones to the mother during pregnancy.

Very rarely is testosterone itself given to the mother. Most of the inciting agents have been progestins which subsequently were found to have androgenic effects. Progesterone itself is not active when administered orally, and a variety of orally effective progestins have been synthesized. The first progestin that was reasonably effective when given orally was 17α-ethinyl testosterone (ethisterone). This compound, discovered in 1938, was used for over 20 years until more powerful progestins were discovered. The 19-nortestosterone compounds (lacking the angular methyl group at carbon 10) were found to be very effective orally after insertion of a methyl or ethyl group in the 17α position (forming 17α-ethyl-19-nortestosterone, or norethandrolone). Unfortunately, all of these agents have androgenic properties. When used in cases of threatened abortion, the danger of masculinizing the female fetus must be considered. The 17α-ethinyl derivative of 19-nortestosterone (norethindrone) is a potent oral progestin with only mild androgenic properties. More recently, it has been possible to obtain powerful progestational agents free of androgenic effects (ethinylestrenol).

Wilkins (1958) reported 15 female infants with varying degrees of virilization whose mothers had been given 17α-ethinyl testosterone before the tenth week of gestation. In another study of 53 female infants born to mothers treated with this drug, 17 were partially masculinized. Occasionally, infants have been reported to be masculinized by progesterone or stilbestrol administered to the mother. Other steroids which have been implicated in masculinization of the female fetus are testosterone, 17-methyl testosterone, 17α-ethyl-19-nortestosterone, 17α-ethinyl-19-nortestosterone, and 17-methyl androstenediol.

In all cases reported, internal duct structure was female and only the external genitalia were masculinized. Androgens alone are not sufficient to induce development of Wolffian duct structures; another substance must be secreted by the fetal testis which "organizes" the Wolffian duct structures, whereupon androgens function to "stabilize" this organization. Therefore, individuals lacking normal testicular tissue would not be expected to exhibit masculinization of the internal ducts.

THE CHROMATIN NEGATIVE PATIENT

Examination of a buccal smear from a patient having only one X chromosome will show few if any Barr bodies. The phenotypic sex of such patients may be either male or female, depending on the presence and activity of the Y chromosome. Some true hermaphrodites are chromatin negative or have low sex chromatin counts, suggesting mosaicism. In true hermaphrodites with the 46/XY genotype, a uterus and vagina may be present. The development of the gonadal ducts depends upon the presence of an ovary, testis, or ovotestis on that side. With an ovotestis, all or part of both ductal systems could develop simultaneously on the same side.

How ovarian tissue can develop in the presence of XY cells and how testicular tissue can develop in the absence of a Y chromosome remain unexplained. Nevertheless, although rare, true hermaphroditism must be considered as a diagnosis in all newborns with ambiguous genitalia and cryptorchidism.

MALE PSEUDOHERMAPHRODITISM

Patients with male pseudohermaphroditism have only testicular tissue but show more or less severe intersexual anomalies in the development of the genital tract. The testis has at least two discrete and quite separable endocrine functions: (1) secretion of a "Mullerian inhibitor" which causes retrogression of the Mullerian ducts and (2) secretion of a masculinizing hormone, testosterone, which stabilizes the Wolffian ducts and masculinizes the external genitalia. In addition, a substance which "induces" or "organizes" the formation of the Wolffian ducts is probably secreted by the human fetal testis. If all endocrine functions are intact, and the target tissues possess receptors for the hormones secreted by the testis, a normal male will develop. If the target tissues cannot respond to testosterone (testicular feminizing syndrome, p. 374), a phenotypic female with testes results. These patients are rarely diagnosed at birth, since there is no ambiguity of the external genitalia.

If there is an absence of or a deficiency in testosterone, the Wolffian ducts are hypoplastic and the external genitalia are feminized or only incompletely masculinized. Mild deficiency of testosterone may result in hypospadias or in female external genitalia with masculine internal ducts.

Absence of only the Mullerian inhibitor results in an otherwise normal male with uterus and tubes. Lack of all endocrine function in the fetal testis permits only female differentiation of internal and external genitalia.

Obviously, not all these conditions produce ambiguous genitalia in the newborn. The male pseudohermaphrodite whose masculinization is incomplete may show underdevelopment of the penis, hypospadias, cryptorchidism, or failure of fusion of the labioscrotal folds; however, if masculinization is completely absent, a seemingly normal female would result. Thus it is usually only in those cases of intersexuality where sexual differentiation is incomplete in one direction or another that the abnormality can be diagnosed at birth.

Hypospadias

This is a fairly common congenital anomaly in which the external urethral orifice is on the ventral surface of the penis instead of at the tip of the glans. In most patients there is no genetic or endocrine abnormality readily discernible; however, in a few cases it may represent the first clue to intersexuality. Certainly if the condition is accompanied by cryptorchidism, or by any defect in scrotal fusion, or if a uterus is palpable by rectal examination, a thorough investigation of genetic sex is indicated. In a chromatin positive patient, one thinks immediately of congenital adrenocortical hyperplasia. In the chromatin negative patient, a failure of normal testicular function should be suspected.

Development of the urethra proceeds from the perineum to the glans penis. If production of androgens is insufficient or ceases prematurely, a feminizing effect will be produced distal to the segment already developed.

In the mildest form of hypospadias—*glandular hypospadias*—the urethra usually opens just proximal to a point where the frenum usually attaches. (In this case the frenum is absent.) This form of hypospadias is not often associated with chordee and in the genetic male no surgical correction is required. In any form of hypospadias accompanied by chordee, the latter should be corrected. The release of chordee can be done at almost any age, but in general the earlier the better.

More severe forms of hypospadias include penile and penoscrotal hypospadias; in the first, the external urethral orifice is located near the penoscrotal junction; in the second, the orifice is located at the penoscrotal junction. The most severe form of hypospadias is perineal hypospadias, in which the urethral orifice is located in the perineum between the unfused labioscrotal folds; this form of hypospadias is suggestive of some form of intersex.

Cryptorchidism

Cryptorchidism is not uncommon in the newborn and of itself is not alarming. Some three percent of full term male infants and 21 percent of premature male infants have one or both testes undescended. Most (about 80 percent) of these testes descend within the first year of life.

The incompletely descended testis may be found anywhere along the normal route of descent—in the abdomen, the inguinal canal, or beyond the external inguinal ring. In the normal male, descent of the testes occurs during the month or two before birth or in the first weeks after birth. The processus vaginalis, which precedes the testis into the scrotum and is in direct communication with the peritoneal cavity, usually becomes obliterated in the first days of life.

By far the most common undescended testis is the *retractile testis*, which may be present for long periods in the inguinal canal but becomes elevated by contractions of the cremasteric muscle. Careful repeated examinations may be necessary to palpate the retractile testis. Sometimes the application of heat to the inguinal, genital, and perineal regions will relax the cremasteric muscle and permit descent of the testis. Spontaneous descent usually occurs before or at puberty and normal function is not impaired.

A testis deflected from its normal path of descent, an *ectopic testis*, is usually normally developed, as is the corresponding side of the scrotum. It may be located in the superficial inguinal area or in the pubic, perineal, or femoral areas. The superficial inguinal testis is readily palpable; however, it cannot be pushed down into the scrotum.

The undescended testis may undergo deleterious changes. The development of the seminiferous tubules may be impaired and the germinal epithelium may fail to mature. Interstitial fibrosis and tubular hyalinization develop if the testes remain undescended after puberty. At one time, injections of hCG were frequently used in the treatment of cryptorchidism; however, many authorities now believe that hormonal therapy will cause descent only of those testes which would descend anyway in the course of time.

FAMILIAL MALE PSEUDOHERMAPHRODITISM

Phenotypic masculinization in utero is a continuous process dependent upon continued testicular function. Inherited defects in masculinization have been reported by several investigators. In a family reported by Lubs, affected offspring were reared as girls since their external appearance was predominantly female. In these patients the testes were small and were located in the labioscrotal folds. In some cases, spermatogenesis was noted. Internal duct structure was incompletely male, with a blind vas deferens. Mullerian suppression was complete. Thus this hereditary disorder represents one of incomplete masculinization of the internal and external genitalia.

In a patient reported by Gilbert-Dreyfus, the phenotype was more masculine and the patient was reared as a male. Masculinization was more complete, for internal differentiation was male and external differentiation was intermediate but more nearly male. The testes presented a normal histologic picture except for slight thickening of the basement membrane of the tubules.

In both the Lubs and Gilbert-Dreyfus patients, the 17KS values were within the normal range. In another kinship reported by Reifenstein, patients were found to have hypospadias, hypogonadism, gynecomastia, and elevated pituitary gonadotropins, along with normal urinary excretion of 17KS. This disorder is limited to males and, like the testicular feminization syndrome, is transmitted either as an X-linked recessive trait or as a sex-limited autosomal dominant. The defective differentiation of the external genitalia may result from some defect in the fetal Leydig cells.

The most troublesome facet of these familial disorders of masculinization is the selection of the sex of rearing. The uncertainty of the degree of further virilization at puberty makes a male role questionable. Although some patients attain a fairly normal-sized phallus at puberty, others do not, and treatment to masculinize the poorly developed genitalia is unsatisfactory. Since reconstructive surgery to provide female genitalia is much easier than that required for a male phenotype, many patients are best reared as females. In most cases, female secondary sex characteristics develop at puberty and pubic hair is of the female type.

The etiology of these disorders is unknown. It is possible that, like the testicular feminizing syndrome, there is a defect in end organ responsiveness to androgens. Other studies, particularly in patients with Reifenstein's syndrome, suggest that the synthesis of androgens may be deficient, but that end organ responsiveness to androgens is normal. Morris and Mahesh reported a patient with this syndrome who responded to exogenous testosterone by deepening of the voice, clitoral enlargement, and growth of sex hair. Obviously, it is much too early to consider these familial disorders as representing manifestations of a single etiology. Suitable metabolic studies should clarify the question regarding synthesis of testosterone and its receptor proteins in these patients.

Congenital adrenocortical hyperplasia

Genetic males with a deficiency in 3β-hydroxysteroid dehydrogenase are unable to synthesize normal amounts of testosterone, and as a result they show incomplete masculinization of the external genitalia. Usually these patients have varying degrees of hypospadias with or without cryptorchidism. When autopsies were performed on patients with a 3β-hydroxysteroid dehydrogenase deficiency, it was found that their genital ducts were male and that there were no Mullerian structures present. This finding provides further evidence that the "Mullerian inhibitor" synthesized by the fetal testis is not a steroid. A defect in 3β-hydroxysteroid dehydrogenase prevents the synthesis of mineralocorticoids as well as glucocorticoids, and symptoms of adrenal crisis are therefore likely to occur. This enzyme defect differs from other forms of adrenocortical hyperplasia in that dehydroepiandrosterone is formed in excessive amounts—in fact, elevated levels in the urine can be diagnostic of the disorder.

Patients with congenital lipoid adrenal hyperplasia are unable to convert cholesterol to pregnenolone and cannot synthesize steroid hormones. Lacking androgens, both male and female patients have a female phenotype.

SYNDROMES OF MULTIPLE CONGENITAL ABNORMALITIES

Genital maldevelopment may occur along with a variety of birth defects. In some instances, there are no obvious chromosomal abnormalities and the defects encompass development of the face, digits, and genitals. In others, an aberration of the autosomes has been noted. For instance, cryptorchidism and abnormal scrotal development occur in some patients having the D trisomy syndrome. Syndromes of multiple congenital abnormalities are found in both genetic males and genetic females.

GONADAL DYSGENESIS

Abnormalities of the external genitalia may be found in either chromatin negative (XY, XO, mosaics) or chromatin positive (XX, mosaics) patients with abnormal gonadal function. The genital anomalies in chromatin negative patients are not usually severe enough to cast doubt about the proper sex of rearing. The testes tend to be hypoplastic and there may be an associated cryptorchidism or hypospadias. More often, patients with gonadal dysgenesis (undifferentiated or "streak" gonads lacking germ cells, p. 381) show no ambiguity of the external genitalia at birth; rather, they develop somatic signs of Turner's syndrome later in life. The patient with this syndrome characteristically has stunted growth and sexual infantilism which is not detected until puberty. Other somatic signs such as webbing of the neck, cubitus valgus, and shield chest may develop. The terms gonadal dysgenesis and Turner's syndrome are often used interchangeably, although in his original paper (1938), Turner referred only to the triad of sexual infantilism, webbing of the neck, and cubitus valgus.

Patients with gonadal dysgenesis may show the somatic signs of Turner's syndrome, although many do not. However, with or without other signs, gonadal dysgenesis (Turner's syndrome) should be suspected if there is unexplained peripheral edema, especially of the feet, in the neonatal period or in infancy. Such gross edema with no other evidence of cardiac or renal disease is almost diagnostic. Most patients with Turner's syndrome are chromatin negative and have a 45/XO karyotype.

Patients with a testis on one side and an undifferentiated "streak" gonad on the other are usually classified as examples of *mixed gonadal dysgenesis.* The internal genitalia are female, but male derivatives of the

Wolffian ducts are sometimes present. The external genitalia range from normal female, through intermediate states, to normal male. At puberty, neither breast development nor menstruation occurs, but varying degrees of virilization are common. The Leydig cells of the single testis are sometimes capable of normal function; however, the adjacent germinal tissue is abnormal, with few or no germ cells and slight thickening and hyalinization of the tubular basement membrane.

All patients with mixed gonadal dysgenesis are chromatin negative, and the incidence of mosaicism is extremely high. The presence of an XO cell line in these patients suggests that this line has a role in the development of the streak gonad, as is the case in the 45/XO patient with Turner's syndrome and bilateral streak gonads. Mosaicism could account for a Y-containing cell line which could be responsible for the development of the testicular tissue. The incidence of tumor of the gonad in this disorder is high. It may occur in the streak, in the testis, or in both, and consideration should be given to early gonadectomy to avert neoplastic change.

ABNORMALITIES OF THE SEX CHROMOSOMES

When more than two X chromosomes are present in addition to the normal set of autosomes, the number of sex chromatin masses (Barr bodies) increases and corresponds to the number of X chromosomes minus one. Each X chromosome in excess of one forms a distinct sex chromatin mass in the nucleus. Presumably, only one X is genetically active, and in different cell lines either the paternal or the maternal X may be the active chromosome.

An excess of X chromosomes does not prevent the morphologic differentiation of testes or ovaries. In females with more than two X chromosomes, ovarian development after birth may be abnormal; however, there is no ambiguity of the genitalia at birth. The most characteristic feature of the multi-X syndromes is mental retardation. In males with more than one X (Klinefelter's syndrome), there may be ambiguity of the genitalia at birth, although more often the disorder is not detected until puberty. Characteristically, the testes are small, and gyncecomastia develops at puberty. In general the severity of mental retardation in these patients is related to the number of excess X chromosomes.

Several types of abnormal X chromosomes have been found in patients with gonadal dysgenesis. Partial deletion of the short or long arm of an X-chromosome has been described. The patients ($X\bar{x}$ or $X\underline{x}$) have signs of Turner's syndrome. The sex chromatin count is usually low, on the order of five percent. An X isochromosome for the long arm of the X chromosome (transverse instead of longitudinal division of the centromere) is usually larger than the normal X chromosome and has more DNA. Patients with a normal X paired to such an X isochromosome have a condition resembling Turner's syndrome. Another abnormality, the ring X chromosome (X_r), apparently forms by simple deletion of parts of both the short and long arms of the X chromosome, followed by fusion of the chromatid ends. Mosaics of XO/XX_r with gonadal dysgenesis have been described; only five percent of the nuclei contained sex chromatin.

Isochromosomes for the Y chromosome have also been reported. For example, patients with an isochromosome for the long arm of Y, XY_i, showed no masculinization and were diagnosed as having Turner's syndrome; however, the somatic stigmata of the syndrome were absent. These findings and others suggest that the male-determining genes are situated on the short arm of the Y chromosome, and that the presence of the long arm of the Y chromosome prevents the development of the somatic signs of gonadal dysgenesis. A patient with ambiguous genitalia has been described who demonstrated three cell lines: XO, XY_i, and XY_iY, with partial deletion of the long arm. Presumably, some male-determining genes were present, since this patient had ambiguous genitalia.

SUMMARY

The presence of ambiguous genitalia in the newborn should suggest to the examiner that an abnormality of sexual differentiation has occurred during intra-uterine existence. The abnormality may be due to an error in chromosome constitution, resulting in dysgenesis of the gonads. Any deficiency in testosterone synthesis (gonadal dysgenesis, 3β-hydroxysteroid dehydrogenase deficiency) or in action at the target tissue site (testicular feminizing syndrome) would result in incomplete masculinization of internal and/or external genitalia. A partial or even complete female phenotype would result. Exposure of the genetic female to androgens in utero (21- or 11β-hydroxylase deficiency, maternal androgens) results in masculinization, usually of the external genitalia only.

The presence of both testicular and ovarian tissue usually produces both masculinized and feminized characteristics. The true hermaphrodite may have a testis on one side and an ovary or ovotestis on the other side, and sexual differentiation of the ducts will reflect the type of gonadal tissue present on that side. Although usually reared as a male, the true hermaphrodite frequently manifests gynecomastia and cyclic hematuria at puberty.

Most schemes for the differential diagnosis of ambiguous genitalia in the newborn include a separation of chromatin positive and chromatin negative patients (Figure 8–2). Chromatin positive patients are most often female, with a deficiency of either 21- or 11β-hydroxylase. Interestingly enough, most true hermaphrodites are chromatin positive. Chromatin negative patients may represent (1) true hermaphroditism, (2) male pseudohermaphroditism, or (3) gonadal dysgenesis.

Careful physical examination should include palpation for (1) a gonad in the inguinal or scrotal region (suggesting presence of testicular tissue) and (2) a uterus (denoting lack of complete testicular function or the presence of both ovarian and testicular tissue). A newborn with ambiguous genitalia and a palpable uterus but no palpable gonads should be considered to have congenital adrenocortical hyperplasia until some other diagnosis is proven.

The newborn with ambiguous genitalia who does not have congenital adrenocortical hyperplasia should have a karyotype determination. Mosaics and abnormalities of the sex chromosomes have now been catalogued extensively, and it is usually possible, by a combination of buccal smear and karyotype, to categorize most patients with chromosomal aberrations.

The importance of carefully choosing the sex of rearing of these children cannot be emphasized enough. The surgeon, pediatrician, endocrinologist, and psychiatrist all play a role in the care and treatment of the sexually malformed child.

SUGGESTED READING

Studies on sex differentiation in mammals, A. Jost, B. Vigier, J. Prepin, and J. P. Perchellet in *Recent Progress in Hormone Research 29*:1, 1973.

An excellent review of our present concepts of hormonal regulation of sexual differentiation. Dr. Jost, an authority in the field, brings the subject matter up to date, providing recent references for the student wishing to pursue this field in depth.

Abnormal Sexual Development, Daniel D. Federman, Philadelphia, W. B. Saunders Co., 1967.

A short, beautifully written approach to disorders of sexual development in the human. The chapter on ambiguous genitalia is particularly appropriate. This book is one of the most helpful for the novice in the field. Appropriate representative cases are discussed.

Disorders of sex differentiation, Melvin M. Grumbach and Judson J. Van Wyk in Williams' *Textbook of Endocrinology,* Philadelphia, W. B. Saunders Co., 1974.

A detailed and authoritative discussion of sexual disorders in the human. The authors cover normal sexual differentiation as well as the clinical syndromes associated with sexual abnormalities. A definitive reference, full of well-presented information.

PART THREE

THE CHILD

CHAPTER NINE

Homeostasis: Water and Electrolytes

The precise adjustment of the ratio of water to solute in the body and the maintenance of an acceptable range of concentrations of sodium and potassium in body fluids are the concern primarily of the kidney. In conjunction with hormones elaborated by the posterior pituitary (vasopressin) and the adrenal cortex (aldosterone), these homeostatic mechanisms are brought into play whenever conditions exist which upset the balance of water and electrolytes. The early immaturity of the kidney makes problems of water and electrolyte homeostasis of special concern in the infant and young child.

HOMEOSTATIC MECHANISMS OF THE KIDNEY

The urinary systems of all the vertebrates are essentially similar. Each is composed of units called *kidney tubules* or *nephrons* which remove wastes from the blood, but the number and arrangement of the nephrons vary in different vertebrates. In the lower vertebrates, the kidney tubules open into the body cavity (pronephric tubules, p. 58), whereas the higher, land vertebrates have developed a dilatation, called Bowman's capsule, which forms the beginning of the uriniferous tubule. The capsule receives fluid filtered through the walls of the capillaries situated within it. Thus the functional unit (nephron) of the mammalian kidney consists of *Bowman's capsule,* which surrounds a spherical tuft of capillaries (the glomerulus), and the coiled, looped *tubules.* The inner wall of Bowman's capsule consists of flat, epithelial cells which adhere closely to the capillaries of the glomerulus, permitting diffusion of sub-

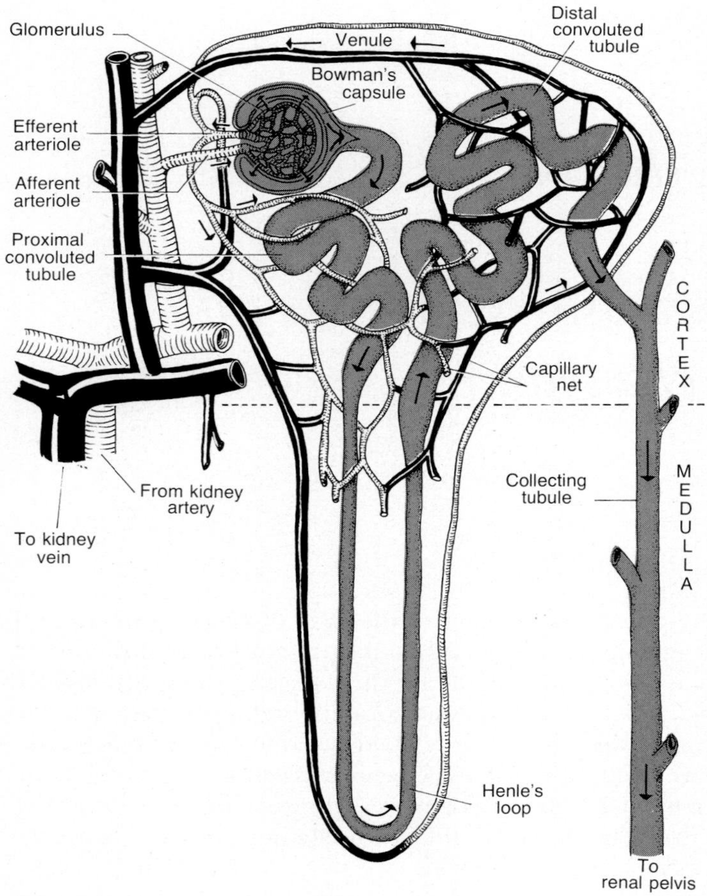

FIGURE 9–1. Diagram of a single kidney tubule and its blood vessels. (From Villee, C. and Dethier, V. *Biological Principles and Processes.* Philadelphia: W. B. Saunders Company, 1971, p. 603.)

stances from the capillaries into Bowman's capsule. Each kidney contains about 10^6 nephrons, each a separate, independent unit for excreting wastes and regulating the composition of the blood.

Approximately 20 to 25 percent of the cardiac output of blood is delivered to the kidneys. Of this, 20 to 35 percent of the *plasma* is filtered through the glomerular capillaries. The filtration process is passive; its driving force is the *filtration pressure.* The arteriole entering the glomerulus, the *afferent arteriole* (Figure 9–1), is larger than the vessel leaving it, the *efferent arteriole,* thus creating a head of pressure. The blood pressure in the glomerular capillaries in the normal individual is about 70 mm Hg. Because of the permeability properties of the glomerular membrane, proteins and other high molecular weight components are virtually excluded from the filtrate. This means that an imbalance exists in the concentration of solutes between that in the fluid of the capillaries and that in the filtrate, such that an osmotic pressure (32 mm Hg) tends to move fluid back into the capillaries. In addition, a hydrostatic pressure of about 14 mm Hg exists in Bowman's capsule. Thus the net force moving fluid out of the glomerulus, the filtration pressure, equals 70 − (32 + 14), or 24 mm Hg. It is well to remember that the rate at which fluid passes from the glomerulus into Bowman's capsule, the *glomerular filtration rate,* rises and falls with the blood pressure, which determines the filtration pressure.

If the composition of the urine ultimately excreted were like that of the glomerular filtrate, excretion would be a wasteful process, and a great deal of water, glucose, amino acids, and electrolytes would be lost. The kidney must reclaim 98 to 99 percent of the filtrate. How is this accomplished? From each Bowman's capsule, located in the kidney cortex (Figure 9–1), the filtrate passes through a *proximal convoluted tubule* (also in the cortex), then through a long *loop of Henle,* passing deep into the medulla and back into the cortex, then through a *distal convoluted tubule,* emptying at last into a *collecting tubule,* through which it passes again through the medulla into the kidney pelvis (Figure 9–1). The efferent arteriole does not pass directly to a vein but connects with a second network of capillaries around the proximal and distal convoluted tubules (Figure 9–1). The route of blood in the kidney is unique; it passes through two sets of capillaries in sequence in passing from the renal artery to the renal vein. The ability of the kidney to regulate the composition of blood depends upon this structural feature.

Although reclamation of filtered substances such as bicarbonate, glucose, potassium, phosphate, and amino acids is crucial to the economy of the body, from a quantitative standpoint the reabsorption of sodium, chloride, and water represents the most important regulatory function of the kidney. Our kidney tubules reabsorb each day about 1200 g of sodium chloride (about 2.5 lb). The reabsorption of sodium by the kidney is an energy-dependent process. Filtered sodium passes freely through the luminal membrane of the cells of the proximal tubules. This passage is actually down an electrochemical gradient, since the tubular cells actively "pump" sodium across the transluminal or basal membrane into the circulation. The energy required for this *sodium pump* is supplied by metabolic processes occurring within the tubular cell. On a stoichiometric basis, sodium reabsorption accounts for about 70 percent of all renal transport activity.

Each cell of the body needs some kind of sodium pump to keep the cell from swelling and bursting. The mechanism of the sodium pump has been studied extensively. Apparently, in one form of transport, sodium ions are exchanged for potassium ions across the cell membrane. Any drugs which inhibit glycolysis or oxidative phosphorylation inhibit Na/K exchange. This suggests a role of ATP in the pumping process. Although the actual mechanism is still unknown, most investigators postulate that (1) special carrier molecules in the cell membrane perform ion transport and (2) the actions of the molecules in binding to and separating from the transported ion are in some way coupled to the hydrolysis of ATP and to metabolic processes. Like most other cells, kidney cells contain a cation-sensitive ATP-ase which is inseparable from the cell membranes and is dependent upon Mg^{++} for activity. The Na-K-ATP-ase of the kidney, although present in the cortex, is most active in the outer medulla and probably plays a role in about 40 percent of renal sodium reabsorption.

The structure of the cells of the proximal tubules is particularly conducive to active transport. These cells and those of the distal convoluted tubules are richly endowed with mitochondria, whereas the tubular cells within the renal medulla (loop of Henle and collecting duct) contain few mitochondria. The inner (luminal) border of the proximal tubule cells is composed of many fine, hairlike processes which extend from the cells into the lumen of the tubule. As the filtrate passes through, this *brush border* provides an extensive surface area for transport across the cell membrane. The actual blood flow is much higher in the cortex than in the medulla, as is the rate of oxygen consumption. Conversely, the rate of anaerobic glycolysis in vitro is two to three times higher in the medulla than that found in the cortex. All of these facts suggest involvement of the renal cortex (proximal and distal convoluted tubules) in active reabsorption of substances from the glomerular filtrate.

The structure of the renal cortex provides a mechanism for monitoring the amounts of substances which have been absorbed. The distal convoluted tubule comes to lie very close to the afferent arteriole serving the glomerulus of that tubule. At the point of contact, the cells of the distal tubule increase in number and become dense, forming a structure called the *macula densa* (Figure 9–2). The smooth muscle cells in the wall of the arteriole adjacent to the macula densa, called the *juxtaglomerular cells,* are swollen and filled with granules. By microinjection under the microscope it is possible to place sodium chloride solutions directly into the distal convoluted tubule and show that the afferent arteriole immediately becomes constricted. It is thus evident that the composition of the fluid in the distal tubule is monitored, presumably by the cells of the macula densa, and this regulates the degree of constriction of the afferent arteriole, presumably via the juxtaglomerular cells. The glomerular filtration rate is of course controlled by the filtration pressure, which depends on the degree of constriction of the walls of the afferent arteriole. In this way, each nephron, by continuously assaying the concentration of salts in the tubular fluid entering the distal tubule from the loop of Henle, regulates its glomerular filtration rate to the optimal value.

So far we have discussed the absorption of sodium. What about water? To become successful on land, man and the other higher vertebrates had to evolve a mechanism to excrete a concentrated urine and thus conserve body water. This ability appears to depend on certain

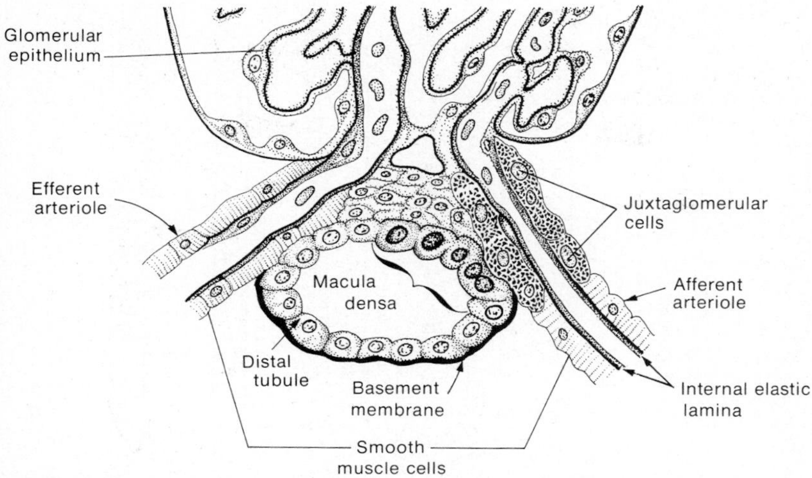

FIGURE 9–2. Diagram illustrating the relationship of the macula densa and the juxtaglomerular cells, muscle cells in the wall of the afferent arterioles of the kidney. The cells of the macular densa monitor the concentration of substances in the glomerular filtrate and stimulate the juxtaglomerular cells to contract or relax, thereby controlling the glomerular filtration rate. (From Villee, C. and Dethier, V. *Biological Principles and Processes.* Philadelphia: W. B. Saunders Company, 1971, p. 607.)

properties of the loop of Henle. The glomeruli and proximal and distal tubules are located in the outer part of the kidney—the cortex—whereas the loop of Henle extends deeply into the central medulla (Figure 9–1). The peritubular capillaries also form long loops, *vasa recta,* that extend down into the medulla. Blood passes down into the medulla and then back up to the cortex in these vasa recta before emptying into the renal veins. As tubular fluid passes through the *ascending* loop of Henle, sodium is actively pumped into the interstitial fluid; chloride ions go along passively, and the concentration of these ions in the interstitial fluid increases. Some of the Na^+ and Cl^- ions diffuse back passively into the *descending* loop. The cycling of Na^+ from ascending limb to interstitial fluid to descending limb results in the establishment of a concentration gradient of Na^+ and Cl^- in the tissue fluid surrounding the loop, with the lowest concentration near the cortex and the highest concentration deep in the medulla (Figure 9–3).

As blood in the vasa recta flows into the medulla, Na^+ and Cl^- diffuse into it, but as the blood flows back up and out of the medulla, Na^+ and Cl^- diffuse out of the blood into the interstitial fluid. This "counter current" flow of blood prevents the loss of Na^+ and Cl^- from the medulla and permits the concentration gradient in the interstitial fluid to be maintained. The active transport of Na^+ out of the tubular fluid in the ascending loop of Henle is so powerful that the fluid reaching the distal convoluted tubule actually has a lower concentration of Na^+ than does the fluid in the glomerular filtrate. The cells of the ascending loop of Henle appear to be impermeable to water, for water does not diffuse

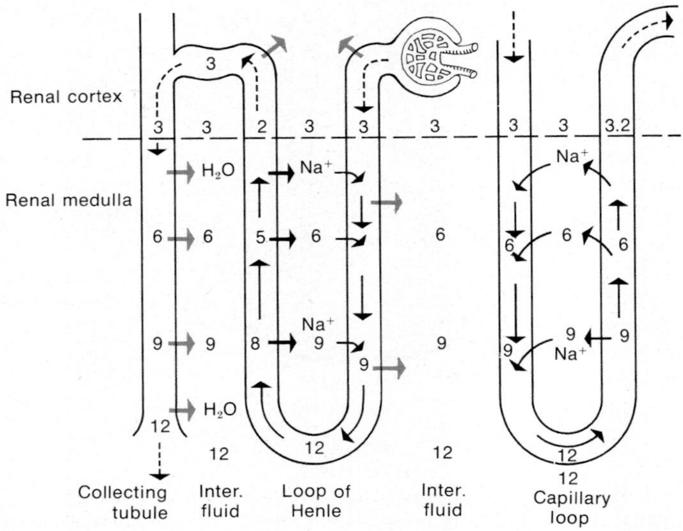

FIGURE 9–3. Diagram of countercurrent flow mechanism of the mammalian kidney. The general direction of fluid movement is shown by dotted arrows; active sodium transport by solid thick arrows; passive sodium transport by solid thin arrows; and the movement of water by light-colored arrows. The numerals refer to the relative concentrations of osmotically active solutes. When two zeros are added they refer to the concentration of solutes in milliosmoles per liter. (From Villee, C. and Dethier, V. *Biological Principles and Processes.* Philadelphia: W. B. Saunders Company, 1971, p. 609.)

out as the sodium is pumped out. As the filtrate passes through the loop of Henle, it loses much sodium but very little water. Then the urine enters the collecting tubules and flows down through the medulla, through an ever-increasing concentration of sodium and chloride in the interstitial fluid. The cells of the collecting tubule *are* permeable to water, and by osmosis water moves from the dilute urine in the collecting tubule to the interstitial fluid with its high concentration of solutes. The urine finally passing into the pelvis is nearly as concentrated as the interstitial fluid deep in the medulla, and it is quite a bit more concentrated than the initial glomerular filtrate.

Built into this system of salt and water reclamation is a means of regulating these processes by hormones. Aldosterone acts on the cells in the distal convoluted tubules to increase sodium reabsorption (p. 215). Its secretion is in turn regulated by the concentration of sodium in the blood. The cells lining the distal convoluted tubules and the collecting tubules are sensitive to vasopressin (antidiuretic hormone). This hormone increases the permeability of these cells to water. The secretion of vasopressin is regulated by the osmolarity (total concentration of solutes) of the blood.

To summarize the functions of the kidney in water and electrolyte balance:

1. Excretion of most substances depends on normal permeability of

the glomerulus and on the filtration pressure. If either of these factors is significantly reduced, the tubules may not be able to maintain a glomerular filtration rate large enough to modulate the composition of blood normally.

2. The proximal tubule reabsorbs almost completely many substances which can be reutilized by the body (glucose, amino acids). About 70 percent of the sodium and water filtered at the glomerulus is reabsorbed at this site, the *active* process being the reabsorption of sodium.
3. The loop of Henle, by means of a counter current system, creates the osmotic pressure which enables hyposmolar or hyperosmolar urine to be formed according to the body's needs.
4. The distal tubule makes further adjustments by additional sodium reabsorption and by regulating the constriction of the afferent arteriolar walls.
5. Final adjustment of water excretion takes place in the distal convoluted and collecting tubules under the influence of vasopressin and is regulated by the osmotic gradient set up by the cells of the loop of Henle.

It is estimated that in the absence of homeostatic mechanisms for reabsorption (both kidney and intestine), the whole of the extracellular water and sodium could be lost in about two hours.

VASOPRESSIN

The octapeptides vasopressin and oxytocin are synthesized in the hypothalamus and transported along the nerve axons to the posterior lobe of the pituitary gland, where they are stored and released on demand (see Chapter Three). A variety of octapeptide hormones from different species have been isolated, and a large body of information is available regarding their chemical structures, their physiologic and pharmacologic actions, and their phylogenetic distribution among the vertebrates. Five functions have been ascribed to these neurohormones: (1) contraction of the smooth muscle of the uterus (oxytocic effect, p. 110), (2) contraction of the myoepithelial cells which surround the mammary alveoli (milk ejection, p. 115), (3) actions upon the kidney to prevent excessive loss of water (antidiuretic effect), (4) contraction of the smooth muscle in the walls of blood vessels (vasopressor effect, p. 210), and (5) regulation of the release of adenohypophyseal hormones (p. 51). Seven naturally occurring octapeptides are known at present: oxytocin, arginine vasopressin, lysine vasopressin, vasotocin, mesotocin, isotocin, and glumitocin. Arginine vasopressin is found in man, monkey, dog, rat, horse, cow, and sheep, whereas lysine vasopressin is found in the pig and the hippopotamus. There is some evidence that arginine vasotocin may be formed in the pineal gland in man.

Because of their similar chemical structures, the octapeptide hormones have overlapping biological activities. Antidiuresis is an adaptation to terrestrial life, and it is therefore not surprising to find that the neurohypophyseal principles have no effect on water conservation in fishes, although they may promote the loss of sodium through the kidneys. Arginine and lysine vasopressins are antidiuretic in mammals, but arginine vasotocin performs this function in amphibians, reptiles, and birds.

Both oxytocin and vasopressin are coupled with small molecular weight proteins (neurophysins) during transport and storage. In the human, there are two immunologically distinct neurophysins, one binding oxytocin specifically, the other binding vasopressin specifically. Each mole of neurophysin binds one mole of vasopressin or oxytocin. The biosynthesis of labeled vasopressin is paralleled by the formation of labeled neurophysin, suggesting that both may arise from a common precursor. The relationship may be much like that of insulin and the C-peptide.

Within the axons of the posterior pituitary are membrane-bound granules of about 160 nm diameter containing the octapeptide hormones, each stored in segregated clusters of granules. In response to a variety of stimuli, the neurohypophyseal hormones are released by a process requiring calcium (p. 328) and are taken up by the capillary plexus in the posterior pituitary. The stimulus for release of vasopressin is normally an elevation in osmolarity of body fluids. Osmoreceptors are located in or near the supraoptic nuclei of the hypothalamus. The system is also designed to respond to changes in blood volume by means of pressure receptors in the left atrium and carotid artery. Volume depletion (for example, hemorrhage) brings about an outpouring of vasopressin. Overexpansion of blood volume or hypotonicity suppresses release of vasopressin.

It is obvious that the renal conservation of water that is stimulated by vasopressin could not alone prevent dehydration. The obligatory loss of water via skin, lungs, and kidney would result in progressive dehydration. Fortunately, a thirst mechanism exists to alert the individual to the need for water. There is a close anatomic as well as physiologic relationship between the thirst and antidiuretic centers. Electrical stimulation (or injection of hypertonic saline) in an area extending from the dorsal into the ventral hypothalamus induces "a conscious urge to drink." This area has been termed the *thirst center.* The interplay of the thirst and antidiuretic centers helps maintain a constant osmolarity of body fluids. Recent studies have strongly implicated the renin-angiotensin system in the control of hypovolemic thirst and in the release of vasopressin.

Once released from the posterior pituitary, vasopressin circulates as the free peptide, disappearing rapidly from the blood with a half time of 10 to 20 minutes. The neurophysins are also found in the blood, suggesting that they are released from the posterior pituitary with vasopressin and oxytocin. Apparently, one neurophysin is sensitive to estrogen and the other to nicotine. In pregnancy, the concentration of the estrogen-sensitive neurophysin in maternal blood is increased. Smoking induces a rise in the nicotine-sensitive neurophysin. Cheng and Friesen have recently reported values for neurophysin (using an immunoassay specific for human neurophysin I) in human serum under basal conditions and in a variety of clinical conditions. The basal level of neurophysin (independent of age or sex) is 2.0 ± 1.0 ng/ml. During pregnancy, it is increased to a mean of 7.6; however, no significant changes were noted before, during, or after nursing. This would suggest that neurophysin I is associated with vasopressin when released from the posterior pituitary. The concentration of neurophysin I in the serum of the newborn was 9.2 ± 6.0 ng/ml, perhaps reflecting the exposure of the fetus to large amounts of estrogen. It is of interest that in patients with diabetes insipidus the serum neurophysin I values were generally elevated.

Both oxytocin and vasopressin are inactivated in the liver, probably by cleavage of the disulfide bond (necessary for biological activity) and deamination. Some vasopressin is cleared unchanged by the kidney.

Mechanism of action of vasopressin

Much of the work on the mechanism of action of vasopressin has utilized the isolated toad bladder. In this tissue, no net movement of water occurs, even in the presence of a water gradient across the bladder, unless vasopressin is added. If the fluid bathing the serosal surface of the bladder is made hypertonic to that bathing the mucosal side, water will move from the mucosal to the serosal side, but only if vasopressin is present. The vasopressin effect is never noted if one measures the movement of water in the reverse direction; presumably, therefore, the barrier exists in the mucosal surface. There is some evidence that a similar condition prevails in the collecting tubules of the mammalian kidney. Thus, although water is freely permeable in the proximal tubules, the cells of the ascending loop of Henle are impermeable to water, and the collecting tubules are impermeable in the absence of vasopressin.

How is the movement of water produced? Apparently vasopressin acts by *removing* barriers to passive transfer, rather than by modifying transport carrier systems. In 1953, Koefoed-Johnsen and Ussing proposed that vasopressin enlarged the radii of pores in the bladder membrane through which the water molecules move. They suggested that many small pores would be converted to a few large ones, with little change in the total surface area of the pores. The large pores would permit water to move rapidly, since they could accommodate the larger, more highly aggregated clusters of water molecules. On the basis of this scheme, Leaf (1961) calculated a mean pore radius for water movement across the toad bladder of 8 Å in the absence of vasopressin and 40 Å in its presence.

There is strong evidence that cyclic AMP is involved in mediating the action of vasopressin, as it is in most peptide hormones. The majority of experiments have been performed on the isolated toad bladder, but results obtained from studies on the kidney are in agreement. Cyclic AMP is itself capable of initiating all the actions of vasopressin in sensitive tissue, and the action of vasopressin (but not that of cyclic AMP) can be blocked by those prostaglandins which inhibit adenyl cyclase. It is of interest that the action of prostaglandin E_1 (in the presence of ATP) on adenyl cyclase of beef renal medullary membranes appears to require the presence of guanosine triphosphate (GTP), whereas the action of vasopressin on such a system is inhibited by GTP. Thus other nucleotides may influence the activation or inactivation of adenyl cyclase, and the whole system is undoubtedly far more complicated than our present knowledge indicates.

The action of vasopressin can also be duplicated by the administration of theophylline, which leads to an increase in cellular levels of cyclic AMP by inhibiting phosphodiesterase. This enzyme catalyzes the breakdown of cyclic AMP to 5′AMP. Both vasopressin and theophylline can elevate the concentration of cyclic AMP in both the kidney and the toad bladder. The adenyl cyclase activity which occurs in response to vasopressin takes place primarily in cells in the renal medulla, as one might have predicted. It is interesting that the adenyl cyclase which responds to parathyroid hormone (p. 114) is concentrated in the renal cortex. There is also an epinephrine-sensitive adenyl cyclase in the kidney.

In addition to its effect on water transport, vasopressin stimulates active transport of sodium in toad bladder preparations. These two effects seem to be distinct, in that the same agent may affect water and sodium transport differently. For instance, 10 mM calcium in the bathing medium decreases the permeability of the bladder membrane to water but does not alter active sodium movement. Fluoroacetate stops sodium transport but increases water permeability produced by vasopressin. In addition, the concentration of vasopressin required to produce an increase in sodium movement across toad bladders is about one tenth that needed for hydrosmotic effect.

Cyclic AMP can mimic vasopressin's effects on the transport of sodium and water. How can the same hormone produce two distinct effects via the same enzyme, adenyl cyclase? Are two different cell types involved? The vast majority of the cells of the toad bladder membrane are "granular" cells which have been shown to be involved in water transport. It seems unlikely that the toad bladder membrane contains enough of another type of cell (such as the "mitochondria-rich" cells) to account for the sodium transport. Possibly more than one adenyl cyclase in the granular cells is activated by vasopressin, or possibly a differential effect on calcium transport produces the separate effects on water and sodium transport. Other cyclic nucleotides may be involved. Clarification of the molecular mechanism of action of vasopressin and the other neurohypophyseal hormones awaits further investigation.

DIABETES INSIPIDUS

Diabetes insipidus, characterized by excessive loss of water, results from decreased secretion or accelerated degradation of vasopressin or from a lack of end-organ response to normal amounts of vasopressin. In children, the appearance of the disease may be accompanied by symptoms of fatigue, irritability, weight loss, disturbed sleep, and poor growth. The classical signs of excessive drinking and urination should alert the physician to the possibility of some form of diabetes. The urine is characteristically of low specific gravity, and dehydration is usually present.

Deficiency of vasopressin

Etiology

Inadequate secretion of vasopressin can result from damage or destruction of the supraoptic and paraventricular nuclei of the hypothalamo-hypophyseal tract. Removal or destruction of the posterior pituitary is not sufficient to produce *permanent* diabetes insipidus. Although the posterior pituitary is the major site for storage and release of the neurohormones, it is not involved in their synthesis. Thus even in the absence of the posterior pituitary, newly formed hormones could still be released into the circulation. A variety of etiologic factors may be involved in the genesis of diabetes insipidus.

Infections. Syphilis and tuberculosis involving the hypothalamus or pituitary were major causes of diabetes insipidus some decades ago; however, the more common infections presently producing diabetes insipidus are meningitis or encephalitis as complications of measles, pertussis, mumps, poliomyelitis, or chicken pox.

Tumors. At all ages the most frequent cause of diabetes insipidus is a tumor involving the suprasellar area, the third ventricle, or the pineal gland. The most frequent infratentorial tumor encountered in children is *craniopharyngioma* (Figure 9–4). This tumor comprises 5 to 13 percent of all intracranial tumors of childhood. It arises from the remnants of Rathke's pouch (p. 37) and therefore is of epithelial origin. The tumor is composed of a solid connective tissue stroma containing epithelial elements. As the tumor outgrows its blood supply, cystic portions may develop. These cysts (frequently the largest portion of the tumor, hence the name suprasellar cyst) are supported by epithelium and contain yellow or dark brown fluid in which an abundance of cholesterol crystals can be found. The tumor varies in size, some tumors attaining the size of an orange. It may extend into the sella turcica.

Depending upon its size and location, the craniopharyngioma usually manifests itself between the ages of 6 and 16 years. If the tumor extends anteriorly, visual field defects and optic atrophy may be noted

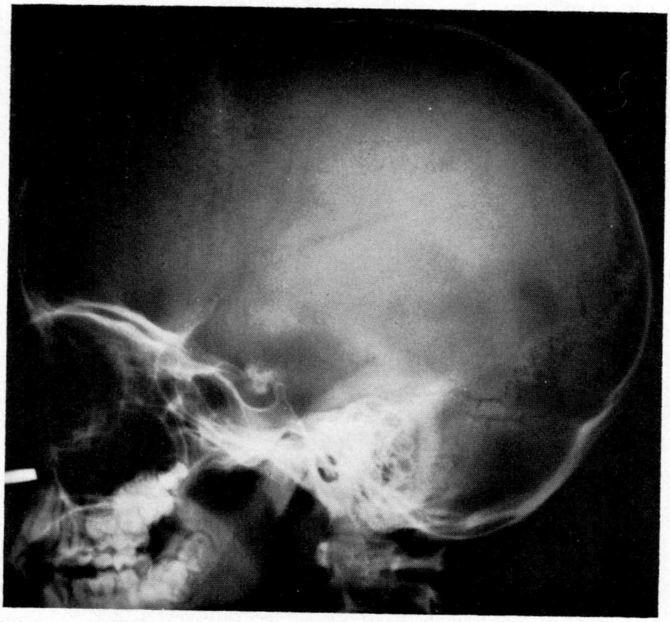

FIGURE 9–4. A lateral skull film of a boy, 11 years and 9 months old, who was of normal height and who showed symptoms of vomiting, lethargy, headaches, and visual field disturbance. There was no evidence of diabetes insipidus. Intrasellar and suprasellar flecks of calcium were evident on the radiograph. The diagnosis of craniopharyngioma was confirmed at surgery. Removal of the tumor produced evidence of diabetes insipidus, TSH deficiency, and ACTH deficiency. (From Gardner, L., ed. *Endocrine and Genetic Diseases of Childhood.* Philadelphia: W. B. Saunders Company, 1969, p. 190.)

from encroachment on the optic chiasma. Pressure on the anterior hypothalamus may affect the centers controlling gonadotropin release. Pressure on the mediolateral hypothalamus can involve the satiety center, producing obesity. More posteriorly the tumor may involve the median eminence, affecting the various hypothalamic centers that regulate release of hormones of the anterior pituitary and the neurons serving the posterior pituitary. Still more posteriorly the tumor may produce symptoms of sexual precocity. Thus craniopharyngioma may manifest itself clinically not only as the syndrome of diabetes insipidus, but also as (1) hypopituitarism with dwarfism and sexual infantilism (p. 277), (2) Fröhlich's syndrome with adiposity, diabetes insipidus, sexual infantilism, and dwarfism (p. 304), (3) a neurological syndrome with increased intracranial tension, vomiting, and retinal changes, or (4) obstruction of the third ventricle causing internal hydrocephalus and papilledema, with weakness of the third, fourth, and sixth nerves, resulting in diplopia.

In any child suspected of having craniopharyngioma, x-ray films of the skull and sella turcica and tests to evaluate visual, neurologic, and endocrine function should be performed. In about 50 percent of cases, the sella turcica is enlarged or distorted. The clinoid processes may be displaced downward. The frequency of calcification in the tumor (occurring in 60 to 90 percent of cases) is helpful in differentiating craniopharyngioma from other pituitary neoplasms (Figure 9–4). There may be increased intracranial pressure with separation of the sutures. In a patient with a history of headache, vomiting, and short stature, and x-rays showing distorted or enlarged sella with suprasellar calcification, the diagnosis of craniopharyngioma is almost certain.

No treatment has a very high success rate. Because of the proximity of the tumor to the internal carotid artery, the optic nerves and chiasma, and the hypothalamus, complete surgical removal is often difficult. Careful attention to glucocorticoid replacement and fluid and electrolyte management have greatly reduced the mortality associated with surgery. Recurrences, however, are frequent, and mortality increases with repeated operations. Surgery tends to exaggerate rather than relieve pituitary dysfunction. Whereas less than 10 percent of patients have diabetes insipidus at the time of diagnosis, up to 50 percent have permanent diabetes insipidus after surgery. Roughly 50 percent have ACTH deficiency, 50 to 80 percent have TSH deficiency, 40 to 50 percent have gonadotropin deficiency, and 10 to 65 percent continue to have a low rate of linear growth. Although recurrences are frequent, the growth of the tumor is characteristically slow, and many years may elapse before symptoms reappear.

Other tumors which can give rise to diabetes insipidus are pinealomas and diencephalic gliomas. In adults (in an age range of 30 to 60 years), adenomas (chromophobic, acidophilic, or basophilic) of the anterior pituitary may exert pressure upon or invade hypothalamic structures, producing a variety of conditions including, rarely, diabetes insipidus.

TRAUMA. Nonsurgical head trauma has been reported as an infrequent cause of diabetes insipidus, presumably via injury to the hypothalamo-pituitary tracts. In most cases the disorder is transient.

DELAY IN MATURATION OF OSMORECEPTOR MECHANISM OR DEFECT IN THIRST MECHANISM. Fanconi (1956) suggested that some infants showing hypernatremia and a lack of thirst may suffer from delayed maturation of the osmoreceptor mechanism. Such children have a fever not attributable to other causes. The disorder may disappear spontaneously or remain permanently.

Derangements of the thirst mechanism may contribute to water loss. For instance, infection or invasive processes (Hand-Schuller-Christian disease, tumors) in the region of the thirst center, as well as surgical trauma of the area during removal of a craniopharyngioma, can produce a defective thirst mechanism, leading to hyperosmolarity.

END ORGAN UNRESPONSIVENESS TO VASOPRESSIN. Unresponsiveness of the end organs to vasopressin is a rare hereditary disease which is transmitted as a sex-linked recessive gene. It occurs in males and results from a failure of the kidneys to respond to vasopressin. The disorder is usually called *nephrogenic diabetes insipidus.* Characteristically, polyuria starts soon after birth and the babies are very thirsty; the body temperature will rise unless sufficient fluids are given, and the electrolytes in both serum and sweat are increased.

Heterozygous females demonstrate a variable concentration defect. Depriving these women of water for a period of 12 hours resulted in an inability to concentrate urine above a specific gravity of 1.018.

DIAGNOSIS OF DIABETES INSIPIDUS

Marked polyuria, reaching an amount of 5 to 10 liters or more daily, accompanied by severe thirst, should always lead to the suspicion of diabetes insipidus. It is important to differentiate true diabetes insipidus from *psychogenic diabetes insipidus* (compulsive water drinking), a condition found most often in young girls with a history of emotional disturbance. In children, primary renal failure may be confused with diabetes insipidus. The direct measurement of vasopressin has recently become possible; however, not many clinical laboratories are equipped for this assay. Therefore, the diagnosis of diabetes insipidus depends upon the demonstration of the failure of kidneys to concentrate the urine in the presence of insufficient water intake (water deprivation test), followed by correction of the condition with exogenous vasopressin (vasopressin test). Testing the ability of the hypothalamic osmoreceptors to react to the stimulus of increased plasma osmolarity (hypertonic saline test) is hazardous and not recommended.

WATER DEPRIVATION TEST

The procedure followed in the water deprivation test is to withhold fluids from the individual being tested (provided the patient is adequately hydrated). The bladder is emptied and the weight and temperature of the patient and the specific gravity of the urine are measured. Adults can undergo an overnight deprivation of water; however, with young children this may be hazardous and a 4 to 6 hour period may be used instead. Urine volumes, specific gravity, and osmolarity (total number of solute particles/kg water) are measured hourly. Excretion of dilute urine (osmolarity less than 150 mosm/kg water; specific gravity less than 1.005), weight loss of 5 percent or more, and an increase in serum tonicity (osmolarity greater than 290 mosm; sodium greater than 150 mEq/liter) are diagnostic of the disease. During the test, patients should be carefully watched for signs of incipient shock. When water is restricted for a period of 12 to 18 hours, patients with psychogenic diabetes insipidus will usually reduce urine volume and increase urinary osmolarity at least to isotonicity.

Vasopressin test

If in the water deprivation test the urine does not reach an adequate concentration, vasopressin should be administered either intramuscularly (0.01 U/kg) or intravenously (0.2 to 0.5 U) before the test is brought to an end. Urine volume and concentration are measured at frequent intervals after vasopressin administration. Patients with deficient hypophyseal function will respond to exogenous vasopressin with decreased urine volume; urine concentration will rise within 30 to 90 minutes. Patients with psychogenic polydipsia and those with nephrogenic diabetes insipidus fail to respond.

TREATMENT OF DIABETES INSIPIDUS

Hormone replacement is the most satisfactory treatment for diabetes insipidus. Unfortunately, vasopressin cannot be given orally because it is quickly inactivated by trypsin. Even when injected, the hormone is rapidly inactivated unless repository forms such as a suspension of vasopressin tannate in oil are used. Intramuscular or subcutaneous injections are effective for 24 to 48 hours. Nasal sprays of an aqueous preparation of vasopressin are available, but the duration of action is brief. Furthermore, local chronic inflammatory changes occur, especially in the nasal mucosa.

Chlorpropamide has been shown to potentiate the action of vasopressin both in vitro and in vivo and it has been recommended by some investigators in the treatment of diabetes insipidus. Its actual mechanism of action is uncertain; however, it is capable of inhibiting cyclic nucleotide phosphodiesterase in vitro and of increasing the excretion of cyclic AMP (as is vasopressin) in urine of patients with diabetes insipidus. In addition, norepinephrine (which decreases cyclic AMP in kidney) inhibits the actions of both vasopressin and chlorpropamide. All these facts suggest a mechanism of action involving increased concentration of cyclic AMP in tubular cells. Chlorpropamide by itself has no effect; however, it is able to potentiate the effect of suboptimal amounts of vasopressin. Undoubtedly some antidiuretic peptides are secreted in patients with diabetes insipidus. Indeed, Coculescu and Pavel have recently isolated material with the characteristics of arginine vasotocin from the cerebrospinal fluid of patients with diabetes insipidus. The mammalian pineal gland contains arginine vasotocin and apparently can secrete this hormone into the cerebrospinal fluid. Since arginine vasotocin is not found in the cerebrospinal fluid of normal individuals, one can postulate that vasopressin deficiency of the hypothalamic neurosecretory system in diabetes insipidus stimulates the pineal to release increased amounts of an arginine vasotocin-like peptide into the cerebrospinal fluid.

Synthetic analogues of vasopressin are becoming available now. Sawyer and Manning have synthesized an analogue of vasopressin* which has about four times the antidiuretic activity of arginine vasopressin in rats, less oxytocic activity, and undetectable vasopressor activity. Most of the undesirable effects of vasopressin are the result of its effects on vascular and visceral smooth muscles. Additional structural modifications have resulted in analogues which resist degradation and thus have a longer duration of action. Synthetic analogues with these properties show great promise for the therapy of diabetes insipidus.

Treatment of nephrogenic diabetes insipidus is more difficult. Attempts to reduce the osmolar load on the kidney (low solute diet) and the use of thiazide diuretics (p. 442) are helpful.

Excess of vasopressin

Just as a deficiency in release or action of vasopressin can lead to water loss, so excessive amounts of circulating vasopressin can impair the excretion of free water and produce hyposmolarity. A variety of stimuli cause the release of vasopressin. When conditions exist which normally trigger vasopressin release—conditions such as hypovolemia, hypotension, or loss of extracellular volume of any cause—the increased secretion of vasopressin is considered "*appropriate.*" Absorption of nicotine from cigarette smoking also triggers vasopressin release. In general, alcohol or emotional stress depresses vasopressin release.

Increased delivery or secretion of vasopressin when the serum osmolarity would not normally call it forth, or when other stimuli are absent, is "*inappropriate.*" One cause of "water intoxication" is excessive treatment of diabetes insipidus with either vasopressin or chlorpropamide, associated with the continued ingestion of water. Such a condition is transient. Surgical damage to the pituitary stalk may also produce a transient excess of vasopressin.

In some conditions, excessive vasopressin release is sustained. Any abnormal stimulation, by disease, pain, drugs, or emotional stress of those areas of the reticular formation, limbic system, or cerebral cortex which have neural connections with the supraoptic nuclei, may cause sustained release of vasopressin. Certain tumors produce an antidiuretic material. George, Capen, and Phillips extracted a bronchogenic carcinoma that had been removed from a patient with the classic syndrome of inappropriate secretion of vasopressin and found large amounts of the hormone in the tissue. They demonstrated the ability of the tissue to form labeled vasopressin from labeled phenylalanine. The tumor cells had many of the ultrastructural features of polypeptide hormone-secreting cells. Adenocarcinoma of the pancreas has also been described as a

*(1-deamino, 4-val,-8-D-arg)-vasopressin.

source of antidiuretic material. Chronic pulmonary tuberculosis can produce "salt wasting," and the presence of vasopressin has been demonstrated in tuberculous lung tissue from a patient with inappropriate secretion of vasopressin.

Not all forms of hyposmolarity are due to excessive secretion of vasopressin. It should be remembered that impaired renal function may prevent delivery of an adequate volume of water to the diluting segments of the nephron. Indeed, iatrogenic hyposmolarity may occur in children (with immature renal function) or adults (with damaged or diseased kidneys) as the result of the injudicious use of intravenous fluids. The inability to excrete a water load in a normal manner is a characteristic of adrenal insufficiency. The effect is due to glucocorticoid deficiency, but the mechanism is unclear.

LOSS OF WATER IN EXCESS OF SODIUM

Diabetes insipidus is just one example of the loss of water in excess of sodium. Any condition in which insufficient water is imbibed (lack of water) or excessive water loss occurs (excessive sweating of a hypotonic fluid; osmotic diuresis as in diabetes mellitus or heavy excretion of urea) will result in an increased concentration of sodium in the serum. Hypernatremia causes water to leave the cell, thus permitting the deficit of water to be shared by all components of the body fluid. In addition, the increased concentration of sodium serves as a stimulus to feedback mechanisms that promote the acquisition and the conservation of water by provoking thirst and stimulating the secretion of vasopressin.

LOSS OF SODIUM IN EXCESS OF WATER

Dehydration due to loss of sodium in an excess of water occurs in many situations characterized by an inability of the kidney to conserve sodium appropriately. The reduced concentration of sodium in the serum creates an osmotic gradient which results in a passage of water from extracellular fluid into the cell. This greatly reduces the extracellular fluid volume. The extracellular compartment—approximately 20 percent of body weight—is comprised of interstitial fluid (15 percent) and fluid that circulates in the vascular compartment (5 percent). Any decrease in extracellular fluid volume will produce a decrease in blood volume.

Renin

Any decrease in blood volume (or *effective* blood volume) will reduce the perfusion pressure in the afferent arterioles of the kidney. The juxtaglomerular cells which surround these afferent arterioles act as stretch receptors. With an increase in the stretch of the wall of the renal afferent arteriole, there is a rise in the number of renin granules in the juxtaglomerular cells; with a decreased stretch, there is a fall in the number of granules. One can experimentally decrease the perfusion pressure by constricting the renal artery as Goldblatt did in 1934, producing persistent hypertension. Clinical conditions such as renal stenosis emulate the Goldblatt kidney. In either the experimental or the clinical model, the increased concentration of plasma renin, secondary to the decreased perfusion pressure, brings about increased formation of angiotensin II, the most powerful hypertensive agent known.

Renin release is also influenced by the transport of sodium across the macula densa in the distal convoluted tubule. The cells of the macula densa act as chemoreceptors sensitive to sodium. A fall in the concentration of sodium in the distal tubules will usually be associated with increased renin output.

The sympathetic nervous system seems to have an important influence on renin. Stimulation of β-adrenergic receptors enhances renin release. Blockade of these receptors with the β-adrenergic blocker propranolol decreases renin release. Humoral catecholamines as well as impulses transmitted by the renal nerves can increase renin secretion; indeed, it appears likely that an intact autonomic nervous system is required for normal release of renin. It is interesting that the two conditions which reduce effective plasma volume (upright posture or mild hemorrhage) also increase sympathomimetic activity.

ANGIOTENSIN

Renin acts as a specific protease to cleave the Leu-Leu bond of a glycoprotein (angiotensinogen) contained in the α_2-globulin fraction of plasma, releasing an inactive decapeptide, angiotensin I (Figure 9–5). This glycoprotein substrate for renin originates in the liver. The rate of the reaction of renin with its substrate has been studied by Krakoff. If one measures the rate of formation of angiotensin I with varying concentrations of renin substrate, one can determine the K_m (concentration of substrate at which the velocity of the reaction is half maximum) of the reaction. Apparently, this K_m is about 1000 ng/ml, or slightly below the normal plasma concentration of renin substrate. Both glucocorticoids and estrogens increase the concentration of renin substrate in the plasma; however, the maximum effect one could obtain by raising the concentration of plasma renin substrate would be a doubling of the rate of formation of angiotensin I. The concentration of renin is probably the more important factor in determining the amount of angiotensin I that is formed. There are antigenic differences among renins in various animal species. Hog renin, for example, will not attack human renin substrate.

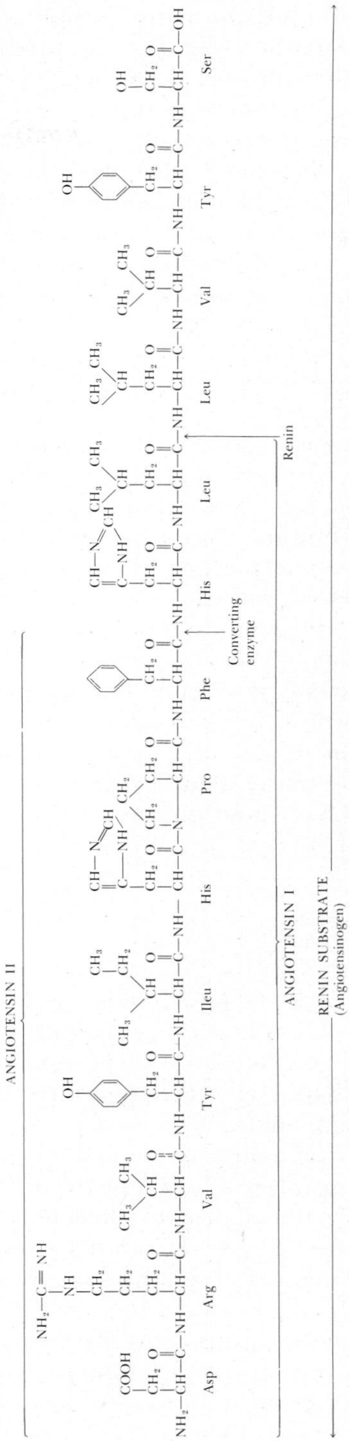

FIGURE 9–5. Amino acid sequences of renin substrate, angiotensin I, and angiotensin II.

A converting enzyme in the plasma removes the two C-terminal amino acids from angiotensin I (Figure 9–5), producing angiotensin II (Asp-Arg-Val-Tyr-Ileu-His-Pro-Phe), a powerful pressor agent which is also a potent simulus to aldosterone production. Angiotensin II, like ACTH and LH, apparently acts mainly in the early phases of steroid synthesis, between the cholesterol stage and the pregnenolone stage. Both angiotensin I and II can be found within the kidney, and the latter, by increasing sympathetic activity, can have direct effects on the kidney (it can act peripherally or in the central nervous system). For example, angiotensin II stimulates thirst and the release of vasopressin.

Potassium

Normally, a rise in serum potassium stimulates aldosterone production, whereas a fall in serum potassium inhibits it. The role of potassium does not depend upon the renin-angiotensin system; indeed, an increased potassium concentration stimulates aldosterone production but inhibits renin release. A small increase in the potassium concentration of the adrenal arterial plasma, with or without a concomitant decrease in sodium concentration, can significantly stimulate aldosterone secretion. An elevation of the potassium concentration by 0.5 mEq/l or less is a potent stimulus of aldosterone production but has no effect on the output of corticosterone or cortisol. It is possible to demonstrate enhanced aldosterone production by rat adrenal tissue incubated in vitro when the potassium concentration of the medium is raised. This effect, however, depends to a considerable extent on the relative concentrations of sodium and potassium in vivo.

ACTH

The regulation of aldosterone secretion is primarily mediated by the renin-angiotensin system and by potassium; however, there is no doubt that under certain conditions ACTH can increase the secretion of aldosterone. Probably it acts to increase the conversion of cholesterol to pregnenolone, and pregnenolone is a precursor of aldosterone as well as of cortisol. ACTH, the renin-angiotensin system, and potassium are all required for optimal control of aldosterone production and release. Sodium restriction is known to enhance the effect of ACTH on aldosterone secretion. The initial effect of ACTH is not sustained, and after about two days of ACTH treatment, the secretion rate for aldosterone will fall below normal values.

It is interesting that the plasma concentration of aldosterone is normal in Cushing's syndrome (p. 293); however, panhypopituitarism or removal of the pituitary gland diminishes aldosterone production and elicits a subnormal response to sodium restriction. This has suggested to some investigators that a special aldosterone-regulating factor (glomerulotropin) may be secreted by the pituitary gland.

ALDOSTERONE

In contrast to the milligrams of cortisol produced daily, aldosterone is secreted only in *microgram* amounts. Some aldosterone is bound to plasma proteins in the vascular compartment, but its affinity for proteins is less than that of the glucocorticoids. About 90 percent of circulating aldosterone is "inactivated" (metabolized to biologically inactive compounds) in a single passage through the liver. A small but significant inactivation occurs in the kidney.

The term *clearance rate* refers to the quantity of a compound *irreversibly* removed from the vascular compartment. The *secretion rate* and *clearance rate* of aldosterone are related as follows:

$$\text{aldosterone secretion rate} = \text{plasma concentration} \times \text{metabolic clearance rate.}$$

Thus the amount of aldosterone in the plasma can rise when the secretion rate increases, when the clearance rate declines, or when both changes occur. To determine the metabolic clearance rate of aldosterone, one can either determine the disposition of an infusion of radioactive aldosterone in the patient or simultaneously measure the secretion rate and plasma levels of endogenous aldosterone.

Active aldosterone molecules leave the vascular compartment and interact with specific receptors located in those tissues in which sodium is actively transported (tubular epithelial cells of the kidney, mucosal cells of the gut, epithelium in the salivary ducts, hepatic parenchymal cells, and brain cells). The biologic activity of aldosterone is determined both by its concentration at a given site and by the site's affinity for the hormone. Thus the activity of aldosterone can be heightened either by an increase in aldosterone concentration at the receptor site or by an enhanced affinity or quantity of the receptor. The mechanism of action of aldosterone was discussed in Chapter Seven.

The most common index of aldosterone metabolism is the urinary excretion of aldosterone (μg per day), although in fact it is the inactive metabolites of aldosterone that are measured. Because techniques of urine collection may be faulty, creatinine excretion should be measured simultaneously. The normal value for the aldosterone excretion rate (on an average salt intake of 80 to 100 mEq sodium per day) is 5 to 20 μg/24 hour urine.

The amount of sodium retained in the body is determined primarily by the action of aldosterone on the distal convoluted tubules of the kidney. Its effects on the proximal tubules and the loop of Henle are only minor. Daily administration of large doses of aldosterone to normal humans results in sodium retention of about 250 to 400 mEq and fluid retention of up to 2 to 3 liters. When these levels are reached, despite the continued administration of mineralocorticoid, no further sodium or water retention will take place. At this point the distal tubule is said to "escape" from the effects of aldosterone.

Although aldosterone is a major factor, it is only one of several affecting the kidney's regulation of sodium. Both glomerular filtration rate (GFR) and plasma volume help control sodium reabsorption in the kidney. When the GFR is decreased, the amount of sodium filtered by the renal glomeruli decreases, and less sodium is excreted in the urine. With a rise in GFR the amount of sodium filtered and excreted is increased. For a time, increased GFR was thought to be the mechanism of the escape from the effects of aldosterone; however, plasma volume appears to be the more likely agent. When plasma volume expands, sodium reabsorption in the proximal tubules falls immediately; however, natriuresis may not occur because distal tubular reabsorption of sodium is actually increased. *Progressively greater* volume expansion finally causes the transport capacity of the distal tubule to be exceeded, and sodium excretion markedly increases. A failure of this escape mechanism is an important factor in edema formation. Patients with edema from heart failure, cirrhosis of the liver, or nephrosis do not manifest this escape phenomenon.

There is some evidence of a humoral substance that can inhibit proximal tubular transport of sodium under conditions of volume expansion. This substance has been variously referred to as the *salt-losing hormone* or the *natriuretic factor*. Such a "hormone" could play a role in the escape mechanism; however, it would have to act solely on the kidney, since the salivary and sweat glands and the gastrointestinal tract do not escape from the sodium-retaining effect of aldosterone.

CONDITIONS OF ALDOSTERONE EXCESS

Excessive amounts of aldosterone may be produced by an adenomatous or hyperplastic adrenal (primary aldosteronism) or as a result of an alteration in extracellular fluid volume as detected by the kidney (secondary aldosteronism). The latter is mediated by the renin-angiotensin system.

Primary Aldosteronism (Figure 9–6)

The clinical syndrome first described by Conn (1955) is due to an aldosterone-secreting tumor. It is characterized by increased production of aldosterone, potassium depletion, and hypertension. The peak incidence of the condition occurs in the third or fourth decades of life; only seven or eight cases have been reported in children under the age of 16 years. The definition of primary aldosteronism has been broad-

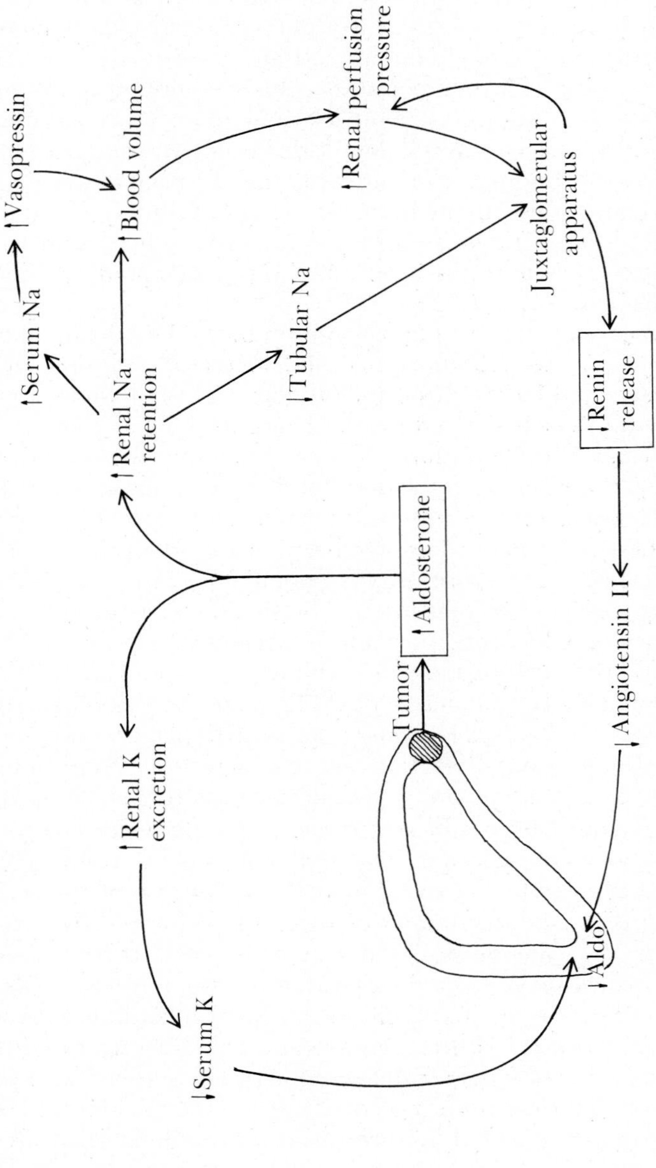

FIGURE 9–6. Primary aldosteronism – a disorder of the adrenal. See text for discussion.

ened by Lauler to include any condition of autonomous hypersecretion of aldosterone occurring in non-edematous hypertensive patients as a result of adrenal disease. The adrenal disease is a single cortical adenoma in 90 percent of cases, but there may be multiple adenomas, carcinoma, or bilateral hyperplasia.

The sequence of events in a condition of excess aldosterone might be predicted from our knowledge of water and electrolyte homeostasis. In the presence of a tumor secreting aldosterone, renal sodium retention occurs. It must be remembered that this secretion of aldosterone is autonomous and not subject to feedback regulation. Thus, although the concentration of plasma renin is low, aldosterone continues to be produced in excessive amounts. We might call this situation low renin aldosteronism to contrast it with the high renin values found in secondary aldosteronism (Figures 9–6 and 9–7). In other words, the renin-angiotensin system has been effectively eliminated as being the causative factor in this condition.

The increased concentration of sodium in the blood stimulates the osmoreceptors in the hypothalamus, and increased amounts of vasopressin are secreted by the posterior pituitary. This, of course, leads to water retention, which will reduce the concentration of sodium in the blood to normal. With continued sodium retention, two conditions develop. Firstly, the retention of sodium and the compensatory retention of water increase the blood volume. Since the osmolarity of the blood is being maintained constant, there is no osmotic gradient between blood and interstitial fluid and therefore no tendency for fluid to pass into the interstitial spaces (edema formation). The steadily increasing blood volume increases the blood pressure and hypertension results.

Secondly, the reabsorption of sodium in the renal tubules is dependent upon a Na/K exchange system. Thus the retention of sodium is at the expense of potassium loss, and potassium depletion develops. The symptoms of potassium depletion are characteristic. Neuromuscular transmission is dependent upon potassium, thus hypokalemia usually brings about symptoms of *muscular weakness* and *hypotonia.* The intracellular pool of potassium becomes depleted in an effort to restore the concentration of potassium in extracellular fluid. Because of the action of the sodium pump, sodium cannot replace potassium in cells in equivalent portions, and the intracellular cation deficit is corrected by hydrogen ions which move from the extracellular fluid into the cells. This hydrogen ion shift occurs in all cells of the body, including those of the renal tubules. More H^+ and less K^+ are available for secretion into the urine and the urine becomes acid. Secretion of H^+ is linked with HCO_3^- reabsorption and the concentration of HCO_3^- in the blood is raised. The loss of H^+ from extracellular fluid results in extracellular alkalosis. Such an alkalosis reduces the ionization of calcium salts and symptoms of muscle cramps or tetany may appear.

Prolonged potassium depletion causes lesions in the renal tubular cells. Severe hypokalemia always carries the danger of cardiac arrest.

Potassium depletion causes typical changes in the electrocardiogram, consisting in a prolongation of the Q-T interval, with widening of the T wave and occasional depression of the S-T segment.

Primary aldosteronism is treated surgically but should be preceded by replacement of body potassium. Potassium chloride is effective in the presence of alkalosis. With unilateral tumors, adrenalectomy is the operation of choice. With adrenal hyperplasia, the choice lies between total and subtotal adrenalectomy.

Secondary Aldosteronism (Figure 9–7)

As we have seen, a variety of factors can stimulate aldosterone production. However, in all cases of secondary aldosteronism, plasma renin activity is elevated. We have already cited the sodium deprived state which leads to increased renin activity in the plasma. Sodium depletion constitutes the most intense physiologic stimulus to aldosterone secretion known.

The plasma renin and aldosterone are increased during pregnancy (p. 101), perhaps by an estrogen-induced increase in renin substrate. In addition, progesterone is a specific competitive antagonist of aldosterone at receptor sites. The resulting sodium loss would activate the renin-angiotensin system in pregnancy.

Renal retention of sodium and water can bring about edema. Certain disorders predispose to the formation of edema. For example, in the *nephrotic syndrome,* the increased permeability of the renal glomeruli to protein leads to enormous losses of albumin. Eventually plasma albumin concentrations fall, with an associated decrease in osmotic pressure. Extracellular fluid then moves from the vascular compartment to the interstitial space, producing edema. Blood volume exerts an important influence on aldosterone release via the renin-angiotensin system; thus, the decreased blood volume in the nephrotic syndrome brings about a decreased renal perfusion pressure which is sensed by the juxtaglomular cells of the kidney. They in turn respond by releasing renin. The subsequent increase in aldosterone secretion causes salt and water retention, thus restoring the intravascular fluid volume.

A similar sequence of events occurs in *hepatic cirrhosis* with *ascites* except that the decreased serum albumin is due to decreased synthesis in the liver. Probably other forms of edema can be explained in a similar manner.

In 1962 Bartter described a condition characterized by hypokalemic alkalosis, polydipsia, polyuria, muscular weakness, and, frequently, stunted growth *(Bartter's syndrome).* In patients with this syndrome plasma renin activity is high and, following open renal biopsy, gross hypertrophy of the juxtaglomerular apparatus (juxtaglomerular cells plus the macula densa) and bilateral hypertrophy of the zona glomerulosa of the adrenals are evident. That these patients do not conserve sodium when receiving a sodium deficient diet suggests a defect in sodium

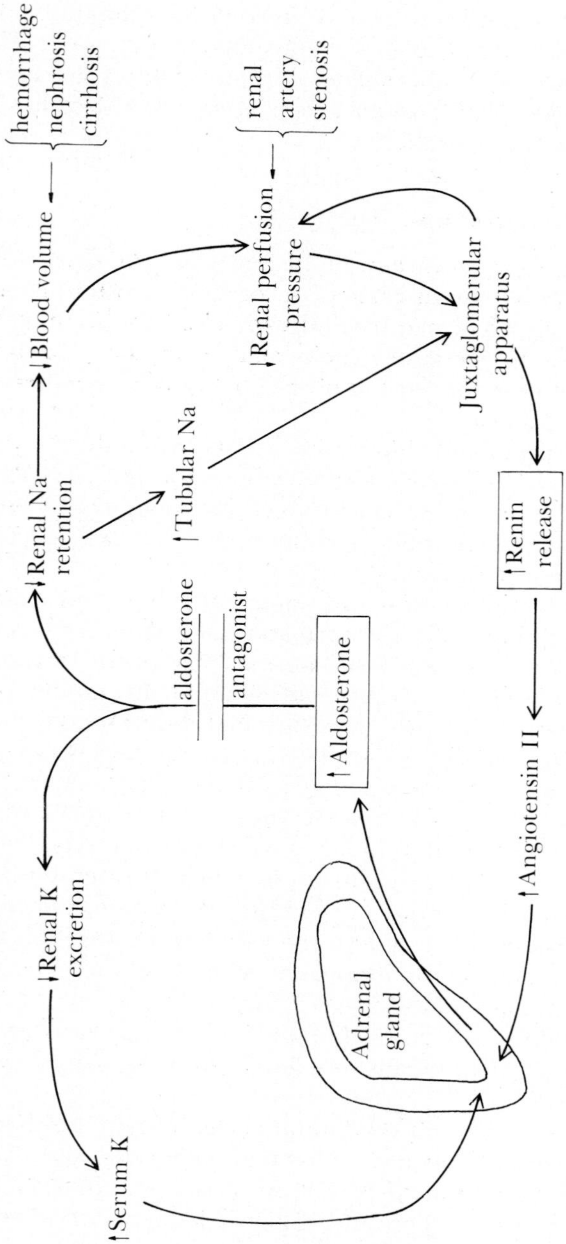

FIGURE 9–7. Secondary aldosteronism – a disorder reflecting stimulation of the renin-angiotensin system. See text for discussion.

reabsorption in the kidney. In addition, they fail to develop a pressor response following infusion of angiotensin II. It is therefore not surprising that these patients are normotensive.

Secondary aldosteronism is a frequent accompaniment of renal disease with renovascular hypertension. It is interesting to note that excess aldosterone, elevated plasma renin values, and slight elevations of both systolic and diastolic pressures have been observed in conjunction with oral contraceptive therapy. As in other cases of secondary aldosteronism, the main manifestation of aldosterone excess is hypokalemic alkalosis.

Differential diagnosis of primary vs. secondary aldosteronism. In both primary and secondary aldosteronism, the aldosterone secretion rate is high (normal equals 50 to 200 μg/24 hours); however, in the former the plasma renin activity is low, whereas in the latter it is high. In addition to the measurement of plasma renin activity, several other tests are helpful in differentiating primary adrenal disease from other conditions which result in excessive production of aldosterone (Table 9–1).

One such test is the measurement of plasma renin activity before and after expansion of the plasma volume with an infusion of saline. A "salt load" suppresses the renin-angiotensin system. If the excessive aldosterone production is due to renin excess, suppression of renin should decrease aldosterone secretion. This occurs in secondary aldosteronism, but in primary aldosteronism aldosterone secretion is independent of circulating levels of renin-angiotensin. Thus further suppression of renin does not materially affect the rate of aldosterone secretion.

Another test involves the administration of deoxycorticosterone acetate to the patient. Much the same principle applies as in the "salt load" test. Deoxycorticosterone acetate is a powerful stimulus to sodium-retention and, in effect, it brings about volume expansion through its sodium-

TABLE 9–1. Differential Diagnosis of Primary vs. Secondary Aldosteronism*

	ASR	PRA	ASR after Salt Load	ASR after DOCA	Response to Spironolactone	Aldosterone Concentration in Adrenal Vein Effluent
Primary Aldosteronism	+	−	+	+	positive	+
Secondary Aldosteronism	+	+	−	−	negative	normal

*Abbreviations and symbols used in the table are as follows:
ASR = Aldosterone secretory rate;
PRA = Plasma renin activity;
DOCA = Deoxycorticosterone acetate;
+ = increased;
− = decreased.

retaining activity. The expanded volume suppresses renin release. Plasma renin activity decreases and aldosterone secretory rate should decrease, unless primary adrenal disease is present.

Specific antagonists to aldosterone, the spironolactones (17-hydroxy-17-propionyl steroid lactones), have found wide clinical use. These steroid lactones occupy aldosterone receptor sites, thereby preempting these sites from aldosterone control. They can be used also for diagnostic tests. In primary aldosteronism one can usually demonstrate a positive response to spironolactones. Thus high doses (400 mg per day in adults) of a spironolactone over three to five weeks will normalize the blood pressure. The response is usually negative in secondary aldosteronism.

Perhaps the clearest diagnostic sign of all is finding a markedly elevated aldosterone concentration in the adrenal vein effluent on one side only. This indicates a unilateral aldosterone-secreting tumor.

TREATMENT OF SECONDARY ALDOSTERONISM. Since increased aldosterone secretion is secondary to primary extra-adrenal disease, the goal of therapy should be control of the primary disease. Nephrotic syndrome and hepatic cirrhosis require medical management to prevent hypoproteinemia. Aldosterone antagonists may be helpful in those cases where clear-cut aldosterone excess is present. Conditions such as congestive heart failure and hypertension often are accompanied by aldosteronism. These disorders are found more frequently with advancing age and will be discussed in Chapter Fourteen. It has been difficult to devise appropriate treatment for Bartter's syndrome. Since the basic defect is probably renal tubular failure to reabsorb sodium, one would expect that a high salt diet might be helpful; however, this measure alone may intensify potassium loss and alkalosis.

Part of the difficulty in treating secondary aldosteronism is the complexity of the homeostatic mechanisms involved and the various entities which can alter electrolyte balance. Nevertheless, our growing knowledge of the renin-angiotensin system and other factors regulating aldosterone secretion will undoubtedly aid in our understanding of clinical syndromes associated with edema, hypertension, and heart failure.

CONDITIONS OF INSUFFICIENT ALDOSTERONE

Just as excessive aldosterone often leads to hypokalemia, alkalosis, and hypertension, so insufficient aldosterone may lead to hyperkalemia, salt loss, acidosis, and hypotension. The deficiency of aldosterone may be due to primary disease of either the pituitary or the adrenal.

Congenital Adrenal Hypoplasia

In most cases of adrenal hypoplasia in which autopsies have been performed, the pituitary gland was absent or hypoplastic, suggesting that the adrenal hypoplasia was secondary to pituitary hypoplasia. Although symptoms may develop acutely in the first 48 hours of life and lead to sudden death, more often a salt-losing syndrome develops during the second or third week of life. The symptoms of the salt-losing syndrome include dehydration, poor feeding, failure to gain weight, intermittent fever, and vomiting. The earliest detectable abnormality of the plasma electrolytes is usually hyperkalemia, but hyponatremia and metabolic acidosis also develop. In addition to adrenal hypoplasia, adrenal *hyperplasia* secondary to a defect in 21-hydroxylase may be a cause of hypoaldosteronism and salt loss (p. 161).

Congenital Hypoaldosteronism

In patients with hypoaldosteronism there is evidence of insufficient aldosterone (dehydration, hyponatremia, hyperkalemia) but no evidence of lack of glucocorticoids. Visser and Cost first suggested a defect in 18-hydroxylation as the underlying abnormality, and this may be the cause in certain cases (p. 163); however, subsequent studies have shown an excessive production of 18-hydroxycorticosterone in many of these patients, suggesting that the final step of aldosterone synthesis—the conversion of 18-hydroxycorticosterone to aldosterone—may be impaired. The enzyme at fault, 18-hydroxysteroid dehydrogenase, only occurs in the cells of the zona glomerulosa. Compensatory mechanisms for these defects frequently develop in later years and steroid therapy may be necessary for only the first few years of life.

Addison's Disease

Destruction of all zones of the adrenal produces the characteristic Addisonian deficiency of both glucocorticoids and mineralocorticoids. In Addison's original patients, the destruction of the adrenal was due to tuberculosis; however, this is now a very rare cause of Addison's disease, at least in the developed countries.

Other causes of Addison's disease may be adrenal hemorrhage in the neonatal period (adrenal function becoming progressively impaired as the child develops), idiopathic adrenal atrophy (possibly secondary to an autoimmune phenomenon), or familial disease which may include other endocrine glands (multiple endocrine disorders, p. 253).

The onset of the chronic form of adrenocortical insufficiency is gradual. Lassitude, muscular weakness, anorexia, weight loss, vomiting and diarrhea may be evident. Dehydration may be marked, and blood pressure is low. Episodes of hypoglycemia are not uncommon. The typical bronze hyperpigmentation is often striking on the extensor surfaces of joints, about the nail beds, on the back of the neck, and particularly about the genitals, nipples, umbilicus, and axillae. Pigmentation in children seldom reaches the degree found in adults.

The sudden onset of adrenal failure in a subject with previously normal adrenocortical function, such as occurs following bilateral adrenal hemorrhage, is commonly known as the *Waterhouse-Friderichsen syndrome.* The features are essentially those of acute shock and peripheral circulatory failure. Patients with chronic adrenal insufficiency may develop acute failure secondary to stresses such as infection, injury, or surgery.

SUMMARY

These discussions have emphasized the many ways in which sodium and water homeostasis are interrelated. The shifts of fluids between intracellular and extracellular compartments, which depend on differences in osmotic pressure, are due mainly to changes in sodium concentration. Aldosterone is the most important factor affecting sodium concentration in body fluids. Thus, factors which control aldosterone secretion are potential regulators not only of sodium homeostasis but also fluid balance. Among the important regulators of aldosterone secretion is the renin-angiotensin system, which in turn is responsive to changes in blood volume.

Vasopressin is the most important factor regulating the water content of the body. Its secretion is controlled by plasma osmolarity, which in turn is determined primarily by the sodium concentration. The close relationship of sodium and water homeostasis is evident from these interacting regulating factors.

Potassium can be readily lost from the gastrointestinal tract and in the urine; however, the body's mechanism for potassium repletion is poor. The ready exchange of sodium for both potassium and hydrogen in all body cells complicates the matter. The loss of intracellular potassium (to make up extracellular deficiency) is replaced partly by sodium and partly by hydrogen. This results in extracellular alkalosis and intracellular acidosis.

Disorders of water and electrolyte balance occur frequently in the childhood years. In some cases, an endocrine cause for the disordered metabolism can be found. In most cases of endocrine disorder, either the pituitary or the adrenal cortex is implicated.

SUGGESTED READINGS

Vasopressin, G. Alan Robison, R. W. Butcher, and E. W. Sutherland, *Cyclic AMP* (Chapter 10), Academic Press, New York, 1971.

A detailed and beautifully developed discussion of the role of cyclic AMP in the mechanism of action of vasopressin. Other factors affecting permeability of membranes are also discussed in relation to the cyclic AMP system. These include theophylline, aldosterone, the catecholamines, prostaglandins, and ions.

Vasopressin-resistant diabetes insipidus, J. Orloff and M. B. Burg, in *The Metabolic Basis of*

Inherited Disease, p. 1567, edited by J. Stanbury, J. B. Wyngaarden, and D. S. Fredrickson, McGraw-Hill Book Company, New York, 1972.
A fine description of water balance, with a particularly lucid discussion of the countercurrent theory. Nephrogenic diabetes insipidus is covered in detail and appropriate references are included.

Mineralocorticoids, I. S. Edelman and D. D. Fanestil, in *Biochemical Actions of Hormones, Vol. 1,* p. 321, edited by G. Litwak, Academic Press, New York, 1970.
Dr. Edelman, a renowned authority in the field, and his coauthor trace the sequence of biochemical events during the action of aldosterone in target cells. The student of biochemical endocrinology will find this chapter most enlightening.

Aldosterone: physiological and pathophysiological variations in man, J. J. Brown, R. Fraser, A. F. Lever, and J. I. S. Robertson, Clinics in Endocrinology and Metabolism, *Vol. 1, No. 2,* p. 397, W. B. Saunders Co., Philadelphia, 1972.
A discussion of both physiologic and pathologic alterations in aldosterone secretion and excretion. The authors attempt to relate clinical conditions to basic pathophysiology of electrolyte homeostasis. An excellent review of the subject, with pertinent references.

PERTINENT SELECTIONS FROM THE LITERATURE

Bartter, F. C. and Schwartz, W. B. The syndrome of inappropriate secretion of antidiuretic hormone. Am. J. Med. *42*:790, 1967.

Cain, J. P. et al. The regulation of aldosterone secretion in primary aldosteronism. Am. J. Med. *53*:627, 1972.

Cheng, K. W. and Friesen, H. G. The isolation and characterization of human neurophysins. J. Clin. Endocrinol. Metab. *34*:165, 1972.

George, J. M., Capen, C. C., and Phillips, A. S. Biosynthesis of vasopressin in vitro and ultrastructure of a bronchogenic carcinoma. J. Clin. Invest. *51*:141, 1972.

Melby, J. C. et al. Diagnosis and localization of aldosterone producing adenomas by adrenal vein catheterization. New Engl. J. Med. *277*:1050, 1967.

Sachs, H. Biosynthesis and release of vasopressin. Am. J. Med. *42*:687, 1967.

Williams, G. H. and Dluhy, R. G.: Aldosterone biosynthesis. Interrelationship of regulatory factors. Am. J. Med. *53*:595, 1972.

CHAPTER TEN

Homeostasis: Glucose

Maintaining the concentration of glucose in the blood within rather narrow limits requires the carefully coordinated actions of a host of physiologic and endocrine mechanisms. This regulation is performed for the fetus in utero largely by the mother. The sensitivity of the pancreatic islets to cyclic AMP-mediated stimuli becomes established in early fetal life (p. 73), whereas sensitivity to glucose develops later and is still somewhat underdeveloped at birth. The infant of the diabetic mother (see Chapter Six) has pancreatic islets which respond readily to glucose, apparently due to intra-uterine exposure to hyperglycemia. Once the β cells have fully matured and can respond to both glucose and other stimuli for insulin release, the concentration of glucose in the blood of the normal individual can usually be maintained within certain limits.

In the postabsorptive state, the concentration of glucose in the blood varies between 80 and 100 mg/100 ml. After ingestion of a meal rich in carbohydrate, it may rise to 120 to 130 mg/100 ml, and during fasting it decreases to 60 to 70 mg/100 ml. Under normal circumstances, the concentration of glucose in the blood is controlled within these limits; however, certain conditions predispose to hyperglycemia or hypoglycemia. Many of these conditions are the result of alterations in the normal endocrine control of intermediary metabolism. Therefore, before discussing diabetes mellitus and the various hypoglycemic states of the young child, let us review the regulation of intermediary metabolism by hormones.

HORMONAL REGULATION OF INTERMEDIARY METABOLISM

In most human diets, carbohydrates account for a large fraction of the total daily caloric intake. The carbohydrates that are ingested provide a source of blood glucose, and, to a variable extent, a source of the fat deposited in adipose tissue. The major significance of carbohydrate in metabolism is that is serves as a fuel—as substrates to be oxidized—and that it provides biologically useful energy to drive other metabolic processes. Cells utilize carbohydrate primarily in the form of glucose, although fructose becomes important if the intake of sucrose (a disaccharide of glucose and fructose) is high. Galactose becomes significant when the milk sugar lactose (a disaccharide of glucose and galactose) is the principal carbohydrate of the diet, as in infancy.

Hexokinase

The first step in the metabolism of glucose within the cell is its enzymatic phosphorylation at carbon 6. Glucose, however, can freely enter only liver cells. Cells of extrahepatic tissues are relatively impermeable to glucose and require the presence of insulin to permit glucose entrance. Once glucose has entered extrahepatic cells, its conversion to glucose-6-phosphate is catalyzed by hexokinase. This enzyme has a rather low Michaelis constant (K_m) for glucose and is inhibited by glucose-6-phosphate, thus providing feedback control of glucose uptake.

The liver is freely permeable to glucose and the rate limiting factor for glucose metabolism in the liver appears to be the activity of the enzyme glucokinase, which catalyzes the conversion of glucose to glucose-6-phosphate. Glucokinase has a higher K_m for glucose (10^{-2} M) than does hexokinase and is specifically concerned with glucose phosphorylation when the concentration of glucose in the blood, and hence in the liver, is high (Figure 10–1). Liver cells also contain hexokinase. Both enzymes, hexokinase and glucokinase, compete for the substrate, glucose. The activity of hexokinase is not affected by hormones or substrate concentration (at physiologic levels), whereas the activity of glucokinase is increased by insulin and high blood glucose concentrations.

The concentration of glucose in the blood can affect the rate of glucose uptake by various tissues, depending upon the K_m values of the enzymes in the tissue. For example, the phosphorylation of glucose

$$\text{Glucose} + \text{ATP} \xrightarrow{Mg^{++}} \text{Glucose-6-phosphate} + \text{ADP}$$

is catalyzed in the liver by glucokinase or hexokinase and in the brain by hexokinase. The term hexokinase implies that this enzyme is relatively non-specific for the kind of hexose phosphorylated. The reaction is essentially irreversible under the conditions prevalent in tissues. The concentration of ATP in liver and brain is maintained at or about 0.001M, considerably greater than the K_m for either enzyme; hence, ATP is not rate-limiting in the reaction.

The glucose concentration in the blood supplying the brain may vary from 0.003M (fasting) to 0.008M (after a carbohydrate meal), but it is always well above the K_m of brain hexokinase ($\sim 5 \times 10^{-5}$M). Actually, the concentration of glucose in blood must drop to nearly 0.001M (18 mg/100 ml) before disturbances of the central nervous system are noted in most humans. Thus the brain hexokinase is always nearly saturated with glucose and is relatively insensitive to fluctuating amounts in the blood.

The situation in the liver is quite different. The K_m of liver glucokinase for glucose is much higher (2×10^{-2}M) and, since the K_m is equal to that substrate concentration at which the reaction velocity is half maximal, at normal glucose concentrations the liver enzyme is operating far below its maximal activity (V_{max}). The liver receives blood from the intestine through the portal circulation as well as from the arterial circulation (Figure 10–1). The portal blood after a meal may have substantially higher concentrations of glucose than does peripheral arterial blood and may be capable of increasing the velocity of the glucokinase reaction. Thus the uptake of glucose by the liver can be enhanced by virtue of the high K_m of liver glucokinase. This is consistent with the physiological role of the liver, which ordinarily produces glucose rather than consuming it. The liver removes more glucose from the blood than it produces only during brief periods of elevated glucose concentration in the portal system after eating.

Glucose, of course, is one of the major stimulators of the synthesis and release of insulin. It is, therefore, of interest to consider how glucose gets into the β cell of the pancreas to produce its effects. Two groups of investigators have concluded, on the basis of kinetic experiments, that mouse pancreatic islets contain hexokinases characterized by two different K_m values for glucose (10^{-5}M and 10^{-2}M). One of these would be analogous to the glucokinase of liver. The low K_m enzyme could function at low concentrations of glucose in the blood, whereas the high K_m enzyme could function during periods of hyperglycemia to facilitate the metabolism of glucose in the β cell and the subsequent release of insulin from the cell. In vitro studies have shown that enhancement of insulin secretion by glucose usually requires a concentration of glucose over 50 mg/100 ml. (3.5×10^{-3}M).

This comparison of glucose uptake in various tissues illustrates the point that substrate concentration itself can control the rate of phosphorylation of glucose. There is some evidence that insulin and/or glucocorticoids may be involved in the synthesis or activation of glucokinase. Weber and others have postulated that insulin induces specific enzymes, such as glucokinase and phosphofructokinase, involved in glycolysis. Glucocorticoids have been used successfully to stimulate the appearance of glucokinase activity in livers of newborn rats. This latter

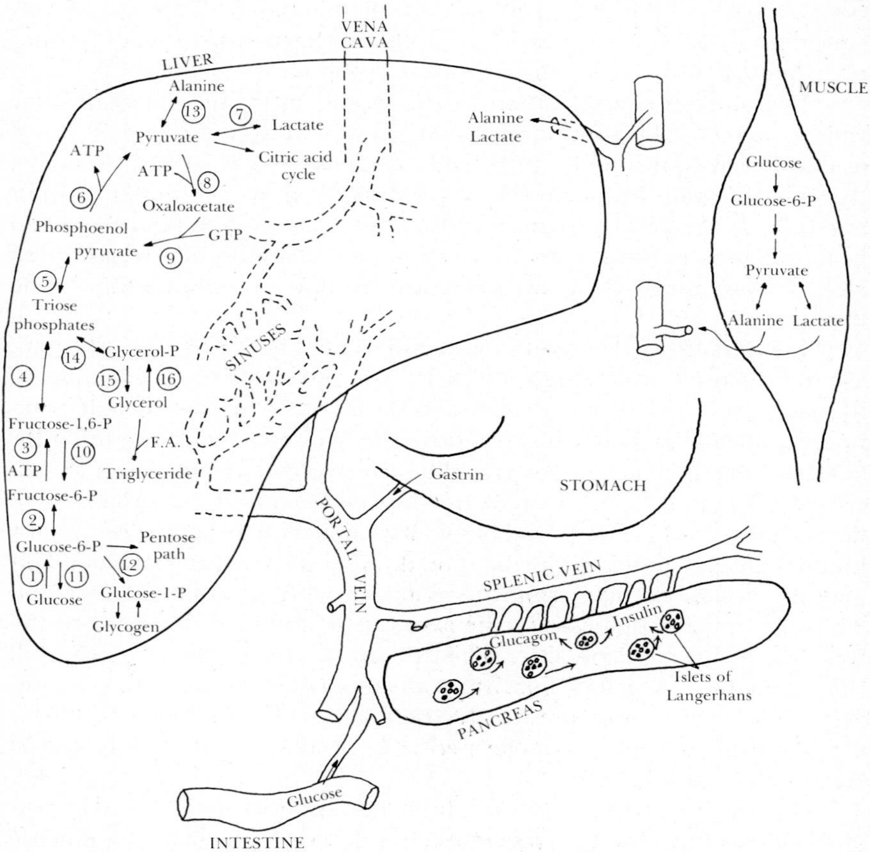

FIGURE 10–1. Glycolysis and gluconeogenesis in liver. The numbers refer to reactions catalyzed by the following enzymes: (1) glucokinase or hexokinase, (2) phosphohexose isomerase, (3) phosphofructokinase, (4) aldolase, (5) sequence of reactions catalyzed in order by 3-phosphoglyceraldehyde dehydrogenase, 3-phosphoglycerate kinase, phosphoglycerate mutase, and enolase (one mole of ATP is formed), (6) pyruvate kinase, (7) lactic dehydrogenase, (8) pyruvate carboxylase, (9) phosphoenolpyruvate carboxykinase, (10) fructose diphosphatase, (11) glucose-6-phosphatase, (12) phosphoglucomutase, (13) aminotransferase, (14) 3-phosphoglycerol dehydrogenase, (15) glycerol phosphatase, and (16) glycerokinase.

effect may be a glucocorticoid function peculiar to the maturation of fetal and neonatal tissues.

GLYCOLYSIS

Glucose-6-phosphate is situated at the branch point of several metabolic pathways (Figure 10–1). Depending on the tissue involved and the conditions prevailing, glucose-6-phosphate may be metabolized by either the glycolytic or the pentose pathway; it may be converted to glycogen for storage; or it may be hydrolyzed to yield glucose. Glycolysis occurs in all cells and is the exclusive pathway for glucose metabolism in red blood cells. The reversal of glycolysis is important in gluconeogenesis.

The conversion of glucose-6-phosphate to fructose-6-phosphate is catalyzed by *phosphohexose isomerase.* A second phosphorylation catalyzed by *phosphofructokinase* requires ATP as phosphate donor. Like the phosphorylation of glucose with ATP, this reaction is exergonic and not reversible. The cleavage of fructose-1,6-diphosphate, catalyzed by *aldolase,* is reversible; indeed, the equilibrium favors the condensation of the resulting two trioses (Figure 10–1). The interconversion of the two trioses, 3-phosphoglyceraldehyde and dihydroxyacetone phosphate, is a readily reversible reaction catalyzed by *triose phosphate isomerase.* Dihydroxyacetone phosphate is in the unique position of serving as substrate for three enzymes: aldolase, triose phosphate isomerase, and *3-phosphoglycerol dehydrogenase.* The latter catalyzes the conversion of dihydroxyacetone phosphate to glycerol-3-phosphate, using NADH as cofactor. In liver the K_m values suggest that the principal role of the enzyme is to generate glycerol for lipid synthesis (Figure 10–1). The isomerase directs dihydroxyacetone phosphate back into the main stream of glycolysis, the further metabolism of 3-phosphoglyceraldehyde. The latter is converted to 1,3-diphosphoglyceric acid (3-phosphoglyceraldehyde dehydrogenase). The phosphate in the 1 position is transferred to ADP (3-phosphoglycerate kinase), yielding 3-phosphoglyceric acid and one mole of ATP. The 3-phosphoglyceric acid is then converted to phosphoenol pyruvate via 2-phosphoglyceric acid (phosphoglycerate mutase and enolase). The conversion of phosphoenol pyruvate to pyruvate is catalyzed by *pyruvate kinase* (Figure 10–1), and in the reaction a mole of ATP is formed.

In the metabolism of 3-phosphoglyceraldehyde to pyruvate, two moles of ATP are formed from ADP and inorganic phosphate. Thus from one mole of glucose (yielding two triose phosphates) four moles of ATP are formed; however, since the initial investment of two ATP's for the phosphorylation of glucose and fructose-6-phosphate must be subtracted, the net energy gain is two moles of ATP for each mole of glucose metabolized via the glycolytic cycle to pyruvate.

Under anaerobic conditions, there is no oxygen to accept the hydrogens of the reduced pyridine nucleotides generated in the glycolytic cycle at 3-phosphoglyceraldehyde dehydrogenase. Instead, the enzyme *lactic dehydrogenase* catalyzes the reduction of pyruvate to lactate, during which hydrogens are transferred from NADH to form NAD. When the lactate production is added to the stoichiometry of the production of pyruvate, the overall reaction is:

$$\text{glucose} + 2\text{ADP} + 2\text{ phosphates} \longrightarrow 2\text{ lactates} + 2H_2O + 2\text{ATP}.$$

Glycolysis therefore represents the dismutation of glucose into two moles of lactate with the concomitant production of two moles of ATP; it does not involve a consumption of oxygen.

This does not mean that glycolysis cannot occur aerobically. In the presence of oxygen, less glucose is utilized and the accumulation of lactate is largely suppressed as pyruvate is metabolized further in the citric acid cycle. This results in a higher yield of energy per molecule of glucose, since the complete oxidation of pyruvate to carbon dioxide and water produces 36 moles of ATP, in contrast to the net gain of two moles of ATP in glycolysis. This effect of oxygen on glucose utilization and lactate accumulation (the *Pasteur effect*) is not exhibited by all tissues. Retina, kidney medulla, and intestinal mucosa continue to form appreciable amounts of lactate even in the presence of oxygen.

Cori cycle

It is possible to convert lactate back to glucose by the reversal of the steps of glycolysis (Figure 10–1). This is an expensive process (six moles of high energy phosphate consumed for each mole of glucose formed); however, the maintenance of a constant blood glucose overrides such considerations. For instance, large amounts of lactate may be produced from glucose by muscle during exercise. This lactate is carried by the circulation to the liver, where it can be converted back to glucose to maintain the concentration of glucose in the blood and to replenish the carbohydrate stores in the muscle. This cycle of glucose to lactate in muscle and lactate to glucose in the liver is called the *Cori cycle.*

How is the reversal of glycolysis achieved? In the liver, lactate is converted to pyruvate. A portion of the pyruvate is oxidized to acetyl coenzyme A, which is subsequently metabolized in the citric acid cycle, and much of the remainder is used to produce glucose. More energy is required to convert pyruvate to glucose than is obtained in the conversion of glucose to pyruvate (Figure 10–1). Pyruvate is initially converted to phosphoenol pyruvate by a pair of reactions, each requiring high-energy phosphate. The first step is a carboxylation of pyruvate catalyzed by the mitochondrial enzyme *pyruvate carboxylase* with biotin as coenzyme. This enzyme is unusual in requiring two metallic ions: Mg^{++} and Mn^{++}. Another unusual and important feature is its absolute requirement for the presence of acetyl coenzyme A. The latter does not participate in the reaction; rather, it seems to act as a modulator. Since pyruvate can diffuse in and out of mitochondria but acetyl coenzyme A cannot, gluconeogenesis in the cytosol is dependent on oxidative metabolism in the mitochondria. The oxaloacetate formed in the first step is converted to phosphoenol pyruvate (Figure 10–1); the reaction is catalyzed by *phosphoenolpyruvate carboxykinase,* but again the price is another high-energy phosphate, this time in the form of guanosine triphosphate (GTP). In contrast to the one-step conversion of phosphoenolpyruvate to pyruvate in which ATP is generated, the reverse reaction is a two-step process which requires two high-energy phosphates (ATP and GTP) to drive it (Figure 10–1).

Phosphoenol pyruvate can be converted to fructose diphosphate readily by a simple reversal of the ordinary glycolytic reactions. The hydrolysis of fructose diphosphate to fructose-6-phosphate controls the rate of gluconeogenesis, whereas the activity of phosphofructokinase (fructose-6-phosphate $\longrightarrow$ fructose 1,6-diphosphate) controls glycolysis. The relative rates of the two reactions are regulated by the concentration of AMP, which inhibits *fructose diphosphatase* and also relieves the inhibition of phosphofructokinase by ATP. This key enzyme, fructose diphosphatase, is present in liver, kidney, and striated muscle.

Another control point for gluconeogenesis is at the enzyme *glucose-6-phosphatase,* which catalyzes the conversion of glucose-6-phosphate to glucose (Figure 10–1). It is present in intestine, liver, and kidney, where it enables these particular tissues to add glucose to the blood.

The activities of these critical gluconeogenic enzymes (pyruvate carboxylase, phosphoenolpyruvate carboxykinase, fructose-1,6-diphosphatase, and glucose-6-phosphatase) are under hormonal control. It has been proposed by Weber that the synthesis of groups of enzymes is controlled by the same functional genetic unit. According to Weber's theory, the glucocorticoids function as stimulators and insulin acts as an inhibitor of the synthesis of the key hepatic gluconeogenic enzymes. Insulin is able to prevent the stimulation of synthesis of new enzymes by glucocorticoids; on the other hand, glucocorticoids have no effect on the activity of glycolytic enzymes (glucokinase, phosphofructokinase, pyruvate kinase) which are sensitive to induction by insulin. Insulin, which is responsive to the concentration of glucose in the blood, directly controls the activity of enzymes responsible for glycolysis and, by preventing their stimulation by cortisol, indirectly controls those responsible for gluconeogenesis. All of these effects, which can be explained on the basis of new enzyme synthesis, can be prevented by agents such as puromycin which block the synthesis of new protein.

Sources of Pyruvate for Gluconeogenesis

Transamination

The interconversion of amino acids and keto acids is catalyzed by *aminotransferases* (or *transaminases).* Bound to the enzyme is the coenzyme pyridoxal phosphate. The amino acid reacts with the pyridoxal phosphate to form a *Schiff base.* A rearrangement within this bound form can produce bound *pyridoxamine,* with the release of the corresponding keto acid. The amino group is transferred from the pyridoxamine to another keto acid. For instance, when alanine undergoes transamination, pyruvate is formed (Figure 10–1), while α-ketoglutarate receives the amino group to form glutamic acid. The equilibrium constant for most transaminase reactions is close to unity; therefore, the reaction is freely reversible. Transamination can function in *both* the synthesis and catabolism of amino acids.

Aminotransferases are specific for the particular amino-keto pair. In the reaction catalyzed by tyrosine-α-ketoglutarate aminotransferase, tyrosine is converted to ρ-hydroxyphenyl pyruvate, while α-ketoglutarate (accepting the amino group from tyrosine) forms glutamate. The synthesis of tyrosine-α-ketoglutarate aminotransferase is increased in mammalian liver by glucocorticoids, glucagon, and epinephrine. Insulin also stimulates the synthesis of this enzyme. The synthesis of alanine-α-ketoglutarate aminotransferase is also increased in mammalian liver by glucocorticoids. Indeed, alanine may play a special role in gluconeogenesis. Studies in man during fasting have shown that alanine is the major glycogenic amino acid. Since amino acids during fasting are derived from the breakdown of protein, and since muscle, the major source of protein, contains relatively little alanine (6 to 8 percent), Cahill has proposed that in the fasting state alanine is synthesized de novo from pyruvate in muscle and provides the major substrate for gluconeogenesis in the liver (Figure 10–1). Direct analysis of arterial-deep venous differences in the forearm has shown that in both the postabsorptive state and prolonged fasting, alanine is the principal amino acid released from muscle.

Oxidative Deamination

Amino acids can be directly oxidized (deaminated) to their keto acids. For example, the removal of the nitrogen (as ammonia) from glutamate, yielding α-ketoglutarate, is catalyzed by *glutamic dehydrogenase.* This enzyme uses either NAD or NADP as cofactor. The reaction is reversible. Since α-ketoglutarate is an intermediate in the citric acid cycle, this reaction provides a way to funnel the carbon chains of amino acids into the cycle to provide oxaloacetate for the synthesis of phosphoenol pyruvate and, ultimately, of glucose.

Glycerol

The cleavage of triglycerides yields free fatty acids and glycerol. A glycerokinase, present in liver and kidney, catalyzes the conversion of glycerol to α-glycerophosphate, which can be oxidized to dihydroxyacetone phosphate (Figure 10–1). Thus liver and kidney are able to convert glycerol to glucose via the triose phosphates. Lipolysis is under hormonal control (p. 424).

Glycogen synthesis and breakdown (Figure 10–2)

Several other metabolic pathways are available to glucose-6-phosphate. In the synthesis of glycogen, the glucose-6-phosphate must be converted to glucose-1-phosphate by phosphoglucomutase, thereafter reacting with UTP to form uridine diphosphate glucose (Figure 10–2). In this form the carbon 1 of glucose can form a glycosidic bond with carbon 4 of a terminal glucose residue of glycogen, a reaction catalyzed by *glycogen synthetase.* In successive reactions, additional glucose residues are added in 1,4 linkages until the chain has been lengthened by 6 to 11 glucose residues. At this point, part of the 1,4 chain is transferred to a neighboring chain in 1,6 linkage, thereby creating a branch point in the glucose polymer (*branching enzyme*).

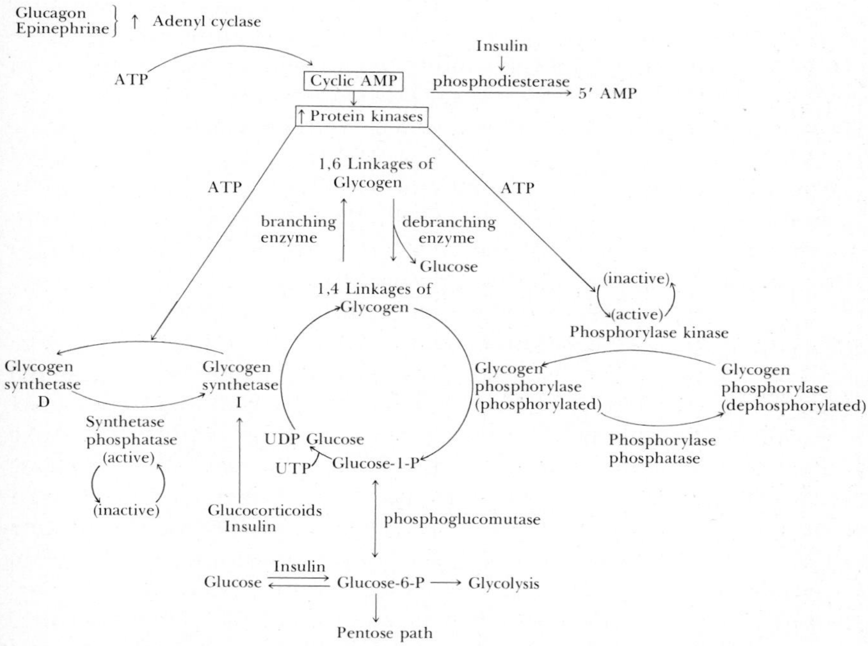

FIGURE 10–2. Regulation of glycogen synthesis and breakdown in liver.

In muscle and liver, glycogen synthetase is present in two interconvertible forms: *synthetase D* (dependent), which is totally dependent for its activity on the presence of glucose-6-phosphate, and *synthetase I* (independent), a form with a K_m for UDPG that decreases in the presence of glucose-6-phosphate. Synthetase D is converted to synthetase I by the enzyme *synthetase phosphatase* (Figure 10–2). During the reaction, one of the serine residues of the synthetase D is dephosphorylated and before the enzyme can act again it must be rephosphorylated. Synthetase I is phosphorylated to form synthetase D, with ATP acting as the phosphate donor and *cyclic AMP-dependent protein kinase (synthetase kinase)* catalyzing the reaction. In resting muscle and in liver that is receiving glucose, the enzyme is in a nonphosphorylated (I), active form; in contracting muscle and in liver that is releasing glucose under the influence of epinephrine or glucagon, the enzyme is phosphorylated (D) and almost inactive. However, in the presence of a sufficiently high concentration of glucose-6-phosphate, the phosphorylated (D) form exhibits almost full activity.

It can be seen that by "activating" or "inactivating" glycogen synthetase, control of glycogen synthesis is achieved. The activity of synthetase kinase is dependent upon cyclic AMP; therefore, hormones which alter the amount of this nucleotide in the cell will exert an influence on the synthesis of glycogen. Glucagon and epinephrine increase the activity of adenyl cyclase in the liver, which leads to an increase in cyclic AMP. The latter activates synthetase kinase, which converts glycogen synthetase from the active (I) to the inactive form (D). The net effect is decreased glycogen synthesis. Insulin increases the activity of synthetase I, possibly by stimulating phosphodiesterase and thus causing a reduction in the intracellular concentration of cyclic AMP (Figure 10–2). Glucocorticoids also increase the amount of active glycogen synthetase; however, the effect appears two to three hours after administration of hormone and involves de novo enzyme synthesis (Figure 10–2).

The reverse process, glycogenolysis, is catalyzed by glycogen *phosphorylase,* which breaks the 1,4 linkages of glycogen to yield glucose-1-phosphate. Phosphorylase is another enzyme which exists in an active and an inactive form. The active phosphorylase *(phosphophosphorylase)* is phosphorylated in an ester linkage with the hydroxyl group of one of the serine residues. By the action of *phosphorylase phosphatase,* the enzyme can be inactivated to *dephosphophosphorylase* (removal of phosphate from serine). Reactivation of the phosphorylase requires ATP and a specific *phosphorylase kinase* which is activated by a cyclic AMP-dependent protein kinase (Figure 10–2). Phosphophosphorylase in muscle is a tetramer containing four moles of pyridoxal phosphate (phosphorylase a). When inactivated, the dimer, dephosphophosphorylase (phosphorylase b), is formed.

The *protein kinases,* activated by cyclic AMP, catalyze the transfer of the γ-phosphate group of ATP to serine hydroxyl groups in proteins. A small protein (MW $\simeq$ 35,000) is the actual catalytic enzyme, associated with a larger protein. The latter inhibits the activity of the smaller catalytic unit. It is the binding of the inhibitor portion to cyclic AMP which results in a conformational change that releases the catalytic unit from the inhibition placed upon it. Thus cyclic AMP serves as a "releaser from inhibition," bringing about the expression of kinase activity.

Glycogen breakdown is as carefully controlled as glycogen synthesis. For example, phosphorylase in muscle is activated by epinephrine, probably via cyclic AMP. The increase in cyclic AMP brought about by epinephrine activates phosphorylase (increasing glycogen breakdown) and inactivates glycogen synthetase (decreasing glycogen synthesis). These controls ensure that the breakdown and synthesis of glycogen will not occur simultaneously. Coordination is achieved by hormonal control of adenyl cyclase and by the reciprocal response to the activity of cyclic AMP-dependent protein kinase.

The 1,6 linkages of glycogen are hydrolyzed by a specific *debranching enzyme,* releasing *free glucose* (Figure 10–2). This enzyme makes possible a rise in blood glucose even in the absence of glucose-6-phosphatase, which releases glucose from glucose-6-phosphate. Since the action of phosphoglucomutase is reversible, glucose-1-phosphate is readily converted to glucose-6-phosphate.

With the breakdown of glycogen to glucose-6-phosphate, why does the liver not metabolize the latter via glycolysis? Another enzyme, lipase, activated by the same hormones which bring about the activation of phosphorylase, catalyzes the breakdown of triglycerides, releasing free fatty acids. Free fatty acids inhibit certain key enzymes of the glycolytic pathway. In addition, the oxidation of fatty acids leads to a rise in acetyl coenzyme A which inhibits pyruvate kinase and activates pyruvate carboxylase, thus channeling pyruvate toward oxaloacetate and phosphoenol pyruvate and favoring gluconeogenesis. In short, the same set of circumstances which enhances glycogenolysis also enhances lipolysis and permits the liver to use the free fatty acids for energy and to "export" the carbohydrate as glucose.

HYPERGLYCEMIA

After a meal (or an oral dose of glucose), glucose is absorbed from the gastrointestinal tract, and the concentration of glucose in the blood rises. This rise in blood glucose (or amino acids) causes a release of insulin from the pancreatic β cells and a decrease in GH secretion from the anterior pituitary.

In addition to glucose itself, the release of gastrointestinal hormones after ingestion of glucose or protein also influences the release of insulin. These hormones include secretin, pancreozymin, gastrin, and a glucagon-like intestinal hormone (p. 120). Unger has suggested that an early enhancement of insulin release by these hormones in response to the ingestion of nutrients could prevent excessive hyperglycemia or hyperaminoacidemia, which might occur if insulin release were entirely dependent upon concentrations of glucose and amino acids in the blood.

Without insulin, blood glucose would continue to rise and, exceeding the renal threshold (170 to 180 mg/100 ml), would be spilled in the urine. In the normal individual, blood glucose reaches a peak at about 1 hour after a meal and falls below 120 mg/100 ml by 2 hours. Thereafter (2 to 4 hours), as the concentration of glucose continues to decrease, the concentration of insulin in the blood falls. Concomitant with the decrease in insulin and glucose, the concentrations of GH and glucagon in the blood rise.

GLUCAGON

The introduction by Unger of a specific immunoassay for glucagon has permitted investigators to study the physiologic role of this hormone in glucose homeostasis. Although interindividual variations in the concentration of this hormone in blood are large, it seems probable that in a given subject, glucagon, like insulin, is important in the moment-to-moment control of glucose homeostasis.

Unger suggests that the juxtaposed α and β cell pair be viewed as a single bicellular functional unit. Through the diametrically opposed actions of its hormones, this bicellular unit controls the movement of glucose and certain amino acids into and out of cells in accordance with energy need and supply.

The nature of this control is best exemplified by a consideration of the alterations in insulin and glucagon during and following a carbohydrate meal. Concomitant with the rise in blood glucose and the rise in blood insulin following ingestion of carbohydrate is a *fall* in the concentration of glucagon. This fall is sharp and is a mirror image of the sharp rise in insulin. Later, as glucose and insulin fall, the concentration of glucagon returns to the baseline value. Blood concentrations of other hormones, such as GH, also rise in response to hypoglycemia; consequently, a lack of glucagon would not be as detrimental to the individ-

TABLE 10–1. Hormonal Responses to Diet and Blood Glucose Concentrations*

	Insulin	Glucagon	GH	Epinephrine
Starvation	−	+	+ or 0	+ or 0
Glucose ingestion	+	−	−	0
Protein ingestion	+	+	+	0
Hypoglycemia	−	+	+	+
Hyperglycemia	+	−	−	0

*The responses are coded as follows:
+ increased;
− decreased;
0 no change.

ual as a lack of insulin. Indeed, no specific endocrine syndrome has been described in association with glucagon deficiency. Tests of α cell function using arginine or alanine as stimulants of glucagon secretion suggest that in nonobese diabetic patients, α cell response is augmented, whereas in obesity, even when accompanied by diabetes, the response is suppressed.

Ingestion of protein (or infusion of amino acids) results in an elevation of plasma concentration of glucagon (Table 10–1). If such a rise in circulating glucagon did not occur, the enhanced insulin release brought

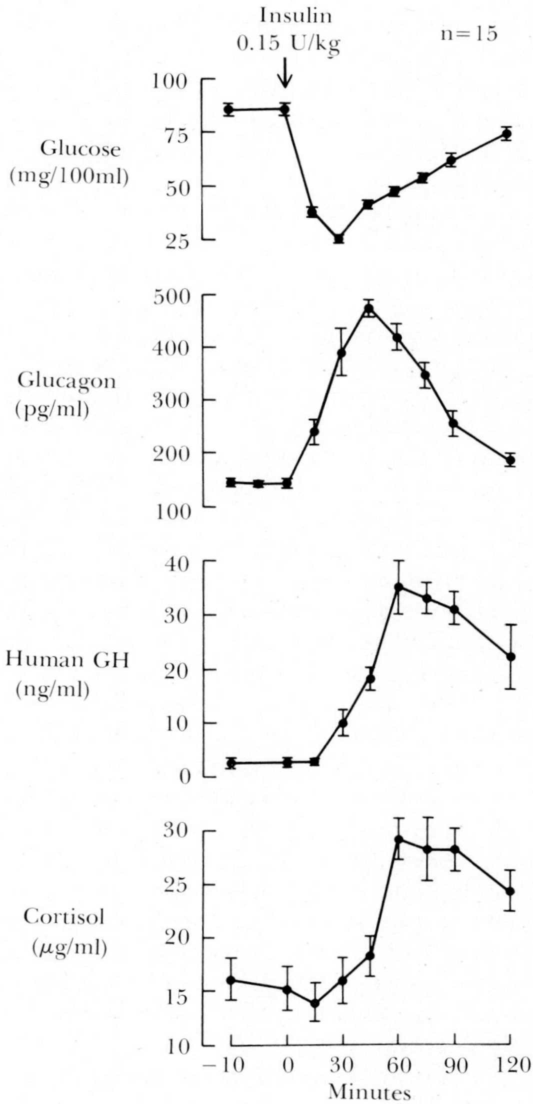

FIGURE 10–3. Changes in plasma concentration of glucagon, human GH, and cortisol in response to insulin-induced hypoglycemia. The values are expressed as mean ± SEM. (From J. Clin. Endocrinol. Metab., *38*:78, 1974, courtesy of Dr. John Gerich.)

about by amino acids would reduce the concentration of glucose in the blood, producing hypoglycemia. Glucagon protects the organism from depleting its circulating supply of glucose and ensures that the liver replenishes any glucose removed by extrahepatic tissues under the influence of insulin. In addition to insulin and glucagon, the release of GH is stimulated by ingestion of proteins (Table 10–1). Under such circumstances, both insulin and GH ensure that the amino acids are used for protein synthesis; glucagon, of course, protects the blood supply of glucose from being depleted.

In starvation, the concentration of plasma insulin falls and that of plasma glucagon rises. The ratio of insulin to glucagon (I/G) in blood falls from the normal value (balanced diet) of 3.8 to a value of 0.4. The liver secretes glucose and maintains the normal plasma concentration. It is aided in this regard by GH, which is secreted in increased amount if blood glucose drops to hypoglycemic levels ($<$ 60 mg per 100 ml). Hypoglycemia also calls forth secretion of ACTH and epinephrine (Table 10–1).

Hypoglycemia can be produced more acutely by administering insulin intravenously to the patient. Such an *insulin tolerance test* serves to provide a means of assessing the individual's ability to respond to hypoglycemia by secreting hyperglycemic hormones. For example, the administration of 0.15 U/kg insulin intravenously to normal nonobese adults will produce a rapid fall in the concentration of plasma glucose as insulin promotes glucose uptake (Figure 10–3). In the studies by Gerich and his colleagues, plasma glucagon rose within 15 minutes after the administration of insulin when the mean plasma glucose concentration was 36 $\pm$ 3 mg/100 ml and was still falling (Figure 10–3). The glucagon response to hypoglycemia preceded the rise in GH and cortisol. Both glucagon and epinephrine probably constitute the more acutely mobilized hormones and act directly on the liver and fat cell adenyl cyclases to promote glycogen and triglyceride breakdown. GH and cortisol function somewhat later as insulin antagonists peripherally, and as stimulators of gluconeogenesis in liver.

Thus the balance of hyperglycemic hormones (glucagon, epinephrine, GH, cortisol) vs. hypoglycemic hormones (insulin) determines the circulating concentration of glucose. Many of the hormonal effects can be related to alterations in concentration of cyclic AMP within the cell. The various effects of these hormones and cyclic AMP on glucose metabolism are summarized in Table 10–2. It is readily seen that insulin stands alone as a hypoglycemic hormone. Thus the importance of the β cell and its response to hyperglycemia cannot be overemphasized. The reactivity of the β cell probably reflects its previous history of exposure to glucose (see Chapter Six) as well as the amount and kind of carbohydrate provoking a given response (see bibliographic entries at the end of this chapter).

A normal response to physiologic hyperglycemia is dependent upon "normal" endocrine balance. There are four endocrine conditions in

TABLE 10–2. Hormonal Effects on Glucose Metabolism

	Gluconeogenesis	Glycogenesis	Glycogenolysis	Peripheral Utilization of Glucose	Insulin Secretion	Net Effect on Blood Glucose
Cyclic AMP	↑ {↑ hepatic lipase → ↑ fatty acids → ↑ acetyl CoA → ↑ pyruvate carboxylation → PEP*}	↓ {glycogen synthetase I → D}	↑ {↑ active phosphorylase kinase → ↑ glycogen phosphophosphorylase}	–	↑	↑
Insulin	↓ {↓ amino acid uptake by liver; ↓ protein catabolism; ↓ pyruvate → PEP}	↑ {↑ glucokinase; ↑ glycogen synthetase}	↓ {↓ liver glycogen phosphorylase}	↑	↓ (by lowering blood glucose)	↓
Cortisol	↑ {↑ synthesis of gluconeogenic enzymes}	↑ {↑ de novo synthesis of glycogen synthetase}	–	↓ (insulin antagonist)	–	↑
Glucagon	↑ {↑ cyclic AMP (see above)}	↓	↑	–	↑ (↑ cyclic AMP in β cell)	↑
Epinephrine	↑ {↑ cyclic AMP (see above)}	↓	↑	↓	↓	↑
GH	↑	↑ in muscle, liver, and heart	–	↓ (insulin antagonist)	↓ acute; ↑ chronic	↑

*PEP = phosphoenolpyruvate.

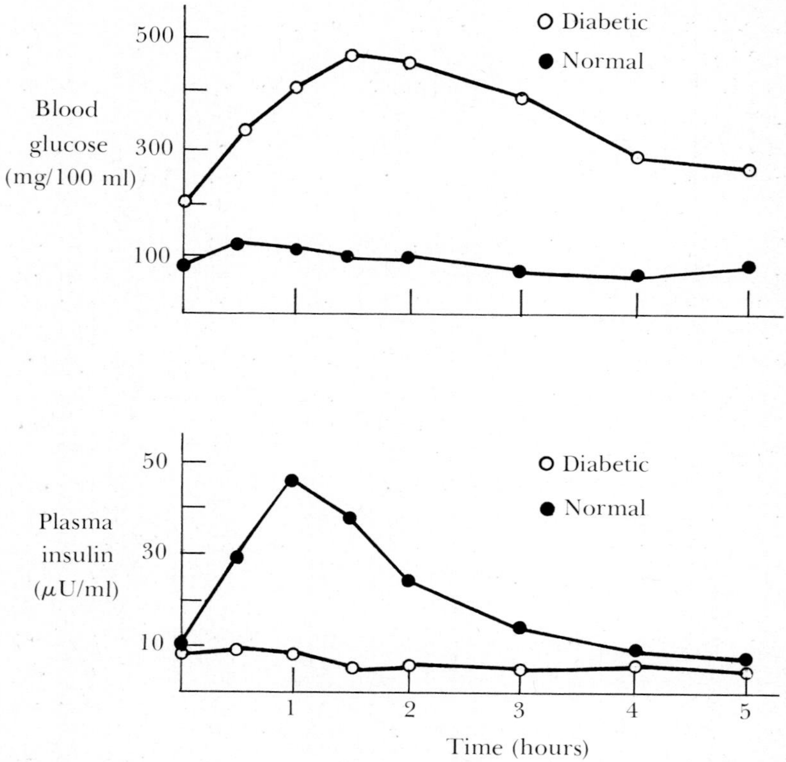

FIGURE 10–4. Changes in concentrations of blood glucose and plasma insulin after oral administration of 100 g glucose at time 0 (mean of 15 normal subjects and 14 nonobese juvenile diabetic patients. (From Parker, M. et al. Juvenile diabetes mellitus, a deficiency in insulin. Diabetes, *17*:27, 1968.)

which hyperglycemia may be sustained or fail to be counterbalanced: diabetes mellitus, GH excess (acromegaly), cortisol excess (Cushing's syndrome) and epinephrine excess (pheochromocytoma).

Diabetes mellitus

Diabetes mellitus was the first of the endocrine disorders to be recognized. It was described over 1800 years ago by Aretaeus of Cappadocia and has served to puzzle and intrigue the medical world ever since. We have already considered the pregnant diabetic and her offspring. Let us now turn our attention to the pathogenesis of the disease and, in particular, to that form occurring in childhood.

The clinical picture of diabetes mellitus is that of insulin deficiency, but the occasional finding of normal or even elevated concentrations of insulin-like activity (ILA) in the plasma of diabetics suggests that lack of insulin may not be the whole problem, at least early in the disease. Nevertheless, in diabetics the β cells react very much more slowly—or not at all—to a given glucose stimulation than do normal β cells (Figure 10–4). Even the high concentrations of insulin present in the blood of certain diabetics are *low* for the degree of hyperglycemia. Cerasi and Luft measured the secretory response of β cells to glucose and found that the normal biphasic curve of insulin release was absent in diabetics. The initial rise in serum insulin was lacking or markedly diminished, and the total insulin response was less than normal. Some healthy subjects also showed a diminished or absent initial rise in serum insulin. These investigators propose that the secretory deficiency of the β cells is the inherited factor responsible for diabetes, but that in most cases *clinical* diabetes will occur only under the effect of additional diabetogenic factors with which the genetically deficient β cells are incapable of coping.

Can the β cells of diabetics synthesize insulin in adequate amounts? In general, diabetics have fewer islets of Langerhans than do normal subjects. Both atrophy and hypertrophy of the islets have been described; however, in so far as it can be estimated, the total mass of insular tissue is less in diabetics than in non-diabetics. In elderly diabetics, this reduction in mass is of the order of 60 percent. It is definitely more pronounced in juvenile diabetics, in whom the majority of islets are atrophic, especially in those patients whose disease has been clinically evident for several years. There seems to be an increased proportion of α to β cells in the diabetic, and many investigators consider that the diabetic has inappropriately high levels of glucagon which exaggerate the consequences of the insulin deficiency. In the initial clinical phase of juvenile diabetes, the pancreas still contains a small number of β cells (10 percent of normal). These cells show cytologic characteristics of secretory hyperactivity.

Is this loss of β cells in the juvenile diabetic congenital, or is it part of a progressive deterioration of islet tissue? Scully found considerable islet hyperplasia in a 13-year-old non-diabetic boy born of diabetic parents. This is suggestive of a compensatory prediabetic phase in the islets secondary to some unknown diabetogenic factor(s). Inflammatory lesions found in the islet tissue of juvenile diabetics may be the result of an autoimmune reaction.

Thus the capacity of the pancreas to produce insulin is severely impaired in the juvenile diabetic, and as the disease progresses, the ability ultimately disappears. The consequences of a lack of insulin can be predicted from our discussion of the action of insulin in various tissues. The transport of glucose into extrahepatic tissues is dependent upon insulin, and therefore the utilization of glucose is impaired and the blood glucose rises. The renal threshold for glucose is exceeded, resulting in *glucosuria.* The excretion of large amounts of glucose requires water; such an osmotic diuresis depletes the body of both intra- and extracellular water. *Dehydration* results and the patient experiences *thirst.* Both *polydipsia* and *polyuria* are common symptoms of diabetes.

The extrahepatic cells of the body are "starved" for glucose and begin to utilize other sources of energy. The breakdown of cellular and plasma proteins to their constituent amino acids proceeds. These amino acids undergo transamination to yield intermediates of the citric acid cycle, which in turn can be metabolized to provide energy for cell functions. Unfortunately, this loss of protein is difficult to replace. The transport of amino acids into extrahepatic tissues and their incorporation into protein are dependent upon insulin. It is not surprising, then, to find *muscle wasting* and *weight loss* as prominent symptoms of diabetes mellitus. In addition, growth is impaired.

One of the major actions of insulin is to enhance the deposition of triglyceride in adipose tissue. Unopposed, lipolytic hormones accelerate the breakdown of fat stores leading to the release of glycerol and free fatty acids. Here, indeed, is a fine source of energy; however, the rate at which free fatty acids appear in the plasma far exceeds the rate at which tissues can oxidize them. In particular, the liver has an active enzyme system for the oxidation of free fatty acids, but even the capacity of this system is exceeded and the excess acetyl CoA which accumulates is converted in the liver to acetoacetic acid, β-hydroxybutyric acid, and acetone. These ketone bodies accumulate in the blood, producing a condition known as *ketosis.* Since these are largely organic acids, a state of metabolic acidosis, or, more exactly, *ketoacidosis,* ensues. To excrete these anions the body must provide cation partners with a resulting urinary loss of Na^+, K^+, Mg^{++}, and even Ca^{++}. The body now has an increased H^+ concentration. Defensive mechanisms such as increased ammonia production or excretion of dibasic salts give temporary relief; however, eventually an uncompensated acidosis results. If the acidosis is severe and left untreated, *diabetic coma* will follow.

Diagnosis of Juvenile Diabetes Mellitus

The classical symptoms of diabetes mellitus in childhood are polyuria and polydipsia, occurring in about 80 to 90 percent of patients. Polyphagia and weight loss are noted in about 50 percent of juvenile diabetics. Impairment of linear growth in the young child may also occur.

A patient with any of these symptoms should have his urine analyzed for glucose and ketone bodies. Glucosuria can occur in renal tubular disease; nevertheless, a glucose tolerance test or a two hour postprandial glucose determination is indicated in any patient with glucosuria. Adequate caloric intake must be ensured prior to these tests. In young children, capillary blood is often used for the analyses of glucose. It should be remembered that in the postprandial period the concentration of glucose in capillary plasma will be 20 to 30 mg/100 ml higher than that in venous plasma. A variety of endocrine disorders can produce abnormalities of the glucose tolerance test, but a child with glucosuria, ketonuria, and hyperglycemia should be considered diabetic.

If the patient gives any indication of acidosis or impending coma (vomiting, deep and rapid breathing, abdominal pain, clouding of consciousness), the extent of the disturbance in acid base balance can be estimated from the individual's blood pH, P_{CO_2}, and bicarbonate. At times the differential diagnosis between diabetic ketoacidosis and acute salicylate poisoning can be difficult. In both there is impairment of carbohydrate metabolism, glucosuria, and acidosis. The metabolic acidosis stimulates the respiratory center, and breathing becomes deeper with a lowering of P_{CO_2}. This compensatory respiratory alkalosis may maintain blood pH within the normal range for a while, but at the cost of a further decrease in the concentration of bicarbonate ion in the plasma. Deep sighing respiration (Kussmaul respiration) with the odor of acetone on the breath is a classical feature of diabetic ketosis.

Complications of Diabetes Mellitus

The complications of diabetes mellitus usually occur after clinical disease has been present for several years (p. 403), and thus they do not constitute a major problem in the childhood years. Nevertheless, it seems well documented that hyperglycemia can lead to the onset of cataracts, increased infections, ketoacidosis, increased atherosclerosis, and even forms of neuropathies.

It has been suggested that the various complications of diabetes may be due to increased metabolism of glucose by pathways which do not require insulin. Normally these pathways account for only a small fraction of total glucose utilization in a tissue; however, in a state of insulin deficiency they appear to operate at increased rates. For example, Spiro noted that glycogen synthesis from glucose in the alloxan-diabetic rat was impaired, but the utilization of glucose for the synthesis of the glucosamine component of hepatic and serum glycoproteins was unimpaired. Spiro has found increased amounts of glycoproteins and mucopolysaccharides in diabetic tissue and suggests there may be a relationship between lack of insulin and increased glycoproteins and mucopolysaccharides via an increase in the glucuronic acid cycle. Thickening of the capillary basement membrane (p. 404), which has been demonstrated in diabetes mellitus, may be related to accumulations of such materials.

Another pathway which is enhanced in the hyperglycemic state is the *polyol pathway* of glucose metabolism. The term polyol, although meaning any organic compound with three or more hydroxyl groups, commonly refers to reduced sugars. The enzyme aldose reductase catalyzes the reduction of these sugars. For instance, glucose is reduced to sorbitol and galactose to galactitol (p. 256). Sorbitol can be converted to fructose by sorbitol dehydrogenase As long as the blood glucose is normal, only 1 percent of glucose goes into the polyol path; however, with hyperglycemia, as much as 10 percent of the blood glucose may be converted to sorbitol. This is particularly true in certain tissues such as seminal vesicle, lens, brain, peripheral nerve, aorta, erythrocyte, and pancreatic islets. Perhaps in these tissues intracellular transport of glucose is not rate-limiting for its utlization by pathways requiring initial phosphorylation. The pathologic consequences of increased polyol pathway activity have been demonstrated in several tissues such as the lens (cataract formation, p. 256) and have been implicated in the etiology of diabetic neuropathy. The polyol pathway is very active in the peripheral nerves of diabetics and results in accumulation of large amounts of sorbitol and fructose (p. 406). Other complications of diabetes may be related to alterations in metabolic pathways brought about by insulin deficiency.

Therapy for Juvenile Diabetes Mellitus

Juvenile diabetics require exogenous insulin because there is an insufficiency—or, a complete absence—of the hormone in their islet cells. Insulin is available as a clear solution of the crystals (crystalline insulin), as a neutral suspension (lente insulin), or as a suspension modified with protamine (NPH and protamine zinc insulin). Crystalline insulin, which is rapidly effective, lasts from 6 to 8 hours, with a peak at 2 to 4 hours. NPH and lente insulin are intermediate, peaking at 10 to 20 hours and lasting 20 to 30 hours. Protamine zinc insulin, lasts 24 to 36 hours; it has an onset of action at 6 to 8 hours, with a peak at 16 to 24 hours. Only crystalline insulin is a clear solution; the others are cloudy. Crystalline insulin can be mixed with NPH or lente insulin to provide more continuous action. The proper combination of insulins usually permits the patient to maintain his blood glucose within normal limits through most of the day.

When diabetes first manifests itself the patient should be hospitalized and a careful assessment of his insulin needs should be made. The proper dose of insulin depends on several factors and may vary from time to time. If the patient is ketotic more insulin will be needed than if he is non-ketotic. The juvenile diabetic may experience periods of remission, and the dose of insulin may need to be decreased. On the other hand, any one of a number of stresses such as puberty may cause intensification of the disease; under such circumstances the dose of insulin must be increased. To monitor control of the diabetes the diabetic must be taught to test his urine for glucose. Commonly used are strips of tape impregnated with reagents which give a color that depends upon the concentration of glucose in the urine. Acetone in the urine can be detected and quantitated by other tapes. In the initial stages of the disease, a certain amount of endogenous insulin is available to the young diabetic; however, as the disease progresses, the β cells become more atrophic and little insulin is released. Thus a constant monitoring of the disease process is necessary. This should be coupled with education of the patient in regard to his disease and its management.

Some children are resistant to insulin and require higher doses to achieve the same control of disease. The basis of this insulin resistance is poorly understood, but it may be due to a humoral insulin antagonist. Acidosis itself can cause insulin resistance, as evidenced by the fact that reducing the pH of an incubating medium from 7.4 to 7.1 causes considerable inhibition of glucose uptake by muscle. This inhibition can be reversed by large amounts of insulin administered either in vivo or in vitro. Increased insulin requirements occur not only in diabetes mellitus but may be an aspect of other conditions (e.g., pregnancy) or other disorders as well. In the presence of infection, increased amounts of glucagon are secreted by the α cells of the pancreatic islets, and more insulin is required by the diabetic to counteract the hyperglycemic action of glucagon.

The diet of the juvenile diabetic is usually restricted to some extent. In general, such diets have less carbohydrate and more protein than the average non-diabetic diet. Diabetics should not eat concentrated forms of carbohydrate such as candy. Such foods could cause marked variations of blood glucose which are not adequately controlled by exogenous insulin.

If too much insulin is given, or the child takes his regular amount of insulin but does not eat or exercises excessively, hypoglycemia will result and, if severe enough, could cause coma. The diabetic must be carefully instructed to recognize the symptoms of hypoglycemia and should be cautioned that whenever he feels hungry, weak, sweaty, dizzy, or drowsy (or feels some combination of these symptoms), glucose is needed. If the patient is conscious, he should drink orange juice or eat several "Life Savers." If he becomes unconscious, glucose must be administered intravenously or intrarectally.

Diabetic ketoacidosis is a medical emergency. The patient may die of acidosis and dehydration. In 15 to 20 percent of children with diabetes mellitus, ketoacidosis was the first manifestation of the disease. Insulin (1.0 unit/kg body weight) should be given, about half intravenously, and repeated as necessary. Adequate fluid replacement must be given. Saline is administered intravenously immediately and, when the blood pH is known, sodium bicarbonate or lactate can be substituted if the acidosis is severe. Initially, the concentration of potassium in the plasma is high; however, as potassium moves into cells with glucose during treatment, the blood level of this cation should be carefully monitored and potassium therapy begun when it begins to fall. Potassium depletion is often severe and may require large amounts of potassium in replacement fluids.

Excess of Growth Hormone

Increased production and secretion of GH can produce either gigantism or acromegaly, depending upon the state of epiphyseal closure in the affected individual. The secretion of GH from the anterior pituitary is under the control of a GH releasing hormone (GHRH) from the hypothalamus. A second hypothalamic factor, GH inhibitory hormone (GHIH), a tetradecapeptide more recently christened *somatostatin*, inhibits the secretion of both newly synthesized and previously synthesized GH.

The daily production rate of GH in man is about 500 μg per day; the concentration of GH in pituitary tissue reaches a peak in adolescence. The concentration in plasma varies considerably but usually lies within a range of 0 to 5 ng/ml. The concentration of GH in blood is increased following stress (pain, cold, severe insulin hypoglycemia) and exercise. The effect of stress may be mediated by ACTH and/or catecholamines; infusion of either agent stimulates GH secretion.

In addition to stress-induced GH secretion, episodic bursts of GH release have been well documented. A particularly prominent burst of GH secretion occurs during the early part of sleep. These episodic releases of GH are probably mediated by higher brain centers. Studies in the rat have shown that GH release can be induced by electrical stimulation of several structures known to have major efferent connections with the ventromedial and arcuate nuclei. The limbic system in particular has been implicated in the modulation of GH secretion. The anterior hypothalamus appears to be involved in inhibition of GH secretion.

Fasting and other conditions which decrease the availability of glucose to the hypothalamus stimulate the release of GH. The administration of 2-deoxy-glucose (a competitive inhibitor of glucose metabolism) causes the prompt release of GH, even though the blood glucose is elevated; therefore, regulation in the hypothalamus is dependent on normal metabolism of glucose rather than simply on the concentration of glucose in the blood. The administration of glucose inhibits GH release, as does the administration of GH itself.

Amino acids, particularly arginine, also stimulate GH secretion. You will recall that amino acids also stimulate insulin release; both insulin and GH are important regulators of protein synthesis.

GH response to insulin-induced hypoglycemia is prevented by α-adrenergic blocking agents such as phentolamine. It has also been shown that β receptor stimulation with isoproterenol inhibits GH release, whereas propranolol, a β adrenergic blocking agent, facilitates GH release in response to certain stimuli such as glucagon. These findings suggest the existence of a central dual adrenergic mechanism for GH regulation that has stimulatory and inhibitory effects opposite to those described for the regulation of insulin secretion by the pancreas.

The exact site of such control is unknown, but it probably exists at a hypothalamic level in order to modulate GHRH release. Many of the stimuli known to cause GH release probably act via central adrenergic mechanisms. GH release induced by exercise, vasopressin, and L-dopa is prevented by administration of phentolamine. It is noteworthy that sleep-related GH release is not affected by either α-adrenergic or β-adrenergic blockade.

Functions of Growth Hormone

The effects of GH are complex and are not well understood. As its name implies, GH stimulates an increased protein synthesis. In addition, however, GH has effects on the metabolism of fats and carbohydrates as well as the indirect effects on growth via somatomedin (to be discussed).

PROTEIN SYNTHESIS. GH stimulates overall protein synthesis in the intact animal, resulting in nitrogen and phosphorus retention. The mechanism of the effect of GH on protein synthesis is discussed in detail in Chapter Eleven, where the regulation of growth is considered.

FAT METABOLISM. Some role of GH in regulating lipolysis has been suspected for many years. In vivo administration of GH is followed 30 to 60 minutes later by an increase in circulating free fatty acids and increased oxidation of fatty acids in the liver.

Studies using adipose tissue in vitro suggest that GH is an ineffective lipolytic agent unless a glucocorticoid is added to the medium. In addition, the effects of GH become evident later than those of other lipolytic hormones. Effects of GH plus dexamethasone, for example, were not significant until after two hours of incubation. When either puromycin or actinomycin D was added to the incubation mixture, the lipolytic effect of GH plus dexamethasone was blocked. From such studies it has been concluded that in all probability the lipolytic action of GH plus glucocorticoids involves DNA-RNA-dependent protein synthesis. Since theophylline potentiates the lipolytic action of GH, it is possible that the synthesis of some protein factor of the adenyl cyclase system is involved in GH action in adipose tissue.

CARBOHYDRATE METABOLISM (Table 10–2). The discovery that diabetic symptoms which appeared in the dog after pancreatectomy could be ameliorated by also removing the pituitary demonstrated convincingly that the hypophysis performs an important role in regulating carbohydrate metabolism. GH was soon implicated as the "diabetogenic" principle of the pituitary. Indeed, permanent diabetes mellitus can be produced in certain species when GH is administered over prolonged periods. The β cells probably become exhausted by the hyperglycemia produced by GH. This hyperglycemia is due to both decreased peripheral utilization of glucose and increased hepatic production of glucose via gluconeogenesis. There is no doubt that prolonged administration of GH results in enhanced release of insulin from the pancreas. This is due in part to stimulation of insulin release by GH-induced hyperglycemia, but, in addition, GH appears to stimulate the synthesis of proteins, including insulin, in the pancreas itself.

In addition to its "hyperglycemic" and "insulinogenic" effects, GH inhibits the action of insulin in muscle, either by inhibiting glucose transport or by impairing glycolysis. The inhibition of glycolysis in muscle may be secondary to the increased amounts of free fatty acids released from adipose tissue due to the lipolytic effect of GH. Free fatty acids are known to inhibit glycolysis. Deposition of glycogen in liver, skeletal muscle, and cardiac muscle is increased under the influence of GH. The effects on cardiac muscle are of particular interest. When the heart works under anaerobic conditions, its glycogen is mobilized rapidly; however, during fasting the glycogen content of the heart is increased, even though that of other muscles becomes depleted. When GH is given to normal animals at the beginning of a fasting period, extremely large amounts of glycogen accumulate in heart muscle. Thus one of the primary functions of GH may be to conserve carbohydrate stores in the heart.

SOMATOMEDIN. GH stimulates the growth of long bones at the epiphyses. Stimulation of growth is mediated by a low molecular weight substance called somatomedin or "sulfation factor," induced by GH in the liver (p. 266). This substance plays a role in the incorporation of sulfate into cartilage.

Hypersecretion of GH

Increased basal GH levels have now been described in several conditions. In disturbances of growth due to excess GH, such as gigantism or acromegaly (see Chapter Eleven), alterations in carbohydrate metabolism are often found. For instance, 12 to 40 percent of acromegalics develop diabetes mellitus. It is quite likely that the diabetogenic stress of chronic hypersecretion of GH produces clinical diabetes in the patient with a predisposition to the disease.

Most, if not all, patients with hypersecretion of GH show diminished response to insulin. The release of insulin from the β cell is not decreased, however. On the contrary, an increased insulin reserve and secretory capacity of the pancreas have been found in these patients. Most patients with acromegaly show an exaggerated insulin response to orally administered glucose.

EXCESS OF GLUCOCORTICOIDS

The administration of glucocorticoids to fasting normal or adrenalectomized animals causes a rise in blood glucose and a striking increase in liver glycogen (Table 10–2). These steroids inhibit glucose utilization and accelerate gluconeogenesis; both actions are antagonized by insulin. Thus, in common with GH, glucocorticoids are insulin antagonists.

Cushing's syndrome represents a disorder of adrenal cortical hyperfunction. Excessive amounts of glucocorticoids are produced; in the adult this is usually secondary to stimulation by excessive amounts of ACTH produced by a pituitary tumor. The disorder is uncommon in young children and when it occurs may be the result of an adrenal tumor (see Chapter Eleven). Iatrogenic Cushing's syndrome, which results from the administration of excessive amounts of glucocorticoids, is rather common and must always be considered in the patient on cortisol therapy.

Whatever the cause, the excessive glucocorticoids produce profound changes in the metabolism of both carbohydrates and proteins. In our discussion of the endocrine control of metabolism, the glucocorticoids were presented as stimulators of the synthesis of gluconeogenic enzymes. This stimulation, together with the decreased glucose utilization produced by glucocorticoids, leads to an increased concentration of glucose in the blood (Table 10–2). The decreased ability of affected patients to utilize glucose can be seen in the diabetic-type glucose tolerance curve which they manifest. These patients may have glycosuria in addition to hyperglycemia.

EXCESS OF EPINEPHRINE

Tumors of the adrenal medulla (pheochromocytoma) are rare, but 80 percent are associated with increased secretion of epinephrine and thus serve as another example of a clinical situation which may produce hyperglycemia (among other things). The effect of epinephrine on glycogen phosphorylase and the resulting breakdown of glycogen explains the rise in blood glucose in patients with adrenal medullary tumors. Epinephrine also inhibits pancreatic insulin release and reduces the sensitivity of peripheral tissues to insulin (Table 10–2).

Tumors which secrete primarily norepinephrine do not usually cause clinically apparent diabetes. In patients with such tumors, however, the glucose tolerance test may be abnormal and insulin secretion is suppressed. Pheochromocytoma is a rare but important cause of hypertension.

Any condition which increases the release of epinephrine (emotional excitement, injury, exercise, anesthetics such as ether and morphine) may, of course, produce an elevation of blood glucose. Epinephrine has an additional, indirect influence on carbohydrate metabolism by stimulating the anterior pituitary to release ACTH. This in turn augments the release from the adrenal cortex of glucocorticoids, which have a hyperglycemic effect.

HYPOGLYCEMIA

Aside from the perinatal causes of hypoglycemia (p. 141), a variety of conditions in the young child and adult are associated with this symptom. Transient episodes of hypoglycemia may be associated with fasting (ketotic hypoglycemia, p. 125), excessive treatment with insulin, or drug intoxication (salicylates, diphenylhydantoin, sulfonylureas, p. 407); however, we shall confine ourselves to a discussion of the causes of relatively permanent decreases in blood glucose.

There may be insufficient glucose circulating in the blood because of excessive removal of glucose from the blood, or decreased secretion of glucose into the blood, or any combination of the two.

EXCESSIVE REMOVAL OF GLUCOSE FROM THE BLOOD

If we consider the factors which might accelerate removal of glucose from the blood, a deficiency of either GH or glucocorticoids and an excess of insulin come immediately to mind. Excess insulin may be due to exogenous administration or to increased secretion of insulin by the β cell secondary to a tumor of the islet tissue or unusual sensitivity of the β cell to glucose or leucine.

Leucine-Sensitive Hypoglycemia

In 1956 Cochrane described certain infants with "idiopathic" hypoglycemia who were sensitive to certain foods. He noted that on a diet rich in casein, the hypoglycemia was aggravated, and, in time, he discovered that the only ingredient of casein implicated in the hypoglycemia was leucine.

Symptoms of hypoglycemia (often a convulsion) occur in the affected patient within the first six months of life. The hypoglycemia probably results from the hyperinsulinism induced by the leucine-sensitive β cell. This disorder should be suspected in an infant who after a protein-rich meal exhibits lethargy, pallor, or convulsions. A low blood glucose at any time, and in particular, within 60 minutes of feeding, is an indication for a leucine-sensitivity test (p. 125).

Early diagnosis and treatment is imperative in order to prevent irreparable damage to the central nervous system. Even at the first examination, the infant may show signs of mental retardation or cerebral palsy or both. The ideal treatment would be a leucine-free diet; however, such a diet is usually unpalatable and inadequate to support growth. A low protein, minimal leucine diet is the usual compromise. In addition, diazoxide (a relative of the thiazide diuretics), which inhibits insulin release, is useful in managing these patients.

Idiopathic Hypoglycemia

This is a catchall classification of hypoglycemic states of unknown etiology. Fortunately, its use is rapidly being eliminated as cases are being diagnosed more specifically. Patients with idiopathic hypoglycemia usually demonstrate symptoms before the age of 6 months. The hypoglycemia tends to come on with fasting. In the majority of infants the pancreas is normal, but in others islet hyperplasia has been reported. The fasting plasma insulin concentration remains high, and mobilization of ketone bodies from the liver is impaired. Frequent feedings may maintain euglycemia in some individuals; however, other patients have required ACTH or glucocorticoids to control the hypoglycemia. Diazoxide may be useful in these patients and has the advantage over steroids in not affecting a child's growth. In patients with severe, persistent hypoglycemia subtotal pancreatectomy has been helpful.

Insulinoma

Instances of insulinomas are *very* rare in children less than 10 years old. Characteristically, the hypoglycemia comes on with fasting or exercise or with a combination of the two. In this respect, it differs from the hypoglycemias brought on by feeding. The diagnosis of insulinoma is usually made by finding a very low blood glucose concentration in the fasting state, but sometimes the fast has to be prolonged (as long as 72 hours), and moderate exercise may be needed to bring on symptoms of hypoglycemia.

In most patients with insulinomas the fasting concentration of immunoreactive insulin is inappropriately elevated. Fractionation of this plasma insulin reveals that proinsulin comprises a much larger portion of the total immunoreactive insulin than is found with comparable studies using normal plasma insulin. Gorden and his colleagues believe that the proinsulin component in insulinomas is a larger molecule than "normal" proinsulin and is specific for islet cell tumors. A test dose of insulin administered to the patient with an insulinoma usually produces little or no effect on the concentration of glucose in the blood.

More than 90 percent of these tumors are benign and all are slow-growing. If surgery is impractical as a form of therapy, diazoxide can be used to reduce the release of insulin.

Multiple Endocrine Adenomatosis

In a review of 85 cases of multiple endocrine adenomatosis, Ballard defined the disorder as the familial occurrence of multiple tumors or hyperplasia of the endocrine organs. Most often affected are the parathyroid glands, the pancreatic islets, and the pituitary gland; less often, the adrenal and thyroid glands are involved. Excessive hormonal activity may or may not be associated with adenomatous glands.

Steiner has proposed that the two main clinical patterns that are evident in this disorder be referred to as multiple endocrine neoplasia type I (multiple endocrine adenomatosis involving the parathyroid gland, pituitary gland, pancreatic islets, and adrenal cortex) and multiple endocrine neoplasia type II (pheochromocytoma, medullary carcinoma of the thyroid, and parathyroid tumors, p. 345). There is also a definite relationship between the total spectrum of multiple endocrine adenomatosis and the Zollinger-Ellison syndrome (excessive gastric secretion and fulminating peptic ulceration in association with noninsulin producing islet cell tumors of the pancreas). Certain forms of the carcinoid syndrome (p. 449) may represent variations of multiple endocrine adenomatosis.

In Ballard's 85 cases, 74 patients had parathyroid lesions, 69 had pancreatic tumors, and 55 had pituitary lesions. The incidence of β and non-β cell tumors in the pancreas was about the same. Peptic ulcer occurred in 49 patients and was associated with pancreatic tumors or clinical hypoglycemia in 43. The syndrome is a familial disorder transmitted by an autosomal dominant gene, affecting mainly adults in the third to fifth decade of life, but it can appear in individuals less than 20 years old.

There is some evidence of pancreatic islet cell dysfunction in both symptomatic and nonsymptomatic members of one family. Vance proposes that the disorder may result from a single genetic defect involving the cytogenesis of the primordial cells of the islet, leading to islet cell hyperplasia and adenomatosis. In 1938 Laidlow postulated that the pancreatic duct cell is the primordial cell of the pancreas and that this totipotential cell is capable of regenerating duct, acinar, and islet cells at any time, if stimulated. The term *nesidioblastosis* was proposed for such islet cell hyperplasia from primitive duct cells. (The term derives from nesidioblast, a Greek phrase meaning "islet builder.") The stimulus for such hyperplasia is unknown. Vance suggests that chronic overproduction of insulin, glucagon, gastrin and/or other polypeptide hormones by hyperactive islet cells could lead to secondary changes in other endocrine glands, resulting eventually in the clinical spectrum of multiple endocrine adenomatosis.

Although rare in children, the possibility of this syndrome must be included in the differential diagnosis of hypoglycemia. Patients who manifest hypoglycemia and who have symptoms of peptic ulcer (or who have a family history of peptic ulcer) deserve further investigation with this syndrome in mind.

GH Deficiency

Children with a deficiency of GH have a tendency to spontaneous hypoglycemia which, if untreated, results in symptoms of sweating, tremor, or even convulsions. This tendency to hypoglycemia may disappear by age five or so, probably due to the development of compensatory mechanisms. These children manifest growth retardation.

Adrenocortical Insufficiency

Chronic glucocorticoid insufficiency is a well-known cause of symptomatic hypoglycemia. The investigation of a child with unexplained recurrent hypoglycemia should always include testing of adrenal function.

Decreased secretion of glucose into the blood

One of the commonest forms of decreased glucose secretion into the blood is a secondary consequence of starvation or malabsorption. Acute starvation rarely causes hypoglycemia because compensatory mechanisms come into play to conserve blood glucose. Prolonged starvation or malabsorption predisposes the individual to hypoglycemia after minor stress. Persistent hypoglycemia in such conditions often indicates a terminal event. Malnourished individuals are more prone to alcohol-induced hypoglycemia.

One of the major sources of glucose other than the intestinal tract is the liver. Thus conditions which disturb liver function may impair the secretion of glucose into the blood. Infections, such as viral hepatitis, may be associated with mild hypoglycemia. Patients with liver disease are often exquisitely sensitive to tolbutamide and may have prolonged hypoglycemia after a tolbutamide test.

Much of the glucose secreted by the liver and the kidney is derived from gluconeogenesis, and any impairment of this pathway would reduce glucose secretion. Deficiency of glucocorticoids would reduce the activity of the gluconeogenic enzymes considerably. Ethyl alcohol, in the process of its metabolism to acetaldehyde (catalyzed by ethanol dehydrogenase), uses NAD. If the amount of alcohol being metabolized is large, the available NAD in the cell becomes depleted. Many enzymes, including some of the enzymes of the Krebs citric acid cycle, require NAD as a cofactor. The NADH which accumulates in the metabolism of alcohol can be converted back to NAD during the conversion of pyruvate to lactate (catalyzed by lactic dehydrogenase). This conversion to lactate reduces the pyruvate available for conversion to oxaloacetate, phosphoenol pyruvate, and so on through the gluconeogenic path. Ordinarily this is not a problem, but in the malnourished alcoholic whose liver glycogen is depleted, hypoglycemia can occur.

A significant number of children with spontaneous hypoglycemia have demonstrated a reduced urinary output of epinephrine during insulin-induced hypoglycemia. These children resemble clinically those with ketotic hypoglycemia, developing hypoglycemia and ketonuria with fasting. It has been suggested that the abnormality may be due to delayed maturation of the mechanisms which trigger adrenal medullary response to hypoglycemia. Some children with ketotic hypoglycemia have been reported to have low concentrations of alanine in the plasma, which suggests that the hypoglycemia may be secondary to an inadequate supply of substrate for liver gluconeogenesis. Both low plasma cortisol concentrations and low urinary excretion rates of epinephrine during insulin tolerance tests have been reported in these children. The ketonuria itself is non-specific and will occur in normal children during fasting. The degree of ketonuria is inversely related to the concentration of glucose in the blood.

Other conditions which impair glucose secretion into the blood are the various deficiencies of enzymes involved in the metabolism of sugars and in the synthesis and breakdown of glycogen.

Fructose Intolerance (Fructosemia)

Patients with fructose intolerance lack fructose-1-phosphate aldolase, which splits fructose-1-phosphate to glyceraldehyde and dihydroxyacetone phosphate. The disorder is characterized clinically by hypoglycemia and vomiting shortly after ingestion of food containing fructose. Children with the disorder fail to thrive, and they develop hepatomegaly.

After ingestion of fructose in the normal individual the concentration of this sugar in the blood rises rapidly. It is utilized far more rapidly than glucose, a large part being converted to fructose-1-phosphate (catalyzed by fructokinase) in the liver. The greater rate of utilization of fructose results from the higher affinity of fructokinase for fructose than of hexokinase for glucose. Fructose-1-phosphate is then cleaved by aldolase.

In the patient with fructosemia, fructose accumulates because its metabolism is blocked. As the level of fructose in the blood rises, the glucose concentration falls; however, the hypoglycemia is not due to hyperinsulinism. The concentration of insulin in the serum is usually unchanged. Apparently, there is a block of glucose release from the liver. The liver does not respond to glucagon by increasing blood glucose concentration.

Other forms of fructose intolerance associated with hypoglycemia have been described recently. One hereditary defect involves a deficiency of liver fructose-1,6-diphosphatase. Patients with this defect have hypoglycemia after fructose ingestion; however, vomiting does not occur, and mental development and growth are normal. In all cases dietary restriction of fructose is the therapy of choice.

The lack of fructokinase results in the relatively benign hereditary condition known as *essential fructosuria.*

Galactose Intolerance (Galactosemia)

In another enzyme deficiency, the lack of galactose-1-phosphate uridyl transferase results in galactose intolerance. This enzyme catalyzes the conversion of galactose-1-phosphate to glucose-1-phosphate. The enzyme deficiency is inherited as an autosomal recessive trait. Infants who lack the enzyme are usually normal at birth but begin to develop symptoms as soon as they are given milk. They fail to thrive and exhibit a variety of symptoms, including vomiting, jaundice, and hepatosplenomegaly. Hypoglycemia occurs in some children but is not a prominent feature.

Either galactose-1-phosphate itself or the metabolite galactitol formed by the reduction of galactose by aldose reductase may be toxic to various tissues. Galactitol accumulates in the lens and may be responsible for the cataracts found in children with galactose intolerance. Both galactose-1-phosphate and galactitol accumulate in the brain and may contribute to mental retardation. Therapy involves the rigid exclusion of lactose from the diet. Failure to do so will result in progressive liver failure and death.

A different mutation at the transferase locus, the *Duarte variant,* leads to the production of an enzyme with only about half the normal activity, but without associated clinical problems. Since all of the cells of galactosemics lack the transferase enzyme, diagnostic assays of the enzyme can be performed using red blood cells, cultured skin fibroblasts, or, for prenatal diagnosis, cultured amniotic fluid cells. Heterozygotes for the galactosemia allele or homozygotes for the Duarte variant have about 50 percent of normal enzyme activity; Duarte heterozygotes have about 75 percent of normal activity.

Glycogen Storage Diseases

Until 1952 only two glycogen storage diseases were recognized, one form being characterized by glycogen accumulation in the liver *(von Gierke's disease),* the other by glycogen accumulation in the heart. At that time Gerti and Carl Cori demonstrated a specific deficiency of glucose-6-phosphatase in a patient with hepatic glycogen storage disease. This was followed by a series of discoveries of deficiencies of each of the enzymes involved in glycogen synthesis and breakdown. At present eight types of glycogen storage disease are recognized.

TYPE I: GLUCOSE-6-PHOSPHATASE DEFICIENCY (VON GIERKE'S DISEASE). Children with this form of glycogen storage disease are short and have massive enlargement of the liver, which produces marked distension of the abdomen. In a child with these symptoms, appropriate biochemical studies of a biopsy of the liver will reveal the enzyme deficiency. In a patient with von Gierke's disease, the amount of glycogen in the liver is increased but the structure of the glycogen molecule is normal. Glucose-6-phosphatase is lacking in kidney and intestinal tissue as well as in liver, and the kidney is enlarged as a result of accumulated glycogen.

The results of a lack of this enzyme are predictable. Hypoglycemia, often severe, is found in affected children, although they may remain asymptomatic even when their blood glucose concentration is less than 10 mg per 100 ml. The brain may have developed the capacity to use alternate types of fuel such as ketone bodies. It is not surprising that the blood glucose changes very little in these patients in response to administered epinephrine or glucagon. Since glucose-6-phosphate cannot be converted to glucose in significant amounts, it is metabolized to other substances. The amounts of lactate, pyruvate, triglyceride, phospholipids, cholesterol, and ketone bodies are increased in the blood, producing a variety of symptoms. The elevated lipids result in xanthomas. Increased concentrations of uric acid in the blood, which result from decreased urinary excretion of uric acid in the presence of lactate and ketone bodies which compete with the uric acid for tubular secretion, may produce gouty tophi. The elevated lactic acid in blood results in a chronic acidosis which in turn produces a negative calcium balance with resulting osteoporosis. Free fatty acids and glycerol are elevated in the serum, probably as a consequence of hypoglycemia. A reciprocal relationship between the concentrations of glucose and free fatty acids in the blood has been noted in a number of conditions, and hypoglycemia itself is a potent stimulus to the release of free fatty acids by adipose tissue.

Frequent feedings, drugs such as diazoxide, and portacaval shunts have been recommended in children with the glucose-6-phosphatase deficiency. The latter procedure is particularly promising, in that glucose-rich blood can bypass the liver and reach peripheral tissues directly. In animals such shunts have reduced liver glycogen by over 50 percent.

TYPE II: α-1,4-GLUCOSIDASE DEFICIENCY (POMPE'S DISEASE). The enzyme which is lacking in this disorder is a lysosomal glucosidase which catalyzes the direct hydrolysis of glycosyl residues from glycogen, forming free glucose rather than glucose-1-phosphate. Hypoglycemia is not a feature of this disorder, and the patient's responses to glucagon and epinephrine are normal. Glycogen tends to accumulate in vacuoles or lysosomes in most tissues: the concentration in heart and skeletal muscle may rise to 100 g of glycogen per kilogram of tissue. Profound hypotonia is the usual symptom, with striking enlargement of the heart; death occurs at an early age, usually brought on by cardiorespiratory failure. The deficiency can be diagnosed prenatally in cells from amniotic fluid; abortion is indicated in the presence of this disorder.

It should not be inferred that a major part of glycogen is normally hydrolyzed by lysosomes, for in other glycogen storage diseases glucosidase activity is normal but glycogen accumulates. This disorder remains a puzzle, but it has suggested some interesting speculations about the role of lysosomes in cellular function.

TYPE III: AMYLO-1,6-GLUCOSIDASE (DEBRANCHER) DEFICIENCY (CORI'S DISEASE). The glycogen molecule undergoes initial breakdown (via phosphorylase) to the *limit dextrin*, which contains four glucose residues in α1,4-linkage attached by a 1,6 link to the glycogen molecule. Three of the four glucoses are removed before amylo-1,6-glucosidase catalyzes the cleavage of the 1,6 link, releasing free glucose. In type III glycogen storage disease, in which this enzyme is lacking, limit dextrin accumulates in tissues which ordinarily have glycogen stores. Thus large amounts are present in liver, producing hepatomegaly, and in muscle, which may cause a chronic progressive myopathy in older patients. The heart is involved, but there is no renal enlargement.

Hypoglycemia may be severe and convulsions have occurred. The clinical disease is typically milder than that found in type I glycogen storage disease. Although lipid levels are often elevated in the serum, uric acid is usually normal. The response of blood glucose to the administration of epinephrine or glucagon is variable. Therapy includes frequent feedings and possible portacaval shunt.

TYPE IV: α-1,4-GLUCAN:α-1-4-GLUCAN-6-GLUCOSYL TRANSFERASE DEFICIENCY (BRANCHING DEFICIENCY). Only seven infants with this disorder have been reported. The accumulation in the liver of abnormal glycogen molecules with long outer chains (similar to those of amylopectin) and much reduced branching produces a clinical picture of progressive cirrhosis. Death occurs at an early age. Carbohydrate metabolism is not disturbed.

TYPE V: MUSCLE PHOSPHORYLASE DEFICIENCY (MCARDLE'S DISEASE). Muscle tissue during ischemic exercise breaks down glycogen and releases large amounts of lactate, which can be reconverted to glucose by the liver via the Cori cycle. The release of lactate can be demonstrated by applying a tourniquet to an arm to shut off the blood supply and measuring the lactate concentration in forearm blood after the fist has been clenched several times. In the normal individual there is a sharp rise in lactate concentration.

McArdle reported a patient who had no increase in venous lactate during ischemic exercise and suggested that there was some defect in the breakdown of glycogen to lactate. In patients with McArdle's disease, the concentration of glycogen in muscle is high, and enzyme studies reveal the presence of phosphorylase kinase but a lack of phosphorylase. These patients can tolerate moderate exercise normally. Liver phosphorylase, which is a very different enzyme in many ways, is normal in these patients. Usually these patients show mild symptoms—or no symptoms at all—during childhood.

TYPE VI: LIVER PHOSPHORYLASE DEFICIENCY (HERS' DISEASE). This group represents a potpourri of disorders found with hepatic glycogen storage disease. There has been a tendency to include in this group those patients who do not fit into type I or type III glycogen storage disease, but who resemble those two disorders clinically. Many have a defect in liver phosphorylase; however, in other patients, clear-cut definition of the enzyme defect has not been possible. Clinically both sorts of patients resemble those with a mild form of type I glycogen storage disease.

TYPE VII: MUSCLE PHOSPHOFRUCTOKINASE DEFICIENCY. Patients with this disorder have clinical histories resembling those of patients with McArdle's disease; however, it is muscle phosphofructokinase which is deficient. The concentrations of glucose-6-phosphate and fructose-6-phosphate in muscle increase. Both glycogen synthetase and UDPG pyrophosphorylase activities are increased. Glycogen can be synthesized and tends to accumulate in muscle cells as in McArdle's disease because of the inability of the cells to utilize it.

TYPE VIII: HEPATIC PHOSPHORYLASE KINASE DEFICIENCY. Hub and coworkers have reported five children with no abnormalities other than hepatomegaly and increased concentration of glycogen in the liver. By in vitro studies with liver biopsies, a 90 percent deficiency of phosphorylase kinase was demonstrated. From our discussion of glycogen breakdown, you will remember that this enzyme activates glycogen phosphorylase, which catalyzes the breakdown of glycogen. The total phosphorylase activity in these children is normal but the activating system is defective. Nevertheless, even a small amount of phosphorylase kinase can be activated by cyclic AMP, so that these patients show a normal response to glucagon. Neither hypoglycemia nor acidosis develops. Many patients originally thought to have a deficiency of liver phosphorylase (type VI) have been shown to be deficient in hepatic phosphorylase kinase (type VIII).

In summary, only patients with type I (glucose-6-phosphatase deficiency), III (debrancher enzyme deficiency), and VI (liver phosphorylase deficiency) show evidence of hypoglycemia. Any child who manifests hypoglycemia, hepatomegaly, and growth retardation in the first year of life may have one of these deficiencies. In these patients the blood glucose fails to rise after administration of either epinephrine or glucagon.

SUMMARY

A careful balance is maintained between the secretion of those hormones which lead to an increased concentration of glucose in the blood (glucagon, GH, cortisol, epinephrine) and the secretion of insulin, which decreases the glucose concentration in blood by enhancing cellular uptake (Table 10–2). Certain natural phenomena may temporarily upset this balance. For example, ingestion of nutrients triggers the release of insulin both via gastrointestinal hormones and via the physiologic hyperglycemia which follows alimentation. The rise in blood glucose also inhibits the secretion of GH and glucagon. In effect, these alterations in hormone secretion return the concentration of blood glucose to normal. Disorders characterized by insulin deficiency (diabetes mellitus) or by GH excess (acromegaly) result in prolonged hyperglycemia. Excessive secretion of ACTH (or cortisol) and epinephrine can also result in a hyperglycemic state.

Hyperglycemia per se is detrimental to many tissues. Many of the pathological changes in tissues which occur after many years of diabetes mellitus may be attributed to altered metabolic pathways. In particular, those pathways which are relatively independent of insulin are increased in activity and may produce abnormally large amounts of normally rare products. The polyol pathway and the glucuronic acid pathway are two systems which have been implicated in the etiology of the complications of diabetes mellitus.

Stress or exercise increases the metabolic rate and the requirement for glucose. Once again hormonal shifts enhance the release of glucose from the liver via glycogenolysis or gluconeogenesis. Both epinephrine and glucagon stimulate adenyl cyclase and increase the concentration of cyclic AMP within the liver cell. Cyclic AMP is necessary for the activity of the protein kinase which "activates" glycogen phosphorylase and "inactivates" glycogen synthetase. Stress also stimulates the release of glucocorticoids which enhance gluconeogenesis. Thus these hormones activate enzymes which increase glucose production by the liver primarily.

Disorders in which either the enzymes are deficient (glycogen storage disease) or the hormones are deficient may produce hypoglycemia. Obviously, excessive amounts of insulin (leucine sensitivity, insulinoma) can also produce hypoglycemia. The central nervous system cannot function normally without a constant supply of glucose. Therefore a condition of low blood sugar is usually heralded by signs of central nervous system dysfunction. The detrimental effects of both hypo- and hyperglycemia suggest that the control of the concentration of blood glucose is of paramount importance for survival.

SUGGESTED READINGS

Glucagon and Insulin, G. Alan Robison, R. W. Butcher, and W. E. Sutherland, *Cyclic AMP*, (Chapter 7), Academic Press, New York, 1971.
A discussion of glucagon and insulin and their respective effects on the adenyl cyclase system. In addition, the authors consider the possible role of cyclic AMP in the etiology of diabetes mellitus.

Endocrine Pancreas, Vol. I of *Endocrinology* (Section 7 of *Handbook of Physiology*), edited by D. F. Steiner and N. Freinkel, American Physiological Society, Washington, D.C., 1972.
This is truly an encyclopedia of the pancreas, covering morphogenesis, chemistry and biosynthesis of pancreatic hormones, mechanism of action of insulin and glucagon, and clinical and experimental disorders of insulin and glucagon secretion. This book is for the student who wants detailed discussions of research and theory concerning the pancreas, its functions and disorders.

PERTINENT LITERATURE REFERENCES

Arky, R. A. and Knoop, R. H.: Evaluation of Islet-cell function in man. New Engl. J. Med. *285*:1130, 1971.

Baruk, S., et al.: Fasting hypoglycemia. Med. Clin. North Am. *57*:1441, 1973.

Donnell, G. N.: Pitfalls in the diagnosis of galactosemia. J. Ped. *83*:515, 1973.

Gerich, J. E. et al: Characterization of the glucagon response to hypoglycemia in man. J. Clin. Endocrinol. Metab. *38*:77, 1974.

Gutman, R. A. et al: Circulating proinsulin-like material in patients with functioning insulinomas. New Engl. J. Med. *284*:1003, 1971.

Hales, C. N.: The role of insulin in the regulation of glucose metabolism. Proc. Nutr. Soc. *30*:282, 1971.

Kreisberg, R. A.: Glucose-lactate interrelations in man. New Engl. J. Med. *287*:132, 1972.

Reaven, G. M and Olefsky, J. M.: Increased plasma glucose and insulin responses to high-carbohydrate feedings in normal subjects. J. Clin. Endocrinol. Metab. *38*:151, 1974.

Thompson, W. J. et al: Effect of insulin and GH on rat liver cyclic nucleotide phosphodiesterase. Biochemistry *12*:1889, 1973.

Unger, R. H.: Glucagon and the insulin: glucagon ratio in diabetes and other catabolic illnesses. Diabetes *20*:834, 1971.

Vance, J. E. et al: Familial nesidioblastosis as the predominent manifestation of multiple endocrine adenomatosis. Am. J. Med. *52*:211, 1972.

CHAPTER ELEVEN

Growth

It has been postulated that growth of the embryo and fetus is "programmed," and that if provided with sufficient nutrients, the organism will grow and develop. There is very little evidence of any hormonal control of linear growth in utero. Perhaps insulin functions as the "growth hormone" of the fetus, ensuring maximum use of available nutrients for anabolism. The infant of the diabetic mother (Chapter Six) provides an example compatible with such a postulate. Thyroid hormone is necessary for normal maturation of fetal bone and brain, and androgens mediate male sexual differentiation. ACTH is probably necessary for normal development of the adrenal gland. With the exception of the hormonal regulation of differentiation of certain tissues, fetal development appears to be regulated primarily by nutritional and hereditary factors.

It is only after birth, in the growing infant and child, that clear-cut growth failure is seen in certain endocrine deficiency states; thus, at some point in development, hormonal regulation is superimposed on the nutritional and hereditary factors which had been regulating growth up to that point. Let us consider the normal pattern of growth before beginning a discussion of endocrinopathies which disturb growth.

NORMAL GROWTH

The process of growth in the child encompasses changes of the body which include not only increase in height and weight but alterations in facial and bodily proportions as well, along with alterations in the growth and maturation of the bones and other organs. It would be quite incorrect to assume that all abnormalities of growth are due to endocrine imbalance. Much more commonly, failure to grow is the result of disease

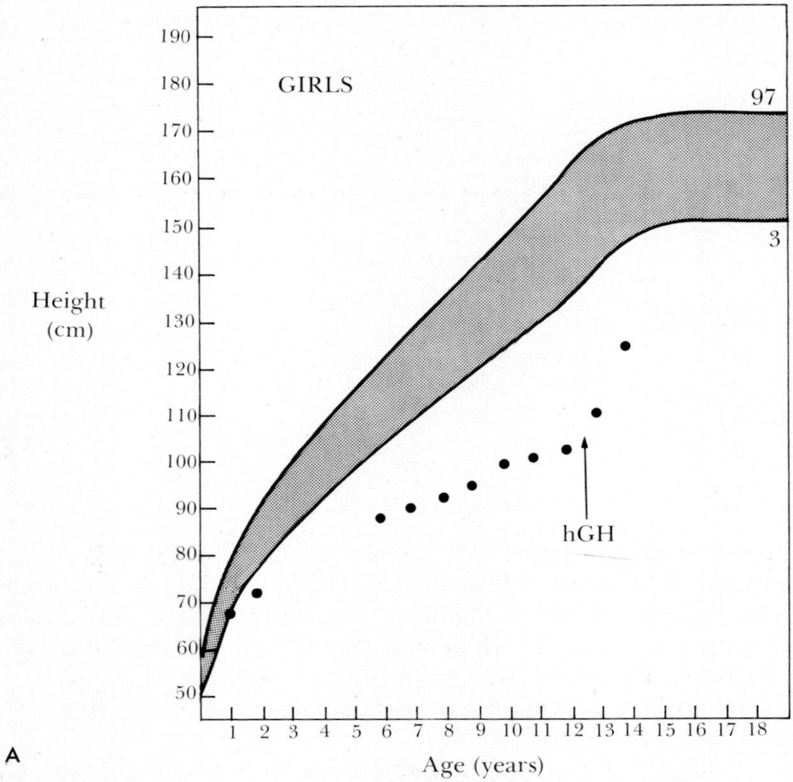

FIGURE 11–1. *A,* Linear growth chart for girls depicting the range between the third and ninety-seventh percentiles. The changes in height of a patient with pituitary dwarfism are shown in solid circles. Therapy with hGH was started at age 12½ years with a dramatic increase in height thereafter. (Data from Dr. John Crigler, Children's Medical Center, Boston, Mass.)

Illustration continued on opposite page.

of a major organ system (respiratory, cardiac, skeletal, renal, gastrointestinal, or central nervous system) or the result of exogenous malnutrition. This should be kept in mind before labeling a disorder of growth as "endocrine' or "metabolic."

Several growth indices are particularly helpful in assessing normal development. Tables of height and weight have been published which depict upper and lower limits of normal growth. These limits represent deviations from the mean or average and are expressed as percentiles (Figure 11–1). Such charts for height and weight are used extensively in following the developmental pattern of the child, and it is customary to refer to the "height age" or "weight age" of the child. Thus if a child is said to have a height age of 4 years, it is meant that he has the mean height (fiftieth percentile) of 4-year-old children of the same sex.

In addition to height and weight ages, other criteria of development, such as the growth and maturation of bones, are useful. Skeletal proportion is in part hormonally determined, and careful measure-

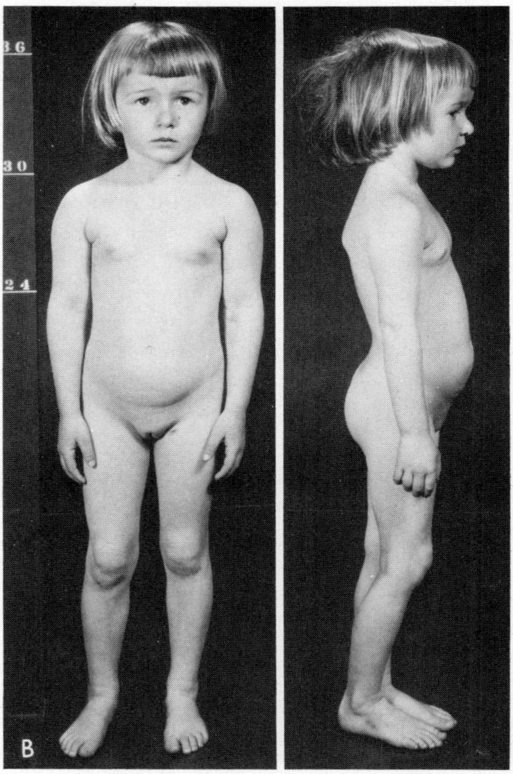

FIGURE 11–1 *Continued.* *B,* Photograph of patient at age 9 years. Her height at that time was 38 inches (95 cm). X-ray films of the skull showed an extremely shallow sella turcica. There was no sexual development during the adolescent years. She was diagnosed as being a pituitary dwarf. At age 16 years, 10 months, she had a height age of 9 years, 3 months and a bone age of 11 years. (Courtesy of Dr. John Crigler, Children's Medical Center, Boston, Mass.)

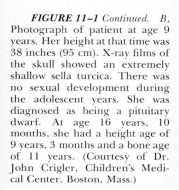

ments of the lower segment and the total height of the body can often provide useful information. At birth the upper:lower ratio is about 1.7:1. In the early years of life the legs grow more rapidly than the trunk; by about age 10 upper and lower segments are of equal length and remain so thereafter.

The maturation of bone is best assessed by studying x-ray films of the epiphyseal centers. A number of tables showing the time of ossification of various cartilages are available. The hand and wrist are most commonly used in determining bone age. The patient's bone age is estimated by comparing his films with the standard plates in the Greulich-Pyle atlas. More recently, a point system has been devised which takes into account the stage of development of individual bones. The scores are added to give a skeletal maturity score for the whole hand and wrist. A percentile status can then be assigned to the child, just as for height and weight.

Facial features change during early development, primarily as a result of growth of the bridge of the nose. Other criteria of development such as head circumference, dental formation, and mental age should be included in the overall assessment of the growing child.

Hormones involved in growth of the child

Somatic growth and development are influenced by at least four hormones: GH, thyroid hormone, glucocorticoids, and the sex hormones (estrogens and androgens). The latter, especially influential at puberty, will be discussed in Chapters Twelve and Thirteen. GH, thyroid hormone, and sex hormones stimulate protein synthesis and nitrogen retention. This is to be expected, for growth connotes increased cell mass, a main constituent of which is protein. About 16 percent of protein is nitrogen, and one would expect increased nitrogen retention with growth. Indeed, a positive nitrogen balance is the classical biochemical expression of growth. Other important constituents of tissue in addition to nitrogen are sodium, chloride, potassium, phosphorus, and calcium.

Increase in cell mass can be achieved either by increasing the number of cells or by increasing the size of individual cells. Which mode of growth will occur depends on the tissue and hormone in question. To increase cell number, DNA synthesis must occur. There is evidence that DNA synthesis ceases in the human brain between 12 and 18 months of age. In contrast, the number of muscle cells can increase through adolescence.

Growth Hormone

In the immature human or experimental animal, removal or destruction of the pituitary gland is associated with a cessation of linear growth. Hypopituitary subjects also show a decrease in the number of muscle cells. If the individual is secreting an adequate amount of thyroid hormone, administration of GH will restore growth and muscle cell number to normal. Virtually all tissues of the body which are capable of growth increase in size in response to GH. Undoubtedly many of these effects are secondary to the known effect of GH on transport of amino acids and incorporation of amino acids into protein.

Linear growth is due primarily to growth of the bones of the extremities. Bones grow as a result of proliferation of cartilage in the epiphyseal plates (p. 322), and this *chondrogenesis* is dependent upon GH. The rate of this process can be estimated by measuring the uptake of ^{35}S-sulfate into the chondromucoprotein of cartilage. In the hypophysectomized rat this uptake is minimal; however, within 24 hours after treatment of these hypophysectomized rats with GH, sulfate incorporation by cartilage is restored to normal. There is no direct effect of GH on cartilage in vitro. Instead it appears that GH stimulates skeletal growth indirectly by induction of a secondary mediator that acts directly on cartilage. This mediator, which is probably formed in the liver, has been named *somatomedin*

Somatomedin is a remarkably stable, neutral peptide of about 8000 molecular weight, which increases the incorporation of ^{35}S-sulfate into chondromucoprotein and the incorporation of labeled thymidine into labeled DNA. These activities were previously believed to be due to separate substances: "sulfation factor" and "thymidine factor." Somatomedin disappears from the serum after hypophysectomy but is restored in hypophysectomized rats by the administration of GH. It has a half-life of about three to five hours. Its action on cartilage involves many aspects of cellular metabolism. Cartilage exposed to somatomedin shows increased incorporation of leucine into protein (after 2 hours), uridine into RNA (after 4 hours), sulfate into chondromucoprotein (after 12 to 24 hours), and thymidine into DNA (after 48 hours).

Purified preparations of somatomedin exhibit insulin-like effects in at least four bioassay systems: the incorporation of amino acids into proteins of rat diaphragm, the utilization of glucose by epididymal fat pads, antilipolytic action in epinephrine-stimulated epididymal fat pads, and stimulation of protein synthesis and cell replication in HeLa cells. In addition, it has been difficult to dissociate somatomedin activity from insulin-like activity during purification procedures. Indeed, at physiological concentrations, somatomedin competes with ^{125}I-insulin for receptor sites on isolated chondrocytes, fat cells, and liver membranes, The relative binding affinities of these two proteins reflect their biological potency in vitro, suggesting a structural as well as functional homology.

Somatomedin can inhibit adenyl cyclase activity in crude preparations of membranes from adipose tissue and liver cells of the rat and from chondrocytes and cartilage of chick embryos. Similar inhibition of adenyl cyclase activity by insulin can be demonstrated using fat and liver cells. Since final purification of somatomedin has not been achieved, it is not known whether its various biological activities can be attributed to a single peptide or to multiple species of closely related peptides. It has even been suggested that somatomedin might represent a portion of the GH molecule, perhaps the "active core." This possibility cannot be excluded until the primary structure of somatomedin is determined.

The effects of GH and insulin are similar in many respects. If GH is administered to a hypophysectomized rat, one can observe increased body weight, skeletal cartilage, muscle mass, and cell number, but *decreased* body fat. Insulin will do all these things, but under the influence of insulin body fat is *increased*. There are other more subtle differences between insulin and GH. The effect of GH on transport of amino acids into cells in vitro is detected within 20 minutes. A similar effect by insulin is detected within five minutes. Caution is advised in interpreting such in vitro studies, since demonstrations of direct GH effects on muscle and fat have required concentrations of GH ten to several hundred times higher than the maximum concentration circulating in vivo.

GH is an insulin antagonist, probably by virtue of its lipolytic action. Free fatty acids are released during lipolysis, and as their concentration in the blood rises, they enter cells and become effective inhibitors of glycolysis. Thus glucose utilization is suppressed and hyperglycemia results. Possibly a different part of the GH molecule is involved in lipolysis, as opposed to that portion which enhances somatomedin production.

GH extracted from plasma and subjected to gel filtration on G-75 Sephadex can be separated into two species of GH which can be detected by immunoassay. Some 65 to 85 percent of the total is the usual GH of molecular weight 21,000. The remainder (15 to 35 percent) has a much larger molecular weight, about 40,000, and has been called "big" or "large" GH. It is not clear whether the "big" GH is a precursor of "little" GH or simply a dimer. When measured for binding to GH receptor sites on cultured human lymphocytes, the larger form has less biological activity than the smaller form.

Many hormones circulate in the blood as "big" and "little" forms. This usually reflects the presence of multiple forms of the hormone in the tissue of origin. The fusion of lysosomes with packaged hormone granules brings about hydrolysis of the large molecule to smaller fragments which are then secreted from the cell. Perhaps there is some optimal size protein molecule for synthesis on the cellular polysomes. These large "prohormones" can subsequently be "cut to size."

Further modification or fragmentation of the hormone molecule may occur in other tissues, yielding peptide moieties of differing biological function. We know so little of the synthesis and metabolism of protein hormones. It is entirely possible that many puzzling effects of protein hormones in vivo are due to multiple forms of the hormone (isohormones) or to peptides produced by cleavage of the original hormone.

Thyroid Hormone

The effects of thyroid hormone (thyroxine or triiodothyronine) on growth of tissue may take several days to become apparent. Presumably, therefore, a series of cellular events must occur prior to net protein synthesis. What are these events? Tata has attempted to determine the sequence of events occurring in the liver of thyroidectomized rats after a single injection (15 to 25 μg) of triiodothyronine. The first effect noted was an increased labeling of nuclear RNA (from labeled uridine), evident after as little as six hours. By 10 to 12 hours, isolated liver nuclei from the rats showed increased activity of DNA-dependent RNA polymerase. By 21 hours, the synthesis of all three forms of RNA (messenger, ribosomal, transfer) had been stimulated. The rapid synthesis of RNA and the increased activity of RNA polymerase both precede the incorporation of labeled amino acids into mitochondrial and microsomal proteins. Eventually the metabolic rate rises (after about 45 hours), and finally the amount of liver tissue increases (after about 70 hours). Some of the most prominent changes occur in the ribosomes. More ribosomes are produced, and they are more tightly attached to microsomal membranes. Amino acid incorporation into ribosomes is increased, and proliferation of microsomal membranes is evident.

In addition to these profound effects on RNA and protein synthesis, thyroid hormone can affect DNA synthesis in actively growing tissues. These effects could be secondary to a primary effect on RNA and protein synthesis. Adequate thyroid hormone is necessary for completely normal growth, and thyroid hormone is exclusively involved in the maturation of brain and bone. Apparently the action of thyroid hormone on growth is a "permissive" one, permitting normal growth and development.

Thyroid hormone has profound effects on oxidative phosphorylation in the mitochondria of the cell. In large quantities, the hormone can uncouple oxidative phosphorylation. Concomitantly water enters the mitochondria, which swell, suggesting an effect of thyroxine on the mitochondrial membrane. Just how these mitochondrial effects relate to the microsomal effects of thyroid hormone is puzzling. Sokoloff has shown recently that in vitro in a cell-free system thyroxine will stimulate the synthesis of microsomal protein and that this effect requires the presence of mitochondria. Inhibitors of RNA synthesis do not abolish this in vitro effect. Thyroxine in high concentration stimulates the synthesis of protein and oxygen consumption in isolated mitochondria. Chloramphenicol inhibits the thyroxine effect on protein synthesis but has no effect on the enhanced oxygen consumption. It is of interest that the increased oxygen consumption in tissues from animals treated with thyroxine can be prevented in large measure by blocking Na^+ transport with ouabain. The maintenance of normal intracellular concentrations of ions such as Na^+, K^+, and Cl^- requires from 10 to 30 percent of the cell's total energy ex penditure. Na-K activated ATPase in plasma membranes from livers of animals treated with triiodothyronine showed considerable increase in activity over that of liver membranes from control animals. Stimulation of this transport system may be a primary effect of thyroid hormone or secondary to a thyroid hormone-induced increase in cellular metabolic rate.

Thus in some fashion thyroid hormone speeds up the metabolic rate of cells, probably by a primary effect on mitochondria, and the synthesis of protein, RNA, and DNA is enhanced. The results of these biochemical perturbations include growth, maturation of target tissues, and physiologic changes in certain tissues of the body. Not all tissues show an increase in metabolic rate on exposure to thyroid hormone. Amongst the major exceptions are the gonads, adult brain, lung, spleen, and thymus.

Other Hormones Influencing Growth

Insulin is a powerful anabolic hormone. It too increases the synthesis of DNA, RNA, and protein in target tissues. Wool has provided strong evidence that there is a deficiency in the functional capacity of ribosomes from diabetic animals. This is not due to a lack of messenger RNA. If one compares the incorporation of amino acids into protein in the presence of a synthetic messenger RNA in muscle ribosomes from diabetic animals with that of ribosomes from normal animals, there is still a deficiency in the capacity of ribosomes from diabetic animals to form proteins. It is not known what change in the ribosome may be brought about by insulin. Wool has some evidence that insulin produces a protein which interacts with the ribosome to increase its protein synthesizing capacity.

There is no question that in addition to its effects on nucleic acid and protein synthesis, insulin has profound effects on the transport of glucose and amino acids across the plasma membrane. These membrane effects could provide the energy and substrates necessary for protein synthesis.

Glucocorticoids act as inhibitors of protein synthesis and stimulators of gluconeogenesis from amino acid moieties of protein. For example, the incorporation of amino acids into protein in the diaphragm of an adrenalectomized animal is greater than the normal rate, and treatment with cortisol reduces this incorporation. Protein synthesis is not uniformly decreased by cortisol. The enzymes involved in gluconeogenesis in liver are induced by cortisol (p. 233). This involves increased protein synthesis to form these enzymes. The effect is probably secondary to stimulation of nuclear RNA synthesis, which is noted as little as 30 minutes after cortisol administration. Nevertheless, the effect of glucocorticoids on the entire body is one of protein catabolism rather than anabolism.

Perhaps most important of all is the intermingling of these hormonal effects. The normal growth response to administered GH requires the presence of thyroid hormone. Many investigators use hypophysectomized animals for study; it should be remembered that such animals lack the tropic hormones of the anterior pituitary (and therefore the hormones of the target glands); in addition, they manifest decreased insulin secretion. Thyroid hormone itself affects the content of GH in the anterior pituitary and probably its secretion as well. Changes in blood glucose affect not only insulin secretion but also the secretions of GH and glucagon. Obviously, any hormone regulating glucose concentration in the blood also influences growth, for the very nature of the biosynthetic process requires a constant supply of chemical energy. In turn, hormones regulating transport of other substances needed for cellular metabolism help regulate growth.

BIOCHEMICAL BASIS OF GROWTH AND ITS CONTROL

In essence, growth of the organism is dependent upon growth and division of cells and an increase in extracellular materials. Most of these extracellular materials (such as collagen, elastin, mucopolysaccharides) are made by cells and secreted into the extracellular spaces. Thus a central feature of growth is the ability of cells to form specific proteins.

Just how are proteins formed? Zamecnik and his colleagues did a series of truly beautiful experiments which helped answer this question. They injected radioactive amino acids into rats, and at different time intervals thereafter they removed the liver, homogenized it, and looked for radioactivity in the various fractions prepared by differential centrifugation. If hours or days elapsed, all liver fractions contained labeled protein, but if the liver was fractionated shortly after the injection of labeled amino acids, only the microsomal fraction contained labeled protein. Thus it was postulated that proteins are first synthesized in those intracellular structures from which the *microsomes* are derived.

It soon became evident that the incorporated radioactivity resided largely in small ribonucleoprotein particles attached to the microsomal membranes. These particles were named *ribosomes.* They can be detached from the microsomal membranes *(endoplasmic reticulum)* by treatment with a detergent such as sodium deoxycholate. In order for ribosomes to form protein, certain essential cofactors must be present in the medium surrounding them. Among these necessary factors are enzymes to activate the amino acids and esterify them and low molecular weight RNA (soluble or transfer RNA). Within the cytoplasm of the cell, amino acids are enzymatically esterified to their corresponding homologous transfer RNA's. The first *aminoacyl transfer RNA,* called the initiator RNA, determines the beginning of the peptide chain. It becomes bound to a 40S component of ribosomal RNA which in turn is bound to messenger RNA (Figure 11–2). A specific triplet of bases in messenger RNA *(codon)* is brought proximate to its appropriate triplet mate *(anticodon)* of transfer RNA. This transfer RNA bears a specific amino acid; therefore, each triplet of bases in messenger RNA ensures that a specific amino acid is "lined up" on the ribosome. Another component of the ribosome (60S) translocates the amino acid bound to the transfer RNA from the attachment to 40S to the growing peptide chain. Peptide bonds are formed between two adjacent amino acids on the ribosome. After the completion of each new peptide bond, both the messenger RNA and the nascent peptide chain (peptidyl transfer RNA) are moved along the ribosome to bring the next codon into position (Figure 11–2). When the peptide chain is complete, it is liberated from the ribosome and the latter is released from its combination with messenger RNA. Several ribosomes are usually attached to a given messenger RNA and form the functional unit of protein synthesis, the *polysome.*

The original messenger RNA, the base sequence of which determines the sequence in which transfer RNA's attach to the ribosome, and which in turn determines the sequence of amino acids, is synthesized in the nucleus according to the pattern of a specific DNA. The entire process of growth must therefore involve *replication* (the process in which DNA is copied to form identical daughter molecules, catalyzed by *DNA*

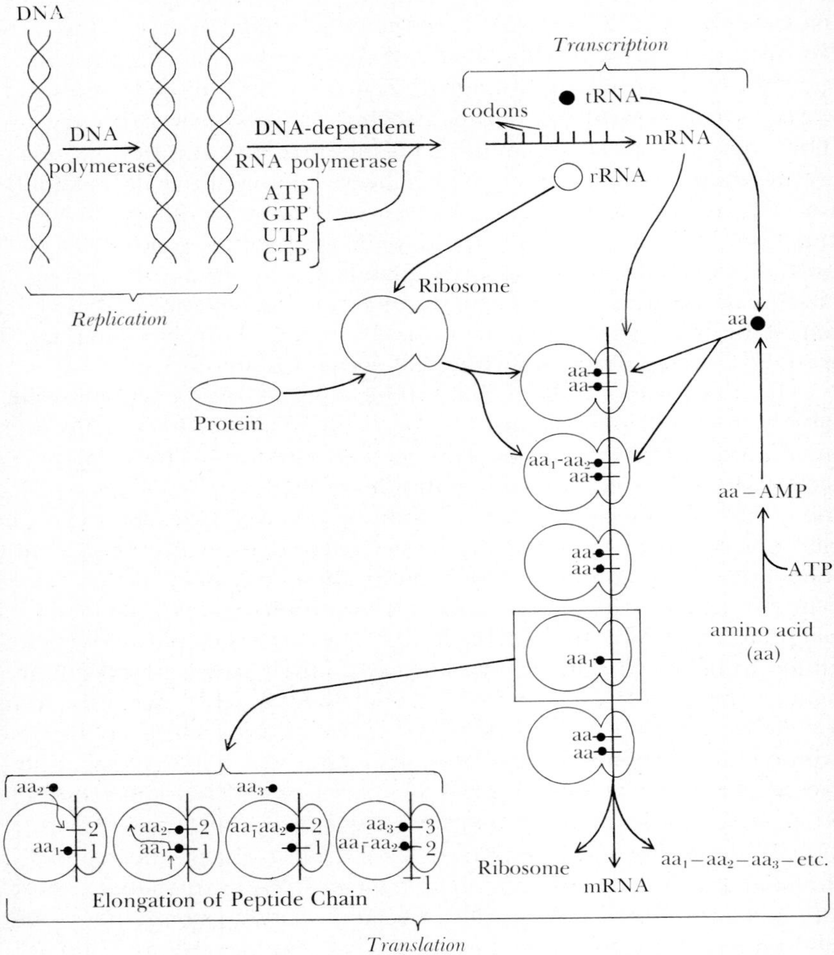

FIGURE 11–2. Biochemical basis of growth showing replication of DNA, transcription of DNA to RNA, and translation of the mRNA code into a linear sequence of amino acids. Not shown is the polyA tail which is attached to the mRNA during its processing in the nucleus.

polymerase), *transcription* (the process in which the genetic message in DNA is transcribed into the form of RNA, catalyzed by *DNA-dependent RNA polymerase*), and *translation* (the process occurring in the *ribosomes* in which the genetic message is decoded and converted into the 20-letter alphabet of protein structure). Biochemical control of growth can occur at any one of these three steps (Figure 11–2).

An increase in the rate at which DNA replicates generally brings about an increased rate of mitosis. Thus the number of cells in a tissue can be regulated by controlling DNA synthesis. No new kind of DNA is formed, however, since each cell has the same complement of DNA molecules. Not all of these molecules are transcribed. In fact, most of the chromosomal DNA is not transcribed; the transcription of large segments is continuously repressed, perhaps by a covering of protein *repressors*.

In regard to repressors, an early proposal by Karlson (1963) suggested that hormones activate genes by acting as inducers, which by combining with appropriate repressors control the synthesis of messenger RNA and thus regulate protein synthesis. It may not be the hormone itself, but a hormone-receptor complex which combines with the repressor. Thus, in effect, the hormone (or hormone-receptor complex) acts as a *derepressor*. An alternative model proposes that the hormone binds to a receptor protein which, in turn, binds to regulatory sites on the genome and promotes transcription of specific genes. Certainly GH, insulin, glucocorticoids, thyroid hormone, and estrogens and androgens all show effects on RNA synthesis in responsive tissues, but we do not know whether messenger RNA is specifically involved. One might suspect this to be the case where specific enzymes are induced, as in the case of the induction of tyrosine-α-ketoglutarate aminotransferase in liver by cortisol.

The actual translation of the base sequence of messenger RNA into the amino acid sequence of a protein is another logical site for hormonal control. Some of the effects of thyroid hormone on ribosomal function as described by Tata serve as examples. The defective ribosomal function in the diabetic animal may be another example of hormonal control of translation.

Still another aspect of the control of protein synthesis and growth involves the adenyl cyclase system. We have referred to this enzyme frequently throughout this book, and the product of its action, cyclic AMP, undoubtedly plays a very important role in cellular metabolism.

Cyclic AMP consists of adenine, ribose, and phosphate in a ratio of 1:1:1 (Figure 11–3). It is remarkably stable to heat and is not inactivated by a number of phosphatases or diesterases. It is, however, converted to

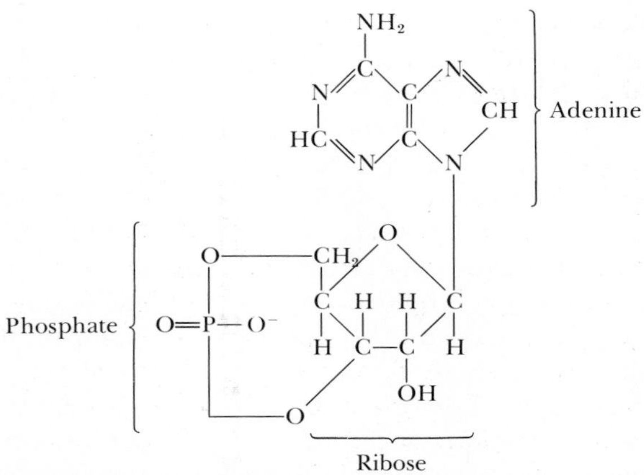

FIGURE 11–3. Cyclic AMP (adenosine 3′,5′-cyclic monophosphate).

5′AMP by specific phosphodiesterases. Cyclic AMP is formed from ATP in a reaction that requires Mg^{++} and that is catalyzed by adenyl cyclase. The actual concentration of cyclic AMP in the cell is determined by the relative activities of adenyl cyclase and the phosphodiesterases. For as yet unknown reasons adenyl cyclase is stimulated by fluoride ion, at any concentration of ATP, increasing the rate of the conversion of ATP to cyclic AMP approximately twenty times over. A comparable stimulation of the enzyme by glucagon occurs in liver, but only if the concentration of ATP is greater than 10^{-4}M. Thus the relative K_m and V_{max} values of these enzyme systems are important in determining the overall effect of a given agent.

The adenyl cyclase of the cell, and there may well be more than one, resides on the inner surface of the limiting plasma membrane. Most peptide hormones interact with a receptor protein on the outer surface of the plasma membrane. The juxtaposition of hormone receptor and adenyl cyclase may be more than just fortuitous; indeed, some investigators believe that the hormone receptor is an integral part of the adenyl cyclase system.

Cyclic AMP is necessary for the activity of a variety of protein kinases within the cell. These protein kinases apparently regulate a considerable number of cellular processes by virtue of their ability to phosphorylate certain critical proteins. We have already mentioned several of these. Phosphorylation by protein kinase activates phosphorylase and lipase and inactivates glycogen synthetase (p. 236). Protein kinases have also been implicated in the phosphorylation of histones, basic proteins which may be involved in the repression of DNA transcription. It is important to remember that as yet there is no direct evidence that transcription is regulated by histone phosphorylation.

Cyclic AMP-dependent protein kinase can phosphorylate ribosomes. Garren has proposed that such a phosphorylation of ribosomal protein may be important in translational control. For example, Gill isolated ribosomes from adrenal cortical cells and incubated them with a cyclic AMP-dependent protein kinase from the cytosol. Extensive cyclic AMP-dependent phosphorylation of ribosomal protein occurred. Hydrolysis of the ribosomal protein and electrophoresis of the products revealed that serine and threonine residues were phosphorylated. ACTH stimulated adenyl cyclase in adrenal cells and also stimulated phosphorylation of ribosomal protein. Thus it is quite possible that the long term growth effects of ACTH on the adrenal gland might be associated with enhanced protein synthesis via phosphorylation of ribosomal protein. This theory would predict that phosphorylated ribosomes are more active in protein synthesis than are nonphosphorylated ribosomes. In all mammalian systems studied, ribosomal phosphoproteins have been identified. Treatment of rats with glucagon resulted in increased phosphorylation of ribosomal proteins in target tissues. Similarly, thyroidectomy resulted in a 35 percent decrease in phosphate content of ribosomal protein; triiodothyronine restored the phosphate content to control levels.

By altering the concentration of cyclic AMP within the cell, the functions of that cell will be altered. In general, the primary function of the cell is increased as the concentration of cyclic AMP within the cell is increased. Let us take an example.

One of the functions of cyclic AMP is to stimulate the production or release of several hormones, including thyroid hormone. The sequence of events for the latter appears to be as follows. Circulating TSH reaches the thyroid gland and there binds to a receptor on the surface of the thyroid epithelial cell. In some way this interaction leads to stimulation of adenyl cyclase, which in turn leads to an increase in the amount of cyclic AMP within the cell. Cyclic AMP is able to increase the rate of endocytosis, and the thyroid cells become full of colloid droplets. These droplets fuse with the lysosomes of the cell. Within the lysosomes are proteolytic enzymes which hydrolyze the thyroglobulin in colloid, releasing thyroid hormones. Other effects of TSH within the cell are noted. The uptake and organification of inorganic iodide is increased, peroxidase and coupling enzymes are stimulated, and proteolysis is increased. The actual relationship of these effects to the cyclic AMP-protein kinase system or to some other cyclic AMP-dependent system has not been worked out. Nevertheless, it seems clear that factors such as LATS and prostaglandin E_1, which can alter intracellular concentration of cyclic AMP, can alter the synthesis and secretion of thyroid hormone.

Cyclic AMP clearly regulates the functions of many types of cells. Does it regulate their growth? Most of the studies of cyclic AMP and growth have utilized cell culture systems. Striking relationships between growth rate and the concentration of cyclic AMP within the cell have been noted in various cell lines. Fibroblasts that grow rapidly in cell culture have very low levels of cyclic AMP intracellularly. The converse is also true; high levels of cyclic AMP are found in cells that are not growing. There is also evidence that cyclic AMP mediates contact inhibition of growth. Certainly with the myriad effects of cyclic AMP on the growth and function of cells it is not surprising that many investigators would attribute all the effects of the non-steroid hormones to alterations in concentration of this nucleotide. They would suggest that the specificity of hormone action resides in the receptors in the target tissues and that the ultimate effect of the hormone-receptor complex is on the concentration of cyclic AMP within the cell. Steroid hormones do not function in this manner. It would seem that steroids act within the nucleus rather than at the cell surface and that their action involves genic derepression, with a subsequent increase in RNA and protein synthesis (p. 99).

RETARDED GROWTH

Although this book is primarily concerned with endocrine relations in development, the central role of nutrition on growth is most germane to that discussion. Even in relatively affluent countries, large numbers of children suffer from malnutrition. This malnutrition is not confined to the poor. Meyer has commented on the poor diets of most adolescents as one example of malnutrition. If the onset is early enough, long-standing malnutrition will be associated with a failure to grow. In addition, the earlier the malnutrition occurs, the more severe the damage in developing organs such as the brain, and the less likely the recovery.

In the human brain the number of cells increases linearly until birth and then increases more slowly until about 12 to 18 months of age. Thereafter there is little if any rise in the number of brain cells. Brain weight, however, increases rapidly in the first two years of life and more slowly thereafter. Thus one would expect the human brain to be vulnerable to nutritional deficits both prenatally and in the first years of life.

Conditions which impair intake of food or promote loss of nutrients can alter the pattern of growth. Most of these are nonendocrine in nature and are not within the scope of this book. A variety of inborn errors of metabolism, congenital defects, chromosomal anomalies, and infectious processes can manifest themselves as disorders of growth. Emotional factors may also be involved in "failure-to-thrive" syndromes. Thus, when presented with a child who is below normal in height age or weight age (or both), the physician must give due consideration to genetic, nutritional, and environmental causes of retarded growth. If adequate nutrients are available to the child and there is no inherited or environmental reason for retarded growth, one must investigate the endocrine system. Deficiency of either GH or thyroid hormone will retard linear growth. Glucocorticoids, insulin, PTH, and gonadal hormones may also influence the rate of linear growth and development of the young child.

Deficiency of GH

Any lesion or congenital abnormality which impairs pituitary function may bring about a state of deficiency in one or more of the hormones of the adenohypophysis. This gland has considerable functional reserve, and clinical features are usually absent until destruction of about 75 percent of the gland has occurred. In general, with progressively severe pituitary damage, deficiencies of GH, gonadotropins, TSH, and ACTH appear.

In many instances pituitary insufficiency is secondary to a lesion or congenital deformity in the hypothalamic area. Some of these conditions, such as *anencephaly,* are incompatible with life. In anencephaly the anterior neuropore fails to close in embryonic life (p. 45), and structures above the level of the basal ganglia are poorly formed or not formed at all. The hypothalamus is among the structures which fail to develop and, in essence, from an endocrine standpoint, anencephalic children represent a state of total lack of the hypothalamic hormones. Although some of these children have pituitaries of normal size, others show varying degrees of pituitary hypoplasia. Studies of a full term female anencephalic infant by Allen and his colleagues showed that the anterior pituitary of this infant contained a readily dischargeable pool of TSH and ACTH; however, both hormones were present in low amounts in the plasma of the infant. GH concentration in plasma was also lower than that reported in normal infants; however, after birth it gradually rose. Thus the fetal pituitary can apparently synthesize ACTH, TSH, and GH in the absence of a hypothalamus. The capacity to increase secretion of ACTH and TSH in response to administered vasopressin and TRH (respectively) was also present. The failure of the target organs to respond to ACTH and TSH in this infant was attributed to functional atrophy of the tissues. Despite adrenal atrophy the plasma concentrations of cortisol were normal; a maternal origin of the cortisol seems likely.

The infant had relatively normal plasma concentrations of T_3 and T_4 despite low plasma TSH concentrations and hypoplasia of the thyroid gland. Since very little maternal T_4 and T_3 reaches the fetus, the investigators suggest that there may be a capacity for some autonomous secretion of T_4 and T_3 in neonates despite low plasma TSH concentrations, or that placental thyrotropin may stimulate hormone secretion of the fetal thyroid to a certain extent. The usual post-delivery increase in plasma TSH (p. 111) was not seen in this anencephalic infant.

The adrenals of the anencephalic are characteristically hypoplastic. In addition, the thyroid gland and testes may show developmental abnormalities, although less frequently than the adrenals do. Certainly, from the evidence available, we must conclude that a certain degree of anterior pituitary function (synthesis of hormones and response to stimuli) exists in the fetus deprived of hypothalamic control. The actual secretion of hormones by the anterior pituitary is undoubtedly impaired and is reflected by the poor development of the adrenals and, on occasion, of the thyroid and testes.

Trauma, tumors (craniopharyngioma, p. 205), infection, or systemic disease may impair pituitary function either indirectly, by altering hypothalamic function, or directly. In some children no readily discernible etiology is apparent, and the term *idiopathic pituitary insufficiency* is applied. This is the most common form of hypopituitarism in childhood, although even as such, it accounts for less than 10 percent of all cases of short stature. It is difficult to diagnose, because localizing central nervous system signs are not present. It must be distinguished from constitutional delays of growth and from various forms of "primordial" dwarfism.

The clinical picture of pituitary insufficiency will, of course, depend upon the hormones involved. If all the anterior pituitary hormones are deficient, the condition of *panhypopituitarism* ensues. In the young child lack of pituitary gonadotropins will not be ascertainable. Such hypogonadal states will be discussed in Chapter Thirteen when the endocrine changes of puberty are described.

The lack of ACTH, TSH, and GH will be readily apparent in the young child. A deficiency of ACTH will produce a picture of glucocorticoid lack. Salt loss is generally not noted, since aldosterone production is not primarily under pituitary control. Symptoms of hypoglycemia may be encountered in children with panhypopituitarism; fasting hypoglycemia is common. This hypoglycemia probably reflects GH lack. Occasionally, hyperglycemia may be found, probably secondary to the insulinopenia found in patients with hypopituitarism.

Characteristically children with pituitary insufficiency grow slowly, deviating from the normal growth curve within the first months of life (Figure 11–1). There is no evidence that GH is needed for fetal growth and development. At birth these children have a normal weight and length. A progressive decrease in growth rate occurs. When this growth is charted, the height is always below the third percentile line and progressively deviates more and more from this line as time goes by (Figure 11–1). Skeletal, dental, and motor development are retarded, probably owing to thyroid hormone deficiency. These children are not typically myxedematous but may have the characteristic dry skin and constipation of hypothyroidism.

Children with pituitary insufficiency manifest proportional growth in general, but the bones of the hands and feet may be small. Obesity is often found, probably because of the lack of the lipolytic activity of GH. The face is rounded and doll-like. A variety of other conditions in childhood can cause growth retardation. Fortunately, many of these conditions, such as Laurence-Moon-Biedl syndrome and Prader-Willi syndrome (p. 304), present certain characteristic features which aid in diagnosis. More difficult to differentiate from pituitary deficiency is hypothyroidism. Cushing's syndrome in childhood retards growth, and uncontrolled chronic diabetes mellitus may do likewise. Girls with short stature should always be suspected of having Turner's syndrome. Thus many endocrine disorders cause impaired growth and must be considered in the differential diagnosis of retarded growth in childhood (Table 11–1).

Hereditary GH Deficiency

Rimoin and coworkers described a deficiency of GH which appeared to be inherited as an autosomal recessive trait. In infancy the patients eat little, but they are sometimes obese. The tendency to hypoglycemia is aggravated by fasting and may necessitate snacks at night. In such children body proportions are normal, but slow growth of facial bones in relation to the skull (already well-developed at birth) and small hands and feet are characteristic. Motor development may be slow. The bone age is retarded but not so much as the height age.

Laron has described several patients with typical signs and symptoms of GH deficiency but with *normal* or even *elevated* concentrations of immunoreactive GH in the blood. These children are dwarfed and obese and have a tendency to hypoglycemia. The concentration of somatomedin in the blood is low and fails to rise following administration of GH. This disorder may represent a deficiency in target cell receptor binding of GH or a defect in the chain of intracellular events between GH binding and somatomedin synthesis.

By observing patients with GH deficiency after administration of human GH (hGH), we can study the effects of this hormone in vivo (Figure 11–1). The younger the patient, the more dramatic the response. Doses as small as one mg administered three times a week produced a growth of seven inches in three months in a 13-month-old boy. Unfortunately, growth is usually less the second year of treatment and still less in the third and fourth years. This may be due in part to the appearance in the patient of antibodies to GH. Even in the absence of antibodies, the potential for growth seems to decline in older children, and their response to exogenous hGH becomes progressively less dramatic.

Tests for Pituitary Reserve of GH

A number of factors trigger the hypothalamus to release GHRH, which in turn brings about the release of GH from the cells of the anterior pituitary. These factors can be utilized clinically to ascertain whether or not the anterior pituitary contains GH and can release it. Exercise brings about a release of GH and is used in many clinics as a test of pituitary reserve of GH. Insulin, arginine, sleep, and L-dopa are also used in testing GH reserve.

Insulin tolerance test (hypoglycemic test). A marked decrease in the concentration of glucose in the blood perfusing the hypothalamus (decreased glucose metabolism, p. 248) is a powerful stimulus for GHRH release, resulting in the discharge of GH from the anterior pituitary (Figure 10–3). Insulin is used to produce such a hypoglycemia. An alternative would be to use tolbutamide, which causes the release of insulin from the pancreatic β cell. Using an appropriate dose of insulin (0.05 to 0.15 U/kg intravenously), the blood glucose concentration can be reduced 40 to 50 percent, which is a sufficient stimulus for GH release. A rise in GH concentration of 5 to 10 ng/ml suggests normal production of the hormone (Figure 10–3). The attending physician must be alert for symptoms of hypoglycemia, since children with hypopituitarism may be particularly sensitive to insulin.

Arginine tolerance test. Arginine is another powerful stimulus for GH release, and in children it usually induces a greater rise in plasma GH than does insulin-induced hypoglycemia. The administration of 10 to 30 g of arginine to normal children intravenously over a 30 to 45 minute period will bring about a rise in the concentration of GH in serum over control concentration values within 30 minutes of the completion of the infusion of the arginine. A sex difference in the response to intravenous arginine has been reported, with some males showing no increase in GH secretion. Prior administration of stilbestrol to these males can convert nonresponding males to responders.

SLEEP. During a normal seven to eight hour sleep period, there occurs a cycle of behavioral and electroencephalographic (EEG) patterns. After two to three hours of sleep, characterized by high voltage, slow wave EEG activity associated with regular respirations and slow eye movements (or no eye movements), a different pattern occurs. This new pattern consists of episodes of irregular respirations, gross conjugate rapid eye movements (REM), and low voltage, fast frequency EEG activity. These periods of REM sleep occur three to five times a night, usually lasting 15 to 20 minutes. This REM sleep occupies 15 to 25 percent of a total night's sleep and has been found to be associated with visual imagery dreaming. Between REM sleep periods the classic slow wave pattern recurs. Characteristically, 50 percent or more of early morning sleep (the two to three hours of sleep prior to awakening) is occupied by REM sleep.

Sleep markedly influences the secretion of GH by the anterior pituitary. GH concentration in the blood rises during sleep, the highest levels coinciding with the first few hours of sleep (slow wave sleep). Measurement of GH concentrations in the blood during sleep have been used as an indication of pituitary reserve capacity for increasing the secretion of GH.

Undoubtedly many biological rhythms exist for secretion of hormones. Some, such as GH secretion, are undoubtedly related to the sleep cycle itself, since a rise in plasma GH will usually occur shortly after the onset of slow wave sleep, regardless of the time of day at which sleep occurs. Other rhythms are controlled by circadian variations, as with ACTH secretion (p. 171). The diurnal variation in ACTH secretion, with the subsequent change in plasma cortisol, constitutes a "biological clock," maximum secretion occurring in the early morning and low secretion in the late afternoon. This clock can be reversed by altering the sleep phase to daytime and the wake phase to nighttime; however, several days of reversal are required before the pattern of hormone secretion changes. Other hormones may have still other patterns of secretion. Present evidence suggests that both circadian and sleep-related fluctuations in the concentration of TSH in plasma occur.

L-DOPA. The adrenergic system modulates the secretion of GH in response to various stimuli. The neurohormone with transmitter functions in sympathetic nerves and ganglia is norepinephrine, and the immediate precursor of norepinephrine is dopamine (3-hydroxytyramine). Both dopamine and norepinephrine have transmitter functions in the central nervous system. From histochemical studies it is concluded that dopamine is the primary amine in the median eminence and that granules containing dopamine are located in close proximity to the capillaries of the pituitary portal system. Thus it has been suggested that dopamine may play a role in the regulation of secretions from the adenohypophysis.

Dopamine does not cross the blood-brain barrier; however, its immediate precursor, L-dopa, does. When administered to humans, L-dopa reaches the brain cells and is decarboxylated to dopamine within them. Boyd and coworkers showed that when patients with Parkinson's disease were given L-dopa orally, they responded with increased GH secretion. Subsequently, L-dopa has been used by some investigators as a means of stimulating GH secretion in adults and children. Following a single oral dose of L-dopa, the concentration of GH in the plasma rises within 60 to 120 minutes. This GH response to L-dopa can be blocked by phentolamine, an α-adrenergic blocking agent, and by hyperglycemia present before the administration of L-dopa. Thus L-dopa can serve as another means of assessing the capacity of the anterior pituitary to secrete GH.

At present, GH is usually measured by radioimmunoassay. Human GH is injected into rabbits (or guinea pigs), and antisera are prepared. The sample of serum to be studied is mixed with radioactively labeled hGH and antiserum. Both the GH in the serum and the labeled GH compete for binding sites on the antibodies in the rabbit antiserum. A serum sample containing large quantities of GH will occupy most of the binding sites, leaving few for the labeled GH. Bound and unbound GH are separated, and the amount of labeled GH in the supernatant fluid or on precipitated antibodies can then be counted. From standard curves it is possible to obtain a precise measurement of the concentration of GH in the original sample of serum. It must be remembered, however, that such values reflect the immunologically active GH and not necessarily the biologically active hormone.

In any of the forms of GH deficiency the basic defect may be hypothalamic. Ideally, one would like to use GHRH to test the presence of a functioning anterior pituitary. A more readily available hypothalamic hormone is TRH. In patients with both GH and TSH deficiency, administration of TRH will produce a release of TSH if the defect resides in the hypothalamus rather than in the pituitary. It is inferred that these same patients would be able to release GH in response to GHRH.

Treatment of GH Deficiency

There is no question that, when available, the ideal treatment for the child with GH deficiency is the hormone itself. Problems arise, however, in differentiating the GH-deficient form of dwarfism from other forms. Human pituitaries obtained at autopsy constitute the only current source of human GH. Indiscriminate use of the hormone for dwarfism would be wasteful and unfair to those patients needing it. In general, other forms of dwarfism respond little if at all to hGH therapy, whereas the child with true GH deficiency responds dramatically with increased nitrogen and calcium retention and increased rate of linear growth. Many investigators have sought other hormones which might accelerate linear growth. Hopefully, in time, a synthetic polypeptide with growth-promoting activity which can be readily manufactured will be discovered and made available to the clinician. It is possible that GHRH or somatomedin will be synthesized and made available for clinical use.

Hypothyroidism

The growing organism is peculiarly dependent on thyroid hormone. Even in fetal life the development of the brain and the appearance of the maturation centers (epiphyses) in bone are dependent on thyroid hormone. The activity of the thyroid gland is controlled primarily by TSH from the anterior pituitary; hence, hypothyroidism may be primary, due to abnormal function of the thyroid gland, or secondary, due to lack of TSH or TRH.

Primary hypothyroidism

The release of TSH is regulated in part by the concentration of unbound thyroid hormone in the blood perfusing the anterior pituitary. If the concentration of thyroxine is high, the release of TSH is suppressed. The converse is true also. Such a classical feedback regulation is not unique to the thyroid system; the release of ACTH and gonadotropins is inhibited by the products of their target organs, cortisol and estradiol (Figure 11–4). In addition to feedback regulation, an autoregulatory mechanism exists within the thyroid gland itself. As the amount of organic iodine within the cell rises, the transport of I^- into the cell is decreased. High concentrations of I^- within the thyroid cell inhibit the release of thyroid hormone from thyroglobulin. Such a tightly regulated scheme speaks for the biological importance of regulating the exact amount of active hormone circulating in the free state in the blood.

A decreased concentration of circulating thyroid hormone is common to all forms of hypothyroidism. In primary hypothyroidism the high concentration of endogenous TSH and the administration of exogenous TSH do not induce a rise in the amount of circulating thyroid hormone. The inability to form thyroid hormone may be due to a lack of thyroid tissue (thyroid agenesis or thyroid hypoplasia), inflammation of the thyroid (thyroiditis), a lack of iodide (endemic hypothyroidism), or a lack of one or another of the enzymes involved in the synthesis of thyroxine (familial hypothyroidism). Any deficiency of thyroid hormone in early life will result in dwarfism and mental retardation.

Thyroid agenesis. In this developmental defect the complete lack of thyroid tissue results in the appearance of severe hypothyroidism soon after birth. Any severe form of hypothyroidism developing at birth is called *cretinism*. Retarded mental development and growth are characteristic of cretinism; these manifestations of the disorder, particularly mental retardation, are often irreversible. It is important that the diagnosis be made as early as possible so that therapy can be instituted in time to prevent irreversible damage.

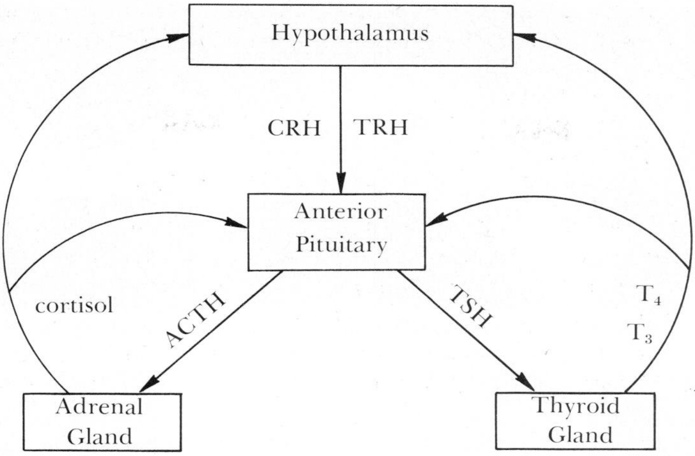

FIGURE 11–4. Feedback controls of adrenal and thyroid function. Pituitary and thyroid form a closed loop negative feedback system. Thyroid hormone can block the response of the pituitary to TRH, thus decreasing the release of TSH required for thyroid hormone synthesis and release. In addition, thyroid hormone may act on the hypothalamus to stimulate (positive feedback) or inhibit (negative feedback) secretion of TRH. Feedback control of thyroid function is exerted primarily at the level of the pituitary. The hypothalamus determines the set-point of the feedback threshold.

Glucocorticoids formed in the adrenal gland under the stimulus of ACTH can exert a negative feedback effect on both the hypothalamus and the anterior pituitary. Both the adrenal and thyroid systems represent examples of the classical negative feedback system or "servomechanism" to regulate hormone synthesis. In such systems the concentration of the hormone in the plasma determines the rate of secretion of the hormone. Both adrenal and thyroid functions are also susceptible to neural control (circadian rhythms, stress for the adrenal, and exposure to cold for the thyroid).

Fortunately, hypothyroidism is one of the most characteristic and readily diagnosed endocrine disorders of childhood. Thyroid dysfunction affects the motility of the gastrointestinal tract and the hypothyroid child may be constipated (Table 11–3). Slow feeding and subnormal caloric intake are characteristic. Affected children suffer both physical and mental retardation, and thus the developmental landmarks of sitting, standing, and walking are delayed and mentation is slow. Linear growth and weight gain are severely impaired; the infant is dwarfed, with disproportionately short limbs. The fontanelles are abnormally patent at birth and closure is delayed. Dentition is also delayed.

The fully developed cretin is readily recognized (Figure 11–5). The nose is broad and flat, the eyes wide-set, the tongue large and protuberant, and the neck short. The skin may be coarse (Table 11–3), with a characteristic pallor. Both skin and hair tend to be dry. The abdomen may be protuberant with an umbilical hernia. The child is dull and apathetic and has a characteristic hoarse cry.

Pathognomonic of hypothyroidism in the child is the radiologic appearance of the epiphyses. Characteristically the bone age is even more severely retarded than the height age. The time in development when the epiphyses ossify varies from one bone to another. Films of the lower

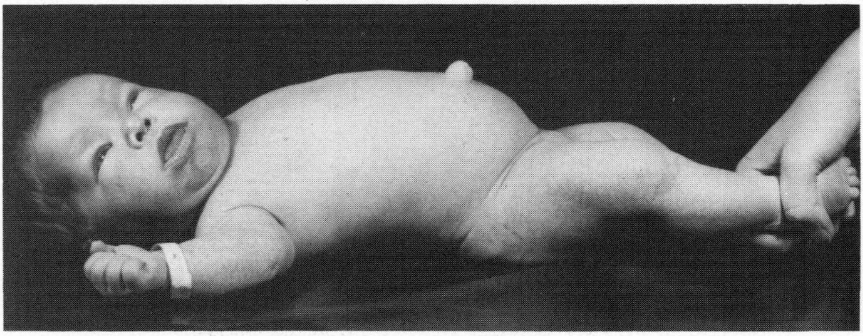

FIGURE 11–5. This two-month-old female cretin shows many of the classical features of cretinism. The nasal bridge is depressed, the tongue is big and broad, and the protruding abdomen has an umbilical hernia. Note also the fat pads around her neck and the shortness of the neck. The thyroid gland was not palpable and the skin felt cool. No ossification of the distal femoral epiphysis could be seen on films of the lower extremities. Her PBI = 1.6, RAI = 6.1, and cholesterol = 300 mg/100 ml. The bone age was less than that of a 36-week-old fetus. (Courtesy of Dr. John Crigler, Children's Medical Center, Boston, Mass.)

extremities of healthy newborns should show ossification of the lower femoral epiphyses (36 weeks gestation) and the upper tibial epiphyses (38 weeks gestation). There may or may not be ossification of the cuboid in the foot (40 weeks gestation). In the cretin at birth, these ossification centers which normally develop in utero may be absent, or, more characteristically, they may be abnormal. A normal ossification center appears on x-ray as a small single area of bone which increases in size in an orderly fashion until the mature epiphyseal end of the bone takes shape. Abnormally developed centers may begin to ossify in several small foci which may later coalesce into one center which is misshapen and has a stippled appearance. Later, the epiphysis may have a flattened appearance, with irregular margins. This disordered radiographic appearance has been called *epiphyseal dysgenesis.* It may be manifest in any of the centers of ossification of cartilage relevant to the patient's age.

Other bony changes, such as abnormalities of the lumbar vertebrae and enlargement of the pituitary fossa, have been described in the cretin. The latter may be due to hyperplasia of the pituitary (thyrotrophs) in response to the deficiency of circulating thyroid hormone.

In hypothyroidism the amount of mucoproteins in interstitial tissue increases. This mucinous edema in the skin is responsible for its coarseness and puffiness. These deposits in other tissues cause, among other things, enlargement of the tongue and thickening of the pharyngeal and laryngeal mucous membranes. This form of edema, classically called *myxedema,* is characteristic of full-blown hypothyroidism. Myxedema is a late sign in children with hypothyroidism and may be absent in mild thyroid deficiency.

Several chemical determinations reflect the amount of thyroid hormone available to tissues. In a cretin, the concentrations of total thyroxine, free thyroxine, and triiodothyronine are low. In the older child with hypothyroidism, the concentration of cholesterol in the blood is usually increased; however, in cretins less than 2 years old, this value is often normal, and the blood urea nitrogen (BUN) is increased. In suspected athyrosis a test of radioactive iodine uptake may be useful. Scanning the thyroid area would reveal no radioactive uptake. However, aberrant thyroid tissue (anywhere along the thyroglossal duct) will take up iodine. Protein-bound iodine (PBI), which measures precipitable iodine, is still used in some hospitals but is rapidly being replaced by measurements of thyroxine, because ingestion of iodine in any form nullifies the value of the PBI.

Thyroiditis. The only common cause of acquired hypothyroidism in childhood is Hashimoto's thyroiditis. This disorder is considered to represent an autoimmune phenomenon. Within the thyroid gland are numerous lymphocytes and plasma cells which may form antibodies to thyroglobulin and other antigenic proteins within the thyroid gland. In Hashimoto's disease, hormone production by the thyroid is decreased, but the gland itself may be hyperplastic, probably secondary to elevated levels of TSH in the blood. The thyroid gland enlarges and produces a goiter which may be smooth, granular, or even lobulated. More or less discrete nodules are sometimes palpable. Not all patients with Hashimoto's thyroiditis have goiters; however, a goiter in a child should suggest thyroiditis.

The impairment of growth is inversely related to the child's age at the onset of the disease. The child with this, or any other form of acquired hypothyroidism, may show fairly abrupt cessation of growth with the onset of the disease (Figure 11–6). Therapy with thyroid hormone brings about growth at a rate similar to that noted prior to the disease. The final height, however, is likely to be below normal in children whose hypothyroidism manifests itself in the preteens, since closure of the epiphyses at puberty prevents further linear growth. Hypothyroid children look "fat" and often gain weight (Table 11–3). With the onset of thyroid therapy it is quite usual to see weight loss, often dramatic. If hypothyroidism manifests itself early in life, the bone age is severely retarded, much more so than the height age. The later the onset of hypothyroidism the less the discrepancy between retardation of bone age and height age.

The peak incidence of Hashimoto's thyroiditis is at 10 or 11 years of age. Over 90 percent of the patients are female; this preponderance of affected females over males is characteristic of all acquired thyroid disorders. Usually the first indication of the disease is the discovery of an asymptomatic goiter (two to five times normal size). Lymph nodes, particularly the Delphian node above the thyroid gland, may be palpable. Early in the course of the disease, symptoms of hypothyroidism may be mild; subsequently, the growth rate decreases and the skin becomes cool and dry. If untreated, patients with this disease will progress to more severe symptoms of hypothyroidism. Rarely, mild to moderate hyperthyroidism may develop in response to the increased secretion of

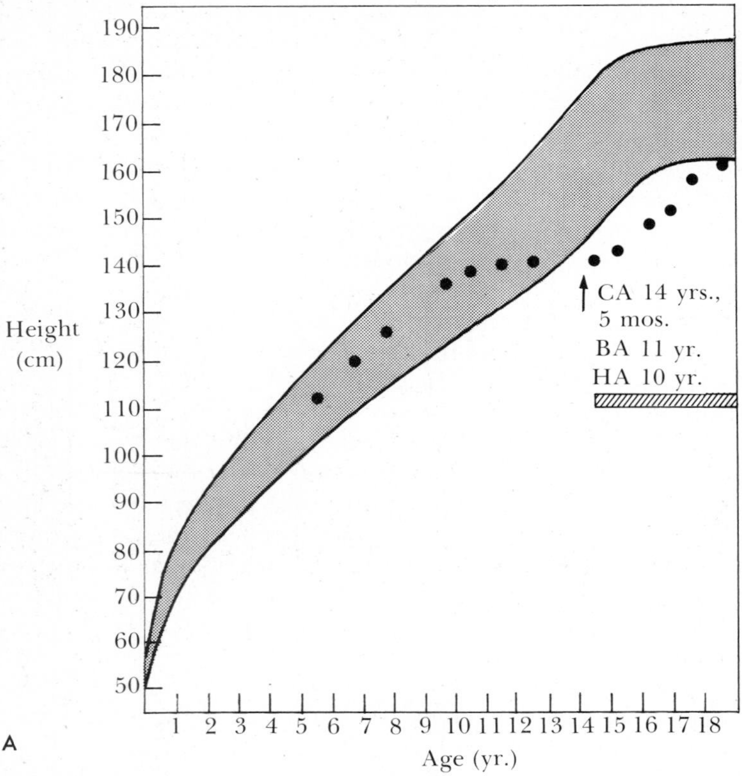

FIGURE 11–6. *A,* Linear growth curve of a young boy with acquired hypothyroidism. Note the cessation of growth followed by the period of growth that took place when the boy was receiving thyroid hormone (hatched bar).

Illustration continued on opposite page.

TSH. Later, in the end stages of the disease, thyroid atrophy and myxedema often appear. The most diagnostic of the laboratory tests available is the demonstration of the presence of antibodies to thyroid antigens in the blood of the patient.

Hashimoto's thyroiditis can coexist with neoplasms of the thyroid. Characteristically a thyroid gland that has been stimulated by TSH over a long period of time takes on a nodular appearance. The nodules may or may not be sharply circumscribed. They may be composed of hyperplastic epithelium with hypertrophic cells, sometimes with papillary formation, or they may be involuted with a flat epithelium enclosing large colloidal spaces. Just what brings about neoplastic change is unknown, although ionizing radiation is considered one causative factor in thyroid carcinoma in childhood. The most common thyroid carcinoma (62 percent) is *papillary carcinoma,* by far the most common malignant thyroid neoplasm in children and young adults. This thyroid neoplasm is characterized by papillae with distinct fibrovascular stalks within the epithe-

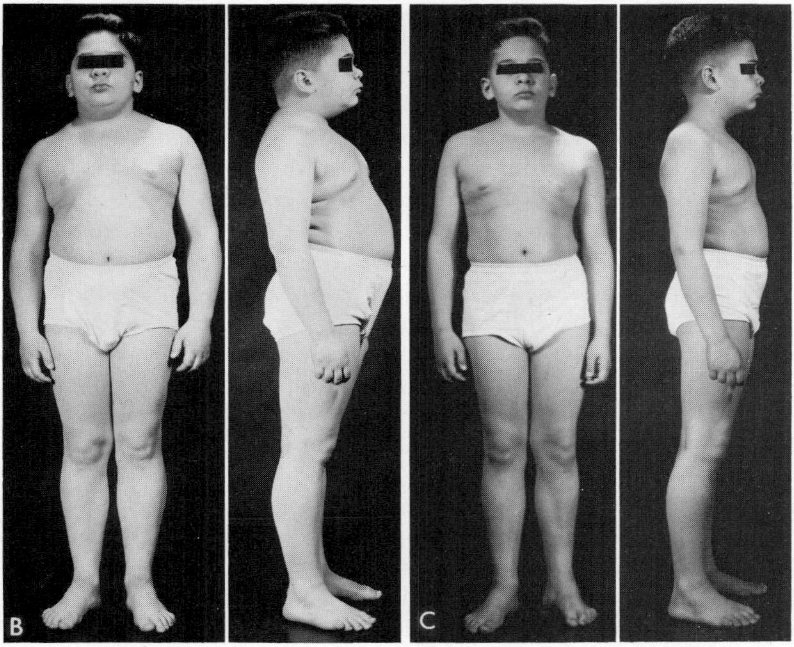

FIGURE 11–6 *Continued.* *B,* Front and profile views of patient before thyroid hormone therapy. At that time he was a short, "obese" boy with dry skin, slow pulse, and low blood pressure. He also showed obvious lassitude, his laboratory values were; PBI, 2.5 mg/100 ml; serum cholesterol, 370 mg/100 ml; BMR, minus 40; radioactive I uptake, 8 percent; Hb, 11 g; and FSH, negative. *C,* Front and profile views of patient after 9 months of thyroid hormone therapy. (Courtesy of Dr. John Crigler, Children's Medical Center, Boston, Mass.)

lial folds. The psammoma body (a concretion in a sclerotic focus of carcinoma) is frequently found and is considered diagnostic of the neoplasm. Papillary carcinoma is a differentiated carcinoma of the thyroid gland, and in contrast to life expectancies with the undifferentiated varieties, survival for 10 or 20 years with this carcinoma is not unusual; however, metastases to vital organs (especially the lung) can occur and cause death. In general, tumors or neoplasms of the thyroid gland do not produce symptoms of excess thyroid hormone. Thus in the euthyroid individual with one or more thyroid nodules or with diffuse hyperplasia, the possibility of neoplasm must be entertained, although by far most goiters in euthyroid individuals are benign.

Malignant nodules tend to be nontender, firm, and sharply demarcated. There may be evidence of infiltration beyond the thyroid capsule with fixation to underlying structures. Local lymph nodes may be enlarged. Nodules in the thyroid can be "scanned." Most malignant tumors of the thyroid do not accumulate radioactive iodine. By surveying the neck region after administration of radioactive iodine, it may be noted that the nodule is "cold" (nonradioactive); such a finding may point to malignancy. Most "cold" nodules are benign, however, and a "warm" (some radioactive uptake) nodule does not necessarily rule out malignancy. Thyroid carcinoma with "hot" nodules is very rare.

Iodine deficiency (endemic hypothyroidism). In certain parts of the world, particularly those areas far from the sea, the limited availability of iodine in the diet renders iodine intake insufficient for normal synthesis of thyroid hormone. The usual result in individuals in such areas is a compensatory increase in TSH secretion from the pituitary which brings about enlargement (goiter) of the thyroid gland. In these regions of the world, goiter is endemic (present in over 10 percent of the population), and many of the inhabitants have low concentrations of inorganic iodide in the plasma. If radioiodine is administered to these iodine deficient patients, it is taken up rapidly by the thyroid gland. Supplementing the diet with iodine will reduce the incidence of goiter.

Familial hypothyroidism (dyshormonogenesis). Six distinct hereditary forms of thyroid dyshormonogenesis are presently recognized. In each, goiter develops and varying degrees of hypothyroidism are found. The gland itself is hyperplastic.

Iodide Transport Defect. In this, the rarest form of dyshormonogenesis, the thyroid gland, the stomach, and the salivary glands are unable to concentrate iodide from the circulation. The diagnosis depends upon the demonstration of either low uptake of radioiodine by the thyroid gland or failure of the salivary glands to concentrate iodide. A biopsy of the thyroid gland reveals hyperplasia and low iodine content. Treating the patient with large amounts of iodine may correct the condition, but the treatment of choice is thyroid hormone replacement.

Organification Defect. In the commonest thyroidal enzyme defect, iodide is trapped rapidly in the thyroid gland, but subsequent reaction with the tyrosine residues on thyroglobulin is impaired. Presumably the peroxidase responsible for converting iodide ion to an iodinating species (Figure 3–12) is defective. Most of the patients with this defect are severely cretinous with profoundly retarded structural and intellectual development.

The most useful diagnostic test for this disorder is the *thiocyanate test.* Radioactive iodine is administered to the patient and accumulates rapidly in the region of the thyroid gland, achieving maximal concentration in one hour. At that time two grams of potassium thiocyanate are given by mouth. In patients with organification defect there is a rapid release of labeled iodine from the thyroid gland after administration of thiocyanate. Since thiocyanate competes in the process of organification with iodide ion, the released labeled iodine represents a store of labeled iodine in the gland which could be readily displaced. In the normal individual virtually none of the accumulated iodine (organic) can be displaced in this way. Since this defect limits or prevents hormone synthesis, compensatory hyperplasia and hypertrophy of the thyroid gland occur. In some patients there is an associated abnormality in the auditory nerves. The combination of goiter with deafness is known as *Pendred's syndrome.* Hypothyroidism may be minimal or absent. One patient with Pendred's syndrome has been shown to have a high concentration of iodide peroxidase in the thyroid. Thus the syndrome may represent a defect in iodination not involving peroxidase activity directly.

Coupling Defect. The thyroid glands of patients with this disorder have an impaired ability to couple monoiodotyrosine (MIT) and diiodotyrosine (DIT) into thyroxine (T_4) and triiodothyronine (T_3). The ratio of iodothyronines to iodotyrosines in a sample of thyroid tissue is low. Since the biochemical mechanisms of coupling are so poorly understood, it is best to refer to this disorder in general terms rather than as a specific enzyme deficiency. The diagnosis is made in part by the exclusion of other defects and in part on the basis of high MIT/DIT ratio with little iodothyronine in the thyroid gland.

Dehalogenase Defect. Patients with this disorder are deficient in the enzyme dehalogenase, which releases iodine from iodotyrosines. This enzyme is present normally not only in thyroid but in liver, kidney, and other organs. Individuals with dehalogenase defect lack the enzyme in these other tissues as well. The continued leak of hormone precursors from the thyroid gland which occurs normally, combined with the failure to retrieve the iodine from these iodotyrosines, results in a gradual loss of iodine from the body. This sets up a vicious cycle of thyroid hyperplasia, increasing amounts of hormone precursors, and increased loss of iodine.

Iodoprotein Defect. This defect may represent an inability to form thyroglobulin, for affected patients have little of this protein in their thyroid glands. In some patients, large amounts of iodinated albumin (but not iodinated globulins) have been found. Most of the iodinated material in plasma is butanol-insoluble, whereas normally at least 90 percent of the protein-bound iodine in plasma is readily removed by extraction with acid butanol.

Protease Defect. A defect in protease would impair the release of thyroid hormone from thyroglobulin (Figure 3–12). In patients lacking protease, partially digested fragments of thyroglobulin are released into the circulation. These iodinated peptide fragments are not extractable into acid butanol as are the iodinated thyronines which normally appear in the peripheral blood.

Diagnosis

Measurements of total thyroxine, free thyroxine, triodothyronine, and TSH are frequently used tests of thyroid function. In hypothyroidism the total thyroxine is usually less than 3 μg/100 ml plasma, and free thyroxine is less than 1 ng/100 ml plasma. Triiodothyronine is less than 50 ng/100 ml plasma. The concentration of TSH in plasma is markedly elevated.

Tests of thyroid function may be normal in the early stages of hypothyroidism if the gland has compensated by increasing the number and size of its cells. A test of thyroid reserve is indicated under such conditions. Failure of the thyroid radioiodine uptake to rise after the administration of TSH is evidence of primary thyroid disease. Measurements of thyroid antibodies and bone maturation are valuable aids in diagnosis. A thiocyanate test will detect the presence of any large pool of inorganic iodine in the thyroid gland and may be a clue to defective organification.

A low concentration of total thyroxine in serum (or a low PBI) does not necessarily reflect a hypothyroid state. A familial deficiency in TBG has been reported recently. Affected males usually show little or no TBG in the serum, whereas in females TBG is detectable but lower than normal. The disorder is inherited as a sex-linked dominant, and consequently in the female one half of the X chromosomes are incapable of causing the synthesis of TBG. The affected individual is *euthyroid*, because the concentration of free thyroxine in the blood is normal. Total serum thyroxine concentration is low, but the T_3 resin uptake is elevated, reflecting the fact that there are fewer TBG binding sites available to absorb the labeled T_3. It is important to remember that alterations in the amount of circulating TBG can change the concentration of total thyroxine in the serum, but it is the free thyroxine which determines the metabolic state of the patient. Thus in a euthyroid patient with low serum thyroxine concentration (or low PBI), either a TBG or a resin T_3 uptake measurement may be helpful.

SECONDARY HYPOTHYROIDISM

Any impairment in TSH synthesis or release will result in secondary hypothyroidism. If the failure is due to hypopituitarism it is important to assess the relative deficiencies of GH and ACTH as well as TSH. With the advent of radioimmunoassays for these hormones, accurate measurements of their concentrations in the blood are feasible. In pituitary failure, the amount of one or more of these hormones in the blood will be decreased. Because a reliable radioimmunoassay for ACTH is still not available widely, the metyrapone test, which indirectly measures the ACTH secreted by the pituitary gland, is used as a test in hypopituitarism.

TERTIARY HYPOTHYROIDISM

Failure of the pituitary gland to release TSH may be due to hypothalamic disease, in which inadequate amounts of TRH may be produced. Such patients, if given TRH, will respond by releasing TSH. In general, it has been shown that a single oral dose of TRH causes a more prolonged elevation of serum TSH than that seen after intravenous administration, with a dose-dependent TSH peak two to five hours after TRH ingestion. Intravenous administration of $50 \mu g$ of TRH gives a rapid rise in serum TSH within 15 to 20 minutes. Prolactin, of course, is also released from the pituitary gland after the administration of TRH.

Treatment of Hypothyroidism

As soon as the diagnosis is made, replacement therapy with orally administered thyroid hormone should be begun. The treatment of choice utilizes L-thyroxine, primarily because the daily use of this hormone permits a more sustained, non-fluctuating level of thyroid hormone to be maintained in the blood. The regimen should be approached cautiously. Because of its prolonged action and the variable needs of the child, the dose of thyroxine should be low initially (0.05 mg daily) and gradually increased each week until the euthyroid state is achieved. It is seldom desirable to give less than 0.1 mg or more than 0.3 mg daily at any age. The bone age should be measured periodically, since overdosage with thyroxine tends to accelerate bone maturity.

Also available for use in therapy is L-triiodothyronine, which is three or four times more potent than L-thyroxine. It has a more rapid peak effect (24 to 48 hours after administration) but a shorter duration of action. The average daily maintenance dose is about 0.1 mg, but there is no real advantage in using triiodothyronine rather than thyroxine. Indeed, there may be disadvantages. Triiodothyronine's more rapid action may cause greater fluctuations in metabolic rate in tissues than the slower, more prolonged action of thyroxine. When given in therapeutic doses, thyroxine, because of its gradual onset of action, is less apt to induce acute cardiovascular responses such as tachycardia. Another replacement hormone available for therapy of hypothyroidism is U.S.P. desiccated thyroid. A dose of 65 mg/day of desiccated thyroid is the equivalent of 0.1 mg thyroxine.

In patients with hypopituitarism who lack ACTH, treatment of hypothyroidism with thyroxine can be dangerous unless the glucocorticoid deficiency is remedied also. In the euthyroid state the metabolism of cortisol is rapid, and the hypothyroid patient who could tolerate cortisol insufficiency can no longer do so when made euthyroid. Thus cortisol or cortisone should be administered with the thyroxine in these patients.

INSULIN DEFICIENCY

Both GH and insulin have a synergistic effect on protein synthesis, and insulin may appropriately be considered a growth-promoting hormone. Years ago Salter and Best claimed that injection of insulin into hypophysectomized rats produced significant growth, with increases in both fat and protein. By measuring cell size (protein/DNA ratio) after hormone therapy it was shown that insulin increases protein synthesis and cell size in rat liver, but there was no change in cell size after GH administration. Clearly, both insulin and GH are important in growth, but insulin appears to increase cell size whereas GH increases cell number. Insulin deficiency leads to decreased protein synthesis and negative nitrogen balance.

Patients with diabetes mellitus, diagnosed before growth is completed, may manifest retarded growth, particularly if their disease is poorly controlled. A form of dwarfism in poorly controlled juvenile diabetics, called *Mauriac's syndrome,* has been described by Traisman.

During routine testing of 190 children with short stature, Karp, Laron, and Doron found 80 children who showed a diminished insulin response to arginine stimulation. These children all had normal plasma values of GH. Clinically, the children manifested growth retardation, retardation of skeletal maturation, and lack of obesity. Both thyroid function and GH responses to provocative tests were normal, and none of the children had any signs of acute or chronic disease. The only common finding was the low insulin response to the arginine infusion test. In 30 out of 36 of these children the insulin response during an oral glucose tolerance test was also low.

Other examples can be cited for a possible role of insulin deficiency in certain forms of short stature. The familial dysautonomia disorder (Riley-Day syndrome) is a congenital disease occurring almost entirely in persons of Jewish ancestry. These patients have a variety of symptoms, including absent lacrimation, excessive perspiration, impaired temperature control, labile blood pressure, and mental and motor retardation. Riley found marked retardation in both height and weight in all 27 of his patients with dysautonomia. In general, these patients are below the tenth percentile, with many being below the third percentile for both height and weight. In a recent study of nine patients with dysautonomia, intravenous glucose tolerance tests revealed insulin values that were significantly below normal at all sampling times during the one hour test. Cole posed the suggestion that the low insulin values might account for the growth failure found in dysautonomia. He could find no abnormality in plasma GH values.

It has been found that children who were malnourished in the fetal stage had low plasma insulin responses to arginine infusion. It is difficult to know what is cause and what is effect in these various clinical entities, but a consideration of the role of insulin in protein synthesis would support the suggestion that insulin deficiency might impair normal growth and development.

Excess glucocorticoids

In discussing cortisol therapy in adrenocortical hyperplasia (Chapter Seven), the danger of impaired growth from excessive treatment was mentioned. This impairment of growth by glucocorticoids (Figure 11–7) may be due, in part, to the diversion of a large part of the pool of amino acids from the formation of proteins toward the synthesis of carbohydrate and fat. It may also be secondary to decreased release of GH, which has been reported in children on high doses of glucocorticoids.

Excessive cortisol, whether exogenously administered or produced by a hyperplastic or tumorous adrenal gland, produces the clinical picture of *Cushing's syndrome.* This disorder is rare in children but should be considered in any differential diagnosis of growth retardation. The outstanding clinical feature of Cushing's syndrome is obesity (Figure 11–7). The excessive fat tends to be deposited over the upper trunk and shoulders (buffalo hump). At times the differentiation of Cushing's syndrome from simple obesity may be difficult, but the unusual distribution of fat in Cushing's syndrome is often helpful in this regard. Furthermore, obesity in childhood is more likely to be associated with increased growth rather than growth retardation.

Besides distinctive obesity, other characteristics of Cushing's syndrome are moon face (fat deposits in the cheeks), easy bruisability, muscular weakness, purple striae (often absent in young children), osteoporotic bones, and decreased ability to utilize glucose ("decreased glucose tolerance"). Hypertension is present in most patients and may lead eventually to congestive heart failure.

The initial complaints in children with the syndrome are often back pain, muscular weakness, impaired growth, and hirsutism (p. 365). The latter may be part of a generalized virilization (pubic and axillary hair, acne, penile or clitoral hypertrophy, and scrotal pigmentation) and is undoubtedly secondary to the secretion of excessive amounts of androgens by the adrenal. Virilization, however, is not always seen in Cushing's syndrome, and when it occurs a tumor of the adrenal should be suspected.

The laboratory findings in Cushing's syndrome include fasting hyperglycemia, glycosuria, osteoporosis, and retarded bone maturation. The plasma cortisol concentration is usually elevated but may be normal; there is usually no diurnal variation in plasma cortisol. It is very important to differentiate between a unilateral cortisol-secreting tumor of the adrenal (adenoma or carcinoma) and bilateral adrenal hyperplasia. Children with adrenal hyperplasia (not congenital adrenocortical hyperplasia, p. 153) are often hyperresponsive to ACTH, showing a three- or fourfold rise in plasma cortisol after ACTH administration in contrast to the doubling of plasma cortisol found in the normal or obese child. Patients with adrenal carcinoma are usually unresponsive to ACTH.

Hyperactive adrenals are usually resistant to the suppressive effect of exogenous glucocorticoids. In contrast, the normal or obese child given 0.5 mg of dexamethasone every six hours for two days will demonstrate a 50 percent or greater fall in urinary excretion of corticosteroids. A higher dose of dexamethasone, 2.0 mg, will usually suppress the hyperplastic adrenal but not the neoplastic adrenal. As it becomes more routine, the direct measurement of the concentration of ACTH in the plasma should be helpful in differentiating hyperplasia from neoplasia of the adrenal.

Another test often used to differentiate adrenal hyperplasia (secondary to ACTH stimulation from the pituitary) from adrenal tumor is the *metyrapone test.* Metyrapone combines with cytochrome P-450 in the mitochondria, thus preventing steroid hydroxylation from occurring in

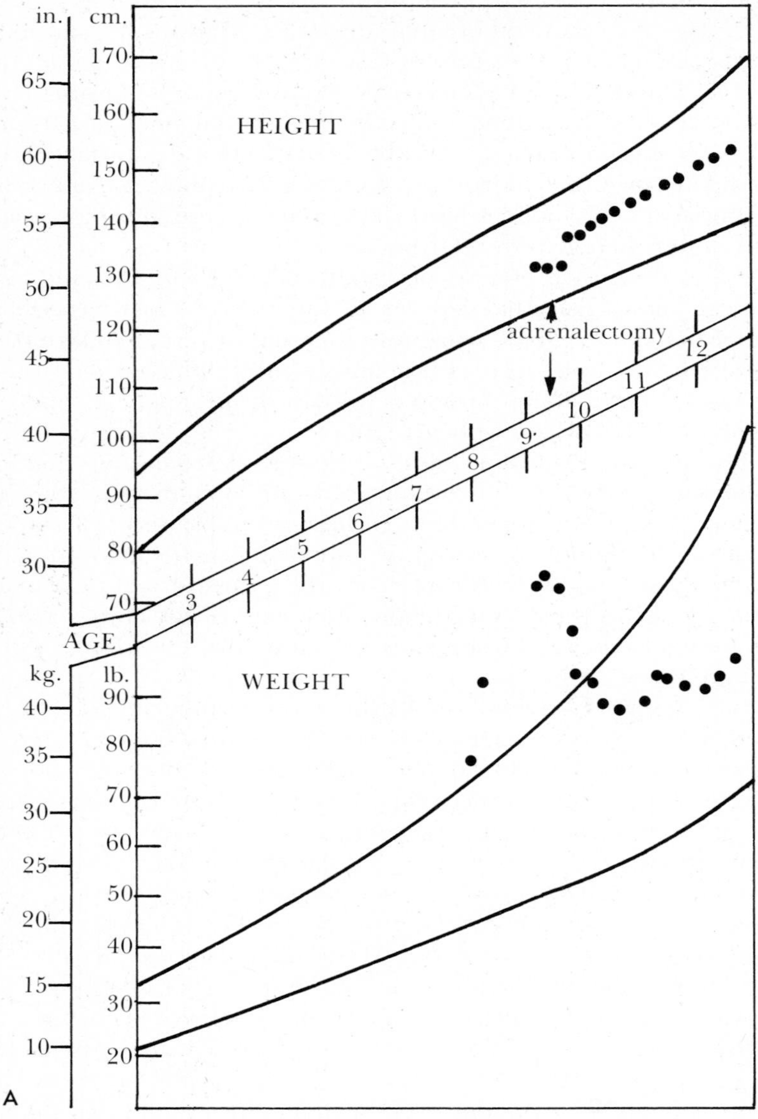

FIGURE 11–7. *A,* Growth chart of a boy with Cushing's syndrome. The normal ranges for height and weight are depicted by the solid lines. The patient grew normally until age 8, at which time he weighed 76 lb. Within three months his weight had increased to 94 lb. At this time roundness of the face, hirsutism, and pubic hair were first noted. He had a prominent interscapular fat pad and truncal and abdominal obesity with striae. At age 9 he weighed 113 lb and was 53 in. in height. Linear growth ceased. The urinary excretion of 17OHCS was suppressed by the administration of 2.0 mg of dexamethasone. A diagnosis of adrenal hyperplasia was made and a bilateral adrenalectomy performed. The patient was subsequently maintained on cortisone. (Data from Dr. John Crigler, Boston, Mass.)

Illustration continued on opposite page.

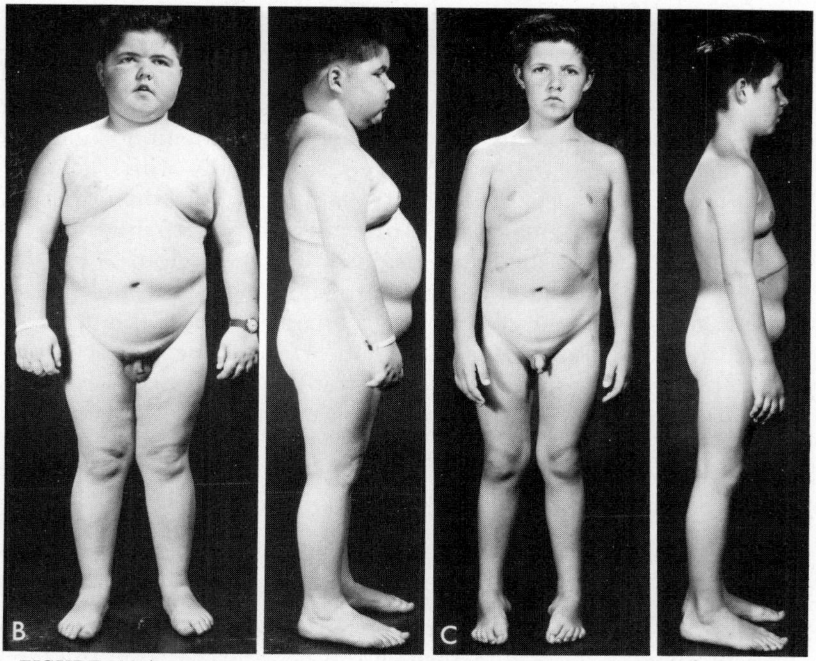

FIGURE 11–7 Continued. *B*, Front and side views of patient at age 9. Note the rounded face and prominent interscapular fat pad. Pubic hair is present and the obesity is central in type leaving relatively normal extremities.

C, Front and side views of patient one year after bilateral adrenalectomy. Note the disappearance of pubic hair, the "moon face," the "buffalo hump," and the truncal obesity. (Courtesy of Dr. John Crigler, Children's Medical Center, Boston, Mass.)

that organelle. As a result, 11-hydroxylation is blocked, and cortisol and corticosterone cannot be secreted by the adrenal gland. The negative feedback to the pituitary gland is disrupted (Figure 11–4) and more ACTH is secreted. The ACTH stimulates the blocked adrenal gland to form increased amounts of 11-deoxycortisol (compound S) and deoxycorticosterone, which can be measured in the blood or urine. More simply, one can measure urinary 17OHCS or 17-ketogenic steroids, since the metabolites of11-deoxycortisol are included among these substances p. 147). In normal subjects, the urinary 17OHCS rise during the day of metyrapone administration and increase still further on the day after. There should be at least a threefold increment. Patients with adrenal hyperplasia usually have an exaggerated response to this test, whereas patients with adrenal tumor usually have little or no response to metyrapone.

When Cushing's syndrome is the result of adrenal neoplasm, it is treated by surgical removal of the tumor. The adrenal that is not involved in the neoplastic process—the normal adrenal—will have been suppressed by the products of the hyperactive adrenal. Therefore, it is essential to prepare the patient beforehand by cortisone administration in order to avoid postsurgical adrenal crisis. Although subtotal adrenalectomy was formerly the operation of choice for adrenal hyperplasia, present day opinion favors total adrenalectomy with replacement therapy. A surprising number of children with adrenal hyperplasia develop pituitary tumors even with adequate substitution therapy. Usually the tumor is a chromophobe adenoma and is suspected when the child develops visual symptoms and/or hyperpigmentation (increased MSH). These tumors are often treated successfully with radioactive implants in the pituitary. One suspects that in children who develop pituitary tumors, the original basis of the adrenal hyperplasia may have been an abnormality in the hypothalamic-pituitary region.

After removal of the abnormal adrenal(s), symptoms of Cushing's syndrome disappear and growth rate returns to normal (Figure 11–7); however, just as in congenital adrenocortical hyperplasia, replacement therapy with cortisol must be "titrated" to the needs of the patient in order to avoid retardation of growth from excessive cortisol.

Differential diagnosis of retarded growth (Table 11–1)

In differentiating the various causes of retarded growth, it is well to remember that most do not involve the endocrine system. Many children are constitutionally short, a fact which can be inferred from the family history. If the parents are short, or have a history of slow development, one might predict that the children would likewise be short in stature. If development is delayed because of constitutional predisposition, the bone age will be less than the height age. This is, of course, also true for hypopituitary dwarfism. Malnutrition will affect the weight age more than the height age; severe malnutrition results in *cachexia*.

Skeletal and metabolic disorders may produce retarded growth. An example of the former would be achondroplasia and of the latter glycogen storage disease (p. 257). Various syndromes of malabsorption will alter growth. Chromosomal aberrations such as Down's syndrome characteristically produce short stature. Even psychological disturbances (emotional deprivation in children) can impede normal growth and development, possibly via alterations in GH secretion. In primordial dwarfs there may be no known etiology (e.g., progeria, p. 449). However, most of these disorders have characteristic signs and symptoms and are not difficult to diagnose. One of the most frequently encountered causes of short stature in the female is Turner's syndrome. In this condition growth is markedly retarded (Figure 11–8). When sexual development is desired, estrogens can be administered and growth will occur. However, the final stature is always below normal.

It is obvious that one needs to know the developmental pattern (height age, weight age, bone age, mental age vs. chronological age) of the patient. This is particularly helpful in sorting out endocrine causes of retarded growth. For example, in GH deficiency the weight age usually exceeds the height age (Table 11–1). A deficiency of thyroid hor-

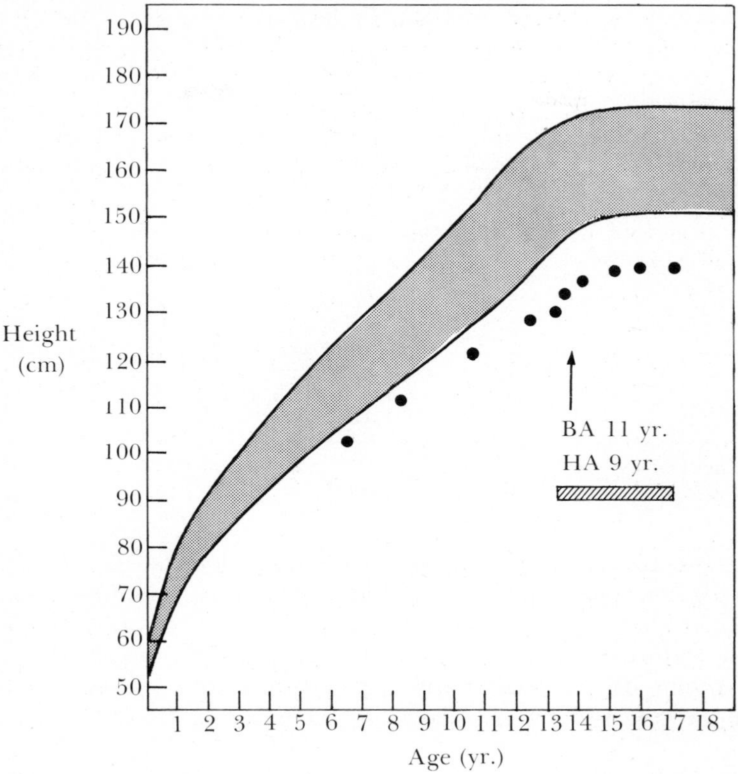

FIGURE 11–8. Linear growth curve for a girl with Turner's syndrome. Estrogen therapy (hatched bar) produced a significant growth spurt. For a description of the clinical disorder and a photograph of the patient, see Figure 13–9.

mone brings about severe retardation of skeletal maturation so that bone age is less than height age. Weight is usually greater than average for height in hypothyroidism. Changes similar to those of hypothyroidism are produced by excessive amounts of glucocorticoids.

The etiology of the hormonal failure or excess may reside at various levels (Table 11–2). Neoplasms of the hypothalamus, for example, may damage neurons producing GHRH or those producing TRH. Stimulation of neurons forming CRH (or failure to respond to the negative feedback control of cortisol) may result in excessive release of CRH. Excessive production of somatostatin will also reduce growth by blocking release of GH. Thus some cases of growth retardation can be ascribed to a hypothalamic disorder. Similarly, conditions which impair the function of somatotrophs and thyrotrophs in the anterior pituitary will produce hypoplasia or atrophy of the target endocrine glands and growth failure. Tumors of the ACTH-secreting cells of the pituitary will produce adrenal hyperplasia and reduced growth. Thus pituitary lesions can cause

TABLE 11–1. Differential Diagnosis of Retarded Growth due to Endocrine Imbalance

	Deficiency of:			Excess of:
	GH	*Thyroid*	*Insulin*	*Glucocorticoids*
Facial features	Immature	Immature	N*	Fat cheeks
Developmental pattern	HA<WA<CA	BA<HA<WA	WA<HA<CA	BA<HA<CA
Dentition	Delayed	Delayed	N	N
GH secretion	↓	↓	N	N
Fasting blood glucose	↓	N	↑	↑
Obesity	+	−	−	+
Plasma T_4	N	↓	N	N
Plasma cortisol	N	N (cortisol secretory rate and metabolic clearance rate ↓)	N	↑

*The symbols used in the table are as follows: N = normal; HA = height age; WA = weight age; BA = bone age; CA = chronological age.

growth retardation. Disease of the target endocrine glands (thyroid, adrenal) can produce primary endocrine growth failure. The GH-mediated formation of somatomedin may be impaired and result in failure of growth. Finally, although the various hormones controlling growth may be synthesized and secreted in normal amounts, a lack of end organ receptors may prevent the biological action of the hormone.

TABLE 11–2. Endocrine Causes of Dwarfism

Level at which Failure Occurs	Hormone Involved	Clinical Condition
Hypothalamus	↓ GHRH (or ↑ Somatostatin)	Hypothalamic hypopituitarism (neoplasms)
	↓ TRH	Tertiary hypothyroidism
	↑ CRH	Hypothalamic Cushing's syndrome?
Anterior pituitary	↓ GH	Hypopituitarism
	↓ TSH	Secondary hypothyroidism
	↑ ACTH	Adrenal hyperplasia secondary to pituitary tumor
Target endocrine gland	↓ Somatomedin	Familial dwarfism of Laron
	↓ Thyroid Hormone	Inborn errors of thyroid hormone synthesis
		Iodine deficiency
		Thyroiditis
	↑ Cortisol	Adrenal tumor
End organ	No response to GH or to somatomedin	African pygmies
	No response to thyroid hormone	Familial resistance to thyroid hormone

An example is the African pygmy, who has normal amounts of GH but does not respond by growing. Similarly, a familial resistance to thyroid hormone has been reported recently.

By careful assessment of genetic, nutritional, metabolic, and endocrine factors, it is usually possible to identify correctly those conditions for which therapy may be helpful. In emotionally deprived children a foster home may be the answer. Those children lacking nutrients or specific hormones require replacement therapy. In still other disorders (progeria, for example) for which there is no therapy our only hope lies in further research to discover the etiology of the condition.

EXCESSIVE GROWTH

Disorders of excessive growth may involve weight (obesity) or height (gigantism, "too-tall girl," precocious puberty) or any combination of the two. Obesity in most children, as in adults (p. 421), is not caused by endocrine disturbances. In contrast, many syndromes of excessive tallness do have an endocrine basis. Problems of excessive weight and height will be discussed separately, but it is important to remember that the two aspects of growth are interrelated.

OBESITY

One of the commonest problems seen in the endocrine clinic in the United States is obesity. The use of the term *obesity* does not mean that these patients are simply overweight, but rather that excessive amounts of adipose tissue can be demonstrated. A glance at the height-weight chart can determine if the child's weight deviates from the normal for his height. If this deviation equals or exceeds two standard deviations above the mean weight for height, the physician can make a tentative diagnosis of obesity. To ascertain whether the excess weight is due to fat or to some other constituent, it is necessary to measure the subcutaneous fat. The amount of subcutaneous fat, which represents about half of the total body fat, is usually measured by estimating skinfold thickness. In particular, the thickness of the triceps skinfold seems to correlate well with total body fat. Standardized calipers should be used and values compared with norms.

It is of some interest that one third of obese adults give a history of juvenile obesity. Indeed, most obese juveniles (80 percent) are still overweight in adulthood. An individual does not usually "outgrow" obesity; rather, obesity tends to become a greater problem with increasing age and constitutes a major aspect of the disorders of senescence.

It is tempting to infer that obesity simply results from eating too much. However, there can be wide discrepancies between food intake and body weight in different individuals; obese persons do not always ingest more calories than the nonobese. Does an obese person simply have less physical activity and, as a result, expend less energy than the nonobese? It has been reported that obese individuals exercise less than the nonobese; however, one must remember that for any given exercise far more energy must be expended by the obese individual. Just moving the excessive body mass uses up energy. Undoubtedly in many obese children the caloric input far exceeds the energy output. However, not all fit into this category and one must invoke alterations in cellular metabolism to account for obesity in these children. It is particularly striking that the tendency to obesity is often familial and may thus suggest either a common environmental or hereditary factor which predisposes to weight gain.

Energy Expenditure

Within each cell of the body are organelles, or mitochondria, for the production of chemical energy (ATP). These small bodies are uniquely designed to coordinate a chain of oxidation-reduction reactions with the generation of ATP. This system transfers electrons from the primary acceptors (NAD, NADP, FAD) in the glycolytic and citric acid cycles (p. 75) to heme-containing proteins (cytochromes) which in turn can react with oxygen to yield H_2O (two H^+ from the primary acceptors plus one oxygen atom). In other words, electrons are transferred from substrate (for example, isocitric acid, Figure 4–2) to oxygen. Depending upon the primary acceptor, either two (FAD) or three (NAD, NADP) energy-rich phosphates (~P) will be generated during this transfer of electrons. Just how the generation of ATP is coupled to electron transfer is still poorly understood, but we do know that it occurs within the mitochondria.

Isolated mitochondria can carry out the entire sequence of reactions in the citric acid cycle, the electron transmitter system, and the oxidative phosphorylation of ADP to ATP. It has been known for some time that mitochondria change shape when they are deprived of substrates, oxygen, Ca^{++}, or ADP. Alterations in shape may have direct implications on function of the mitochondria. For example, when ACTH is administered to rats, or added to tissue cultures containing rat adrenal cells, the structure of the adrenal mitochondria changes dramatically; they become enlarged and vesicular, and concurrently the production of corticosteroids by these cells is enhanced.

The structure of the normal mitochondrion can be observed under the electron microscope (Figure 11–9). The membrane is double-layered, the outer, smooth layer encircling the entire organelle. The inner layer is folded repeatedly, forming projections within the mitochondrion called *cristae.* This inner layer has much greater surface area, and undoubtedly much of the cell's biologically useful energy, ATP, is generated by enzyme systems located in this layer. A single cell may have a thousand or more mitochondria, and the function of each

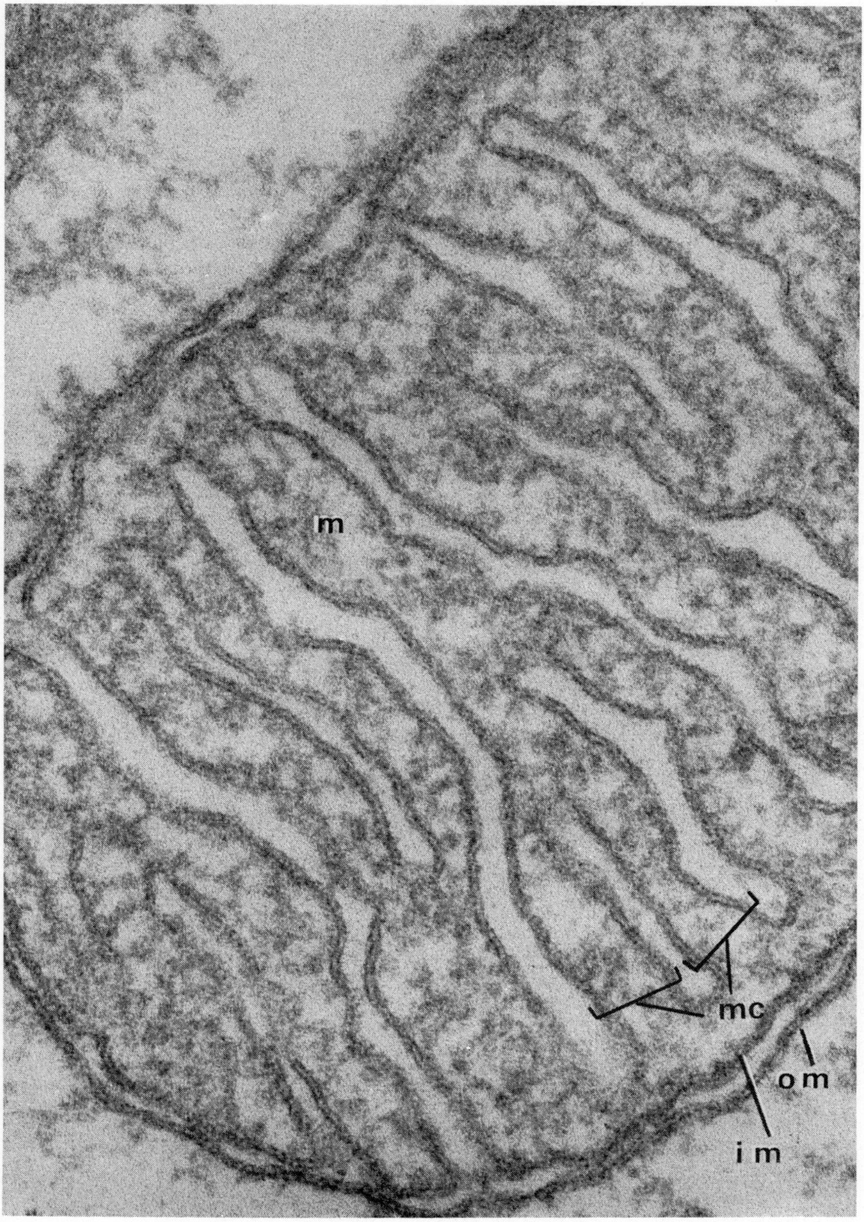

FIGURE 11–9. Electron micrograph of a mitochondrion from a pancreatic acinar cell. The double-layered unit membrane is evident in the smooth outer membrane (om) and in the inner membrane (im) which folds to form the cristae (mc) Magnified 207,000 ×. (Courtesy of G. E. Palade; from De Robertis, E. D., Nowinski, W. W., and Saez, F. A. *Cell Biology.* Philadelphia: W. B. Saunders Company, 1970.)

one must be controlled appropriately to generate the amount of energy required by the cell at any given moment.

The generation of ATP in the mitochondria depends upon the consumption of oxygen. When considered in terms of body surface area, the basal oxygen consumption of the obese is normal or low. However, when expressed as volume of oxygen consumed per unit of time, it is high. It is possible to estimate the active cell mass (thus excluding the inactive fat stores), and when oxygen consumption is expressed on this basis, there is no difference from normal control values. Therefore, we must conclude that in obesity oxygen consumption is at a normal rate when related to active body mass.

The tissue most directly involved in the deposition of fat is adipose tissue. Contrary to previous concepts, this tissue is very active metabolically and accounts for a considerable portion of the total daily energy expenditure in the human. The turnover of free fatty acids occurs at a rapid rate and involves the expenditure of ATP. The accumulation of fat will depend upon the relative rates of lipogenesis and lipolysis, both under endocrine control. Even a slight change in the rate of either lipogenesis or lipolysis would predispose, respectively, toward accumulation or breakdown of triglyceride. Such alterations in rate might well be secondary to hormonal changes.

Is there any evidence for this? Some studies indicate that GH secretion may be altered in obese subjects. Concentrations of GH in the plasma showed no rise after a 14-day fast in one study; normally, plasma GH rises after 48 hours of fasting. The GH response to hypoglycemia appears to be significantly decreased in the obese individual. El-Khodary proposes that altered GH secretion may be the primary phenomenon in obesity.

Other studies suggest that obese individuals are relatively resistant to insulin and that hyperinsulinism tends to accompany obesity. The insulin response following glucose administration in obese subjects is exaggerated. It has been proposed that there may be a defect in peripheral (but not adipose tissue) utilization of glucose in obese individuals, such that a compensatory rise in insulin secretion is necessary to maintain normal blood glucose concentration. The high insulin concentrations would augment glucose entry into the adipose tissue cell and therefore increase lipogenesis. In addition, insulin increases the activity of extracellular lipoprotein lipase, which catalyzes the hydrolysis of circulating triglycerides, thus providing more fatty acids for adipose tissue cells to utilize as substrates for the synthesis of triglyceride.

In addition to the relative rates of lipogenesis and lipolysis in the adipose tissue cell, the number of fat cells will determine the extent of deposition of fat. The number of adipose tissue cells is largely determined by the nutrition of the individual during that period of life when these cells are still increasing in number. This period covers the prenatal and early years of postnatal existence. Experiments with animals have shown that offspring given large amounts of food in the early postnatal period develop far greater numbers of adipose tissue cells than do littermates on normal diets. Such overfed offspring may have two or three times as many adipose tissue cells as their normally fed littermates. Once cell division of adipose tissue cells ceases, that number of cells remains constant through life. Each cell is capable of storing triglyceride. Thus the individual with three times as many adipocytes can theoretically store three times as much fat. When such individuals lose weight, they lose fat but not fat cells. These cells remain, waiting for the next surfeit of food to lay down more triglyceride.

Aside from possible defects in GH secretion or in peripheral utilization of glucose, there is only scanty evidence of other hormonal imbalance in obesity. Migeon has some evidence that adrenocortical function is increased in 30 to 60 percent of obese individuals. There is no good evidence that abnormal thyroid function plays any role in the etiology of obesity. It is rare to see classical signs of hypothyroidism in obese children. Physicians may be misled by basal metabolic rates (BMR) which are characteristically low in obesity (because of different body composition) as well as in hypothyroidism.

Psychological Obesity

Emotional problems are common in obesity, particularly in obese adolescents, and it is difficult to determine which came first—the obesity or the emotional disturbances. Certainly, once obesity is established, embarrassment and perceived (or imagined) disapproval by our weight-conscious society may aggravate the condition. The belief in psychological causes of obesity is based on surveys indicating that people tend to eat more when nervous or worried, or when they are bored or have nothing to do.

Appetite is stimulated by pleasant sights, tastes, smells, or recollections. Conversely, unpleasant associations decrease the desire for food. Undoubtedly these cerebral influences play a role in certain forms of obesity. The patterns of eating differ in different individuals and may reflect psychological differences. Night eaters eat little or no breakfast and lunch, but their evening meal is heavy, and eating often continues for several hours. Binge eaters are apt to eat throughout the day without a sensation of satiation. Marked fluctuations in weight may occur because of alternate "binges" and "crash diets."

The incidence of psychopathology seems to be no different in obese and nonobese populations. Thus the obese individual cannot simply be dismissed as neurotic or psychologically disturbed. Our knowledge of factors which regulate hunger and satiety in centers of the brain is still incomplete, and the influence of slight metabolic or endocrine deviations on these control centers is largely unknown. With full appreciation of psychological factors in the etiology of obesity, it would be appropriate to reserve judgment in a particular individual until knowledge in this area permits differentiating psychological and metabolic (or endocrine) causes of obesity.

Effects of Obesity

Most of the secondary effects of obesity on the cardiovascular system, on carbohydrate metabolism, and on aging are discussed in Chapter Fourteen. There is, however, a rare syndrome in children which demonstrates the effects of severe obesity on respiratory function. The *Pickwickian syndrome* is named after the fat boy in Dickens' *Pickwick Papers*: "and on the box sat a fat and red-faced boy in a state of somnolence." In these children, as obesity becomes marked, respiratory exchange in the lungs is severely impaired. Carbon dioxide is retained and arterial oxygen saturation decreases. A state of lethargy and somnolence ensues. It is difficult to wake these children and, indeed, they seem to do little but eat and sleep. Eventually heart failure develops.

Endocrine Conditions with Associated Obesity

A primary endocrinopathy—a disorder of hypothalamic, pituitary, or adrenal function—may be responsible for gain in weight. True obesity is generally not associated with thyroid disease; however, the accumulation of myxedematous material in the hypothyroid child may confuse the issue. This material is *not* fat and should not be confused with it.

HYPOTHALAMIC DISORDERS. Disorders of the hypothalamus are a rare cause of obesity. Tumors, trauma, infections, or infiltrative disease may involve the appetite center of the hypothalamus and produce obesity, among other symptoms. Fröhlich, in 1901, described a 14-year-old sexually infantile boy who was moderately obese and retarded in growth. He had diabetes insipidus and signs of a hypothalamic tumor (headache, vomiting, loss of vision). Subsequently such a tumor was found. The particular combination of obesity and sexual infantilism is often referred to as *Fröhlich's syndrome.*

Another disorder which may reflect a congenital defect of the hypothalamus is the *Laurence-Moon-Biedl syndrome.* This is an inherited condition characterized by obesity, mental retardation, polydactyly, syndactyly, sexual infantilism, short stature, and retinitis pigmentosa. The *Prader-Willi syndrome* is characterized by obesity, short stature, muscular hypotonia, mental retardation and typical facies. These patients frequently develop the adult-onset type of diabetes mellitus.

PITUITARY AND ADRENAL DISORDERS. Cushing's syndrome can result from an ACTH-secreting tumor of the pituitary or from adrenal tumor or hyperplasia. Tumors of the adrenal gland are quite common, appearing in up to five percent of autopsies. Often the tumors are nonfunctioning, single adenomas. Adenomas which function to produce adrenal hormones are most often single but may be multiple ("nodular cortical hyperplasia"). Both glucocorticoids and androgens may be produced in excess to give a clinical picture of Cushing's syndrome with virilization. The androgens may prevent the usual excessive protein breakdown seen in unalloyed Cushing's syndrome.

Adrenal hyperplasia may be secondary to a chromophobe adenoma of the pituitary. Since such tumors secrete both ACTH and MSH, the patient may show increased pigmentation in addition to the symptoms of Cushing's syndrome. ACTH-like or CRH-like peptides may be formed by nonendocrine tumors and result in secondary adrenal hyperplasia and Cushing's syndrome. This is often referred to as the "ectopic ACTH syndrome." Whatever the source of ACTH—whether pituitary or non-endocrine tumor—the adrenal responds by secreting excessive amounts of cortisol. A variety of tests (dexamethasone, ACTH, metyrapone) provide aid in differentiating primary adrenal disease from secondary adrenal hyperplasia. Hypercortisolism, whether exogenous or endogenous, produces characteristic changes in the pituitary gland (Crooke's changes), consisting of nests of basophilic cells often containing hyaline deposits.

The differential diagnosis of exogenous obesity and Cushing's syndrome can be difficult. One might think that an elevation of urinary 17OHCS would be an indication of Cushing's syndrome; however, one third of obese subjects have such a finding. Values of urinary 17OHCS greater than 10 mg/m^2/24 hours are suggestive of Cushing's syndrome. The administration of dexamethasone markedly decreases the output of 17OHCS in patients with exogenous obesity, whereas the patient with Cushing's syndrome is unresponsive. Occasionally the ACTH test may be helpful in differentiating obesity from Cushing's syndrome.

Excessive height

An increase in the linear growth rate above normal will result in a height age exceeding the chronological age. Just as with short stature, the too-tall boy or too-tall girl may represent hereditary or environmental influences on growth. The social problems of the very tall girls are far more pressing than those for the tall boys, and often considerable pressure is exerted on the physician to prevent further linear growth in these girls. The judgments involved in deciding whether or not therapy is indicated are complex and cannot be fully explored in this book. The psychosocial problems of the very tall girl may be severe and necessitate therapy of some sort. Estrogens have been used to limit further growth by accelerating fusion of the epiphyses; this therapy is recommended by some physicians, but is never indicated unless the patient's ultimate height will exceed six feet.

GH Excess

Tumors of the pituitary or the hypothalamus can result in excessive production and secretion of GH. Very rarely this occurs prior to fusion of the epiphyses and results in *gigantism.* More often these tumors occur in adults, bringing about skeletal overgrowth, particularly of the hands, feet, cranial sinuses, jaw, and supraorbital ridges (Figures 11–10). Overgrowth of soft tissues manifests itself as coarsening of the features, thick heel pads, and enlarged viscera. This condition of GH excess in adults is called *acromegaly* (Gr., *akron* = extremity, *mega* = large). Gigantism and acromegaly may occur together in adolescents.

Such tumors produce both endocrine effects (from altered secretion of pituitary hormones) and local effects. Headache is a common symptom and has been reported in 57 percent of patients with acromegaly. Abnormalities of the visual fields, papilledema, and atrophy of the optic nerve may result from local compression by the tumor. Most commonly, pressure is exerted on the inferior medial aspects of the optic nerves and chiasm. This is followed by loss of peripheral vision in one or both eyes (temporal hemianopsia). Almost all patients will show enlargement of the sella turcica or erosion of its margins. Eosinophilic adenomas

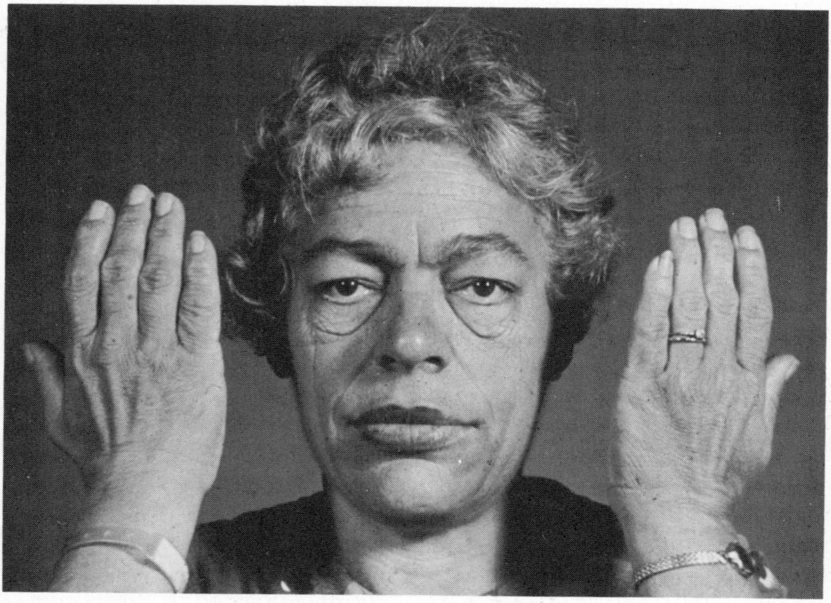

FIGURE 11–10. A 51-year-old woman with acromegaly showing typical features of thick-set facies with prognathism and large hands. Ten years prior to her admission to the hospital she developed hypertension. Over the ensuing years she noted increase in shoe and glove sizes, excessive sweating, and fatigue. Skull films showed an enlarged sella turcica, thickening of the cranial vault, and a prominent mandible. A diagnosis of pituitary adenoma was made and the patient received x-ray therapy. (Courtesy of Dr. Leslie Rose, Peter Bent Brigham Hospital, Boston, Mass.)

frequently erode the anterior clinoid processes, possibly because eosinophils are located mainly in the superior, lateral portions of the human pituitary.

Compression of the hypothalamus may produce diabetes insipidus and damage to the cells that produce gonadotropin releasing hormone. The hypogonadism that results is responsible for the delayed closure of the epiphyses in gigantism, and for loss of libido and impotence in men and for amenorrhea in women. Damage to the hypothalamus can release the prolactin-secreting cells of the anterior pituitary from the normal influence of prolactin inhibiting hormone. The resulting persistent lactation (galactorrhea) may actually precede other features of acromegaly.

DIAGNOSIS. In most patients the diagnosis is obvious. It is helpful to look at serial photographs; the change in the facies, with thickening of the zygomas and widening of the nasal bridge, can be striking (Figure 11–10). The increase in hand and foot sizes is usually noted by the patient. In contrast to craniopharyngiomas, intracranial calcification does not usually occur.

Tests of carbohydrate metabolism are often indicative of GH excess. The glucose tolerance test is abnormal in about 25 percent of affected patients. Administration of glucocorticoid prior to the glucose tolerance test increases the number of patients manifesting abnormal results to 50 percent. Most acromegalics are resistant to insulin. The concentration of GH in peripheral plasma is elevated in acromegaly and is not suppressed by the administration of glucose. Some but not all patients will show a rise in plasma GH concentration in response to hypoglycemia. Many acromegalics also release GH in response to TRH and to GHRH.

TREATMENT. Extension of the tumor beyond the sella turcica calls for partial or complete hypophysectomy in order to protect the optic nerves. The operation is usually followed by external radiation, since total removal of the tumor is not always possible. Postsurgical pituitary insufficiency must be treated according to the tropic hormones involved.

Implantation of radioactive seeds (^{198}Au or ^{90}Y) transnasally will often control the disease; however, there is always the danger of radiation damage to surrounding structures. Irradiation with a proton beam has been used by others.

The medical management of acromegaly is as yet unsatisfactory. Catecholamines are known to be involved in the process of GH release. The administration of chlorpromazine to acromegalics to block catecholamines and suppress GH release has been attempted. A 13-year-old girl with acromegaly was treated recently with chlorpromazine; however, she showed no change in her fasting serum GH or in the release of GH after appropriate stimuli. In this patient, conventional radiation therapy (5000 rad) delivered to the pituitary over a six week period was successful in decreasing the plasma concentration of GH. The studies by Alford et al., in which the effect of chlorpromazine on the secretion rate of GH in acromegalics was measured, suggest that the drug is ineffective.

A far more promising possibility for the medical therapy of acromegaly is the use of somatostatin. Studies in England have provided some evidence that the administration of somatostatin to patients with acromegaly can lower the plasma concentration of GH dramatically. The availability of somatostatin, however, is very restricted at present.

Cerebral Gigantism

Sotos described a group of infants of very large size at birth, weighing 5 to 6 kg after a gestation of normal length. These infants continued to grow rapidly, and osseous development was accelerated, but less so than that of height. Mental retardation was present in most cases. GH secretion was normal in these children and somatomedin levels were paradoxically low. Also, the extremities had none of the changes seen in acromegaly; thus this would not appear to be a syndrome of GH excess. The rapid growth slows after about the fourth year of life, but height curves remain above the 97th percentile. The characteristic facies of these children (prognathism, hypertelorism, depressed nasal bridge, highly arched palate, and dolichocephaly) suggest a discrete syndrome which Sotos has called *cerebral gigantism.*

Hyperthyroidism

Most evidence suggests that hyperthyroidism in childhood and adolescence is associated with accelerated growth. Hyperthyroidism, or *thyrotoxicosis,* is uncommon before puberty and is nearly always due to *Graves' disease.* This condition, first recognized in the early nineteenth century by Parry, Graves, and Basedow, is characterized by the classical triad of goiter, thyrotoxicosis, and exophthalmos, and usually by the presence of long-acting thyroid stimulator (LATS) in the patient's serum.

The intravenous injection of LATS into thyroxine-treated guinea pigs stimulates the discharge of thyroid hormone. However, the effect is prolonged and a maximum discharge is not reached until 16 to 24 hours after the injection. In contrast, a maximum discharge is obtained 1½ to 3 hours after intravenously administered TSH. Like TSH, LATS increases thyroid uptake of ^{131}I and alters thyroid histology, but appears to be a more powerful stimulator of the thyroid gland than TSH. Both TSH and LATS stimulate thyroidal adenyl cyclase, although, here again, the effect of LATS is later than that of TSH. Unlike TSH, the concentration of LATS in the serum is not suppressed by thyroxine.

LATS is present in the γ-globulin fraction of the serum and is itself an IgG γ-globulin and as such can cross the placenta, resulting in neonatal thyrotoxicosis (p. 106). It is virtually certain that LATS is a thyroid autoantibody, and therefore Graves' disease may well join the growing ranks of autoimmune disorders. It must be remembered, however, that LATS has not been found in all patients with Graves' disease and that the correlation between LATS activity and the extrathyroidal manifestations of the disease is not impressive. Thus to ascribe the disorder to LATS is premature at this time.

The stimulatory effect of LATS on the thyroid gland brings about the development of goiter. The goiter, however, is usually small. The thyroid gland is enlarged uniformly and has a firm, somewhat rubbery, consistency. Because of the associated thyrotoxicosis these goiters are referred to as *diffuse toxic goiters.* Viewed under a microscope, the follicles are small and lined by hyperplastic columnar epithelium. Little colloid is present. Vascularity is increased and occasionally a bruit can be heard (the latter is more common in adults).

The symptoms of hyperthyroidism include nervousness, irritability, weight loss, heat intolerance, heightened reflexes, and palpitations (Table 11–3). The child, almost always a girl, is thin, with flushed, warm,

Table 11–3. Features of Hypothyroidism and Hyperthyroidism

	Hypothyroidism	Hyperthyroidism
General	Fatigue and lethargy ↓ Activity ↑ Sleep Intolerance to cold Impaired growth and development	Fatigue and constant activity Poor sleep Intolerance to heat Accelerated growth
Skin	Cool, dry, coarse Carotenemic Hair coarse	Warm, moist Hair fine (Graves' disease: pretibial myxedema)
Eyes	–	Lid lag, stare, poor convergence Widened palpebral fissures (Graves' disease: exophthalmos)
Cardiovascular	Cardiomegaly Slow pulse	Arrhythmias Rapid pulse ↑ Pulse pressure
Gastrointestinal	Constipation ↓ Appetite ↑ Weight	↑ Frequency of bowel movements ↑ Appetite ↓ Weight
Neuromuscular	Muscle cramps Paresthesias Delayed relaxation phase of deep tendon reflexes	Proximal muscle weakness Tremor Brisk deep tendon reflexes
Psychological	Depression, apathy	Nervous, emotional lability
Laboratory tests:		
T_4	↓	↑
Free T_4	↓	↑
Radio I uptake	↓	Normal or ↑
TSH	Primary ↑ Secondary or tertiary ↓	↓ –

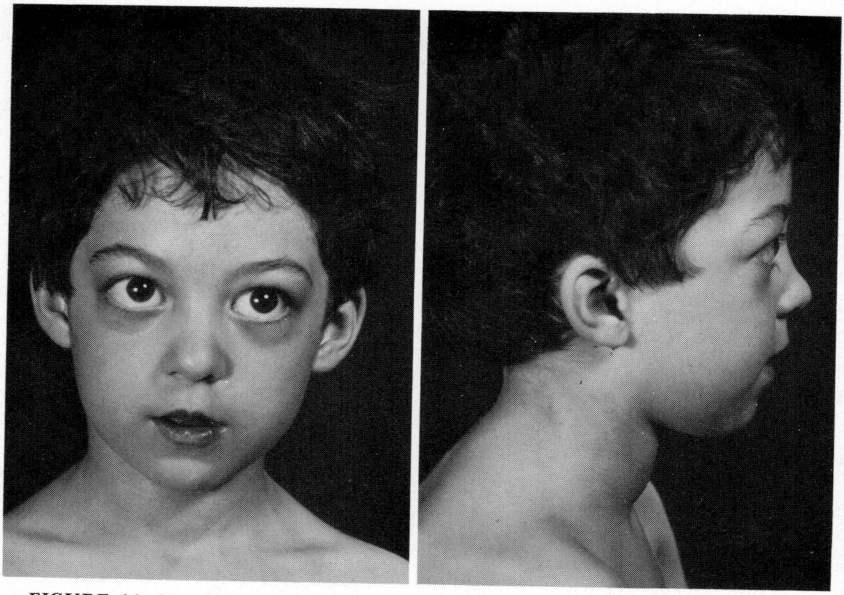

FIGURE 11–11. Front and side view of a four-year-old girl with hyperthyroidism. She had a history of bulging eyes, excessive fatigue, failure to gain weight, and a mass in the neck. On physical examination she had bilateral exophthalmos, lid lag, and a goiter with a loud bruit. Her laboratory values were: PBI, 19 mg/100 ml; T_4, 13.6 μg/100 ml; resin T_3 uptake, 52 percent; radioactive I uptake at 4 hours, 45 percent, and at 24 hours, 50 percent; serum cholesterol, 176 mg/100 ml; bone age, 5 years, 9 months; and height age, 5 years, 5 months. She was given propylthiouracil therapy. (Courtesy of Dr. John Crigler, Children's Medical Center, Boston, Mass.)

moist skin and palms. In five percent of patients (usually adults), accumulations of myxedematous material are observed in the pretibial region. In patients with exophthalmos, the total bulk of the orbital contents is increased, owing partly to edema and possibly to an increase in orbital fat, but mostly to an increase in bulk of the extraocular muscles. This causes proptosis of the eyes, which may eventually lead to inflammation and corneal damage. The extraocular muscles show swelling, loss of striation, fragmentation, and lymphocyte infiltration. Ultimately they undergo marked degeneration, fibrosis, and hyalinization. Superimposed upon the ophthalmopathy of Graves' disease may be the typical ophthalmic complications of hyperthyroidism: widened palpebral fissure, stare, lid lag, an poor convergence (Figure 11–11). Graves' disease is more than just a disorder of excess thyroid hormone. The findings in the eye cannot be reproduced by any amount of thyroid hormone administration. In addition, the pretibial myxedema, lymphadenopathy, and splenomegaly seen in Graves' disease are not found in other causes of hyperthyroidism. In the usual case of Graves' disease, TSH is undetectable even after TRH administration.

Unique to childhood is the acceleration of growth and advancement of bone maturation seen with hyperthyroidism. The relationship of bone age to height age, however, falls within the normal range for proportionate growth. There is no evidence that the hyperthyroidism alters either the plasma concentration or clearance rate of GH.

Hyperthyroid patients typically have a concentration of serum thyroxine above 12 μg per 100 ml, and an elevated triiodothyronine concentration in the blood (Table 11–3). Thyroidal iodide clearance rate is increased in Graves' disease, and therefore the thyroidal ^{131}I uptake is increased over normal. There is an increase in both the proportion and absolute concentration of free thyroxine in the blood (Table 11–3). The uptake of ^{131}I-labeled T_3 by red cells or resin is abnormally high, reflecting saturation of thyroxine binding globulin. The BMR is high also.

TREATMENT. Most physicians prefer a trial of medical therapy in children before resorting to surgery; others advocate immediate surgical removal of the thyroid. Of the several antithyroid drugs available, the ones used clinically belong to the category of the thioamides, such as thiourea, thiouracil, carbimazole, and propylthiouracil. The usual dose of propylthiouracil is 100 mg every 8 hours orally. The spacing of administration of the drug throughout the day is necessary because each dose is fully effective for only a few hours. There may be no discernible clinical improvement for several days or even a week or more. If signs of hypothyroidism appear, the dose should be reduced. Persistent hyperthyroidism may require higher doses of antithyroid drug or surgical intervention.

Remissions of disease can occur spontaneously on or off therapy, but there is no way of predicting which patients will eventually achieve a lasting remission and which will relapse. When therapy has been continued for about a year, about one half the patients remain well for long periods thereafter. If the treatment is stopped, about 20 percent of patients relapse within two months. Others experience remissions lasting several months or years. During treatment a reduction in the size of the goiter is a sign that remission may have taken place. Another favorable sign is freedom from symptoms of hyperthyroidism on a small maintenance dose of antithyroid drug. One can test normality of thyroid function by measuring the uptake of radioactive iodine after three weeks on suppressive doses of thyroxine. If the uptake of radioactive iodine is suppressed by thyroxine, one can assume normal feedback controls exist once more. Unfortunately, hyperthyroidism in children is particularly obstinate, and drug therapy usually must be continued for several years.

Adrenergic blocking agents such as propranolol are often used for temporary suppression of the cardiac complications of hyperthyroidism. Certain ionic inhibitors, such as thiocyanate or perchlorate, block the concentration of iodide ion by the thyroid gland. Thiocyanate is present in cabbage, and ingestion of large quantities of this vegetable could produce impairment of thyroid function. Iodide itself produces a rapid and striking effect in the hyperthyroid patient. The BMR falls and signs and symptoms of hyperthyroidism are greatly improved. The thyroid gland changes; vascularity is decreased and the gland becomes harder and firmer. The effects of iodide, however, are not permanent and the beneficial effects seem to wear off. Therefore, iodide therapy is most often used to prepare the patient for thyroidectomy. Like the stable iodine, ^{131}I is rapidly and efficiently trapped by the thyroid gland and stored organically bound in the colloid. Here the destructive β rays can act almost exclusively upon the parenchymal cells of the thyroid, with little or no damage to surrounding tissues. This form of therapy for hyperthyroidism is indicated for older patients and in patients with heart disease. It has no place in the treatment of children with hyperthyroidism because of the dangers of inducing myxedema or neoplastic change. Many clinics reserve the use of radioiodine for patients over 40 years of age.

T_3 TOXICOSIS. The hyperthyroid state may be produced by isolated hypersecretion of triiodothyronine. Patients with T_3 toxicosis, as this condition is called, have all the usual clinical features of hyperthyroidism, but laboratory tests reveal normal total and free thyroxine concentrations in the blood. The concentration of T_3 in the blood is elevated.

Excess Sex Hormones

A variety of endocrine disorders can bring about increased secretion of androgens or estrogens, which in turn will accelerate the rate of linear growth and skeletal maturation. These conditions may originate in the brain, adrenals, or gonads.

Tumors, malformations, or infiltrative processes of the pineal gland or hypothalamus can cause sexual precocity. Symptoms relating to the nervous system are usually present. However, in a large majority of all cases of sexual precocity, it is not possible to detect any abnormality other than the early onset of puberty. These cases are referred to as *idiopathic sexual precocity*. This should not imply, however, that pathology within the hypothalamus or pineal gland does not exist. We simply do not know enough about the "biological time clock" which triggers the onset of puberty.

ADRENAL HYPERPLASIA AND ADRENAL TUMORS. Untreated congenital adrenocortical hyperplasia is characterized by rapid linear growth (p. 161). The early fusion of the epiphyses results in eventual dwarfism in affected patients. Adrenal tumors may cause androgen production. Virilizing tumors of the adrenal in children are commonest in girls between 4 and 8 years of age. Particularly large amounts of dehydroepiandrosterone are secreted by these tumors. Peripheral conversion of this steroid to androgens occurs readily. In females, these androgens produce clitoral enlargement; in males, the penis enlarges. Sexual hair grows and acne develops. The rate of linear growth and epiphyseal maturation and fusion is accelerated in both sexes. Three fourths of these tumors are unilateral and well encapsulated. Tumors of the adrenal may be benign adenomas or carcinomas.

Carcinomas of the adrenal, most often seen in adults, frequently manifest impaired 11-hydroxylation. Thus immediate precursors accumulate, such as 11-deoxycortisol and deoxycorticosterone. The latter may cause hypertension. Large amounts of estrogen are often produced by these tumors, and the patient may become feminized. In women, amenorrhea and ovarian atrophy may occur secondary to suppression of gonadotropin release by the estrogens. Like other carcinomas, these adrenal tumors can produce, on occasion, inappropriate polypeptide hormones.

OVARIAN TUMORS. One to two percent of girls with sexual precocity have been shown to have ovarian tumors. Some of these tumors (granulosa cell tumors, theca cell tumors) produce estrogen, whereas others (teratomas, dysgerminomas) produce gonadotropins which stimulate the secretion of estrogens by the normal ovarian tissue. The most frequent early symptoms and signs are breast development, increased growth rate, and advanced bone age.

TESTICULAR TUMORS. Virilizing tumors within the testis may be of Leydig cell origin or "adrenal rest" origin. It is not unusual to discover nodules of adrenal-like cells in normal testicular tissue or in patients with congenital adrenocortical hyperplasia. Indeed, a review of the origins of the gonadal and adrenal cells (p. 58) would predict the occurrence of such "aberrant" cells. These cells cannot be differentiated histologically from Leydig cells; however, these adrenal rest tumors are capable of 11-hydroxylating in vitro both deoxycorticosterone and 11-deoxycortisol to form corticosterone and cortisol respectively. Normal testicular tissue cannot perform these transformations. Testicular adrenal rest tumors from patients with 21-hydroxylase deficiency either are unable to 21-hydroxylate progesterone or 17-hydroxyprogesterone or do so at rates far below those found in normal adrenal tissue. That these testicular tumors constitute aberrant adrenal tissue is supported by their response to ACTH. The tumors visibly enlarge with ACTH administration to the patient and regress with glucocorticoid therapy.

Leydig cell tumors of the testis are rare in childhood. They are usually unilateral. The secretion of testosterone by these cells (or of androstenedione by adrenal rest cells) produces the clinical picture of virilization with accelerated growth.

SUMMARY

Linear growth in man does not continue throughout life. The bones mature under hormonal influence (thyroid hormone) and eventually the epiphyses fuse (sex hormones), preventing further longitudinal growth. The anabolic process is aided and abetted by growth-promoting hormones such as GH, insulin, and thyroxine and is hindered by other hormones (cortisol). Just when do these controls first appear? The fetus is exposed to large amounts of estrogen in utero and apparently does possess estrogen receptors in certain tissues, such as the vagina, uterus, and breast. At birth, estrogenization of these tissues is clinically evident. Fetal bones and brain undergo a maturation process under the influence of thyroid hormone.

With the exception of thyroid hormone and possibly insulin, there is no good evidence that fetal hormones regulate growth in utero. In contrast, within a short time after birth, endocrine deficiency syndromes manifest themselves. A surprising number of hormones influence "growth"; the progress of a child's gain in height and weight is, therefore, a valuable clue to the normality of the endocrine system. Unfortunately, nothing is ever as simple as we might wish. The roles of emotional and nutritional factors in growth cannot be ignored. The physician must keep in mind the overall problem of cellular growth: are sufficient nutrients reaching the cell?; moreover, does the cell have the appropriate genetic machinery to utilize these nutrients? The first question is one of supply and can involve any of the stages of food transport, from diet (malnutrition, emotional disturbances) to absorption in the gastrointestinal tract (malabsorption syndromes) to transport across the cell membrane (structural or hormonal deficiencies). The second question is often more difficult to answer and many of our present cases of "idiopathic failure to thrive" probably belong in this category of "abnormal cellular machinery."

The beautiful balance of normal growth in the child is not easily disturbed, but when it is, whether by emotional, nutritional, endocrine, or genetic factors, the child may not be able to "catch up" later. The growth potential is not the same at one age as another, even in early childhood, and a permanent deficit of cells may be the fate of such a child. Efforts to maintain normal gains in height and weight in the formative years of the child are critical to the child's physical and emotional well-being. Appropriate therapy should be instituted as early as possible to circumvent permanent cellular deficiency.

SUGGESTED READING

Human Pituitary Growth Hormone, Allen W. Root, Charles C Thomas, Springfield, Illinois, 1972.

This book discusses the chemistry, biological action, and clinical disorders of growth hormone. An excellent reference book with full bibliography for the reader interested in pursuing in depth any of these aspects of growth hormone. The discussions of hypopituitarism and acromegaly are particularly appropriate.

Iodine Metabolism and Thyroid Function, edited by K. Mashimo and H. Suzuki, Hokkaido University School of Medicine, Sapporo, Japan, 1973.

A collection of recent papers by Japanese workers on iodine metabolism. In particular, discussions of effects of excess iodide in Graves' disease and the alterations of cortisol metabolism in hyperthyroidism are of interest. For those interested in the oxidative mechanisms involved in thyroid hormone synthesis, there are several worthwhile papers.

The role of cyclic nucleotides in the secretion of pituitary growth hormone, Glenn T. Peake, in *Frontiers in Neuroendocrinology,* edited by W. R. Ganong and L. Martini, Oxford University Press, 1973.

An up-to-date discussion of the regulation of GH release. Both cyclic AMP and cyclic GMP are discussed as well as the special roles of Ca^{++} and prostaglandins. A chapter by Carlos Gual in the same book discusses the clinical uses and effects of hypothalamic releasing factors. The TRH test of pituitary reserve is of special interest.

SELECTED REFERENCES FROM THE LITERATURE

Alford, F. P. et al. Temporal patterns of integrated plasma hormone levels during sleep and wakefulness. J. Clin. Endocrinol. Metab. *37*:841, 1973.

AvRuskin, T. W. et al. T_3 toxicosis in adolescence. Ped. *52*:649, 1973.

Bitensky, M. W. and Gorman, R. E. Cellular responses to cyclic AMP. Progr. Biophys. and Mol. Biol. *26*:411, 1973.

Blackwell, R. E., and Guillemin, R. Hypothalamic control of adenohypophyseal secretions. Annu. Rev. Physiol. *35*:357, 1973.

Burger, M. M. et al. Growth control and cyclic alterations of cyclic AMP in the cell cycle. Nature *239*:161, 1972.

Daughaday, W. H.: Regulation of skeletal growth by sulfation factor. Adv. Intern. Med. *17*:237, 1971.

Elders, M. J. et al. Laron's dwarfism: studies on the nature of the defect. J. Ped. *83*:253, 1973.

Hintz, R. L., Clemmons, D. R., Underwood, L. E., and Van Wyk, J. J.: Competitive binding of somatomedin to the insulin receptors of adipocytes, chondrocytes and liver membranes. Proc. Nat. Acad. Sci. *69*:2351, 1972.

Kaneko, T., Zor, U., and Field, J. Stimulation of thyroid adenyl cyclase activity and cyclic AMP by long-acting thyroid stimulator. Metabolism *19*:430, 1970.

Karp, M., Laron, Z., and Doron, M.: Insulin secretion in children with constitutional familial short stature. J. Ped. *83*:241, 1973.

Laron, Z. et al. Insulin, growth and GH. Israel J. Med. Sci. *8*:440, 1972.

Reichlin, S. et al. Neural control of TSH Secretion. Recent Progress Hormone Research *28*:271, 1972.

Schlesinger, S., MacGillivray, M. H., and Munschauer, R. W. Acceleration of growth and bone maturation in childhood thyrotoxicosis. J. Ped. *83*:233, 1973.

Sledge, C. B. Growth hormone and articular cartilage. Fed. Proc. *32*:1503, 1973.

Tell, G. P. et al. Somatomedin: inhibition of adenylate cyclase activity in subcellular membranes of various tissues. Science *180*:312, 1973.

Vasques, A. M., Drash, A. L., and Kenny, F. M. Diurnal patterns of secretion of cortisol and growth hormone in normal adolescents, in patients with exogenous and endogenous Cushing's syndrome, in patients with diabetes mellitus, and in a fasting subject. J. Ped. *83*:578, 1973.

PART FOUR

THE ADOLESCENT

CHAPTER TWELVE

Maturation: Skeletal

In the course of the maturation process which the skeletal system undergoes, condensed mesenchyme is converted into cartilage, and either mesenchyme (membranous bone) or cartilage (cartilaginous bone) can be transformed into bone. Cartilage first appears in embryos at about 5 weeks. Mesenchymal cells in developing bones differentiate into chondroblasts or osteoblasts, which can form a *matrix*. The organic portion of the matrix, called *osteoid*, consists of collagen embedded in a ground substance composed of proteins, mucopolysaccharides, and mucoproteins. This matrix subsequently becomes calcified to form cartilage or bone.

Skeletal maturation begins with the appearance of *ossification centers* visible by x-ray. Characteristic of mammalian skeletal development is the formation of separate diaphyseal and epiphyseal ossification centers in the long appendicular bones. The first ossification centers appear in the diaphyses of the long bones at 8 weeks gestation (Table 12–1). A cylindrical sheath of membranous bone, the periosteum, appears first and confers structural rigidity to the early limb. Cartilage cells within the shaft increase in size, the matrix becomes calcified, and the cartilage cells die. The calcified cartilage is invaded by vascular connective tissue from the periosteum. The cartilage is broken up and replaced by bone *(primary ossification center)*. Other mesenchymal cells differentiate into hematopoietic cells to form the primary bone marrow. The central core of cartilage in the humerus is completely replaced by bone and marrow by the middle of the third month of gestation. The mineralization of osteoid involves the orderly formation of crystals of the bone mineral hydroxyapatite, $Ca_{10}(PO_4)_6(OH)_2$. Crystals of hydroxyapatite bind water, forming a "hydration shell" on the crystal surface.

New ossification centers appear according to a definite time sched-

TABLE 12-1. Chronology of Bone Development in the Human Fetus as Measured by Roentgenograms

Fetal Age (in weeks)*	Ossification Centers
8–9	Diaphyses of humerus, radius, ulna, femur, and tibia; terminal phalanges of hand
9–12	Metacarpals; metatarsals; terminal phalanges of foot; basal phalanges of hand
12–16	Basal phalanges of foot; middle phalanges of hand
20–35	Middle phalanges of foot; fibula; os calcis
35–40	Distal epiphysis of femur
40	Proximal epiphysis of tibia; astragalus

*The ages are approximate and should serve only as a guide. More precise tables of skeletal maturation are available in standard textbooks of radiology.

ule, which provides the basis for standard tables and atlases of skeletal growth (p. 265). In the human fetus 90 mm in length the ossification of clavicles, vertebrae, ribs, iliac bones, and jaws is well advanced. In addition, the progress of ossification of the shafts of the long bones toward both metaphyses is readily visualized on x-ray.

Certain cartilage cells occupying the area where the epiphyseal cartilage will later be formed do not undergo hypertrophy. Their matrix remains uncalcifiable, and without calcification vascular penetration is prevented. These cells organize themselves in close parallel columns (Figure 12–1). They undergo proliferation, and growth of the long bones occurs at these diaphyseal-epiphyseal junctions. Ossification centers (secondary) occur in most epiphyses postnatally (Table 12–2). The progress of development is much the same as in the fetal diaphysis, with hypertrophy of the epiphyseal cartilage cells, calcification of the matrix, invasion of vascular connective tissue, and ossification.

Linear growth can continue as long as the epiphyses of long bones are separated from the diaphyses by a plate of cartilage *(cartilage plate)*. When this plate disappears and epiphyses and diaphyses unite (epiphyseal fusion), growth ceases. Epiphyseal fusion occurs in various bones in an orderly sequence, starting usually at or after puberty, and this sequence provides another indication of skeletal maturity (Table 12–2).

Aside from the growth of the skeletal system, a process of bone remodeling is taking place constantly. Bone is resorbed in discrete areas by cells called *osteoclasts* (Figure 12–1); later, osteoblasts appear in these areas and fill in the space with osteoid, which subsequently calcifies.

Bone remodeling takes place on both outer (periosteal) and inner (endosteal) surfaces as well as within the central portion of the bone cortex.

The growth, maturation, and remodeling of bone is controlled by the complex interaction of several hormones. Bone formation is stimulated by GH and depressed by glucocorticoids. Bone resorption is stimulated by PTH in the presence of vitamin D. Calcitonin, mechanical stress, estrogens, androgens, inorganic phosphate, and fluoride all reduce bone resorption (Table 12–3). Linear growth of bones continues throughout childhood, and with the approach of adolescence a truly remarkable increase in the rate of linear growth occurs. This adolescent growth spurt and the subsequent fusion of the epiphyses are under hormonal control. In this chapter we shall explore the hormonal controls of bone metabolism and try to relate these controls to the phenomena of linear growth and epiphyseal fusion. Finally we shall discuss briefly the various endocrine causes of disordered bone metabolism.

THE PROCESS OF OSSIFICATION

Linear growth is primarily dependent upon growth in the length of long bones. The bones of the extremities, pelvis, and vertebral column, and those at the base of the skull, are called *cartilage bones* because they

TABLE 12–2. Chronology of the Postnatal Development of Bone in Humans as Measured by Roentgenograms

Postnatal Age (in years)*	Joint	Ossification Center	Postnatal Age of Complete Ossification (in years)
0–1	Ankle	Calcaneus	15–16
	Wrist	Capitate, hamate, distal epiphysis of radius	15–16
	Shoulder	Epiphysis of head of humerus	18
	Hip	Epiphysis of head of femur	16
1–2	Shoulder	Greater tuberosity of humerus	5
	Elbow	Capitellum of humerus	15
	Ankle	Distal epiphysis of fibula	16
2–3	Wrist	Epiphyses of phalanges and metacarpals	15–16
	Ankle	Epiphyses of metatarsals	15
3–4	Wrist	Lunate	15
	Knee	Proximal epiphysis of fibula	17
	Ankle	Middle cuneiform, navicular	15
4–5	Elbow	Proximal epiphysis of radius	15
	Knee	Patella	

*The ages are approximate and should serve only as a guide. More precise tables of skeletal maturation are available in standard textbooks of radiology.

replace cartilage. This cartilage is transformed into bone by *endochondral ossification.* In the middle of the shaft (diaphysis) of a long bone, the cartilage cells (chondrocytes) enlarge, glycogen accumulates within them, and the cytoplasm becomes vacuolated. These cells form a precursor of collagen, *protocollagen.* Certain amino acids (proline and lysine) of this molecule are hydroxylated, and carbohydrate moieties are attached at these hydroxylated sites. The molecule (now called *procollagen*) becomes more soluble and can be extruded into the intercellular spaces. Procollagen is converted to *tropocollagen* (loss of a portion of procollagen), which in turn undergoes further maturation to form the less soluble collagen. Hydroxyproline and hydroxylysine are unique to collagen and provide a convenient marker for this protein. Indeed, when bone is resorbed increased quantities of hydroxyproline are present in the urine. The growth process involves a constant remodeling of bone and a continuous breakdown of collagen; hence the excretion of hydroxyproline in the urine becomes an indication of growth. In the child who is not growing, the excretion of hydroxyproline is very low, usually less than 10 mg per 24 hours.

In the epiphyseal plate there is a progression from a zone of actively proliferating cells to a zone of maturing cartilage cells, giving way to a zone of hypertrophied cells, culminating finally in a region of calcified cartilage (Figure 12–1). The proliferative zone in these columns of cells accounts for all subsequent growth in the length of the long bones. Under normal conditions, the rate of multiplication of cartilage cells in this zone is matched by the rate of removal from the diaphyseal ends of the bones. The cartilage cells continually grow away from the shaft and are replaced by bone. The result is an increase in the length of the shaft, but the epiphyseal plate maintains approximately the same thickness. Hypophysectomy in young rats reduces the width of the epiphyseal plate, whereas GH restores it to normal. The effect on chondrogenesis forms the basis for one of the most commonly used bioassays for GH (rat tibia test).

Before bone can be formed in endochondral ossification, the cartilage must be removed. Blood vessels grow into the area and invade the calcified cartilage, carrying with them mesenchymal cells. Some of these cells differentiate into hematopoietic elements of the bone marrow. Those cells which come into contact with the cartilage differentiate into osteoblasts (Figure 12–1). These latter cells form a layer on the surfaces of spicules of calcified cartilage matrix and deposit bone matrix upon them. This matrix becomes calcified, forming bone.

The mechanism of calcification remains unclear. It is probable that, as Glimcher has proposed, the initial seeding or nucleation of apatite crystals requires a specific stereochemical configuration present in collagen. Electron microscopy and x-ray diffraction studies indicate that formation of the bone mineral crystal lattice is initiated within the collagen fibers. Phosphorylation of collagen appears to be required before mineralization will occur. The enzyme phosphokinase, which

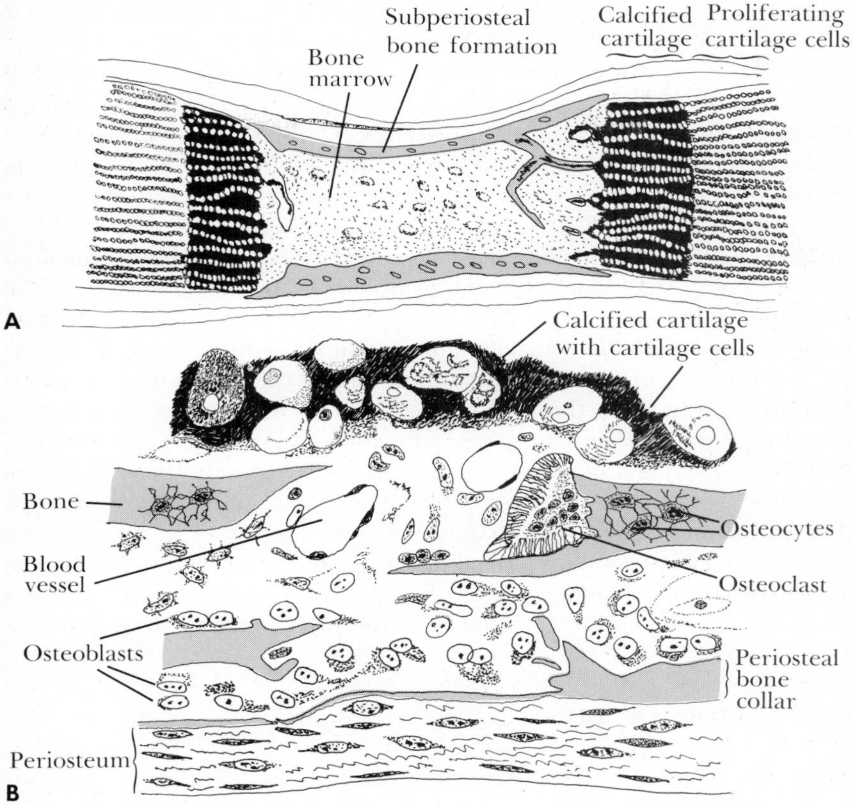

FIGURE 12–1. (a) Drawing of diaphysis of typical long bone showing proliferation and calcification of cartilage cells and development of periosteal bone. (b) Detail of endochondral ossification. Connective tissue cells (osteoblasts), together with blood vessels, pass through the spaces in the periosteal bone collar and invade the calcified cartilage, resorbing it and replacing it with bone. Remodeling of newly formed bone occurs continuously.

catalyzes the attachment of phosphorus to the hydroxyl of serine in many proteins, has been found in significant concentrations in connective tissues, in bone enamel, and in other collagen-rich tissues. Osteoblasts are unusually rich in alkaline phosphatase, but the relationship of this enzyme to the calcification process is not clear. Perhaps it acts to bring about a local increase in the concentration of phosphate and a decrease in the concentration of pyrophosphate. The latter can inhibit mineralization in vitro even though the solutions are supersaturated with respect to Ca^{++} and phosphate.

Any cell that survives its own formation of a matrix which calcifies is an osteoblast. The chondroblast, in contrast, dies. When calcification of the matrix occurs, the osteoblast becomes an *osteocyte* (Figure 12–1). Apparently the survival of osteoblasts in a calcified matrix is due to the establishment of cytoplasmic processes. A syncytium is formed, linking osteocytes to osteoblasts and to precursor (progenitor) cells. If these cytoplasmic connections are damaged (from a fracture of osteoporotic bone, for example), the osteocytes beyond the break die.

Trabeculated bone (spongy bone) consists of a three-dimensional lattice of branching bony spicules or trabeculae. The intercommunicating spaces are occupied by bone marrow. Compact bone appears as a solid continuous mass; however, microscopic spaces exist within it. The periosteum of long bones is osteogenic and forms a cylinder of compact bone surrounding the central medullary cavity. The increase in thickness of the shaft of long bones is the result of progressive thickening of the periosteal band. The deposition of bone on the outside of the shaft is accompanied by the appearance of osteoclasts on the inside and by erosion of bone from within to enlarge the marrow cavity. The adjustment of bone formation and resorption is such that the cylindrical shaft expands rapidly while the thickness of its walls increases more slowly.

At the end of the growing period, chondrogenesis slows and finally, when the epiphyseal plate has been replaced by spongy bone and marrow, ceases. At that point the epiphysis and diaphysis are continuous. Further linear growth is impossible. The two epiphyses of a long bone do not contribute equally to growth. For example, growth in the length of the femur takes place primarily at the distal epiphysis, whereas growth of the tibia occurs primarily at the proximal epiphysis.

RESORPTION OF BONE

In the process of bone resorption, calcium, phosphate, and products of digested collagen (hydroxyproline) are released into the extracellular fluid. Coincident with bone resorption is the presence of cells called *osteoclasts.* These giant multinucleated cells are often seen enveloping the tip of each spicule of bone undergoing resorption. This association has led to the view that these cells are actively involved in the resorptive process. Certainly the evidence to date would support this view. The origin of the osteoclast is of some interest. The most prevalent theory is that the osteocytes, being capable of some bone resorption, are released from their bony lacunae during the resorptive process and assume the form of osteoblasts once more, or are incorporated into a multinucleated osteoclast. Osteoclasts are also produced by fusion of *preosteoclasts* formed from mesenchymal cells. The osteoclast presumably can secrete proteolytic enzymes which degrade the organic matrix. Parathyroid hormone increases both the number of osteoclasts and the osteolytic activity of individual osteoclasts (Table 12–2). Thyroid hormone increases the rate of bone resorption, probably by stimulating the rate of cellular metabolism.

If bone resorption is increased, as, for example, by administering PTH or thyroid hormone, bone formation increases also. As a result, the turnover or remodeling of bone is accelerated, but the net effect is a decrease in bone mass. The reverse is also true: if bone resorption is slowed down (by calcitonin or by sex hormones, for instance), bone formation decreases. In such cases, the net effect is a reduction in the rate of loss of skeletal mass. Thus the two processes, bone formation and bone resorption, are coupled.

The release of PTH and calcitonin is regulated by the concentration of ionic calcium in the blood. The latter, in turn, is maintained within a very narrow range (9 to 11 mg/100 ml serum) by the actions of PTH, calcitonin, and vitamin D. The role of calcium in bone formation is just one of the many biologically important facets of this remarkable cation. The regulation of calcium concentration and metabolism constitutes one of the most important of the body's homeostatic mechanisms.

CALCIUM HOMEOSTASIS

Presumably, when life first developed on this planet the primordial sea was rich in K^+ and Mg^{++}. With the passage of eons of time the composition of the sea shifted, becoming rich in Na^+ and Ca^{++} and poorer in K^+ and Mg^{++}. If the functional integrity of the cell was to depend on a milieu like the primordial one, some means of retaining K^+ and Mg^{++} and exporting Na^+ and Ca^{++} had to be found. The solution was the evolution of the semipermeable cell membrane and its ion pump.

The control of sodium takes place largely at the cell surface, where the sodium pump is located. In contrast, calcium is regulated not only at the cell surface but also within the mitochondrial and microsomal membranes inside the cell. Ca^{++} has a marked tendency to form complexes with both organic and inorganic anions; this property is the basis for the biological significance of calcium. Its combination with phosphate in the formation of bone is of obvious significance in the development of the skeletal system. However, this mineralization process is an extracellular event. Of equal if not greater importance are the roles of calcium in various intracellular functions. Rasmussen has proposed an interesting model of *cell activation*, connecting the adenyl cyclase-cyclic AMP system with alterations in calcium within the cell. A number of cellular systems require both calcium and cyclic AMP for response to a given stimulus. Parathyroid hormone activates kidney and bone cells by stimulating adenyl cyclase and by increasing calcium entry into these cells. As a result of increased calcium concentration in bone cells, (1) cellular systems of bone resorption are activated, (2) the rate of conversion of precursor cells into both osteoblasts and osteoclasts is increased, and (3) collagen synthesis by osteoblasts is inhibited. All three of these effects can be produced by infusion of calcium into parathyroidectomized animals.

Apparently both PTH and calcitonin can act on all types of bone cells. Calcitonin can block the effect of PTH on bone cells both in vitro and in vivo. Rasmussen suggests that calcitonin acts by decreasing the concentration of calcium within the target cells. The effect of PTH on bone resorption is partially responsible for the hypercalcemic action of this hormone.

MEMBRANE PERMEABILITY

How does the concentration of calcium within or outside the cell influence cellular function? Several functions of cells are thought to be dependent upon Ca^{++} concentration. Two of these functions, irritability and muscle contractility, are probably secondary to changes in the permeability of membranes to calcium.

Calcium is biologically active only in the ionic state, and the concentration of Ca^{++} in blood is determined by the dissociation constant, K.

$$K = \frac{[Ca^{++}]\,[Protein^{=}]}{[Ca - Protein]} = 10^{-2.2}$$

The calcium is present almost entirely in the plasma, at concentrations ranging from 2.3 to 2.5 mM. Human red cells were found to be associated with calcium at a level of 0.63 μg per ml of packed red cell volume. This calcium is associated with the red cell membrane. In plasma at pH 7.35, the free (diffusible) Ca^{++} is about 60 percent of the total concentration of calcium. The non-diffusible calcium is complexed to protein. The permeability of membranes varies indirectly with the concentration of Ca^{++} in extracellular fluid. Elevation of extracellular Ca^{++} concentration reduces membrane permeability and the rate of transport of various substances (particularly Na^+ and K^+) across the membrane. Decreasing the concentration of Ca^{++} enhances membrane permeability.

Probably as a direct consequence of these effects, Ca^{++} changes the electrical properties and the excitability of nerves and other membranes. If the concentration of Ca^{++} is too low, nerves fire spontaneously, muscle cells show lowered threshold to stimuli, cardiac contractility is augmented, and relaxation is retarded. Thus, a characteristic symptom of hypoparathyroidism is sustained and painful contractures of various sets of muscles (tetany).

The stimulus for muscle contraction is an electrical impulse arriving from the motor neuron at the neuromuscular junction. This impulse is transmitted to the muscle cell and rapidly spreads over the *sarcolemma* (the plasma membrane of muscle cells). In the resting state, there is a difference of potential on the two sides of the membrane; however, as the impulse spreads, the membrane is *depolarized.* This depolarization is probably due to a sudden increase in the permeability of the membrane to cations such as Na^+, K^+, and Ca^{++}, and these cations flow across the membrane. The sarcolemma has a structure of repeated tubular invaginations that are in contact with the myofibrils within the cell. The depolarization of the outer membrane is rapidly followed by depolarization of the double-membraned *sarcoplasmic reticulum,* which surrounds the *sarcomeres* (longitudinal repeating units of the myofibrils). The reticulum becomes more permeable, and Ca^{++} ions, which had been sequestered in cisternae of the reticulum, escape. The extremely rapid discharge of Ca^{++} from the reticulum into the sarcoplasm (intracellular matrix of muscle) is accompanied by the synthesis of ATP and is believed to trigger the interaction of ATP with the myofilaments of the myofibrils. Ca^{++} specifically activates the ATPase of myosin, which hydrolyzes ATP.

During relaxation of the muscle, calcium ions are once again segregated within the sarcoplasmic reticulum. The transport of calcium across the sarcoplasmic reticulum is assumed to involve the formation of a phosphoprotein intermediate. ATP is bound to the membrane, after which the binding of calcium and the release of ATP occurs. This process occurs on the outside of the membrane surface. The transport of calcium to the inside of the membrane involves a conformational change of a calcium-carrying phosphorylated protein. On the inside of the membrane, calcium is released and the protein is dephosphorylated. Calcium efflux from the sarcoplasmic reticulum probably is mediated by the same carrier protein, with a reversal of the process just discussed.

Calcium can also accumulate in mitochondria in massive amounts. The process of accumulation may be similar to that seen in the sarcoplasmic reticulum (which involves hydrolysis of ATP). Calcium stimulates both respiration and hydrolysis of ATP in mitochondria in a stoichiometric relationship. Thus calcium transport may be driven either by electron transport provided by respiration, or by the hydrolysis of ATP, or by both. Mitochondria have a high affinity for calcium, and calcium uptake takes precedence over oxidative phosphorylation in these organelles. This suggests that calcium plays an essential role in mitochondrial function.

In addition to triggering muscle contraction, increased intracellular calcium ions enhance the conversion of phosphorylase b to phosphorylase a in muscle cells. Indeed, it seems clear that the activation of phosphorylase by cyclic AMP requires the presence of a certain minimal level of free Ca^{++}. Rasmussen has proposed that hormonal activation of cells increases Ca^{++} concentration within the cell both by increased entry of Ca^{++} across the plasma membrane and by a cyclic AMP-mediated shift of calcium from mitochondria to cytosol. Thus, according to his theory, both "second messengers"—Ca^{++} and cyclic AMP—are necessary for cell activation, and simultaneous changes in their intracellular concentration must be closely coordinated to obtain the optimal physiological response. The activation of phosphorylase in cardiac muscle also requires calcium. Apparently, the calcium is required for the conversion of phosphorylase b to phosphorylase a, and not for the activation of phosphorylase b kinase.

Another cellular function that apparently requires calcium is secretion in response to specific stimuli. The best documented example of such a calcium-dependent function is the secretion of catecholamines from the chromaffin cells of the adrenal medulla in response to stimulation by acetylcholine. The granules in chromaffin cells contain an ATP-Mg-dependent catecholamine pump, much like the calcium pump in muscle. Calcium is concentrated within these granules, and it has been suggested that the granules control intracellular calcium concentration in a way similar to that of the sarcoplasmic reticulum of muscle. The influx of calcium has been assumed to occur as a result of increased membrane permeability resulting from depolarization by acetylcholine. This calcium influx in secretory cells may depend upon the intracellular sodium concentration. Adrenal cells perfused with ouabain (which inhibits Na^+-K^+-ATPase) show increased intracellular sodium concentration and an enhanced response to acetylcholine. Decreased intracellular potassium has a similar effect.

The secretion of vasopressin and oxytocin also requires calcium. Indeed, the rate of secretion is directly related to the concentration of calcium in fluids surrounding the cells. The secretion of both catecholamines and neurohypophyseal hormones is stimulated by ouabain. There is now strong evidence that the secretion of ACTH, prolactin, LH, TSH, and insulin all require calcium. Thus the release of hormones and transmitter substances appears to be brought about by the influx of calcium occurring with stimulation of the target cell. The resultant increase in intracellular Ca^{++} (or redistribution of intracellular Ca^{++} via cyclic AMP) provokes hormone release by contraction of tubular elements within the cell, much as muscle myofibrils contract. In turn many of the effects of these hormones on their target cells are dependent upon calcium. An increased concentration of calcium appears to be required for the activation of the phosphorylated proteins or enzymes produced by protein kinase activity (i.e., phosphorylase).

Among their other biological activities, calcium ions are essential for the cohesiveness of cells, for enzyme activation, for blood coagulation, and for fertilization.

The Absorption of Calcium

Calcium is absorbed along the entire length of the small intestine. The total amount of calcium that is absorbed will equal the dietary calcium (about 800 mg per day) plus the calcium in intestinal secretions (about 600 mg per day) minus the calcium lost in the feces (about 600 mg per day). The total calcium absorbed in a day amounts to about 800 mg. Brine and Johnston calculated the fecal endogenous loss of calcium in adults to be about 75 mg per day, and as the calcium intake rose from 400 to 1200 mg per day the absorption percentage fell from 43 to 28 percent. More recently, Parsons et al. found that calcium absorption in adults ingesting about 1000 mg of calcium per day ranged from 15 to 34 percent and did not vary with calcium intake or age of the patient. In general, however, there is an adjustment to low calcium intake. Calcium deprivation increases active transport of the cation, particularly in the duodenum. This effect is not changed by thyroparathyroidectomy, hypophysectomy, or adrenalectomy.

When the gut is unable to absorb calcium normally, an unusually large amount is lost in the feces. Among conditions impairing calcium absorption are (1) alkalinization of the gut contents (2) dietary factors which form insoluble salts or complexes with calcium, (3) administration of Mg^{++} salts (Mg^{++} and Ca^{++} share a common transport system), (4) malabsorption disorders such as diarrhea and steatorrhea, and (5) vitamin D deficiency.

The hormone which enhances calcium absorption in the gut is a metabolite of vitamin D. As with other steroid hormones, this vitamin D metabolite is specifically bound to a receptor protein in target cells (intestinal and bone cells) and accumulates within the nuclei of these cells. Here the hormone either influences genetic transcription directly or acts on the release or transport of nuclear RNA. The vitamin D metabolite induces the formation of proteins in the cytoplasm (calcium-binding protein) or in the brush border (calcium-dependent ATPase) which are concerned with calcium translocation.

Calcium-binding Protein

Using the reversed intestinal loop method, Schachter and Rosen showed that a relatively specific process existed for the absorption of calcium against a concentration gradient. Giving vitamin D to the animal before the intestine was removed greatly increased the calcium transport. Vitamin D had no effect on the system in vitro. Thus a metabolite of vitamin D was implicated. In 1966 Wasserman and his coworkers discovered a calcium-binding protein which is induced by the administration of vitamin D. Four high affinity sites exist for calcium per molecule of the protein. It is found in all segments of the small intestine, in the surface coat of the microvilli. It is also found in the kidney, but is absent from plasma, liver, pancreas, and bone. All available evidence suggests this calcium-binding protein is involved in the transport of calcium across intestinal cells.

Calcium-dependent ATPase

A calcium-dependent ATPase in the brush border of intestinal cells is susceptible to induction by vitamin D. The enzyme appears at the same time that calcium absorption is increased in response to vitamin D and may function in the transfer of calcium from the lumen to the mucosal cell. The enzyme is closely associated with alkaline phosphatase activity. Haussler and coworkers noted an increase in both calcium-dependent ATPase activity and alkaline phosphatase when vitamin D was given to rachitic chicks. From inhibitor studies these investigators have concluded that both of these enzyme activities are properties of the same enzyme molecule.

The metabolism of vitamin D

The naturally occurring form of vitamin D, cholecalciferol, or vitamin D_3, is formed in the skin from its precursor, 7-dehydrocholesterol, by ultraviolet radiation (Figure 12–2). It can also be supplied in the diet. After absorption in the intestinal tract or formation in the skin, vitamin D is metabolized in the liver. The most biologically active of these metabolites, 25-hydroxycholecalciferol (Figure 12–2), has 40 percent more biological activity than does cholecalciferol and for a time was thought to be the active form of vitamin D.

In recent years our understanding of vitamin D has been increased. Independently, Lawson and his colleagues and DuLuca et al. identified a polar metabolite of 25-hydroxycholecalciferol from incubations of kidney homogenates. This metabolite, 1,25-dihydroxycholecalciferol, is formed only in the kidney and is the form of vitamin D with the greatest biological activity (Figure 12–2). The activity of this metabolite in intestinal calcium transport is many times greater than that of cholecalciferol, and it has a potent direct effect on the mobilization of bone calcium. Recent studies suggest that the metabolite 24,25-dihydroxycholecalciferol may be important in regulating intestinal absorption of calcium. When administered to rats on a low calcium diet deficient in vitamin D, there was a pronounced and long-lasting increase in intestinal calcium absorption. This metabolite had no effect on mobilization of calcium from bone. When nephrectomized rats were used, the effect of 24,25-dihydroxycholecalciferol on calcium absorption was completely abolished. A further metabolite formed in the kidney, 1,24,25-trihydroxycholecalciferol has been identified recently and may be a biologically active steroid for calcium absorption.

DeLuca found that if the parathyroid glands are removed from experimental animals, the kidneys form 24,25-dihydroxycholecalciferol—not 1,25-dihydroxycholecalciferol. If PTH is given to these parathyroidectomized animals, 1,25-dihydroxycholecalciferol is formed, and the formation of 24,25-dihydroxycholecalciferol is suppressed. Thus PTH increases the synthesis of an active form of vitamin D, which may explain the observation that in the absence of vitamin D PTH cannot increase calcium absorption in the gut or mobilize calcium from bone. We may, therefore, consider vitamin D a *prohormone*, PTH a *tropic hormone*, and 1,25-dihydroxycholecalciferol (and possibly 1,24,25-trihydroxycholecalciferol) a true *steroid hormone*.

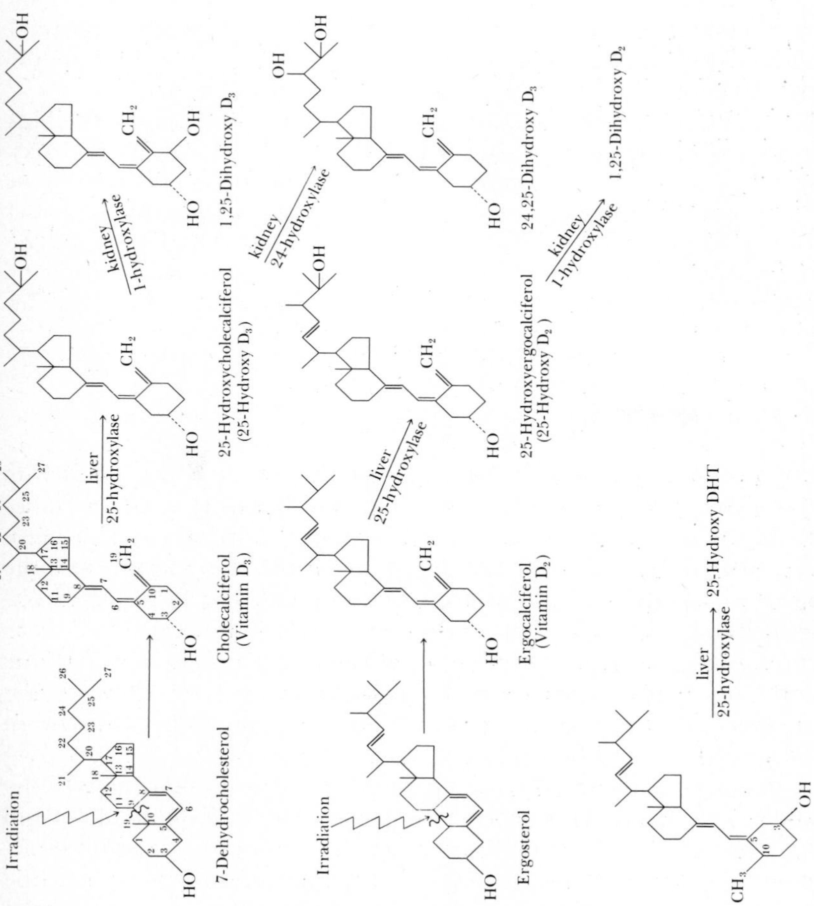

FIGURE 12–2. Formation and metabolism of vitamin D's.

Another form of vitamin D, ergocalciferol (vitamin D_2), can be produced by irradiation of ergosterol (Figure 12–2). Vitamin D_2 is added to many foods and, indeed, so much is present in our diet that much of our circulating and stored vitamin D is likely to be D_2. Vitamin D_2 is converted to biologically active 25-hydroxy and 1,25-dihydroxy metabolites. The hydroxylated forms of D_2 and D_3 enter the circulation, where they are carried by a specific binding protein. Both D_2 and D_3 are subject to other transformations in liver, particularly if the microsomal hydroxylating system has been activated by drugs such as phenobarbital and diphenylhydantoin. Patients receiving these drugs usually have low serum concentrations of 25-hydroxy D_2 and 25-hydroxy D_3.

Certain forms of vitamin D do not require hydroxylation in the kidney to be active. Dihydrotachysterol and the trans isomer of 25-hydroxy D_3 are active in nephrectomized animals. Because the ring is rotated in these compounds, the hydroxyl at C_3 may sterically replace the hydroxyl function that is located at C_1 in other forms of vitamin D (Figure 12–2). The dihydrotachysterols act for the most part on the mobilization of bone mineral and have much less effect on calcium transport across the intestine.

VITAMIN D DEFICIENCY

Mineralization of bone requires adequate concentrations of calcium and phosphate in extracellular fluid. Vitamin D, acting via its metabolites, plays a major role in maintaining plasma calcium concentration within normal range. The absorption of calcium by the intestine and the mobilization of calcium from bone are both regulated by 1,25-dihydroxycholecalciferol. In addition, 1,24,25-trihydroxycholecalciferol may function as an alternate regulator of calcium transport in the intestine. Recently, it has been shown that 25-hydroxy D_3 or 1,25-dihydroxy D_3 will produce increased reabsorption of both calcium and phosphate in the proximal tubules of the kidney.

A deficiency of vitamin D (or unresponsiveness of end organs to the metabolites of vitamin D) results in diminished mineralization of osteoid tissue. When defective mineralization occurs in nongrowing adult bone, the condition is known as *osteomalacia.* During periods of growth, the defect in mineralization also involves the epiphyseal cartilages, and the term *rickets* is applied. In both conditions the total amount of uncalcified osteoid tissue in the skeleton is increased. We may look upon these disorders as disturbances in bone quality rather than bone quantity (osteoporosis, p. 409); however, in time, the quantity of bone is affected also.

Rickets

The disease called rickets, in which bones do not form properly, probably first appeared when our ancestors started wearing clothes and living in houses. By greatly reducing the amount of ultraviolet irradiation of the skin, the conversion of 7-dehydrocholesterol to vitamin D_3 was reduced. As a result, this compound became a "vitamin"—something that was required in the diet. At one time rickets was widely prevalent in Northern Europe and North America. Our understanding of rickets began in 1919 when Sir Edward Mellanby first produced experimental rickets in dogs by feeding them oatmeal in the absence of sunlight. Mellanby was able to prevent this disease by administering cod liver oil, and he incorrectly concluded that this must be due to the newly discovered fat-soluble vitamin A, shown by McCollum to be present in cod liver oil. However, in 1922 McCollum showed that it was not vitamin A, but a different fat-soluble vitamin, which he named D, which was antirachitic. In 1919 Huldshinsky had reported that he could cure rachitic children by exposing them to sunlight. Then it was discovered that the livers of rats irradiated with ultraviolet light would cure rickets when fed to rats deficient in vitamin D. The next step was the discovery by Steenback and his coworkers that irradiation not only of the skins of animals but of their *diet* could prevent or cure rickets. The material activated by ultraviolet light was shown to be a sterol, and this led in the early '30's to the isolation and identification of Vitamin D_2 from plant sterol fractions.

Dietary deficiency as a cause of rickets has been largely eliminated in many countries, particularly in those countries where milk is fortified with vitamin D. The minimum daily requirement for infants and children is 100 to 400 IU of vitamin D daily. Children living in industrialized areas where air pollution is high, particularly in the winter, may not receive enough ultraviolet radiation to form adequate amounts of vitamin D. Various malabsorption syndromes may produce vitamin D deficiency. Anticonvulsant drugs which interfere with the conversion of vitamin D to its active metabolites may also produce a deficient state.

The rachitic infant develops slowly and his growth is retarded. Normal endochondral ossification is disturbed in children with rickets, and the replacement of cartilage by bone does not take place. Hypertrophied cartilage cells accumulate and produce the widening of the epiphyseal cartilage which is so characteristic of this disorder. The muscles are hypotonic, and the child becomes potbellied. Evidence of bone disease is not usually manifest until the vitamin D deficiency has been present for several months. Bone pain and muscle weakness are characteristic symptoms.

The early rachitic lesions of bone involve softness of the skull (craniotabes) and enlargement of the costochondral junctions (the "rachitic rosary"). Later, widening of the epiphyseal cartilages becomes evident, especially at the ends of long bones, such as at the wrists. Ossification centers at wrists, ankles, and the epiphyses of long bones fail to calcify, giving an appearance of greatly retarded bone age. The long, weight-bearing bones become bowed in the young child. The overall aspect of the bones on x-ray film takes on a "ground glass" appearance.

In vitamin D–deficient rickets, hypocalcemia and/or hypophosphatemia are almost invariably present. Secondary hyperparathyroidism is probably responsible for the hypophosphatemia. Normal or slightly depressed serum calcium concentrations may be found in some infants—again, probably due to secondary hyperparathyroidism. This increased PTH secretion may also alter renal tubular transport of amino acids; generalized aminoaciduria is a common finding in vitamin D deficiency. Calcium excretion in the urine is markedly reduced or is absent. As in other bone disorders, the concentration of alkaline phosphatase in serum is usually elevated.

Treatment for vitamin D–deficient rickets involves, principally, the administration of vitamin D. Large doses of vitamin D hasten the healing process, and doses of 1,000 to 10,000 IU are given daily for several months. Hypocalcemia frequently occurs during initial treatment. This may be due to a sudden influx of calcium into bones, or it may result from an abrupt cessation of PTH secretion. Usually, within one to three weeks, the concentrations of phosphate and calcium in the serum rise toward normal, and evidence of healing of bone lesions can be seen on x-ray. Serum alkaline phosphatase values require much longer to return to normal.

HYPOPHOSPHATEMIC RICKETS. Some patients with rickets or osteomalacia are refractory to the usual doses of vitamin D. Patients in this category are usually classified as having refractory or vitamin D–resistant rickets. Another term that has been used is *hypophosphatemic rickets*. This form of rickets, the most commonly encountered among children, probably results from impaired renal conservation of phosphate. Usually the disorder is associated with a familial sex-linked dominant trait. Marked skeletal deformity and stunted growth are evident in affected children, and hypophosphatemia can be persistent and severe. The concentration of calcium in the serum is within the normal range, and tetany therefore does not occur. The proportion of dietary calcium that is absorbed is definitely decreased, which has suggested to some that there is a defect in intestinal absorption. The primary defect does not lie in the bone, for bone from affected patients calcifies normally in normal serum in vitro.

Treatment of hypophosphatemic rickets involves the restoration of phosphate balance. If serum phosphate concentration is sustained by continuous administration of phosphate, healing of bone occurs, as is visible by x-ray in 7 to 10 days. Apparently, phosphate is the limiting factor in the mineralization of bone. Large doses of vitamin D aid mineralization but do not restore bone quality or growth to normal. Neither 25-hydroxycholecalciferol nor 1,25-dihydroxycholecalciferol is capable of correcting the hypophosphatemia, although both agents enhance intestinal calcium absorption. Therefore, there is no evidence that either the synthesis or action of 1,25-dihydroxycholecalciferol is impaired in this disorder. In addition to vitamin D, orally administered phosphate is recommended for the therapeutic regimen of affected patients. It must be remembered that vitamin D can accumulate in the body and produce toxic effects.

Disorders of tubular function such as Fanconi's syndrome and renal tubular acidosis may produce rickets. The former is characterized by phosphaturia, glucosuria, aminoaciduria, and refractory rickets. As the name implies, renal tubular acidosis represents a disorder of tubular base conservation. For some unknown reason phosphate transport is affected also, and hypophosphatemia occurs.

Disorders of vitamin D metabolism may produce a form of rickets *(pseudodeficiency rickets).* The defect in this inherited disorder seems to involve conversion of 25-hydroxycholecalciferol to 1,25-dihydroxycholecalciferol, as suggested by the fact that the administration of minute quantities of the latter compound corrects hypocalcemia and promotes healing of the rickets.

Hypocalcemia

A deficiency of vitamin D can produce a hypocalcemic state with characteristic bone lesions. Aside from vitamin D, several other hormones can influence the concentration of ionized calcium in circulating blood. Among these endocrine causes of hypocalcemia we shall consider hypoparathyroidism, calcitonin-secreting tumors, and glucocorticoid excess. It should be remembered that diminished protein levels in the blood, as for example in the nephrotic syndrome and in hepatic cirrhosis, can cause hypocalcemia; however, symptoms do not arise since the concentration of *ionized calcium* in the plasma remains normal.

If the concentration of Ca^{++} in extracellular fluid is subnormal, the threshold of sensory nerve receptors is lowered, and spontaneous activity may occur. Paresthesias and muscular spasms may result. Eventually, if the hypocalcemia is severe enough, the symptom complex called *tetany* develops. This consists of paresthesias, carpopedal spasm, positive Chvostek sign (unilateral contraction of facial muscles on percussion of the facial nerve anterior to the ear), and positive Trousseau sign (muscle spasm induced by ischemia). Hypocalcemia may be accompanied by seizures; increased intracranial pressure and papilledema are common in chronic hypocalcemia. Emotional disturbances such as irritability, lability, depression, confusion, and hallucinations may be associated with hypocalcemia; often affected patients are suspected of being psychotic. Prolonged hypocalcemia in children may produce mental retardation.

Hypoparathyroidism

The parathyroid glands secrete a protein hormone—PTH—that is composed of 84 amino acids in a single peptide chain. A small amount of proPTH (a larger parent molecule) is also found in parathyroid glands, and the conversion of proPTH to PTH normally takes place within parathyroid cells. In human plasma several distinct immunologic forms of PTH are found. In particular, three species have been identified: PTH (predominant form in parathyroid gland, M.W. 9500), a smaller species (M.W. 7000), and another still smaller form (M.W. 4500). Of the total circulating PTH, only about 50 percent is the 9500 species of PTH. It is still uncertain which of the species is responsible for the biologic activity of PTH. (PTH acts on three tissues: bone, kidney, and intestine.) One view states that only the 9500 species is biologically active; however, there is much evidence that the smaller species may be formed by peripheral conversion from the 9500 species and constitute the active form(s) of the hormone.

The hypercalcemia noted after injection of PTH in animals deprived of food is undoubtedly due to the calcium-mobilizing action of PTH on bone. The feedback regulation of PTH release is rapid; therefore, any rise in serum calcium is opposed by suppression of endogenous PTH output and increased secretion of the hypocalcemic hormone calcitonin. The latter inhibits calcium mobilization from bone.

It is interesting that one of the earliest responses to PTH is a small *uptake* of calcium into bone. The permeability of the membranes of bone cells is increased specifically for calcium. The calcium entering bone cells in response to PTH may then serve as a second messenger. In addition, the effect of PTH on adenyl cyclase of bone may alter the intracellular distribution of calcium via a cyclic AMP-mediated shift of Ca^{++} from mitochondria to cytosol. The net effect in osteoclasts is increased activity of several lysosomal enzymes, including collagenase, hyaluronidase, and acid phosphatase. These enzymes are undoubtedly responsible for the bone resorption in response to PTH.

Parathyroid hormone also has an effect on osteoblasts. The metabolic activity of these cells is depressed by PTH, and as a result bone formation is inhibited (Table 12–3). From the known effects of PTH on bone, one might expect that the hypoparathyroid patient would show increased bone formation and decreased bone resorption. However, hypoparathyroidism is characterized by a decrease in both bone formation and resorption. The overall rate of skeletal remodeling is greatly reduced (Table 12–3). The bones are similar in appearance to those of patients with calcitonin excess caused by medullary carcinoma of the thyroid.

Parathyroid hormone has two separate renal actions: phosphaturia and the enhancement of calcium reabsorption. Phosphaturia is a nonspecific response and can be elicited by more than one mechanism. For example, an increase in the glomerular filtration rate or a decrease in tubular reabsorption of phosphate can cause phosphaturia. Parathyroid hormone produces phosphaturia by inhibiting the reabsorption of phosphate; however, Goldberg and his colleagues argue that this effect is secondary to a primary effect of PTH on sodium reabsorption in the proximal tubules. The sodium rejected by the proximal tubule is reabsorbed distally whereas phosphate is not. The enhancement of calcium

TABLE 12–3. Effects of Hormones on Bone Metabolism

Hormone	Effects	Net Result on Bone and Blood
PTH	Increased number and activity of osteoclasts; decreased number and activity of osteoblasts	↑ serum calcium R > F*
Cortisol	Decreased number and activity of osteoblasts; decreased biosynthesis of collagen; antagonist of vitamin D	R > F ↓ Serum calcium
Thyroid hormone	Increased bone turnover	R > F
Calcitonin	Increased number of osteoblasts (acute); decreased number and activity of osteoclasts	F > R (acute) Decreased skeletal remodeling
GH	Increased biosynthesis of collagen	F > R
Sex steroids	Anti–PTH effect	F > R

*R = resorption of bone; F = formation of bone.

reabsorption by PTH takes place in the distal tubules of the kidney. In hypoparathyroidism the urinary excretion of phosphate is decreased, and the percentage of filtered phosphate which is reabsorbed by the renal tubule is abnormally high. Despite the lack of PTH to enhance calcium reabsorption, urinary excretion of calcium is also decreased in affected patients. It should be recalled that changes in renal calcium excretion are due to changes in the amount of calcium that is filtered or to altered renal tubular reabsorption, or to both. The amount of calcium that is filtered is a function of the GFR and the calcium concentration in the ultrafiltrate. In hypoparathyroidism the concentration of calcium in the plasma (and hence in the ultrafiltrate) is low. As a general rule, calcium disappears from the urine when the concentration in plasma is less than 7.5 mg/100 ml. However, metabolic acidosis can markedly increase calcium excretion in the urine even in hypoparathyroidism.

Apparently PTH also enhances the absorption of calcium in the intestinal tract either by a direct effect or by its effect on the 1-hydroxylase of the kidney. Thus in hypoparathyroidism malabsorption of calcium is noted. It has been observed that hypoparathyroidism is also often accompanied by poor absorption of fat and/or vitamin B_{12}. These abnormalities can be corrected with PTH or vitamin D.

CAUSES. Neonatal hypoparathyroidism may be due to congenital absence of the parathyroid and thymus glands, or secondary to maternal hyperparathyroidism. In any case, the onset of symptoms of tetany should alert the physician to the condition.

Idiopathic and hereditary forms of hypoparathyroidism tend to appear later in life. One familial form of hypoparathyroidism is associated with adrenocortical insufficiency and mucocutaneous monoliasis. Another cause of hypoparathyroidism, which should always be considered, is damage to or removal of the parathyroid glands in the course of surgical thyroidectomy.

In 1942 Albright first described *pseudohypoparathyroidism*, a rare (usually familial) condition that results from resistance to the action of PTH. It occurs more often in girls than in boys and always manifests itself in early childhood. The patients are generally mentally retarded and of small stature. The face is rounded and there is frequently bilateral shortening of one or more metacarpals or metatarsals (Figure 12–3). Soft tissue calcification—in addition to the involvement of the basal ganglia, which is common to all types of hypoparathyroidism—is seen in most cases of pseudohypoparathyroidism. The parathyroid glands are hyperplastic.

The low concentration of plasma calcium and high concentration of plasma phosphate are similar to the values seen in hypoparathyroidism. Tubular reabsorption of phosphate is high. The conditions are differentiated by testing for response to PTH given intravenously (Ellsworth Howard Test) or by measuring the concentration of circulating PTH (which is high in pseudohypoparathyroidism).

Patients with the skeletal features (and other identifying aspects) of pseudohypoparathyroidism who have normal plasma calcium and phosphate concentrations are said to have *pseudopseudohypoparathyroidism.* Since both pseudohypoparathyroidism and pseudopseudohypoparathyroidism occur frequently in the same kindred, it would seem that they represent variants of the same genetic disease. The sex incidence and frequency of both disorders would seem to indicate that they are transmitted by an x-linked dominant, although recently four cases of apparent male-to-male transmission were reported.

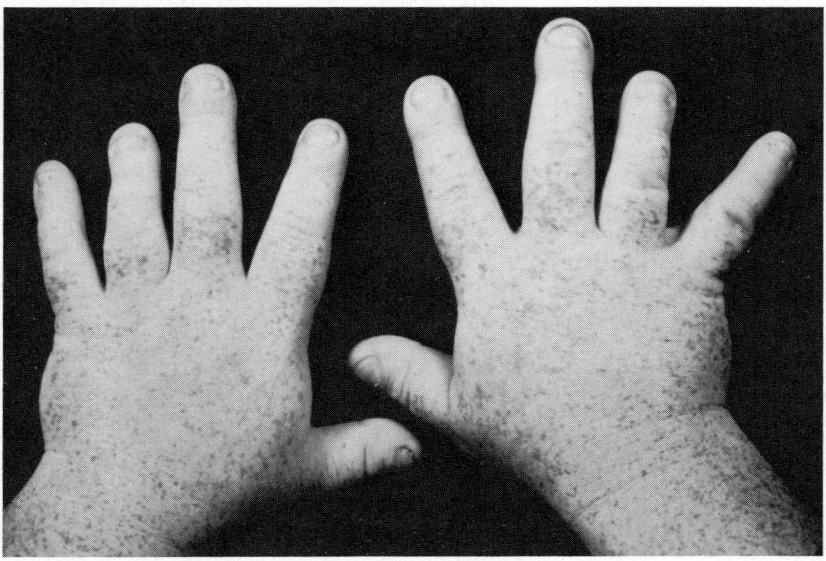

FIGURE 12–3. Hands of a patient with pseudohypoparathyroidism showing the shortened fourth finger (shortened fourth metacarpal). (Courtesy of Dr. Leslie Rose, Peter Bent Brigham Hospital, Boston, Mass.)

In normal subjects administration of PTH causes an increased urinary excretion of cyclic AMP. When PTH is administered to patients with pseudohypoparathyroidism, there is a blunted rise—or no detectable rise at all—in urinary cyclic AMP; however, one patient with pseudopseudohypoparathyroidism showed a normal cyclic AMP response to PTH. Thus pseudopseudohypoparathyroidism may constitute an incomplete form of the disease.

Recently Drezner et al. described an infant with pseudohypoparathyroidism, hypocalcemia, and elevated concentration of PTH in the serum. This child had increased urinary excretion of cyclic AMP and showed a marked rise in urinary cyclic AMP in response to exogenous PTH. Neither the renal tubular handling of phosphate nor the serum calcium concentration responded to PTH, suggesting to the authors a failure in the intracellular reception of the cyclic AMP "message." Obviously, a disease state of "hypoparathyroidism" can result from any interruption along the sequence of PTH secretion, PTH binding to target cell receptor, activation of adenyl cyclase, increased intracellular concentration of cyclic AMP, and mediation of cyclic AMP effects within the cell. As our technology improves and more precise diagnoses can be made, words such as pseudohypoparathyroidism and pseudopseudohypoparathyroidism can be abandoned for more informative terms.

Diagnosis. The manifestations of hypoparathyroidism are largely secondary to the hypocalcemia produced by the disease. Nevertheless, certain symptoms persist even if the hypocalcemia is corrected by high calcium intake and vitamin D. Despite normalized concentrations of calcium and phosphate in the plasma, hypoparathyroid patients have a high incidence of severe mental depression and frequent occurrence of tetany. Perhaps PTH is needed to provide "normal" calcium distribution within the nervous system. Nearly 50 percent of hypoparathyroid patients have cataracts. Moreover, a specific effect of PTH on calcium permeability in the lens capsule has been noted. Teeth which erupt during PTH deficiency remain permanently abnormal.

Hypoparathyroidism must be distinguished from other causes of hypocalcemia and tetany. The presence of psychoneuroses, psychoses, or epilepsy is suggestive of the disorder, and patients with such psychological symptoms should have their serum calcium concentrations measured. Hypoparathyroid patients may manifest marked diarrhea or steatorrhea which may be difficult to differentiate from primary idiopathic steatorrhea.

Treatment. Unfortunately, PTH must be injected in order to be effective, and this fact plus the expense of parenteral PTH preparations has virtually eliminated the hormone as a form of therapy. One can correct the hypocalcemia that accompanies hypoparathyroidism by using vitamin D and calcium; the success of the therapy can be assessed by frequent measurements of serum calcium. At no time should the physician base the therapeutic regimen for his patient on urinary calcium measurements. Calcium supplementation alone may be sufficient to maintain the patient in a normocalcemic state. More often, vitamin D is needed also. The latter can be given in the form of D_2 (25,000 to 200,000 IU daily). It is important to remember that the maximum effect of vitamin D is often not achieved until five to six weeks after the start of therapy. Therefore, it is unwise to increase the dose of vitamin D more often than every six to eight weeks. Dihydrotachysterol may be used in preference to D_2 because of its more rapid onset and shorter duration of action.

Even with great care, vitamin D intoxication is a frequent complication of the treatment of hypoparathyroidism. To make matters worse, vitamin D intoxication can develop suddenly in patients who had been well controlled for years on a given dose of vitamin D. Even slight degrees of hypercalcemia can produce severe and irreversible renal damage.

Calcitonin-secreting Tumors

The only primary endocrinopathy involving hypersecretion of calcitonin is *medullary carcinoma of the thyroid.* The tumor cells contain large amounts of calcitonin, and the concentration of the hormone in the plasma of patients having such tumors is high. This thyroid neoplasm is uncommon, accounting for approximately 6 per cent of all thyroid carcinomas. Surprisingly enough, patients with medullary carcinoma of the thyroid show no overt skeletal abnormalities, and irregularities in plasma calcium are rare. The commonest clinical feature is diarrhea. In addition, patients may have other tumors, such as neuromas, pheochromocytomas, and ACTH-secreting tumors.

Studies of bone specimens from affected patients have yielded interesting results. The extent of bone surface at which either active bone formation or active bone resorption was occurring was found to be drastically reduced. Apparently, chronic excessive circulating calcitonin leads to a profound reduction in the rate of activation of new bone remodeling units. As a consequence, both resorption and formation surfaces are equally reduced (Table 12–3). Thus there is no apparent disorder of bone, but the overall rate of skeletal remodeling is reduced.

How does this fit our concept of calcitonin as a hormone which inhibits bone resorption? Rasmussen emphasizes the need to distinguish between transient and steady-state changes. Certainly calcitonin may lead to transient increased bone formation – *acutely*. But what about the long range effects of calcitonin? When calcitonin is administered to young rabbits, the number of multinucleated osteoclasts is decreased markedly within 15 minutes. The osteoclasts do not die, according to Rasmussen; rather, they undergo fission into mononucleated cells. These *preosteoblasts* can become osteoblasts. In turn, osteoblasts, after they have completed their synthetic function, can become osteocytes. The original osteoclasts are produced by fusion of *preosteoclasts* formed from mesenchymal cells. Thus in a bone remodeling unit, formation is preceded by resorption, and the two aspects of bone metabolism are always coupled. Frost described such a unit of bone surface remodeling as an "active bone metabolic unit." Calcitonin causes an immediate increase in the modulation of osteoclasts to osteoblasts, but it simultaneously blocks the differentiation of mesenchymal cells into preosteoclasts. The average lifetime of a remodeling unit is two to three months, and unless new osteoblasts can be formed, no new remodeling unit can develop. Consequently, enhanced bone formation may be an early effect of calcitonin; however, chronic excess calcitonin greatly reduces the total rate of skeletal remodeling. In contrast to calcitonin, PTH increases the formation of new preosteoclasts and reduces the rate of modulation of osteoclasts to osteoblasts. It is not surprising that the appearance of bone in conditions of excess calcitonin (medullary carcinoma of the thyroid) and deficient PTH (hypoparathyroidism) should be similar, because the two hormones have directly opposite effects on the bone remodeling unit.

The concept of an active bone metabolic unit is an attractive notion; however, it must be remembered that proof of the cellular transformations involved is lacking. In particular, the conversion of osteoclasts to osteoblasts is questioned by many investigators who propose that the daughter cells of the osteoprogenitor cells can proceed directly to either osteoclasts or osteoblasts. Thus only with appropriate reservations should modulation of cell types be accepted as a working model.

In its familial form, medullary carcinoma of the thyroid appears to be transmitted as a Mendelian dominant. Thus although it is a rare disorder, its familial incidence creates important epidemiological considerations among relatives of affected individuals; genetic counseling may be required. The inherited nature of the disorder should make possible an early diagnosis. Most physicians caring for families with a high risk of medullary carcinoma of the thyroid utilize a calcium infusion test annually. A small but progressive rise in basal serum calcitonin secretion and increasing responsiveness to calcium infusion suggest C-cell hyperplasia, an early stage in the disease. The prognosis for patients with medullary carcinoma of the thyroid is fair. Five years after surgical treatment, 48 percent of the patients in Fletcher's series were alive and well; only 16 percent were known to have died of carcinomatosis.

The etiology of the disorder has been attributed to a defect in a single cell system, originating in the neural crest. It has been suggested that the thyroid, parathyroid, ultimobranchial body, and adrenal medulla all share a common stem-cell component derived from the neural crest early in embryonic development. Weichert postulates that the neuroectodermal stem-cells migrate into the primitive gut, forming the enterochromaffin system and contributing to the endocrine glands that are derived from the pharyngeal pouches. The stem-cells also, of course, form the chromaffin system, including the adrenal medulla. These cells have the potential to form non-steroidal hormones. Chromaffin cells have been found in medullary tumors of the thyroid, and these tumors have been known to secrete serotonin. We might therefore speak of a syndrome of medullary carcinoma of the thyroid in which neuroectodermal dysplasias of other tissues may develop concomitantly.

Glucocorticoid Excess

Glucocorticoids have a dramatic effect in lowering serum calcium in situations characterized by vitamin D overdosage and/or hypersensitivity to vitamin D. The mechanism of the glucocorticoid hypocalcemia is still unclear. Cortisol has been shown to inhibit the uptake and incorporation of precursors of both RNA and protein by isolated bone cells in culture. This might explain the osteoporosis that often occurs in conditions of cortisol excess. Cortisol at 10^{-6} M significantly inhibits bone resorption produced by prostaglandin E_1 and dibutyryl cyclic AMP; cortisol less effectively inhibits the resorption produced by PTH or 25-hydroxy D_3. This is puzzling in view of the increased bone resorption evident by x-ray in patients on large doses of glucocorticoids. In general, glucocorticoids tend to produce osteoporosis at any age; but what of the effect of excess glucocorticoids on *lowering* the concentration of calcium in the plasma?

One intriguing theory suggests that cortisol affects the metabolism of vitamin D. In four adult subjects, Avioli and coworkers found that prednisone induced a decrease in the half-life of labeled vitamin D_3 and decreased the accumulation of 25-hydroxy D_3. If less biologically active vitamin D is formed, the intestinal absorption of calcium and the reabsorption of calcium in the kidney could, presumably, be impaired.

There is little doubt that patients on corticosteroid therapy suffer impaired intestinal absorption of calcium. Kimberg found in animal experiments that cortisol affects both steps in calcium transport: uptake at the mucosal surface, and transfer to the serosal medium. Vitamin D_3 or 25-hydroxy D_3 could not reverse the cortisol effects; however, other investigators have been able to reverse the steroid effect with large doses of vitamin D, suggesting that cortisol may compete with intestinal receptors for vitamin D. The most active substance, 1,25-dihydroxy D_3, should be tested in this system. It remains an open question as to whether an effect of cortisol on the liver hydroxylating system could alter the rate of vitamin D metabolism sufficiently to impair calcium absorption and balance.

HYPERCALCEMIA

A variety of conditions may produce a hypercalcemic state. The concentration of calcium in the blood which brings about symptoms of such a state varies greatly from individual to individual. General symptoms of hypercalcemia include easy fatigue, weakness, headaches, and thirst. The latter is secondary to dehydration occasioned by polyuria. The polyuria is a manifestation of impaired renal concentrating ability. The high calcium concentration may interfere with sodium transport across the tubular cell membranes by forming a tight complex with intracellular ATP. This complex is a potent inhibitor of Na-K-ATPase, the enzyme responsible for ATP hydrolysis and for providing energy for sodium transport.

As the concentration of calcium in the blood rises, increasing amounts are found in the kidney ultrafiltrate, and hypercalciuria develops. The site of the maximal concentration of calcium is the renal medulla, where the early lesions of renal calcification develop. The cells become necrotic and calcified and then slough away. The sloughed material obstructs the lumen of the tubule and may lead to hydronephrosis. Hypercalcemia also produces thickening and calcification of the basement membranes of the proximal tubules.

Gastrointestinal symptoms including anorexia, nausea, and vomiting frequently accompany chronic hypercalcemia. There is also a high incidence of psychiatric disturbances in hypercalcemic patients. In mild hypercalcemic states, memory may be impaired. Hypercalcemia diminishes neuromuscular excitability, producing hypotonia and decreased tendon reflexes.

If the serum calcium concentration exceeds 16 mg/100 ml, severe mental disturbances may develop, with psychoses, delirium, stupor, and even coma sometimes occurring. The patient's condition may deteriorate rapidly, marked by intractable vomiting, severe dehydration, and impaired consciousness.

More often than not the cause of the hypercalcemia is nonendocrine. In the older age group, one thinks immediately of metastatic bone disease. In particular, neoplasms of breast and lung tend to form bone metastases. Multiple myeloma, lymphomas, and leukemia may also result in hypercalcemia. These disorders usually involve bone destruction, which has been suggested as the etiology of the hypercalcemia. Some tumors seem to produce a lytic substance which acts on bone in much the same fashion as PTH. Parathyroid hormone itself, or a closely related polypeptide, may be produced by certain tumors.

Patients with sarcoidosis appear to have an increased sensitivity to vitamin D, as do hyperthyroid patients. In both instances hypercalcemia is a frequent development. Overdosage of vitamin D can, of course, produce hypercalcemia. Excessive intake of calcium, found often in patients with peptic ulcer who take large amounts of milk or absorbable alkali, may result in hypercalcemia. The latter has been termed the *milk-alkali syndrome.*

Another important cause of hypercalcemia is immobilization. In bone that is rapidly turning over (as in childhood or in adolescence), the amount of calcium released during resorption induced by immobilization may exceed the kidney's excretory capacity, and hypercalcemia may result. Newborn infants with prolonged anoxia and subcutaneous fat necrosis may also develop severe hypercalcemia.

The endocrine causes of hypercalcemia include hyperparathyroidism, hypervitaminosis D, adrenocortical insufficiency, and hyperthyroidism.

Hyperparathyroidism

The symptoms of this disease may be due to hypercalcemia and hypercalciuria per se, or to the bone changes and calcification of tissue which occur in these disorders. In any case, the clinical picture is so variable and sometimes so bizarre that it is impossible to present a standard description. The gastrointestinal symptoms, dehydration, and mental changes have already been discussed. Muscle hypotonia is extremely variable in hyperparathyroidism and may affect all muscle groups or only the proximal muscles.

Calcium may be deposited in many tissues, but it is most readily seen in the eye. Examination of the eye by slit lamp may show band keratitis. Deposition of calcium may occur in the capsules around joints, in tendons, and in articular cartilage. Calculi in the renal tract may be due to hyperparathyroidism. The calcification in the kidneys may be so extensive that it can be seen as streaks or masses on x-ray film; such a condition, termed nephrocalcinosis, is a bad prognostic sign.

The changes in bone in hyperparathyroidism are characteristic, the hands and skull being most often involved. There is a moth-eaten appearance to the middle phalanges, and a diffuse decalcification (ground-glass appearance) in the bones of the skull may be evident. If hyperparathyroidism persists, bone cysts occur, most typically in the short bones of the hands and feet, in the ribs, and in the bony pelvis. Vertebrae may decalcify and collapse.

The classic form of bone disease in hyperparathyroidism is *osteitis fibrosa cystica*. Subperiosteal resorption is characteristic and particularly evident in the middle phalanges of the hand (Figure 12–4). For practical purposes, such changes are diagnostic of either primary or secondary hyperparathyroidism. Osteitis fibrosa cystica typically causes bone pain and pathologic fractures.

DIAGNOSIS. The most consistent biochemical abnormality in primary hyperparathyroidism is hypercalcemia; however, many patients have only a slight elevation of serum calcium. An occasional normal serum calcium may be found, particularly in those few patients with fluctuating hypercalcemia. The serum alkaline phosphatase is elevated, usually in proportion to the extent of the bone disease.

Hypophosphatemia commonly accompanies the hypercalcemia but may be absent in the presence of acromegaly or renal insufficiency. When these conditions co-exist with hyperparathyroidism, the concentration of serum phosphate may be normal or even elevated. Measurement of this concentration is often a valuable diagnostic point in differentiating hyperparathyroidism from other causes of hypercalcemia. In the absence of renal insufficiency or acromegaly, primary hyperparathyroidism is an unlikely diagnosis if the serum phosphate concentration is above 3.5 mg/100 ml and chloride is below 102 mEq/liter. If renal function is impaired, the serum creatinine concentration will rise.

Another diagnostic test which has been found useful in differentiating the hypercalcemia of hyperparathyroidism from that associ-

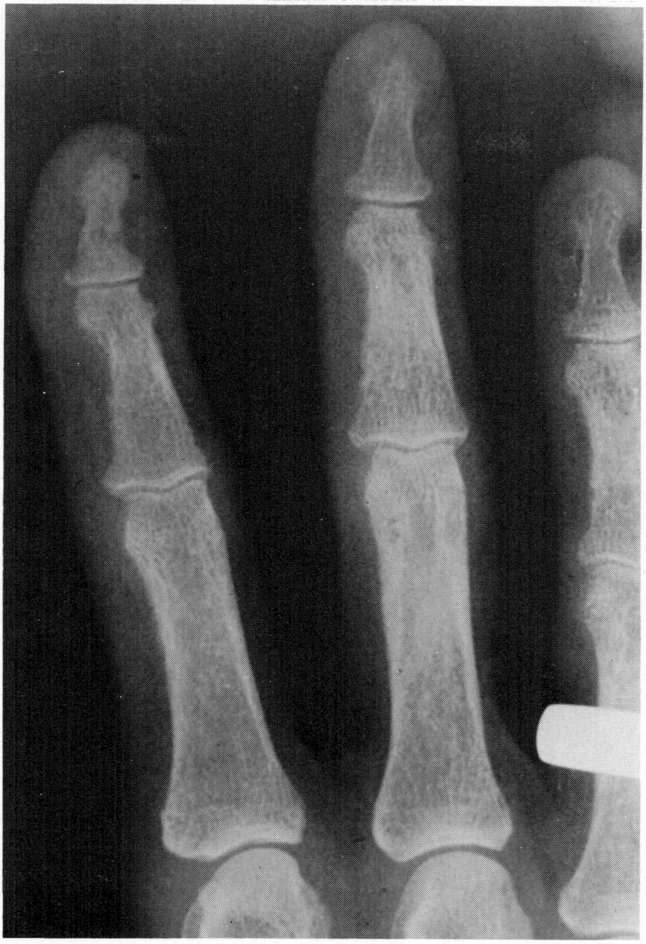

FIGURE 12–4. Portion of a hand film of a patient with hyperparathyroidism. Note the subperiosteal resorption in the phalanges. (Courtesy of Dr. Leslie Rose. Peter Bent Brigham Hospital, Boston, Mass.)

ated with sarcoidosis; multiple myeloma, vitamin D intoxication, and some malignant diseases with osseous metastases involves the administration of glucocorticoids to the patient. Glucocorticoid treatment for ten days or so will often reduce the serum calcium concentration in these latter disorders, whereas the hypercalcemia of hyperparathyroidism tends to be resistant to steroids.

ETIOLOGY. Over 80 percent of reported cases of primary hyperparathyroidism are due to single adenomas of the parathyroid glands. Ten percent of the cases are due to hyperplasia of all four glands. Localization of the tumor(s) can sometimes be achieved by catheterization studies in which the concentration of PTH is measured in the venous effluent and compared to that in the peripheral circulation. Carcinoma of the parathyroid gland is a rare cause of hyperparathyroidism. Hyperparathyroidism may be a feature of multiple endocrine adenomatoses.

These are usually familial and may involve adenomata of the pituitary gland, the pancreatic islets, and the adrenal glands (p. 253). Hyperparathyroidism is also associated with pheochromocytoma and medullary carcinoma of the thyroid.

Primary hyperparathyroidism is approximately twice as common in females as in males and manifests itself most commonly in postmenopausal women. The loss of estrogen, which antagonizes the action of PTH on bone (Table 12–3), may permit symptoms of pre-existing mild hyperparathyroidism to become clinically evident.

Secondary hyperparathyroidism may be due to chronic renal insufficiency or to vitamin D deficiency or resistance. Hypercalcemia is not usually encountered, because the normal feedback control regulates PTH secretion.

Hypervitaminosis D

Prolonged intake of vitamin D will produce symptoms of vitamin D intoxication. Usually, intoxication results when the daily dose has been over 50,000 units. Calcium absorption in the gut is enhanced, and, at such high concentrations, vitamin D may cause the release of calcium and phosphate from bone. If renal damage from hypercalcemia occurs, the concentration of serum inorganic phosphate may rise. Nephrocalcinosis, renal stones, and kidney failure may ensue.

Glucocorticoid Insufficiency

The hypercalcemia of glucocorticoid insufficiency may be due to a prolonged half-life of vitamin D, or to improved calcium absorption in the gut, or to decreased competition of glucocorticoids for binding to the hydroxycholecalciferol receptors in the kidney and gut mucosa.

Hyperthyroidism

The majority of patients with hyperthyroidism have plasma concentrations of calcium and phosphate within the normal range, but the mean plasma calcium concentration of these patients tends to be higher than that found in normal subjects. Plasma inorganic phosphate is also reported to be higher than average in hyperthyroid patients, but, again, most values are within the normal range. Urinary calcium excretion is frequently increased in hyperthyroidism, and the tubular reabsorption of phosphate tends to be raised.

There is no doubt that marked bone changes occur in patients with severe, prolonged hyperthyroidism. Bone turnover is increased, and histologically the bone resembles that seen in hyperparathyroidism. The bone loss is due to an excess of resorption over formation and is attributed to the direct effects of thyroid hormone on bone (Table 12–3). Both the hypercalcemia and increased turnover of bone can be corrected by antithyroid drugs; however, osteoporosis, once developed, tends to persist.

SKELETAL MATURATION AND THE SEX HORMONES

We may define skeletal maturation as that sequence of events which changes the cartilaginous and membranous skeleton of the fetus into fully ossified adult bone. The first phase of this process, the ossification of the diaphyses of the long and short bones, is practically complete in utero (Table 12–1). The second phase, beginning just before birth, involves osteogenesis in the epiphyses of the shafted bones and in the round bones (Table 12–2). This phase is complete by puberty. The third and final phase involves the functional destruction of the growth cartilage plates, followed by the bony fusion of epiphysis and diaphysis. This process starts at puberty and is completed in the appendicular skeleton of the female by about the seventeenth year. In the male the process is completed by about age 19 or 20 (Table 12–2).

A variety of factors determine the rate and pattern of skeletal maturation. Some are sex-specific, some have an autosomal origin, and some are hormonally mediated. The sex differences in skeletal maturation may be due to inherited factors associated with the X chromosome, or to the difference in the predominant sex hormone. There is no doubt that skeletal maturation in the female occurs earlier than in the male. The difference is present even in fetal life, but it is accentuated during the ninth or tenth year.

Clinical and experimental studies of hormonal regulation of skeletal maturation indicate that osteogenesis in skeletal cartilage is initiated and maintained by thyroid hormone until the time of puberty. At that time, apparently, thyroid hormone cannot complete the process of skeletal maturation without the increasing influence of the sex hormones secreted by the gonads.

There is additional evidence that sex hormones are involved in skeletal maturation. The epiphyses of the eunuch remain unfused, and, in fact, growth may continue slowly in many of his cartilage plates through the third and fourth decades of life. The administration of testosterone rapidly induces epiphyseal fusion and cessation of growth. In patients with ovarian dysgenesis the epiphyses may remain unfused into the third or fourth decade. Fusion can be induced by estrogen therapy. Children who exhibit sexual precocity show advanced skeletal maturation; unless the sex hormone production is suppressed, epiphyseal fusion occurs early, and ultimate stature is shortened.

In 1946 Bayley proposed that given the skeletal maturity of a child and his standing height, it should be possible to predict his adult height. Subsequent studies have shown that within reasonable confidence limits such predictions can be made, at least for children over 7 years of age. The proportion of total stature gained per unit increase in skeletal maturity is relatively constant, depending chiefly on the sex and skeletal age of the child. Tables have been compiled that cite the percentage of his mature height that a child should have gained at each skeletal age. These data are then incorporated into tables for converting present height to predicted height on the basis of these percentages.

SUMMARY

Normal growth and maturation of bone requires normal endocrine function. Lack of thyroid hormone in utero impairs skeletal maturation, and the cretin at birth shows a severely retarded bone age. Both thyroid and growth hormones are necessary for linear growth in childhood, and the additional influence of sex hormones is necessary for epiphyseal fusion.

The process of ossification begins in utero with the formation of diaphyseal ossification centers. Epiphyseal growth of bones takes place throughout childhood, and with fusion of diaphysis to epiphysis, growth ceases. The actual ossification process involves calcification of either mesenchymal tissue or cartilage. Optimal amounts of calcium and phosphate in the surrounding fluids are necessary, as is previously formed osteoid. The osteoid of bone, which is primarily collagen, is formed and secreted into extracellular spaces to be subsequently calcified.

The maintenance of calcium homeostasis involves the interaction of at least three hormones: PTH, calcitonin, and 1,25-dihydroxycholecalciferol. A fall in serum calcium stimulates the parathyroid glands to secrete PTH. The actions of this hormone on bone (resorption) and on kidney (absorption of calcium, induction of the synthesis of 1-hydroxylase) serve to restore the serum calcium to normal. The 1-hydroxylase of kidney catalyzes the conversion of 25-hydroxycholecalciferol to 1,25-dihydroxycholecalciferol, the active form of vitamin D. This "new" hormone enhances calcium reabsorption and facilitates the action of PTH on bone. If the concentration of calcium in serum exceeds normal values, PTH secretion is suppressed (through feedback inhibition) and calcitonin secretion is stimulated. Calcitonin acts to reverse the actions of PTH on bone. Calcium is deposited in bone, lowering the serum concentration of this cation.

Vitamin D deficiency and disorders of PTH secretion and calcitonin secretion produce characteristic alterations of bone metabolism. In addition, renal and/or gastrointestinal alterations may be prominent. Aside from effects on these known target tissues, the role of calcium as a "second messenger" in many cells suggests that other systems may be involved as well. Particularly intriguing is the possibility that disturbances of mental function associated with hypercalcemia or hypocalcemia indicate direct effects of PTH or calcium in neural functions.

The concentration of phosphate in serum is largely dependent upon renal function and the effects of PTH on decreasing the renal reabsorption of phosphate. Thus PTH tends to increase serum calcium and decrease serum phosphate. The reciprocal relationship of calcium and phosphate is maintained under normal circumstances. Serum inorganic phosphate itself may play some role in regulating the synthesis of 1,25-dihydroxycholecalciferol. At serum inorganic phosphate values below 8 mg/100 ml, the kidney makes 1,25-dihydroxycholecalciferol; at values above that, 24,25-dihydroxycholecalciferol, an inactive metabolite of vitamin D, is made. Thus the ability of PTH to decrease renal reabsorption of phosphate helps lower the serum value and stimulate 1,25-dihydroxycholecalciferol synthesis.

The close control of serum calcium concentration is another example of homeostatic mechanisms regulating a vital element. With the addition of 1,25-dihydroxycholecalciferol to the list of hormones, we must add another tissue—kidney—to the ranks of the endocrine glands.

SUGGESTED READINGS

The Physiological and Cellular Basis of Metabolic Bone Disease. H. Rasmussen and P. Bordier, Williams and Wilkins, Baltimore, 1973. See the remarks on the next reading, by the same authors.

The cellular basis of metabolic bone disease. H. Rasmussen and P. Bordier, New England Journal of Medicine, *289*:25, 1973.
A beautiful description of the bone remodeling unit and its hormonal control. Specific disorders of bone metabolism, such as primary hyperparathyroidism. hypoparathyroidism, and postmenopausal osteoporosis are discussed in terms of bone remodeling. This review of a difficult subject will be very helpful to the student of endocrinology.

The kidney as an endocrine organ: production of 1,25-dihydroxyvitamin D_3. Hector F. DeLuca, New England Journal of Medicine, *289*:359, 1973.
The author brings this rapidly changing area of investigation up to date. The metabolism of vitamin D and the roles of liver and kidney in calcium homeostasis are considered. The regulation of 1-hydroxylase in the kidney is also discussed.

Calcium Metabolism and Bone Disease, edited by Iain MacIntyre, Clinics in Endocrinology and Metabolism, *1*:1, W. B. Saunders Company, March, 1972.
In chapters by Rasmussen, Copp, and Parsons and Potts, this volume proceeds from the basic biology and chemistry of calcium homeostasis to discussions of clinical disorders of calcium regulation. An excellent opportunity to learn in depth from experts in the field.

Hard Tissue Growth, Repair, and Remineralization, Ciba Foundation Symposium II (new series), 1973.
This volume, based on the proceedings of a symposium on hard tissue growth, repair, and remineralization held in London in 1972, is definitely for the more advanced student. Among the topics covered are osteogenic precursor cells, calcium-accumulating vesicles in bone, the biochemistry of collagen from mineralized tissues, bone remodeling, and vitamin D.

Metabolic Bone and Stone Disease, B. E. C. Nordin, Williams and Wilkins, Baltimore, 1973.
The author discusses the various disorders of bone and calcium metabolism. The various osteoporoses and osteomalacias are discussed, as are hypercalcemia and hypocalcemia. The final chapter deals with medullary carcinoma of the thyroid.

Parathyroid Hormone, Calcitonin, Vitamin D, Bone and Bone Mineral Metabolism, J. T. Potts, Jr. and L. J. Deftos in *Duncan's Diseases of Metabolism,* seventh edition, P. K. Bondy and L. E. Rosenberg, W. B. Saunders Company, Philadelphia, 1974.
An encyclopedic approach to bone metabolism and calcium homeostasis is offered in this work. Detailed discussions of skeletal homeostasis, mineralization, bone turnover, vitamin D metabolism, and the mechanisms of action of PTH, calcitonin and vitamin D are presented. Disorders of parathyroid function and metabolic bone disease are covered, and ample references are included on all materials. An up-to-date and inclusive work.

CHAPTER THIRTEEN

Maturation: Sexual

The period between childhood and maturity, frequently referred to as *adolescence,* is defined as beginning with the gradual appearance of secondary sex characteristics and ending when somatic growth ceases. In girls this generally spans the period between ages 10 and 18 and in boys between 12 and 20 years. Both physical and psychological changes occur during this time. One facet of adolescence, the growth and maturation of bone, was discussed in Chapter Twelve. Many other somatic changes occur during adolescence, and the gonads complete their maturation. The acquisition of the capacity to procreate characterizes the onset of *puberty.*

The long interval between weaning and puberty and the growth spurt that accompanies adolescence are characteristic of primates. It has been suggested that the high degree of social interaction associated with mating in humans may require that psychosocial maturation occur prior to sexual maturation.

NEURAL CONTROL OF SEXUAL MATURATION

The involvement of several areas of the central nervous system in the regulation of reproductive function appears almost certain. There seems little doubt that the hypothalamus plays a dominant role in the onset of puberty, and the limbic system has been implicated in the regulation of sexual function in certain species. Higher brain centers undoubtedly play an important role in the behaviorial aspects of sexual function.

Hypothalamus

One of the current and widely held theories of sexual maturation associates the onset of puberty with age-related changes in the sensitivity of the hypothalamus to sex hormones. The theory states that during the prepubertal period, the hypothalamus is very sensitive to the normal, relatively low concentrations of circulating sex hormones. By negative feedback control, these low levels of sex hormones inhibit gonadotropin release. A subsequent decrease in the sensitivity of the hypothalamus to the negative feedback control is the presumed trigger for the increased release of gonadotropins and the onset of puberty. Thus, during childhood, the pituitary secretes a small amount of gonadotropin, chiefly FSH, and the gonad responds by releasing small amounts of estrogen or androgen. The hypothalamic "set-point" is so low that the low concentration of sex hormones is sufficient to maintain the secretion of gonadotropin below the level required to stimulate gonadal maturation.

The pattern of gonadotropin release in the female is cyclic, whereas the release of gonadotropins in the normal male is non-cyclic. In the rat, these patterns of gonadotropin release are determined in early postnatal life. The hypothalami of both male and female rats will develop a female (cyclic) pattern of gonadotropin release unless exposed to androgens early in postnatal life. Similar results have been obtained in studies using mice, hamsters, and guinea pigs. In contrast, sexual differentiation of the central nervous system mechanism that mediates gonadotropin secretion in primates has not been confirmed. Indeed, there is some evidence that the female pattern is not eliminated by exposure to androgens in early life. Females with congenital adrenocortical hyperplasia, exposed to large amounts of androgen in utero, subsequently develop normal ovulatory cycles if treated adequately with cortisol. Both men and male monkeys respond to an acute rise in serum estradiol concentration with a surge of LH, indicating that the female pattern remains intact in the male primate. The low concentrations of estrogen and the high concentrations of androgen in the normal adult male produce the male non-cyclic pattern of gonadotropin release.

The cycling center of the human female must "awaken" before ovulatory cycles can begin. We must postulate some system whereby a surge of LH release by the pituitary can bring about ovulation. Such a surge of LH is probably brought about by a positive feedback control of LH secretion via an effect of estrogens on the hypothalamus and perhaps on other parts of the brain, such as the limbic system.

Limbic system

A series of structures including the subcallosal, cingulate, and hippocampal gyri, the hippocampal and septal nuclei, and the amygdala forms a border (limbus) around the brainstem. Formerly called the rhinencephalon ("nose brain"), this limbic system is now known to have important functions other than olfaction, including the regulation of sexual function. The experimental work, largely performed in the rat, has involved the placing of specific brain lesions, followed by observations of the effects of the lesions on sexual behavior and other functions.

Timiras and his colleagues found that electrical stimulation of the amygdala and hippocampus leads to ovulation in several species. They found that in the rat the seizure threshold (the minimum stimulus necessary to elicit a seizure response) was high at birth in both the amygdala and the hippocampus and decreased as the animal developed, reaching a nadir at about 20 days of age. At this age these areas of the rat brain are electrophysiologically, biochemically, and morphologically mature. In the amygdala a transient but pronounced fall in threshold occurs two to three days before vaginal opening and first ovulation. Thus a significant change in the excitability of the amygdala seems to be coincident with the onset of sexual function. Similar but smaller changes occur in the hippocampus.

Experimental results that have been achieved after neonatal ovariectomy and hormonal treatment are consistent with the hypothesis that estrogen regulates the cyclic activity of the amygdala and the hippocampus in certain species. The amygdala sends fiber tracts to the septum and to the preoptic and anterior hypothalamic regions. It is well documented that the amygdala is sensitive to the concentration of circulating estrogens, and many investigators believe it is a site of positive feedback action of estrogen. Thus a rising level of estrogen secreted by the graaffian follicle stimulated by FSH could stimulate the amygdala. In some way this stimulation would prevent or circumvent the negative feedback control, with the result that the hypothalamus releases GRH and the pituitary in turn produces the LH surge.

Knobil has devised a surgical technique of isolating ventromedial and arcuate nuclei from the rest of the hypothalamus in the rhesus monkey. His experiments show that these two hypothalamic nuclei and the pituitary stalk and gland are all that is necessary for the production of an LH surge after a single large dose of estrogen. Thus in the rhesus monkey the anterior hypothalamus and the limbic system are not obligatory components of the positive feedback system. Individual species variation is great; therefore the regulation of sexual function in the human cannot be extrapolated from experimental results that are obtained with rodents or even with subhuman primates.

The details of the neural controls of ovulation are far from clear; however, all present evidence is compatible with a positive feedback circuit capable of inducing LH release (Figure 13–1). At the same time, it is known that prolonged treatment with either estrogen or progesterone can block ovulation; apparently it is the sharp rise in estrogens in midcycle which affects the positive feedback center. This is supported by the observation that a single injection of estrogen can induce ovulation in

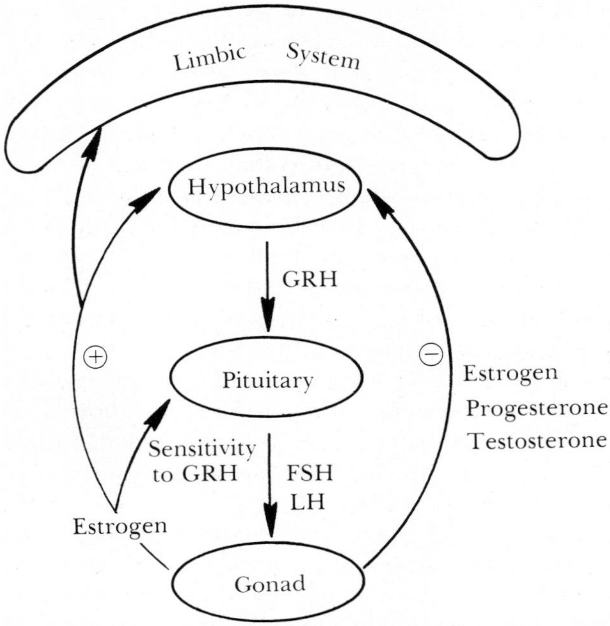

FIGURE 13–1. Regulation of gonadotropin release by steroid hormones. The plus sign denotes positive feedback and the minus sign negative feedback control.

ovaries previously primed with suitable doses of FSH and LH. It is concluded, therefore, that it is the rapid rise in circulating estrogen which accounts for the LH surge in the human menstrual cycle.

Although in some lower animals reproductive function is intact even in the absence of the cerebrum, in the higher animals, and in particular in primates, a mature neocortex is required for normal sexual function. In the course of evolution sexual activity has become increasingly dependent on neural function, as can be seen in the number and diversity of stimuli needed to elicit sexual activity and in the forms in which sexual behavior may be expressed.

Most of the structures thought to have a role in the regulation of sexual activity have other important functions as well. The anterior hypothalamus, involved in the cyclic release of pituitary gonadotropins, also governs some aspects of thyroid control, temperature regulation, and mating behavior. Neurons in the lateral hypothalamus respond to a variety of stimuli, including pain, cold, and uterine contraction. The amygdala is involved in integrative activity with the rest of the nervous system, in fear-rage responses, in feeding behavior, and in autonomic activity. Factors which affect any one of these functions may also alter reproductive function indirectly.

The pineal gland produces melatonin, which appears to inhibit gonadotropin secretion. The administration of pineal extracts or of melatonin has been shown to delay sexual maturation in several nonprimate species. In immature animals constant exposure to light seems to accelerate the onset of puberty by inhibiting the synthesis of melatonin.

Clearly, the complexities of the neural control of reproduction are great, and results from experimental studies using rats are not necessarily applicable to the human. In particular, studies of the sexual dimorphism of the rat hypothalamus, which indicate male and female behaviorial patterns as well as cyclic vs. non-cyclic release of hormones, cannot be applied directly to primates. Primates are sexually receptive throughout the menstrual cycle; they therefore do not have an estrous stage as found in the non-primate. Nevertheless, a number of behavioral as well as functional changes are associated with estrus in nonprimates and with ovulation in primates. The nonprimate female in estrus becomes passive in the presence of the male, and with mounting she depresses her abdomen and rotates her pelvis upward in a lordosis. During estrus female animals increase their physical activity. There is some indication that women walk more at ovulation. At ovulation, the vaginal mucus becomes more fluid and forms fernlike patterns on drying; it is also more acid. Just after ovulation, progesterone secretion from the corpus luteum begins. This steroid has mild thermogenic properties, and a sustained postovulatory rise of basal body temperature (0.4°F or more) indicates a functioning corpus luteum.

In summary, the hypothalamus regulates the release of gonadotropins from the anterior pituitary by means of gonadotropin releasing hormone. The basic pattern of release of GRH is probably cyclic and in most species is regulated by neurons in the anterior hypothalamus and preoptic areas. At some point in development in rodents these areas of the hypothalamus are sensitive to androgens, and if exposed to hormone at this time they change their pattern of GRH release. There is as yet no evidence that this occurs in the human, however. In a sense, the nervous system of the female (or non-androgenized male) is neutral, with an inherent rhythmicity. Testosterone alters the nervous system in some subtle way, whereupon a non-cyclic pattern of GRH release is displayed. In addition, although far from certain in the human, exposure of the nervous system to androgens in prenatal life may subsequently alter the behavioral pattern.

The ventromedial and arcuate nuclei are tonic regulators of gonadotropin secretion. The cyclic discharge of GRH from the anterior hypothalamus and preoptic area is probably brought about by a positive feedback system. In some species the limbic system and the anterior hypothalamus are involved in this positive feedback system.

GONADOTROPINS AND GONADAL MATURATION

The gonadotropin-secreting cells of the anterior pituitary respond to GRH by increasing the synthesis and secretion of FSH and LH. Labrie and his coworkers treated cells of the anterior pituitary cultured in monolayers with synthetic GRH and showed that the synthesis of FSH and LH was markedly stimulated within 24 hours. Exposure to the neurohormone for six days led to a fourfold increase in the total content (cells plus medium) of LH and a threefold increase in the total content of FSH. These same investigators showed that exposure of anterior pituitary cells to GRH stimulated the intracellular accumulation of cyclic AMP. The rates of release of FSH and LH corresponded closely to the observed changes in the intracellular concentration of cyclic AMP. Apparently the changes in concentration of cyclic AMP were secondary to stimulation of adenyl cyclase. Indeed, administration of monobutyryl cyclic AMP to cells in culture brought about increased gonadotropin synthesis. Either cyclic AMP in a cell-free system or dibutyryl cyclic AMP with intact cells could stimulate phosphorylation of proteins associated with the ribosome complex, suggesting that cyclic AMP may act at the translational level to enhance protein synthesis in cells of the anterior pituitary.

Estrogens apparently can modulate the responsiveness of gonadotropin-secreting cells to GRH. In particular, the release of LH in response to GRH is enhanced (Figure 13–1). This may explain why anterior pituitary cells, which presumably contain both LH and FSH, release a greater amount of LH than of FSH in response to GRH. There seems no doubt that a negative feedback system also plays a role in gonadotropin release. The release of both FSH and LH is increased during the menopause or after castration. Although large amounts of progesterone or androgens can diminish gonadotropin release, the primary negative feedback effect is exerted by estrogens. This negative feedback effect of estrogens is rapid and evident within hours.

The studies of Kaplan, Grumbach, and Shepard have shown that gonadotropins are synthesized and secreted by human fetal pituitaries. As early as the end of the first trimester, immunoreactive FSH and LH are detectable in fetal pituitaries and sera. The amounts of these gonadotropins in the fetus are rather large and are generally higher in females than in males of comparable gestational ages. A decrease in the concentration of gonadotropins in the blood is noted at birth. For example, the content of fetal pituitary LH rises steadily from 0.06 μg (per pituitary) at 90 days' gestation to a mean peak of 1.5 μg at 200 days; at term the value falls to 0.9 μg. The peak of FSH in fetal pituitaries at 200 days was 5.9 μg for females and 0.5 μg for males. There is evidence that when LH and FSH reach their maximum content in fetal pituitaries, the number of Leydig cells in the testis of the male fetus increases, and active formation of primordial follicles in the ovary of the female fetus takes place.

Grumbach has proposed that early in gestation gonadotropin release in the fetus is unrestrained, and that maturation of the negative feedback mechanism occurs gradually during the last trimester. Intrauterine fetal androgens may enhance the maturation of the negative feedback system, as suggested by the fact that males in both the fetal *and* infant stages of life show lower gonadotropin values than do females at these stages. The higher incidence of cryptorchidism and gonadal hypoplasia in anencephalic and apituitary infants suggests that fetal gonadotropins may play a role in the development of the fetal gonads.

If a negative feedback system develops between hypothalamus, pituitary, and gonad during fetal life, it should be demonstrable in children. Researchers with this in mind have studied patients with gonadal dysgenesis. Penny and coworkers noted abnormally high concentrations of FSH in sera from 5- to 10-year-old patients with this condition; their mean serum LH concentration was significantly higher than control values. Grumbach and Kaplan observed significantly elevated plasma FSH concentrations in patients with XO gonadal dysgenesis as early as two months after birth.

Prepubertal children respond to exogenous estrogen by a decrease in urinary gonadotropins. Gonadectomy in children (4 months to 9.8 years of age) results in increased gonadotropin excretion. Thus the negative feedback system seems to be working in the prepubertal child. A progressive increase in mean FSH and LH concentrations in serum occurs in relation to age and stage of sexual development. There is a greater correlation between gonadotropin concentrations and stages of sexual development than between gonadotropin concentrations and chronological age.

The mean chronological ages at which the serum concentrations of FSH and LH begin to rise in girls are 9.8 and 10.9 years, respectively; the corresponding ages in boys are 11.5 and 12.0. Thus the rise toward adult levels of both hormones begins one to two years earlier in girls. Appreciable, although variable, sexual maturation was noted by all investigators to have occurred by the time that the plasma concentrations of FSH and LH had begun to increase. There seems no doubt that in females, at least, gonadotropin secretion exhibits intermittency, if not periodicity, long before the menarche.

The intermittency of gonadotropin release is even more striking if measurements are made over a 24 hour period. There is an impressive increase in LH secretion that is synchronous with sleep in normal prepubertal children. Most children in early puberty have significantly higher mean FSH concentrations during sleep, but the findings are not as dramatic as those for LH.

Mechanism of Action of Gonadotropins on Gonads

Gonadotropins regulate three functions of gonads: (1) the growth and maintenance of the tissue structure, (2) the formation of spermatozoa and ova, and (3) the biosynthesis of steroid hormones.

Ovary

During fetal life primordial germ cells multiply in number, forming several million oogonia. Some of these oogonia undergo meiosis and become oocytes. When in attenuated prophase of the first meiotic division, these primary oocytes are surrounded by a single layer of flattened granulosa cells; this represents the most immature stage of follicular development and is referred to as the *primordial follicle*. The flattened granulosa cells become cuboidal and begin to divide, forming the *primary follicle*. The division of granulosa cells forms a concentric ring several layers thick; this is the zona granulosa, and its secretion—the zona pellucida—separates the oocyte from the granulosa cells. Adjacent stromal cells become specialized, envelop the granulosa, and form the *theca*.

Examination of ovaries obtained from fetuses late in gestation reveals many primary follicles, some of which have become filled with fluid (graafian follicles). Follicles of both types undergo atresia. From birth to puberty the ovary continues to undergo follicular development and atresia. Ovarian weight increases progressively with age, primarily as a result of increase in ovarian stroma. As the ovary matures, this stroma invades the cortical region of the gland, separating individual follicles.

Follicle growth can proceed to a certain extent in the absence of pituitary hormones, but FSH is required for normal follicular develop-

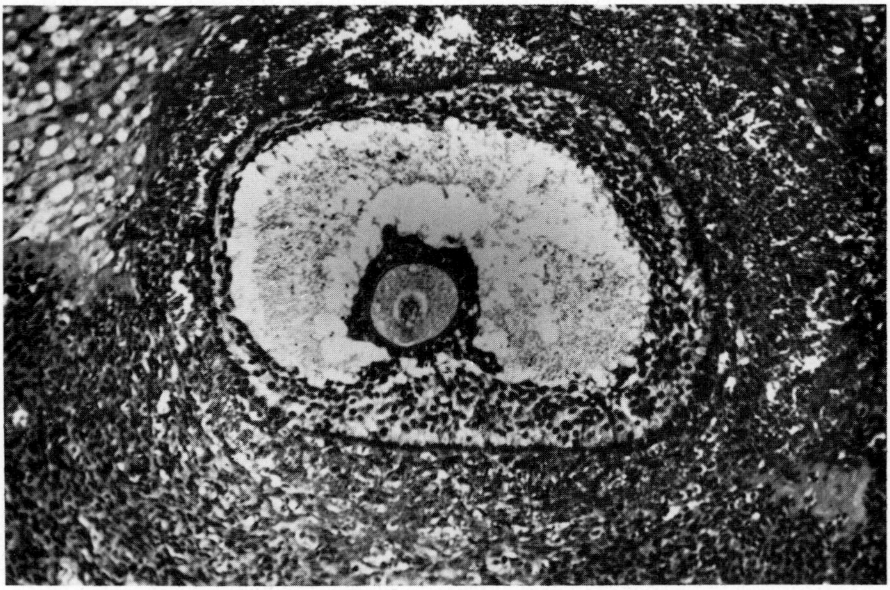

FIGURE 13–2. Mature follicle showing granulosa cells and follicular fluid. (Courtesy of Dr. Shirley Driscoll, Boston Hospital for Women, Boston, Mass.).

ment. FSH stimulates the proliferation of granulosa cells and the accumulation of follicular fluid (Figure 13–2). In addition to promoting follicular growth, FSH in some way prepares the follicle for the action of LH and enhances the release of estrogen induced by LH. The action of FSH in the growth and maturation of the follicle involves stimulation of mitotic activity and consequent growth of three different cell types: (1) connective tissue cells that form the outer layers of follicles, (2) theca cells in the middle layer, and (3) granulosa cells in the innermost layer. There is no good evidence that FSH per se stimulates steroid production in the ovary.

Testis

The development of Leydig cells in the fetal testis is well documented. Sometime shortly after birth they disappear; however, Forest has found that in males, after the first week or two of life, there is a sharp increase in the concentration of testosterone in plasma. Maximal values (265 ± 31 ng/100 ml) were reached by the second month of life, then decreased to reach prepubertal values (7 ± 4 ng/100 ml) by the seventh month. These findings suggest postnatal testicular activity despite a decline in the number of Leydig cells. It is interesting that Faiman and his colleagues found that serum LH values in male children reached adolescent levels at one month of age and declined thereafter to the normal childhood range by four months. They found a similar pattern in females but with much lower values. A postnatal rise in the concentration of FSH in plasma was also noted, the values for females being greater than the values for males. Faiman et al. suggest that the postnatal rise in gonadotropins represents a response to removal of the negative feedback effects of placental hormones. Presumably, the postnatal rise in testosterone in the male is in response to increased LH secretion.

Some growth of the testis occurs between age six and puberty. The seminiferous tubules develop lumens and the spermatocytes proliferate, but there is little or no change in the interstitial cells during this period. At puberty, with increased exposure to FSH, the seminiferous tubules initiate and maintain spermatogenesis. It has been proposed that the Sertoli cells are the principal target of FSH action. Sertoli cells, fixed to the basement membrane of the seminiferous epithelium, are supporting cells, surrounding the differentiating germ cells and probably participating in their nutrition.

Protein synthesis in the seminiferous tubules is stimulated by FSH, an effect attributed to the Sertoli cells because there is apparently no specific binding of FSH by germ cells. Although the testis binds FSH specifically, it is still far from certain what cells within the testis may be stimulated by this gonadotropin. Mancini has demonstrated the localization of fluorescein-labeled FSH in Sertoli cells, whereas LH was localized to the interstitial cells.

Recent work has shown that Sertoli cells, in response to FSH, produce an androgen-binding protein which is secreted into the testicular fluid and concentrated in the caput epididymis. This protein has high affinities for dihydrotestosterone and for testosterone. It has been suggested that this androgen-binding protein could facilitate transfer of androgens into the germinal epithelium, where they could stimulate meiotic division of primary spermatocytes to form spermatids. Luteinizing hormone apparently has no effect on the formation of androgen-binding protein.

Castration of the adult male leads to an elevation in the concentration of circulating gonadotropins within about 72 hours. The administration of androgens to normal males results in a marked decrease in plasma LH but no suppression of plasma FSH. Data such as these have led to the suggestion that FSH secretion in males may be controlled by a non-androgen factor. This speculation is supported by the fact that testicular irradiation, which destroys the germinal epithelium but not the interstitial cells, results in elevation of plasma FSH, while values for LH remain normal. This leads to the inference that some product of the seminiferous tubules controls FSH release. It has been proposed that mature spermatozoa alter the secretory function of Sertoli cells, resulting in the release of estrogen into the circulation which in turn inhibits FSH; however, as yet no direct correlation has been shown between sperm count or germinal cell population and concentration of FSH in the plasma. Some researchers have proposed that the germinal epithelium secretes an inhibitor of FSH or that Sertoli cells secrete an estrogen that controls FSH secretion.

Research by Naftolin has shown that small amounts of testosterone can be converted to estradiol by rat hypothalamus in vitro. Thus even the testosterone-mediated fall in plasma LH concentration may be due to estrogen formed in the hypothalamus from circulating androgen. Certainly at pharmacologic levels either androgens or estrogens can inhibit the secretion of both FSH and LH, but the physiological control of gonadotropin secretion in the male still remains somewhat unclear.

Steroidogenesis

LH can stimulate steroidogenesis in both ovary and testis. Before discussing the mechanism of this effect, let us review the biochemical steps. LH depletes ovarian cholesterol and stimulates estrogen formation, but not in the presence of aminoglutethimide, an inhibitor of the conversion of cholesterol to pregnenolone. In this connection, studies of the testis have indicated an effect of LH on the conversion of cholesterol to pregnenolone.

The rate-limiting step in the conversion of cholesterol to steroid hormones involves oxidative attack (hydroxylation) at C20 and C22, with a subsequent side-chain cleavage catalyzed by desmolase to form pregnenolone. In common with other hydroxylases, this reaction requires NADPH and molecular oxygen. The enzyme system is located in the mitochondria, as are 11β-hydroxylase and 18-hydroxylase. All these hydroxylation reactions are dependent on cytochrome P_{450} (p. 159). Apparently there are at least two forms of cytochrome P_{450} in the adrenal cortex, one involved in 11β-hydroxylation, the other in cholesterol cleavage.

Treatment of immature male rats with LH increased the cholesterol side-chain cleavage by the mitochondrial enzyme system prepared from the testes. The rate of cholesterol cleavage declined markedly after hypophysectomy. Thus the cholesterol side-chain cleavage reaction is markedly dependent upon LH. Similar results have been obtained using ovarian tissue. Comparable effects on cholesterol side chain cleavage in adrenal tissue are found by treating with ACTH.

Present evidence suggests that the effects of tropic hormones on cholesterol cleavage in target tissues are mediated by cyclic AMP. Marsh and Savard have studied the relationships between cyclic AMP and steroidogenesis in bovine corpus luteum. Luteinizing hormone increased cyclic AMP concentration in luteal cells before progesterone synthesis was increased. The increase in cyclic AMP was shown to be due to activation of the adenyl cyclase system. Hall and Koritz showed that LH and exogenous cyclic AMP were acting on the cholesterol cleavage reaction. Comparable studies with ACTH and the adrenal gland have yielded similar results. In short, the mechanisms of action of LH on corpus luteum and of ACTH on the adrenal cortex are virtually identical, with the exception that the final steroid products are different because different steroid-metabolizing enzymes are present in each tissue. Apparently LH affects steroidogenesis in interstitial cells in a similar manner.

Dorfman has suggested that the mechanism whereby cyclic AMP enhances cholesterol cleavage may be similar to the mechanism originally proposed by Haynes and Berthet for ACTH. Cyclic AMP increases glycogen phosphorylase activity, which in turn increases the conversion of glycogen to glucose-6-phosphate. Adrenals and gonads have very active pentose pathways which can utilize glucose-6-phosphate to generate NADPH. The latter is an important cofactor in the rate-limiting step (cholesterol cleavage) for steroidogenesis. Such a mechanism presupposes that: (1) NADPH is rate-limiting for the cholesterol side-chain cleavage reaction and (2) sufficient glycogen is present in the tissues to provide the necessary amounts of glucose-6-phosphate to generate NADPH. It is quite possible that other effects of cyclic AMP may be involved in the mechanism of action of LH. There is evidence that certain effects of ACTH on protein synthesis in the adrenal cortex may be independent of cyclic AMP.

Progesterone

The conversion of pregnenolone to progesterone, catalyzed by a $\Delta 5$-3β-hydroxysteroid dehydrogenase, can occur in any of the cells that secrete steroid hormones. Many of these cells can metabolize progesterone further: it is converted to corticosteroids by adrenal cells, to testosterone by Leydig cells, and to estrogens by theca cells. The granulosa cells of the human ovary, however, secrete primarily progesterone. Apparently LH stimulates this secretion of progesterone by granulosa cells. Whether in vitro or in vivo, granulosa cells can undergo a process of luteinization under the influence of LH. In the usual reproductive cycle, luteinization follows ovulation (brought on by LH). The cells of the granulosa layer enlarge, accumulate lipid, and become plump, pale-staining polygonal (lutein) cells. The follicle becomes filled with cells and is called a corpus luteum. The same phenomenon can be observed in vitro. Granulosa cells from follicles of various species have been harvested and grown in culture. If previously exposed to LH, and the LH receptors of the cells are (presumably) saturated, the granulosa cells will undergo spontaneous luteinization in vitro. Granulosa cells from follicles of immature animals can respond to LH in vitro and undergo the histological and ultrastructural changes of luteinization; concomitantly, they can secrete large amounts of progesterone. Clearly, LH receptors are present on the granulosa cells long before sexual maturation occurs. In culture systems, dibutyryl cyclic AMP, theophylline, and prostaglandins can mimick the LH effects, suggesting that prostaglandins may play some intermediary role in the cyclic AMP-mediated effects of LH.

Progesterone secretion rises steeply during the luteal phase of the menstrual cycle, and its effects on target tissues are profound. These effects are thought to involve a series of cellular events, including (1) an interaction with a receptor protein located in the cell cytoplasm and (2) a temperature-dependent and ionic strength-dependent transformation of the receptor that permits (3) binding to some chromatin component, with subsequent derepression of genetic material.

The first step, the specific binding of progesterone to target tissues, was at first difficult to demonstrate, until it was realized that this binding is estrogen-dependent. For example, the ability of the vagina of the ovariectomized mouse to bind progesterone is markedly increased after treatment with estrogen. The uterus of the ovariectomized guinea pig shows a small uptake and retention of progesterone in vivo; this incorporation is increased sevenfold by pretreatment of the animal with estrogen. Estrogen priming significantly increases the concentration of uterine receptor molecules for progesterone. Other tissues that specifically bind progesterone include the chick oviduct and the mammary gland.

The transfer of progesterone from cytosol to nuclear binding sites is markedly temperature-dependent. When tissues are incubated at 0°C in vitro with labeled progesterone, the label appears almost exclusively in the cytosol; if these tissues containing extranuclear progesterone are then incubated at 37°C, the label shifts steadily, until, at 30 minutes, 75 percent of the label has entered the nucleus. How the steroid induces the receptor protein to move to the nucleus and how the hormone leaves the nucleus and the cell once its function is completed are unknown. Somehow, via steroid-receptor complexes, a regulatory message is delivered to the target cells (Figure 5–1).

In response to progesterone, the oviduct of an estrogen-primed chick synthesizes a specific protein, avidin, which appears in the white of the egg. O'Malley has shown that progesterone added in vitro to minced estrogen-primed chick oviduct brought about the synthesis of avidin. Indeed, messenger RNA extracted from oviduct pretreated with progesterone will also cause avidin synthesis. Actinomycin D and cycloheximide added in vitro inhibit this induction. The time course of synthesis is interesting. Avidin synthesis was first noted about six hours after exposure to progesterone, a delay that suggests that other effects, such as nuclear derepression, had to precede the protein synthesis. In the complete absence of progesterone, no avidin is synthesized.

In general, progesterone exerts its effects on target tissues previously primed with estrogen. These effects are quite dramatic in the vagina (desquamation of superficial cell layers and infiltration with leukocytes), the cervix (flattening of cells and changes in viscosity of cervical mucus), the endometrium (conversion of proliferative cells to secretory cells), and the fallopian tubes (flattening of cells and altered secretion). These morphologic changes undoubtedly are secondary to changes in enzyme activity brought about by progesterone.

The effects of progesterone on smooth muscle are also of interest, for in some way this hormone decreases the amplitude and interval of contractility of smooth muscle. These effects are manifest in myometrium, fallopian tubes, and ureters. This quiescent effect on the myometrium may be involved in the maintenance of pregnancy; in the absence of progesterone, pregnancies are quickly terminated.

The decidual reaction of the endometrium is dependent upon progesterone. In the uterus of an intact animal that has been primed with estrogen and treated with progesterone, implantation (or traumatic injury to the uterine lining) causes the cells surrounding the implant (or injury) to undergo differentiation and to proliferate. These decidual cells become packed with glycogen granules and eventually form the maternal portion of the placenta (see Chapter Two).

Progesterone is essential for the development of the mammary gland. In the estrogen-primed gland, acini and lobules develop. Progesterone also may have effects on the central nervous system. Cyclic temperature changes have been ascribed to this hormone, as has the negative feedback control of LH secretion. The competitive inhibition by progesterone of the aldosterone effect on renal sodium reabsorption has already been mentioned.

ANDROGENS

Gonads and adrenals can form androgens, and the peripheral conversion of dehydroepiandrosterone and androstenedione to testosterone provides another source of biologically active androgen. The major androgen of the adrenal is dehydroepiandrosterone and of the ovary androstenedione; only the testis forms testosterone in large amounts.

Adrenal Androgens

The main androgens secreted by the adult adrenal are dehydroepiandrosterone, dehydroepiandrosterone sulfate, and 11β-hydroxyandrostenedione. Smaller quantities of androstenedione are also secreted. From about the age of seven, the concentration of these androgens in blood rises steadily. Just before puberty, the values are about one third of the normal adult level. The urinary excretion of these steroids increases comparably over this period.

The three major urinary 17KS are dehydroepiandrosterone, androsterone, and etiocholanolone. The values for androsterone and etiocholanolone at age twelve are about five times greater than at age five, and at adolescence the excretion of these 17KS undergoes a further steep rise. The fact that the same amount of 17KS is excreted by boys and girls suggests that the 17-ketosteroids originate in the adrenal.

There seems little doubt that the adrenal rapidly increases its secretion of androgens at adolescence. This prepubertal increase in adrenal function has been called *adrenarche* by Wilkins. There is a particularly striking increase in the concentration of dehydroepiandrosterone sulfate in the blood at this time. Usually, adrenarche begins at about age seven. Peripheral conversion of dehydroepiandrosterone to biologically active androgens has been noted. This conversion is particularly important in considering the control of hair growth. Both androstenedione and dihydrotestosterone have been shown to stimulate amino acid uptake and protein synthesis in intact human scalp hair follicles in vitro. Human skin and scalp hair follicles of both sexes can metabolize dehydroepiandrosterone to 7α-hydroxydehydroepiandrosterone, 7-ketodehydroepiandrosterone, 5-androstene-3β,17β-diol, 5α-androstane-3,17-dione, and androstenedione. The latter could function to promote hair growth in early puberty; the far greater hair growth in the male at puberty may be the result of testosterone secretion by the maturing testis.

Forest and coworkers found no difference in the total testosterone in peripheral blood in prepubertal boys and girls (6.62 ± 2.46 ng/100 ml for boys and 6.58 ± 2.48 ng/100 ml for girls). This might be explained by assuming that testosterone arises in prepubertal children from peripheral conversion of adrenal androstenedione, dehydroepiandrosterone, and dehydroepiandrosterone sulfate. The marked sex difference in testosterone values in the newborn (68 ± 59.5 ng/100 ml of plasma for boys and 12.0 ± 6.2 ng/100 ml of plasma for girls) can probably be attributed to activity of the fetal Leydig cells.

The term precocious adrenarche or pubarche refers to the development of sexual hair with no other manifestations of sexual maturation. The syndrome is more frequent in girls than in boys (85 percent of the cases reported involve girls). The increased production of weak adrenal androgens may result, by peripheral conversion to powerful androgens, in the precocious development of sexual hair. This theory is supported by the observation that the increased urinary 17KS in patients with precocious sexual hair growth is suppressed by dexamethasone.

The threshold of response to hormonal stimulation may vary from one area of the body to another. The skin of the pubis appears to have the lowest threshold and responds to the increasing levels of androstenedione and dehydroepiandrosterone which occur early in puberty. Axillary hair has a higher threshold, and in precocious adrenarche axillary hair is increased far less commonly than pubic hair. The beard has a still higher threshold for response to androgens. Excessive growth of hair may be generalized over the whole body (hypertrichosis) or confined to the sexual areas: pubic, axillary, abdominal, chest, and facial (hirsutism). Evidence of these conditions may become manifest during adolescence. In 55 percent of women with hirsutism or hypertrichosis, the excess hair developed before 20 years of age.

Hirsutism may be encountered in the adolescent girl with disorders of the adrenal or ovary. Three adrenal disorders may produce hirsutism with or without other signs of virilization: adrenocortical hyperplasia due to a hydroxylase deficiency, adrenocortical tumors, and Cushing's syndrome.

Adrenocortical hyperplasia. The details of the specific enzyme deficiencies were discussed in Chapter Seven. Mild or latent forms of hydroxylase deficiency may not become apparent until puberty, at which time failure of menarche may be the first sign.

Adrenocortical tumors. In the presence of a virilizing adrenocortical tumor in the adolescent girl, menstruation is usually delayed. If menstruation has already begun, the menstrual periods tend to be irregular and eventually may cease. Hirsutism frequently occurs, and male pattern baldness may be noted. The patient may develop clitoral enlargement, decreased breast size, and a low-pitched voice. Urinary 17KS are usually markedly elevated (25 to 75 mg per 24 hours), and dehydroepiandrosterone may be present in large amounts in the urine.

Cushing's syndrome. Although this syndrome is classically associated with an excess of glucocorticoids, excessive amounts of androgen may be produced by the hyperplastic or tumorous adrenal cortex. Hirsutism is a rather frequent accompaniment to this syndrome. Cushing's syndrome, however, is relatively rare in the teenager.

Ovarian Androgens

Androgens are precursors of the estrogens, and thus it should not come as a surprise that in conditions such as the Stein-Leventhal syn-

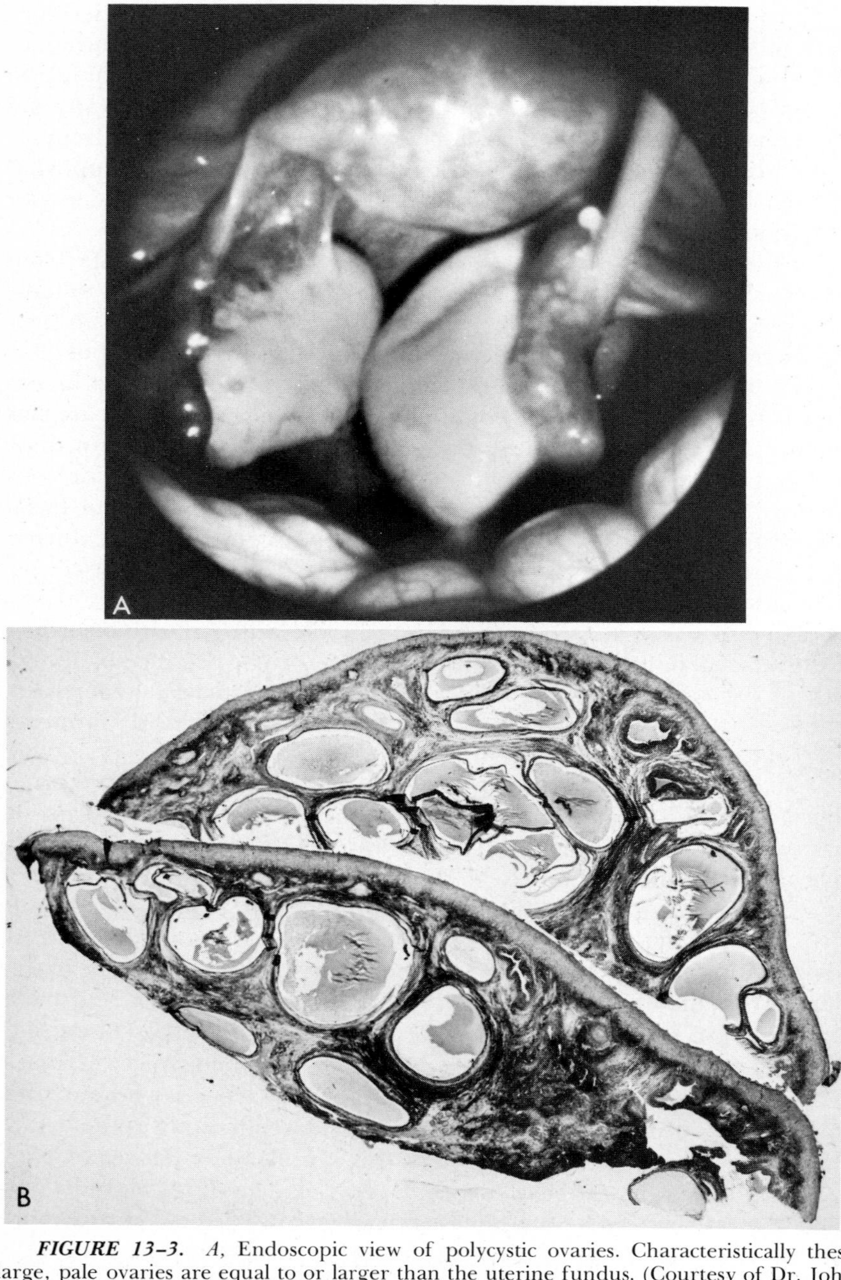

FIGURE 13-3. *A,* Endoscopic view of polycystic ovaries. Characteristically these large, pale ovaries are equal to or larger than the uterine fundus. (Courtesy of Dr. John Leventhal, Boston Hospital for Women, Boston, Mass.). *B,* A wedge resection of polycystic ovaries. The patient was a 27 year old female with amenorrhea, hirsutism, and obesity. Note the thickened capsule of the ovary and the many cystic follicles. (Courtesy of Dr. Shirley Driscoll, Boston Hospital for Women, Boston, Mass.).

drome and virilizing tumors of the ovary, excessive amounts of androgen may be produced by the ovary.

STEIN-LEVENTHAL SYNDROME. Menstrual dysfunction is the cardinal symptom of this disorder. Although occurring more often in the third or fourth decade of life, it is not uncommon in late adolescence. The patient notices longer and longer intervals between periods or a complete absence of periods (amenorrhea). The ovaries are enlarged and cystic, and the stroma is dense (Figure 13–3). Mahesh found large quantities of androstenedione and dehydroepiandrosterone in these ovaries. Urinary 17KS may be elevated, and removal of part (wedge resection) or all of the ovaries causes a marked decline in 17KS excretion. Thus the source of the androgens is considered to be the cystic ovaries. The hirsutism associated with this syndrome may be severe, but in 50 percent of the cases reported, patients showed no degree of hirsutism at all. Obesity is a common feature of the syndrome also. The patient is feminine in appearance with normal breast development.

VIRILIZING TUMORS OF THE OVARY. The incidence of such tumors is low, but they must be suspected in any virilized female. The tumor cells may resemble testis (arrhenoblastoma), adrenal, or ovary (thecoma, luteoma). Removal of the tumor may not reverse the hirsutism or may decrease the hairiness only slightly.

The presence of excessive hair growth when no abnormality of ovary or adrenal can be demonstrated and no androgen excess is present is often referred to as *idiopathic hirsutism.* Individual and racial differences in sensitivity to normal amounts of androgen have been invoked as the etiologic factor in these cases. Equally possible would be a difference in the rate of conversion of weak adrenal androgens to the more biologically active steroids.

Testicular Androgens

In most nonprimates the prepubertal state is associated with relatively high values for circulating androstenedione and rather low values for testosterone. The ratio of androstenedione to testosterone changes dramatically at puberty in the male, with a reversal from the prepubertal state. More testosterone than androstenedione circulates in the blood. Experiments in which blood was obtained from the spermatic vein in the bull and the concentration of testosterone compared with that in peripheral blood suggested that this increased amount of testosterone is coming from the testis.

A similar change occurs in the human at puberty. The ratio of androstenedione to testosterone in the blood of prepubertal boys and girls is about 2, whereas in adult men this ratio falls to about 0.08. In adult women the ratio rises to 3.5. At puberty, the Leydig cells of the testis convert androstenedione to testosterone in much larger amounts. The enzyme catalyzing the interconversion of these two steroids is 17β-

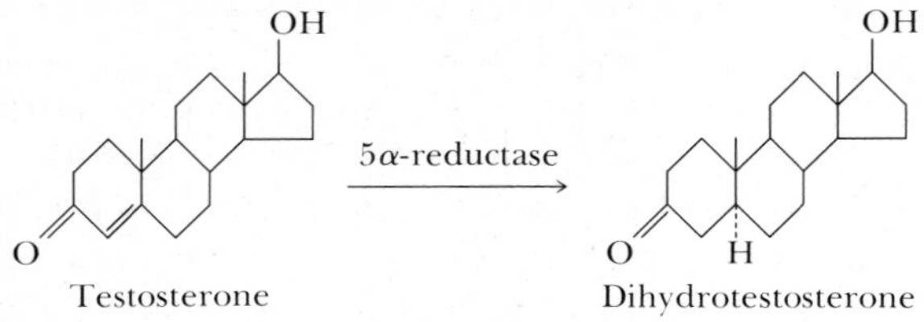

FIGURE 13–4. Conversion of testosterone to dihydrotestosterone.

hydroxysteroid dehydrogenase. The relationship between LH and the Leydig cells is such that when the cells are damaged to the degree that the concentration of testosterone in the blood declines, LH secretion from the pituitary rises. On the other hand, when testosterone secretion rises, LH secretion falls. In the normal adult male the mean testicular production rate of testosterone is about 7.0 mg/day.

It is estimated that about 97 to 99 percent of circulating testosterone is bound to protein (albumin or sex hormone binding globulin). The metabolic clearance rate of testosterone is high. It is metabolized in the liver primarily to 17KS. In addition, hydroxylation of testosterone can occur, yielding weakly androgenic metabolites. Increases in the activity of liver hydroxylating enzymes (microsomal hydroxylases) due to administration of drugs such as phenobarbital can profoundly depress the androgenic activity of exogenous testosterone. In adult men, the testes account for about one third of the total urinary 17KS, and the adrenal cortex accounts for the remainder. Although testosterone itself is biologically active in muscle and bone, the active steroid in seminal vesicle and prostate is the 5α-reduced metabolite 5α-dihydrotestosterone (Figure 13–4).

Dihydrotestosterone. If animals are infused in vivo with labeled androstenedione or testosterone—or if the prostate gland itself is perfused with such precursors—the principal products are 5α-androstane-17β-ol-3-one (dihydrotestosterone) and 5α-androstane-3α,17β-diol. Tritiated testosterone injected directly into rat ventral prostate is rapidly bound to the nuclear chromatin as dihydrotestosterone. Anderson and Liao found that dihydrotestosterone formed from testosterone was retained by the rat ventral prostate for at least six hours, long after radioactive steroid had disappeared from blood and other non-target tissues.

There are proteins in the nuclei and cytosol of rat ventral prostate that have a high, specific affinity for dihydrotestosterone. As with the estrogen receptors, androgen receptors interact spontaneously at 0°C with their ligand, dihydrotestosterone. Apparently a temperature-dependent process in the cytosol permits the dihydrotestosterone receptor complex to enter the nucleus and be bound. Thus the intracellular progress of dihydrotestosterone in androgen-sensitive tissues is similar to that of the estrogens in estrogen-sensitive tissues (Figure 5–1).

The interaction of androgen and nucleus in the target cell produces profound changes. For example, DNA polymerase in the ventral prostate is increased 50 times over within three days of the administration of testosterone to castrated rats. Within 15 hours there is a doubling of prostatic RNA polymerase. Another striking enzyme change is the tenfold increase in S-adenosyl-L-methionine decarboxylase activity in the prostate within seven days of the administration of testosterone to castrated rats. The only enzyme that is involved directly in the metabolism of steroids which is altered by testosterone treatment is 5α-reductase, which shows a twelvefold increase in activity in the ventral prostate.

Like the prostate, the seminal vesicle converts testosterone to dihydrotestosterone, with effects on tissue growth and function similar to those noted with the prostate. A third tissue—the kidney—probably utilizes dihydrotestosterone as its "active androgen." The conversion of testosterone to dihydrotestosterone in skin suggests that this tissue may also utilize the reduced androgen for masculinizing effects. A 5α-reductase has been described in the hypothalamus, and hypothalamic receptors for dihydrotestosterone have been found in the rat.

Not all androgen target tissues possess a 5α-reductase. There is evidence that testosterone itself is the active androgen in muscle and bone. At this time it would be unwise to rule out the possibility, suggested by Baulieu, that other metabolites of testosterone may possess growth-promoting or virilizing effects. Shimazaki and coworkers have shown that 5α-androstane-3,17-dione, formed from testosterone by dog gluteal muscle in vivo, has androgenic activity, although less than that of testosterone.

In addition to the Leydig cells, cells in the seminiferous tubules and epididymis are capable of synthesizing testosterone. It is suggested that such transformations in these sites ensure a high local concentration of testosterone. A 5α-reductase has been described in adult testis; dihydrotestosterone may, therefore, be the active androgen in the tubules and epididymis.

Whatever the mechanism, there is no doubt that testosterone (or dihydrotestosterone) promotes the growth and function of the epididymis, vas deferens, prostate, seminal vesicle, and penis. Androgens also contribute to growth of muscle, bone, and kidney. Part of the effect of androgens on the kidney is increased production of erythropoietin, which in turn enhances erythropoiesis.

Influence of Androgens on Behavior

Aside from the obvious way in which androgens may affect behavior by virtue of their influence on physical stature, musculature, and strength, there is evidence that in rodents androgens may influence the central nervous system directly. Administration of androgen to neonatal female rats will permanently alter not only the pattern of gonadotropin release but also the sexual behavior of the animal. There appears to be a critical time in development when patterns of behavior and hormone release are established, for treating the female with androgen later in development is without effect. The female pattern will develop unless androgens are present and active at this critical time. Other androgen-responsive tissues may have a comparable critical period in development when the subsequent response to androgens is determined. In Whalen's experiments to determine the influence of androgen on penile development in the rat, neonatal castration resulted in reduced penile development even if the rats subsequently received androgen in infancy. Treatment of these animals in adulthood with testosterone caused an increase in shaft and glans length and in total weight of the phallus; however, this androgen effect in adulthood was greatly enhanced if the animal had received a single dose of androgen on day one or day four of life.

The consequences of such androgen imprinting are obvious. Unfortunately, most of the evidence in this regard stems from studies of non-primates. Is there any evidence of a similar imprinting in primates? The experiments by Goy and Resko on subhuman primates suggest that there may be such imprinting, but to a different degree. These investigators postulate that androgens that are present before birth act upon the neural circuits that mediate the effects of experience as well as upon the neural circuits for masculine and feminine behavior. Thus experience may play an important role in sexual and social behavior in primates. This seems to be especially true in humans, as the observations of Money and Ehrhardt suggest. These investigators have studied "experiments of nature" in an attempt to assess the effect of prenatal exposure to androgens on postnatal behavior. Genetic females who had been prenatally androgenized (by congenital adrenocortical hyperplasia) showed an increased incidence of tomboy behavior and bisexual imagery, but the gender identity was always female. Girls with Turner's syndrome show completely feminine behavior patterns. There may well be prenatal hormonal influences on the developing brain; however, experience to date indicates that postnatal influences are equally if not more important. In general, gender identity coincides with the sex assigned in rearing, irrespective of prenatal events. The possible influence of prenatal sex hormones on the subsequent development of homosexuality and transsexuality has excited a great deal of interest. The "nature vs. nurture" theories for the etiology of these conditions may soon be resolved. Quite possibly a combination of both prenatal imprinting (or lack of it) plus environmental influences is necessary for the development of the homosexual and transsexual.

Androgen Deficiency Syndromes

Provided the Leydig cells function normally, the male in adolescence shows progressive pubertal changes, normally beginning sometime between ages 9 and 16. These changes encompass many systems. Growth prior to puberty (about 5 cm per year) is probably regulated by the thyroid and GH; the increased linear growth rate in early adolescence (7.5 cm per year) has been ascribed to androgens. An increase in GH secretion occurs in early adolescence and often precedes the rise in testosterone secretion. It is quite possible, therefore, that at least part of the adolescent growth spurt is due to enhanced GH secretion. The overall increment in growth found in males can quite appropriately be ascribed to testosterone action. Fusion of the epiphyses is dependent upon sex hormones.

The anabolic effects of testosterone are manifested at puberty in many tissues. Both muscle mass and bone tissue are increased under the influence of testosterone. The genital organs increase in size. The prostate and seminal vesicles enlarge; the voice becomes low pitched, owing to enlargement of the larynx and thickening of the vocal cords. The scrotum enlarges, becomes pigmented, and develops rugal folds. Pubic hair grows upward in a typical diamond-shaped pattern (male escutcheon). Hair appears at the axilla, on the body, on the extremities, and around the anus. Facial hair develops, and the scalp line undergoes the typical male recession. The production of sebum by sebaceous glands is increased under the influence of androgens. The psychological changes in the adolescent are equally profound.

If the Leydig cells fail to function at the usual age of adolescence, the pubertal changes normally brought on by testosterone will fail to appear. Most often the androgen deficiency is due to a constitutional delay in the onset of adolescence. The concentrations of gonadotropins in the blood are low, and the hypogonadism is secondary to delayed function of the hypothalamic-pituitary-gonadotropin system. In time the onset of Leydig cell function will occur.

In the teenager who fails to manifest sexual maturation one must consider the possibility of primary gonadal failure. By far the most common example of male hypogonadism is *Klinefelter's syndrome* (see Figure 13–5).

KLINEFELTER'S SYNDROME. The fundamental etiology of this disorder is the presence of supernumery X chromosomes; most often the patients are XXY. It is characterized by tubular failure and decreased Leydig cell function. In 1942 Klinefelter described nine men with aspermia, gynecomastia, small testes, and elevated urinary gonadotropins. Leydig cell function was obviously present to some degree, since each patient had a phallus of normal size and moderate amounts of pubic hair; however, diminished facial and body hair suggested some impairment of testosterone secretion.

The incidence of this disorder is surprisingly high—it occurs in 1 of 400 liveborn males. Apparently the presence of one or more extra X chromosome(s) in testicular tissue brings about the typical Klinefelter's testicular dysgenesis. At birth the testes of affected patients appear nor-

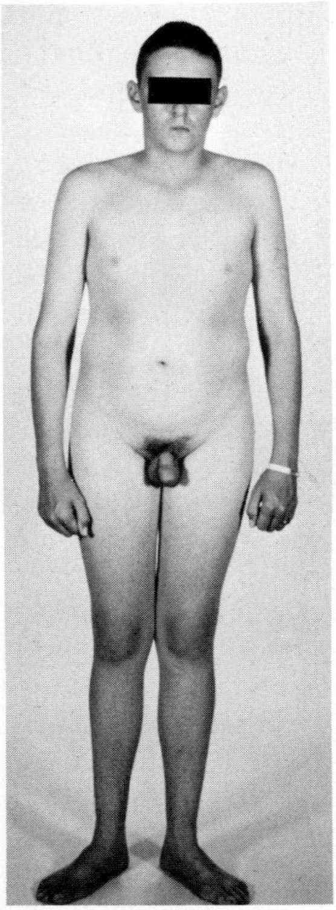

FIGURE 13–5. Patient with Klinefelter's syndrome. Note small testes, decreased pubic hair, sparse body hair, mild gynecomastia, and length of long bones. (Courtesy of Dr. Leslie Rose, Peter Bent Brigham Hospital, Boston, Mass.)

mal, and during the prepubertal years the growth and histological appearance of the testes are normal, although there is some evidence of a gradual loss in germ cells. At puberty the rise in gonadotropins brings about a progressive hyalinization and fibrosis of the seminiferous tubules. The tubules, which make up about 85 percent of the volume of the normal testis, fail to develop, and the testis remains small in size. Rarely does the testis of a patient with Klinefelter's syndrome exceed 2.0 × 1.5 × 1.5 cm in dimensions. Normally the adult testis measures 4.6 cm in length and 2.6 cm in width. The small, *firm* testes of Klinefelter's syndrome are characteristic.

It is interesting that many patients with Klinefelter's syndrome show excessive long bone growth prior to puberty (Figure 13–5); the bone age, however, is appropriate for the chronologic age. The growth of long bones is greater in the lower extremity than in the upper extremity, resulting in a ratio of arm span to height of one or less. In patients who are eunuchoidal (lacking androgen), the bones in the upper and lower extremities grow comparably, resulting in an arm span at least five cm greater than height, giving an arm span to height ratio greater than one. The etiology of the differential skeletal growth in Klinefelter's syndrome is unknown, but it is probably not related to androgen deficiency per se.

Explanations for other aspects of Klinefelter's syndrome are also lacking. The gynecomastia is bilateral and involves hyperplasia of the interductal tissue. In contrast, estrogens produce ductal hyperplasia. Subnormal intelligence (I.Q. less than 80) and characteristic behavioral alterations are found in many patients. Individuals with Klinefelter's syndrome have an increased incidence of conditions such as diabetes mellitus, chronic bronchitis, neoplasia, and autoimmune disorders.

More than two X's may be present in cells from patients with Klinefelter's syndrome. Variants include XXXY, XXXXY, and mosaicism. Mental retardation in the XXXY and XXXXY patients is usually severe, whereas the mosaic patients, particularly those with an XY cell line, show far less severe symptoms and may even have normal gonadal function. Rarely, a patient with XY genotype will manifest Klinefelter's syndrome ("chromatin negative" Klinefelter's syndrome). Some of these cases may represent unrelated disorders, such as mumps orchitis, which produce similar testicular pathology. It is important to ascertain the gonadal genotype since only supernumery X's in *testicular* tissue produce testicular dysgenesis. Buccal smears and karyotyping of skin and blood will not necessarily reveal the abnormal genotype.

A testicular biopsy is important in the diagnosis of Klinefelter's syndrome. The tissue should be examined histologically, and the testicular cells should be karyotyped. The classical features of the disorder are: (1) hyalinization of the seminiferous tubules and (2) clumping of the Leydig cells. Compared with the tissue of normal subjects, the Leydig cells tend to be less granular and contain less lipid material.

Azoospermia is also a classical finding in Klinefelter's syndrome. There are no unique changes in seminal fluid volume; however, with severe androgen deficiency, the volume of ejaculate is small, and the concentrations of fructose and phosphate are reduced.

The concentrations of both serum and urinary gonadotropins are usually elevated. Serum FSH values generally exceed 0.024 IU/ml; urinary FSH may range from 56 to 205 IU/24 hours. The mean serum LH concentration ranges from 16.5 to over 128 mIU/ml. The concentration of testosterone in plasma ranges from 50 to 860 ng/100 ml, overlapping in part the range of values for normal men (230 to 1440 ng/100 ml).

The only treatment for affected patients is correction of the androgen deficiency. Replacement therapy produces adequate sexual maturation. The infertility is irreversible, and the gynecomastia, if embarrassing, requires plastic surgery. Although there is an increase in the incidence of testicular neoplasms in other conditions involving dysgenetic gonads, such is not the case in Klinefelter's syndrome.

Errors in the synthesis of testosterone. We have already discussed certain enzyme deficiencies which result in impaired testosterone synthesis (cholesterol 20α-hydroxylase deficiency, 3β-hydroxysteroid dehydrogenase deficiency, and 17α-hydroxylase deficiency, all detailed in Chapter Seven). In addition, deficiencies of the 17,20-desmolase and 17β-hydroxysteroid dehydrogenase have been described. Patients with any of the various deficiencies manifest a form of male pseudohermaphroditism. Provided they benefit from early detection of their disorder, affected patients can be reared as males and treated with testosterone to induce male sex characteristics.

Reifenstein's syndrome (p. 187) may belong to the category of inborn errors of testosterone synthesis. This hereditary disorder is characterized by hypospadias of varying degree and incomplete fusion of labioscrotal folds. Atrophy of seminiferous tubules occurs after the onset of puberty, and gynecomastia develops. The karyotype is XY. Testosterone concentrations are usually reduced, possibly owing to a defect in the conversion of androstenedione to testosterone (17β-hydroxysteroid dehydrogenase deficiency). Gonadotropins are usually elevated. Affected patients respond to androgen therapy.

TESTICULAR FEMINIZATION SYNDROME. This disorder does not represent a failure of testosterone synthesis; rather, in all probability, it is the result of a genetic defect in androgen receptors in target tissues. In addition, some patients have reduced 5α-reductase activity in androgen target tissues. The patient is chromatin negative and the karyotype is 46XY; however, the phenotype is completely female (Figure 13–6). At puberty the breast development is marked, but pubic and axillary hair are scanty, and no menses occur. Culdoscopy reveals a small vagina but no uterus, tubes, or ovaries; the testes are either abdominal or inguinal.

Patients with the testicular feminization syndrome fail to respond to androgen at any time in life, and fetal development reflects this. The external genitalia are female. The fetal testis secretes both Wolffian duct inducer and Mullerian inhibitor, and response to these substances is normal. Thus the male genital ducts develop, but because of the lack of response to androgens they tend to be hypoplastic. As mentioned, the female genitalia are incomplete: the uterus and tubes are absent, and the upper portion of the vagina does not develop. The shallow vagina ends in a blind pouch.

The testis is capable of forming testosterone and estrogens. Indeed, after removal of the testes the breasts regress, suggesting that testicular estrogens are implicated in the gynecomastia. Usually the testes are removed because of the increased incidence of testicular malignancy in affected patients. After orchiectomy the patient is maintained on estrogens.

As one might predict, affected patients are totally feminine in behavior, dress, and attitudes. Indeed, they are amongst the most strikingly feminine individuals one is likely to encounter. The disorder is transmitted by the heterozygous female to half her male offspring. As for her female offspring, half will carry the trait.

Recently Wilson and his colleagues reported an extensive study of a single family in which there were 11 members with familial male pseudohermaphroditism. The phenotypic expression of the disorder in this

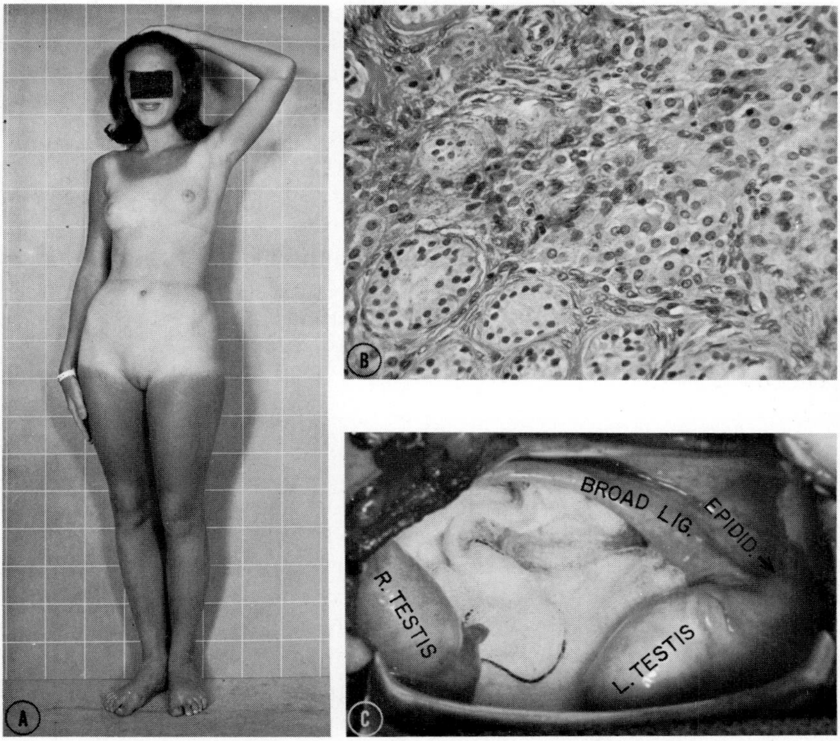

FIGURE 13–6. Testicular feminization syndrome. *A,* Seventeen-year-old patient with complete syndrome. This girl is chromatin-negative and has total absence of sexual hair with feminine secondary sexual development. A small vagina ends blindly. *B,* The testes exhibit Leydig cell hyperplasia, and the seminiferous tubules lack germinal elements (× 400). *C,* At laparotomy abdominal testes and male genital ducts were found. The structure resembling a broad ligament contained no identifiable müllerian derivatives. The epididymes connect with normal vasa deferentia. (From Williams, R., ed. *Textbook of Endocrinology,* Fifth Edition. Philadelphia: W. B. Saunders Company, 1974, p. 486.)

family varied from minimal defects in virilization (microphallus and bifid scrotum) to more severe defects (perineoscrotal hypospadias) to complete male pseudohermaphroditism (perineoscrotal hypospadias, absent vas deferens, and vaginal orifice). Wilson suggests that the various syndromes of defective virilization described by Reifenstein, Lubs, and Gilbert-Dreyfus (p. 187) may represent variable manifestations of the same mutant gene transmitted as an apparent X-linked recessive trait. The concentrations of testosterone and LH in the plasma of affected members was elevated, suggesting that the failure to fully virilize might be due to defective androgen action rather than defective synthesis of testosterone.

Estrogens

Transformation of androstenedione to estrone involves the elimination of (1) the angular methyl (C19) group and (2) the hydrogens from

C1 and C2. The sequence of reactions is thought to proceed as follows: (1) the hydroxylation of carbon 19 to form 19-hydroxyandrostenedione, (2) oxidation of this compound to 19-oxoandrostenedione, and (3) elimination of hydrogens from C1 and C2 in concert with the removal of the C19 oxygenated group (Figure 7–4). A similar series of reactions will convert testosterone to estradiol-17β. Estrone and estradiol-17β are interconvertible by the reaction catalyzed by 17β-hydroxysteroid dehydrogenase.

Estrogens are formed by granulosa and theca cells of the ovary under the influence of both FSH and LH. The cyclic release of gonadotropins and gonadal hormones becomes established at puberty; however, several changes precede the actual onset of menstruation (menarche).

Sexual Maturation in the Female

Most often the earliest change noted in the adolescent girl is the onset of breast development. Marshall and Tanner (1969) made a longitudinal study of 192 English girls to observe the sequence of physical changes in adolescence (Table 13–1). They tabulated breast and pubic hair development according to stages. For breast development stage 1 is considered to be the lack of palpable glandular tissue. Breast buds may appear as early as 8 years of age in normal puberty. In a condition called *premature thelarche,* premature breast development without other signs of precocious puberty occurs. The typical age range for this condition is 1½ to 4 years. Affected children subsequently undergo normal adolescence. It has been suggested that their breast tissue may be hypersensitive to normal amounts of secreted hormones.

TABLE 13–1. Pubertal Development in the Female

Tanner Stage	Breast Development	Pubic Hair
I	No palpable glandular tissue	None
II	Palpable glandular tissue; nipple and breast project as a single mound	Occasional wispy strands
III	Increased glandular tissue; areola increased in diameter and more pigmented	Darker, coarser hair over pubis
IV	Increased areolar pigmentation; second mound of nipple and areola above mound of glandular tissue	Dark, coarse, curly hair in adult pattern
V	Areola and nipple no longer project above gland; smooth contour in profile	Extension of hair down the medial aspects of the thighs

At stage 2 of breast development, glandular tissue is palpable, and the nipple and breast project as a single mound from the chest wall. As the breast continues to develop, increased glandular tissue can be palpated. The areola increases in diameter and becomes more darkly pigmented (stage 3). Eventually a secondary mound of nipple and areola forms above the mound of the increased glandular tissue (stage 4). Finally the nipple and areola recede to make a smooth contour in profile view (stage 5).

Similarly progressive development of pubic hair occurs, from no hair at all (stage 1), to occasional wispy strands along the labia (stage 2), to darker, coarser hair extending over the pubis (stage 3), to dark, coarse, curly hair covering the pubis in an adult pattern (stage 4), to extension of the hair down the medial aspects of the thighs (stage 5). The completion of all five stages usually takes about three years. Complete breast development usually takes longer (four years) but tends to start about six months before the onset of pubic hair.

About one year after the appearance of the breast bud the young girl usually reaches the peak of the adolescent growth spurt. One to one and a half years later menarche begins. Frisch and Revelle have found that the onset of the adolescent growth spurt in girls occurs one year before the appearance of secondary sexual characteristics. Furthermore, the mean weight at the time of the onset of the growth spurt (31 kg), at the time of maximum weight gain (39 kg), and at menarche (48 kg) does not differ significantly between early and late maturing girls. These investigators have postulated a "critical body weight" that is associated with menarche.

Menarche has been appearing at progressively earlier ages since the middle of the nineteenth century, undoubtedly owing to improved nutrition. This would fit the concept of a critical body weight, for with improved nutrition, such a weight would be attained at an earlier age. But how do nutritional and metabolic factors affect the timing of puberty? In discussing these questions, Ruf has called attention to the alleged structural and functional similarity between nerve growth factor and proinsulin. The extent of secretion by the pancreas is a function of food intake and body mass; thus proinsulin or some other pancreatic component might theoretically trigger central adrenergic neurons once a critical rate of secretion has been reached. Ruf believes that the resetting of the "gonadostat" during puberty might be caused by increased terminal arborization of adrenergic neurons synapsing directly or indirectly with neurons releasing GRH. Similar adrenergic neurons would cause increased GHRH secretion, with subsequent GH release and the adolescent growth spurt. This is an attractive theory, for in postulating a pancreatic material similar to nerve growth factor, it ties in the known adrenergic effects on GH and GRH secretion with (1) "maturation of the hypothalamus at puberty" (in actual fact growth and maturation of adrenergic neurons) and (2) the body composition. Whatever the explanation, the hypothalamus is directly or indirectly attuned to the body composition (critical weight) and releases increasing amounts of GRH. Consequently, secretions of LH and FSH increase, stimulating the ovary, and a new level of steroid-hypothalamic interaction is attained. Present studies indicate that the adult level of hypothalamic sensitivity to estrogen may be present by mid-puberty.

The Menstrual Cycle

For each cycle a new set of follicles must grow under the influence of pituitary FSH (Figure 13–7). Thus the initial phase of the cycle is characterized by rising concentrations of FSH and early follicular growth. As the follicles grow, they produce more estrogen, which exerts a negative feedback effect on FSH secretion. During this second phase the follicles are maturing and are secreting increasing amounts of es-

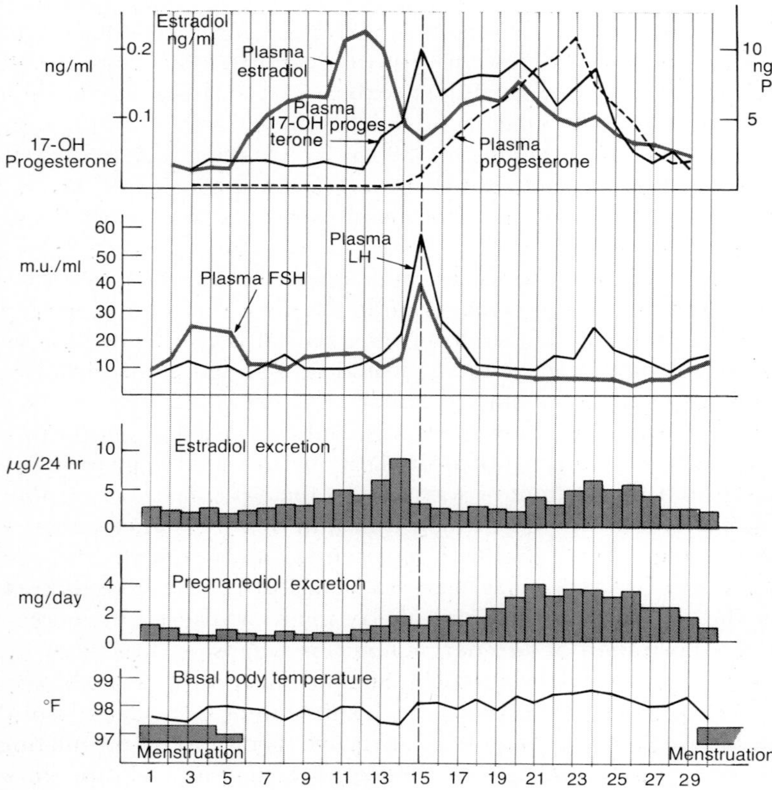

FIGURE 13–7. Diagram illustrating the concentrations of gonadotropins, estrogens, and progestins in the plasma during a single human menstrual cycle. The urinary excretion of estradiol and pregnanediol and the changes in basal body temperature are also shown. (From Villee, C. *Biology.* Philadelphia: W. B. Saunders Company, 1972, p. 517.)

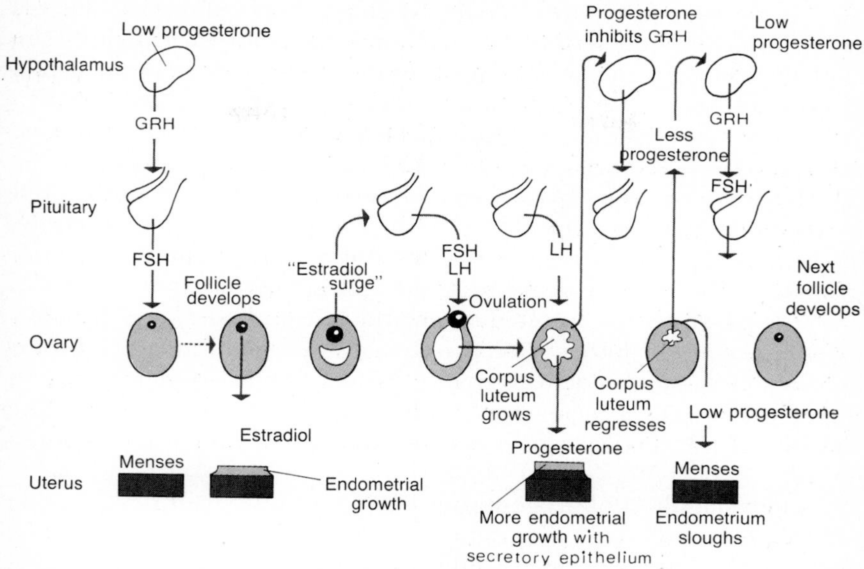

FIGURE 13–8. Interrelations of hypothalamic, pituitary, and ovarian hormones in regulating the events of the menstrual cycle in women. (From Ville, C. *Biology.* Philadelphia: W. B. Saunders Company, 1972, p. 518.)

trogen while the FSH concentration in blood falls. One follicle grows on to full maturity and the other follicles become atretic.

The estrogens produced during the preovulatory part of the cycle originate principally in the theca interna of the growing follicles. The estrogens produce changes in the uterine endometrium that are largely proliferative (Figure 13–8). Cells of the epithelium and stroma undergo mitosis; the mucosa thickens, and the tubular glands lengthen but remain straight.

Proliferative changes also occur in other epithelial cells, including those of the vaginal and urethral epithelia. As the concentration of estrogens in blood rises, the vaginal epithelium becomes thicker and keratinized. The endocervical cells secrete much larger amounts of mucus under the influence of estrogens than they do otherwise, and qualitatively this mucus is more watery, viscous, and elastic than it is when estrogen levels are lower.

The rising titer of estrogen triggers the LH surge (positive feedback) which completes the maturation of the follicle. The LH surge stimulates follicle rupture and expulsion of the oocyte (Figures 13–7 and 13–8). There is a more modest rise in FSH concentration concomitant with the LH rise. When the LH surge occurs, estrogen production falls precipitously while progesterone synthesis increases (Figure 13–7). The high levels of LH persist for about 24 hours. It has been suggested that the abrupt decline in estrogen production shuts off LH secretion (Figure 13–7).

Ovulation occurs 16 to 24 hours after the beginning of the LH surge; however, not all cycles are ovulatory. Only a follicle of sufficient maturity will rupture in response to an LH surge. Indeed, anovulatory cycles are common for the first year after menarche.

LH initiates luteinization in the follicle(s) that has ruptured and expelled its oocyte (Figure 13–8). The luteinized granulosa cells secrete increasing amounts of progesterone and estrogens. This part of the cycle is called the *luteal phase,* in contrast to the *follicular phase,* which precedes ovulation. The corpus luteum reaches full maturity 8 or 9 days after ovulation. Thereafter it regresses unless pregnancy occurs.

The progesterone secreted during the luteal phase exerts physiologic effects on the uterus. The glands become coiled, and the stroma becomes increasingly edematous and vascular. The glycogen content of the epithelial cells is increased. In addition, the quantity, viscosity, and elasticity of the cervical mucus declines under the influence of progesterone.

The rising titers of progesterone exert a negative feedback effect on LH secretion, and circulating values of LH decline. In turn, the function of the corpus luteum declines, and the plasma concentrations of progesterone and estrogens start to fall. No longer maintained by these hormones, the uterine mucosa undergoes necrotic changes. Cells are exfoliated, and necrosis of blood vessels opens up vascular channels, with resultant menstrual bleeding.

Metabolic Effects of Estrogens

Aside from their effects on reproductive organs, estrogens produce alterations in metabolism elsewhere in the body. Under the influence of estrogen, the liver forms increased amounts of certain proteins such as TBG, transcortin, and renin substrate. In the plasma, lipoprotein lipase activity is decreased and pre-β-lipoproteins are increased by estrogens (see Chapter Fourteen). Plasma proteins that bind copper and iron are increased by estrogen; there is a characteristic sex-linked difference in the erythrocyte count and hemoglobin concentration, women having fewer erythrocytes and less hemoglobin than men. The alterations in bone metabolism produced by estrogens are discussed in Chapters Twelve and Fourteen.

Disorders of Estrogen Deficiency: Hypogonadism

Deficient production of estrogen by the ovary may be due to primary or secondary hypogonadism. Any interruption of the hypothalamic-pituitary-ovarian axis will produce secondary hypogonadism. Whatever the cause of hypogonadism, one of the major symptoms is amenorrhea. If menstrual periods have never occurred, the condition is called *primary amenorrhea.* The abnormal cessation of menstrual periods that are already established is called *secondary amenorrhea.* Infrequent menstruation is termed *oligomenorrhea.* Periods accompanied by cramps *(dysmenorrhea)* occur only in ovulatory cycles, and the cramps are due to effects of progesterone on the uterine musculature.

If a girl has not menstruated by age 15 and has not matured physically, an investigative study should be initiated. One half of all girls who have not menstruated by age 18 have primary ovarian failure or a congenital anomaly of the reproductive system. Primary ovarian failure can result from congenital disorders (gonadal dysgenesis) and from acquired conditions (ovarian neoplasms), either of which may involve defective steroidogenesis and/or germ cell failure.

CONGENITAL OVARIAN FAILURE. Although occasionally a child is born with total absence of the gonads (gonadal agenesis), more often gonadal function is present for some time in fetal life and subsequently becomes impaired (gonadal dysgenesis). The variety of phenotypes associated with gonadal dysgenesis can create problems in diagnosis. Most affected patients are short, but some are normal in height—or even tall. Other stigmata may be present, such as webbed neck, wide carrying angle (cubitus valgus), short metatarsals, and coarctation of the aorta. There is a tendency to regard the patient with XO karyotype, streak gonads, short stature, webbed neck, and cubitus valgus as an example of Turner's syndrome (Figure 13–9). This phenotype is not difficult to recognize. At the other end of the spectrum is the genetically normal (46XX or 46XY) individual with streak gonads and no somatic anomalies. This is known as *pure gonadal dysgenesis* and the individuals with this form of gonadal dysgenesis invariably have normal stature. Primary amenorrhea is associated with all of the variants of gonadal dysgenesis.

Singh and Carr studied 45XO human embryos in early development and found that germ cells migrate into the genital ridges. However, the primary oocytes undergo rapid attrition during the latter part of intrauterine and early neonatal life. The cause of the degeneration is unknown. It would appear that not all primordial follicles are destroyed in all patients; individuals with streak gonads have been described with degrees of ovarian function ranging from development of secondary sex characteristics to sporadic menses and even pregnancy.

Apparently the incidence of somatic anomalies is positively correlated with the loss of genetic material. Thus the XO individual is likely to have the classical Turner phenotype and almost invariably has short stature. Individuals with mosaicism (45XO/46XX) may show less severe anomalies and less severe stunting of growth in general. Individuals with the 45XO/46XY karyotype may have one testis and one streak gonad (*mixed gonadal dysgenesis*) and may show evidence of virilization (large phallus, urogenital sinus).

The Turner phenotype may be present in an individual with a normal karyotype (46XX, 46XY). The somatic features of Turner's syn-

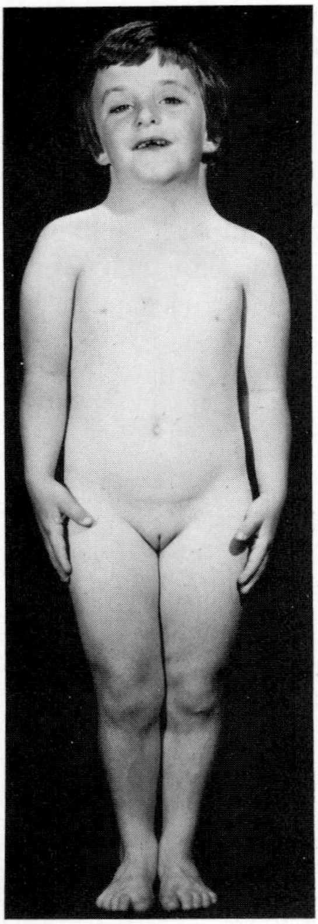

FIGURE 13–9. Thirteen-year-old patient with Turner's syndrome showing web neck, low set ears, and widely spaced nipples. In the first few months of life the patient was noted to have edema of the feet which disappeared spontaneously. Her growth rate (see Figure 11–8) fell below the third percentile. Her buccal smear was chromatin negative, and the karyotype was 45/XO. Urinary excretion of FSH was high; 17KS were 1.4 to 1.6 mg per 24 hour urine. No evidence of sexual maturation could be seen. An exploratory operation was performed. Streak gonads and a very small uterus were found and removed. Estrogen therapy was instituted. (Courtesy of Dr. John Crigler, Children's Hospital Medical Center, Boston, Mass.).

drome, particularly webbing of the neck, low posterior hairline, and prominent, low set ears, are present. The facies are characteristic and the stature is small. Hypogonadism may be present. In contrast to cases of XO Turner's syndrome, in which the most frequently occurring cardiovascular defect is coarctation of the aorta, XX or XY patients tend to have pulmonary valvular stenosis and atrial septal defects. Patients with this form of gonadal dysgenesis have been described by a variety of eponyms, including *Noonan's syndrome* and the *Ullrich-Noonan syndrome.*

Diagnosis of Gonadal Dysgenesis

The very diversity of phenotypes in this disorder makes diagnosis a challenge. In any girl with primary amenorrhea, gonadal dysgenesis should be considered in the differential diagnosis. Certain tests are helpful.

Buccal Smear. Not only should the presence or absence of Barr bodies be noted, but the number of Barr bodies per cell should be observed as well. If some cells possess one or more Barr bodies and others have no Barr bodies, the individual may be a genetic mosaic. Chromosomal karyotyping of white cells from peripheral blood may be helpful.

Bone Age. Maturation of bone requires gonadal hormones; thus, measuring the bone age can help to date the gonadal failure. In most affected patients the bone age is commensurate with chronological age until about age 12 or 13. The iliac epiphysis normally begins to appear (calcify) within six months of endocrine menarche; this ossification center grows and fuses at about age 21. Any alteration in this ossification pattern that may be revealed in an x-ray film of the pelvis indicates altered ovarian steroid secretion. Individuals lacking gonadal steroids will show no ossification center on the x-ray. If the epiphysis has begun to ossify, gonadal steroids are being or have been secreted.

The same x-ray film may show calcification in the region of the streak gonads. One of the two most common tumors occurring in streak gonads is the gonadoblastoma, which frequently calcifies. This rather distinctive tumor tends to occur bilaterally either in streak gonads or in intra-abdominal testes. Rarely has such a tumor been identified in a normal ovary. The gonadoblastoma characteristically secretes androgens.

Vaginal Smear. A pool of mucus and desquamated epithelium accumulates in the posterior vaginal fornix. These secretions can be aspirated, transferred to a clean microscopic slide, spread as a thin film and fixed in 50 percent ether-alcohol. In childhood, when the circulating estrogen is at a low level, such a smear is composed chiefly of round or oval *basal cells* with vesicular nuclei comprising about one third of the total area of the cell. The cytoplasm is basophilic.

Under estrogen stimulation desquamated cells become *cornified* and are recognized by the presence of small, deeply pigmented, homogenous nuclei. They are polygonal in shape, and the cytoplasm is acidophilic. Under the influence of progesterone, *precornified cells* with folded edges are seen on smear. The nuclei of these cells are vesicular and may be elongated or oval. The cytoplasm is basophilic.

Clearly, the appearance of cells in the vaginal smear provides evidence of ovarian hormone secretion; this evidence may be helpful in the diagnosis of patients with gonadal dysgenesis.

Laboratory Measurements. In patients with primary ovarian failure, both serum FSH and serum LH values are elevated. The urinary 17KS are only slightly reduced. Some patients with gonadal dysgenesis have poor adrenal function which becomes manifest only under stress (this is particularly important on any occasion when surgery may be contemplated).

It is critical to evaluate the cardiovascular and renal systems in any patient suspected of having gonadal dysgenesis. The incidence of renal anomalies and of coarctation of the aorta is high in affected patients. These conditions may pose a serious threat to life and should be evaluated and treated as early as possible. There is a positive association between gonadal dysgenesis and obesity, hypertension (due to causes other than coarctation of the aorta), diabetes mellitus, Hashimoto's thyroiditis, precocious aging, cataracts, and corneal opacity.

Therapy for Gonadal Dysgenesis

Aside from estrogen therapy, one of the most important aspects in the management of girls affected by gonadal dysgenesis is careful counseling. The short stature is often a difficult condition to accept and must be discussed with honesty. The question of sterility must also be explained, usually at a later date. Breast development, growth of pubic hair, and menstrual periods can be achieved by hormonal therapy; this usually results in an improved outlook on the part of young girls with the disorder.

The physician should see the affected patient at reasonable intervals to oversee the hormonal therapy. Pelvic examination should be included, and if a mass is palpable, or calcification is seen on x-ray examination of the pelvis, surgical exploration is indicated. Neoplasms of the streak are not uncommon. If surgical removal of one or both gonads is performed, the question of hysterectomy at the same time should be considered.

One of the unfortunate byproducts of gonadal dysgenesis is osteoporosis. This disorder is usually attributed to lack of estrogen and is similar to the osteoporosis that develops after the menopause (p. 411). The osteoporosis tends to develop early in life in affected girls.

Acquired primary ovarian failure. Any process that destroys or displaces normal ovarian tissue may result in ovarian failure. Infectious processes and tumors are the most commonly encountered causes of acquired primary ovarian failure. The tumors may be primary to the ovary or metastatic. Many but not all ovarian tumors secrete hormones, and a convenient classification system differentiates these tumors as estrogen-producing, androgen-producing, or gonadotropin-producing tumors.

The estrogen-producing tumors are the most common functioning ovarian neoplasms and are composed of cells morphologically similar to granulosa and theca cells of normal follicles (Figure 13–10). These granulosa-theca tumors account for 15 to 20 percent of all solid ovarian neoplasms. The most common symptom is irregular bleeding. There may be excessive bleeding alternating with periods of amenorrhea. These tumors in the premenarcheal child are associated with sexual precocity.

Among the several androgen-producing ovarian tumors are arrhenoblastomas, gonadoblastomas, and lipoid cell tumors (adrenal rest and hilar cell tumors). Such tumors result in signs of virilization. Tumors that produce testosterone, such as the arrhenoblastomas, may not cause an elevation of the urinary 17KS. In contrast, patients with adrenal rest tumors are more likely to have increased excretion of 17KS. The cell that secretes androgens in the adrenal rest tumors and hilar cell tumors has not been conclusively identified. Indeed, Lipsett rejects the concept that lipoid cell tumors originate from adrenocortical cells.

Occasionally, tumors of the ovary (dysgerminoma, teratoma) may secrete gonadotropins resembling hCG. Other teratoid tumors occasionally contain chromaffin tissue and thyroid tissue (struma ovarii) and

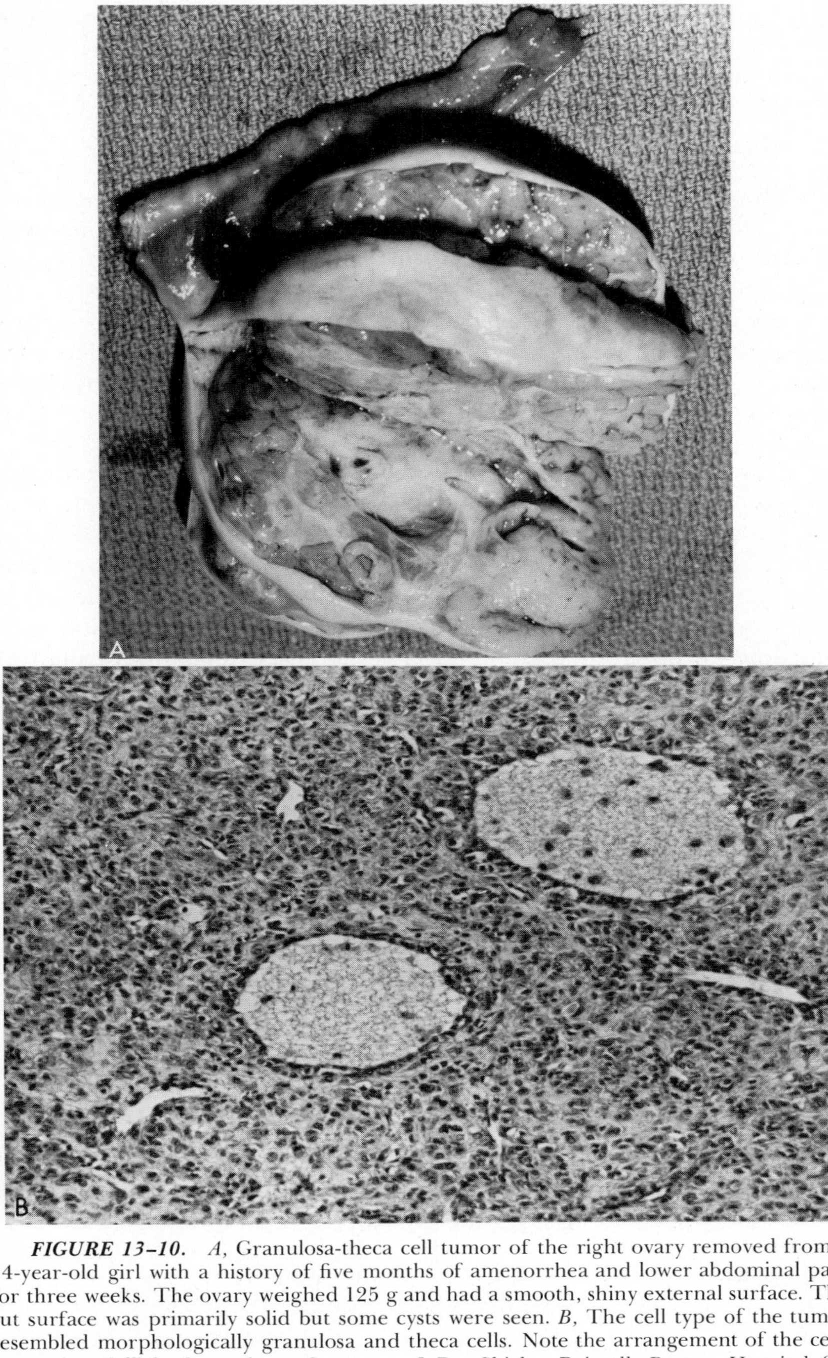

FIGURE 13-10. *A,* Granulosa-theca cell tumor of the right ovary removed from a 14-year-old girl with a history of five months of amenorrhea and lower abdominal pain for three weeks. The ovary weighed 125 g and had a smooth, shiny external surface. The cut surface was primarily solid but some cysts were seen. *B,* The cell type of the tumor resembled morphologically granulosa and theca cells. Note the arrangement of the cells suggesting follicle formation. (Courtesy of Dr. Shirley Driscoll, Boston Hospital for Women, Boston, Mass.).

secrete serotonin and thyroxine respectively. The production of serotonin can result in a *carcinoid syndrome,* whereas thyrotoxicosis very rarely may be due to struma ovarii.

Disorders of Estrogen Excess: Precocious Puberty

The onset of pubertal changes at an earlier age than normal is secondary to increased sex hormone production. The lower normal limit for the onset of pubertal change in American girls is approximately eight years of age. The increase in sex hormones may be due to increased gonadotropin (from some pituitary or extrapituitary source) or to primary disease of either the adrenals or the ovaries. In all cases, a thorough examination for drug exposure should be made, as estrogens may be present in skin creams and vitamins as well as in oral contraceptives.

GONADOTROPIN EXCESS. The most commonly encountered cause of precocious puberty is premature activation of the hypothalamic-pituitary axis. The increased circulating FSH and LH lead to increased gonadal hormone secretion and to precocious development consistent with the sex of the individual *(isosexual precocity).* Certain anomalies of the central nervous system, such as tumors in the hypothalamic region, postinfectious encephalitis, craniopharyngioma, hydrocephalus, or neurofibromatosis, may result in precocious puberty. If careful investigation reveals no anomaly of the central nervous system, the term *idiopathic isosexual precocity* is used. This is the most common form of premature puberty in girls.

OVARIAN NEOPLASMS. Granulosa-theca cell tumors are the most common form of ovarian tumor causing sexual precocity. These tumors are usually large and easily felt. They may recur many years after resection.

The clinical signs are similar whether the hormone excess is due to hypothalamic-pituitary stimulation or to ovarian neoplasm. The precocity may begin at any time after birth. Pubescent changes progress and within about two years menstruation begins. Ovulatory cycles occur, and even pregnancies have been recorded. The most famous case on record is that of Escomel, who delivered a normal infant born to a 5-year- 7-month-old girl.

The premenarcheal growth spurt occurs early, as expected, and may result in early epiphyseal closure and subsequent short stature. Dental development usually corresponds to the chronological age.

Gonadotropins are often elevated in hypothalamic-pituitary disorders, whereas in the presence of autonomous estrogen secretion gonadotropins are suppressed. Vaginal smear, bone age, and specific analyses for estrogen in the blood are helpful. Girls with isosexual precocity show an increased percentage of cornified cells on vaginal smear.

The treatment for sexual precocity is operative removal of the hormone-secreting tumor, if such is possible. Hypothalamic tumors are only rarely amenable to curative surgery. At present, excessive gonadotropins are most often suppressed with 6-methyl, 17-hydroxyprogesterone (medroxyprogesterone acetate), which has no estrogenic or androgenic properties. Unfortunately, although menses can be prevented with low doses of this steroid, little or no deceleration of bone maturation has been achieved.

CONTROL OF HUMAN REPRODUCTION

It is rather remarkable that man should reproduce at all. Every stage of development from growth of the egg and spermatozoon through embryonic and fetal life seems fraught with peril. Thus it is not surprising that some couples fail to reproduce. Still others only bear children after considerable delay. Another aspect is the increasing social pressure to restrict population increase. The fertile female who wishes to delay having children, or to have none at all, must employ some form of contraception. Whether the problem is infertility or superfertility, an understanding of the control of human reproduction is essential.

INFERTILITY

Primary gonadal failure (Turner's syndrome, Klinefelter's syndrome) results in sterility which is not amenable to hormonal or surgical therapy. Affected patients must be made aware of the fact that they are permanently sterile. However, if germ cells are present, infertility may be due to other anomalies of the reproductive tract. Complete or partial obstruction of the fallopian tubes following infection of the reproductive tract can be alleviated surgically in about 20 percent of cases. Endometriosis may produce infertility and may be treated medically or surgically. Cervical secretions may be hostile to spermatozoa, reducing their viability. In this case, hormonal therapy is indicated.

Infertility may be due to oligospermia (less than 30×10^6 spermatozoa per ml) or to azoospermia (no spermatozoa). Infection of the male reproductive tract can block the vas deferens, and surgical removal of the stenosed portion may rectify the situation. Sometimes artificial insemination can correct oligospermia. Ejaculates can be collected and stored at low temperature until sufficient spermatozoa are accumulated. If the husband is azoospermic, semen from a donor can be used for artificial insemination.

Since gonadotropin secretion is regulated by the hypothalamus, infertility may be due to pituitary or hypothalamic failure. A large proportion of men with hypogonadotropic hypogonadism have no evidence of pituitary disease. In men with *Kallman's syndrome,* a primary neurogenic disorder is likely. These patients have anosmia or hyposmia associated with the hypogonadism. In some patients pathologic examination of the brain has shown agenesis or maldevelopment of the olfactory lobes. This disorder is thought to be inherited as an x-linked dominant gene with incomplete penetrance. The trait is transmitted through females who are normal or who show partial or complete anosmia.

Infertility in women may be due to lack of gonadotropins. If the pituitary can form gonadotropins but lacks the stimulus of GRH from the hypothalamus, the latter can be supplied. Although still limited in supply, GRH is rapidly becoming more available and should be clinically useful for patients with hypothalamic infertility. A dose-response relationship between circulating gonadotropin levels and synthetic LHRH has been established in both men and women. In addition to its possible therapeutic value in patients with hypothalamic forms of infertility, synthetic LHRH has already been shown to be of value in identifying pituitary failure and in differentiating between various causes of infertility in the human. Another compound which has been found effective in treating hypogonadotropic infertility is clomiphene. In appropriate dosages, clomiphene causes the release of endogenous gonadotropins from the pituitary. It has both estrogenic and anti-estrogenic properties and its mode of action is unknown; however, administration of clomiphene often results in ovulation, and many infertile patients have conceived and have had babies after treatment with this drug.

If the pituitary gland cannot form gonadotropins, the hormones can be supplied. Usually FSH (or human menopausal gonadotropin) is used to stimulate follicular development, followed by hCG (which is rich in LH activity) to trigger ovulation. The dosage and timing of administration of these hormones is critical; multiple ovulation is frequent. One pregnancy with fifteen fetuses has been reported. One set of sextuplets survived to term.

Contraception

The truly frightening data and graphs of the demographers have brought us to a realization of the reckless rate at which we are threatening the world we live in by overpopulation. Certainly the dramatic decrease in mortality rates, primarily through the control of infectious processes, has increased the number of people reaching and surviving the reproductive age. At present, approximately 98 percent of children in developed countries reach reproductive age. In 1798 Malthus stated that "the power of population is infinitely greater than the power in the earth to produce subsistence for man." He foresaw but one inevitable consequence of the clash between population increase and food restriction: a degradation in the quality of human life, marked by widespread misery and vice. Roger Short, writing on this subject, states that "more terrifying than Malthus' concept of a finite limitation to population growth imposed by the available food supply would be the development of an infinite capacity for food production." The effects on our environment of unlimited population growth would be intolerable.

Is it possible to stem the relentless tide of population growth? There are many who believe we have already passed the point at which we can depend on individual motivation. Governmental decree may be forthcoming, if not in this century, surely in the next. A person's sexual behavior is not purely a personal affair if procreation results. If the world's population continues to grow at its present rate, doubling every 35 years, we must eventually reach a condition where life is not just intolerable, but impossible.

The methods for controlling population growth involve interrupting procreation before conception (contraception) or afterward (abortion). The subject of abortion is not entirely within the scope of this book, but suggested readings are provided. Contraception does merit detailed discussion in an endocrinology text. The emphasis will be placed on hormonal methods of interrupting the reproductive cycle, with brief coverage of other methods included.

Coitus Interruptus

This is the oldest and probably the most widespread of contraceptive methods. It is widely used in Europe and appears to be reasonably effective. There is no objective clinical evidence that its use is psychologically harmful.

Condoms

The use of condoms is the most common method of family planning in many developed countries. Modern condoms are mass produced and tested routinely for defects. More recently, they have been lubricated with silicones. Their use provides a simple, reasonably reliable method of contraception. One advantage is a reduction in the risk of venereal infection, and a possible reduction in the risk of cancer of the cervix in the female partner.

Vaginal Spermicides and Diaphragms

Unfortunately, the fitting of a diaphragm requires a trained person, and motivation is required in the user. Various spermicidal jellies may be used alone or in conjunction with the diaphragm. These methods are less effective than other means of contraception and are being used less often now than formerly.

Rhythm Method

For the rhythm method to be most effective, the individual must chart the length of her menstrual cycle for at least a year, noting daily basal body temperatures. The irregularity of the adolescent cycle, especially in the first years following menarche, makes this method rather ineffective in the teenager. Even in the adult, restriction of intercourse to the "safe period" is not a particularly effective means of contraception (Table 13–2).

Although menstrual cycles are more regular between ages 20 and 40, two thirds of all cycles will vary in length as much as six days, and in one third the variability will be even greater than this. The fact that an abnormally short or long cycle can occur at any time means that a woman using the rhythm method is never completely free from the risk of pregnancy. In the four years before the menopause the variability in cycle length is extreme, and the rhythm method becomes almost useless.

In measuring the effectiveness of contraception, the term "women-years" is used. This is based on 13 cycles per year for one woman, or one cycle for 13 women, or any combination thereof. The rhythm method at its *most effective use* will produce about 14 pregnancies per 100 women-years, a rate considerably above that for patients using other contraceptive methods (Table 13–2).

Intra-uterine Contraceptive Device (IUD)

It has been known for a long time that a foreign body placed in the uterus causes infertility. Such devices do not prevent fertilization. Present evidence suggests that a foreign body reaction occurs, with a migration of leucocytes into the uterine lumen creating a hostile environment in which blastocysts cannot survive or implant. The IUD is a highly effective method of contraception; however, pregnancies have occurred with the device in situ and after unnoticed expulsion. Women who have never borne a child (nulliparous women) are more likely to

TABLE 13–2. Failure Rates (Pregnancies per 100 Woman-years) for Various Types of Contraception*

Method	Percent	Method	Percent
No contraception	75–100	Suppositories	8–15
Withdrawal	20– 35	Diaphragm and Jelly	6–15
Douche	20– 30	IUD	2– 4
Rhythm	14– 25	Oral contraceptives:	
Foam	10– 20	Sequential	1.0
Condom	10– 16	Combined	0.5
Jelly alone	8– 15		

*From Page, E., Villee, C., and Villee, E. *Human Reproduction.* Philadelphia: W. B. Saunders Company, 1972, p. 84.

expel the IUD, and discomfort, pain, and bleeding occur more frequently in this group.

The IUD must be inserted under aseptic conditions by a physician or other trained personnel. Although it is less effective than hormonal contraception, the IUD is being used on a large scale in countries where the dependable use of steroids is unrealistic.

The IUD may have unfortunate sequellae. The uterus may be perforated at the time of insertion, and the IUD may be found subsequently in an extra-uterine location. The Dalkon shield has a particularly high incidence of extra-uterine placement, with the additional disadvantage of a greater reactivity in cases of peritoneal position. The manufacture of this IUD has been discontinued. The risk of infection in the upper genital tract is another problem for the IUD user.

Recently, copper coils have been added to IUD's in hopes of reducing the pregnancy rate among users. The presence of copper in the endometrial cavity causes an outpouring of white blood cells. This tissue reactivity may explain the observed decrease in pregnancy rate and in expulsion rate in patients using copper IUD's. Silastic IUD's which release progesterone are also being used clinically on a trial basis. Apparently the progesterone renders the endometrium unsuitable for implantation.

Interference with Testicular Function

At present, extensive research is in progress to find contraceptives for males that either will prevent the process of spermatogenesis or will act upon the mature spermatozoa in the epididymis. Inhibition of gonadotropins is probably not acceptable, for androgen production would be diminished, as would be the libido.

The spermatogenic process is accurately timed and thus lends itself to manipulation. In man the process takes 10 to 11 weeks, with an additional 1 to 2 weeks for sperm maturation and transport through the epididymis. Therefore, inhibition of this process could result in the absence of spermatozoa in the ejaculate at any time from two weeks at the earliest to some two to three months.

After proliferation of the spermatogonia, the resulting spermatocytes undergo a long phase of growth in preparation for the crucial meiotic stage. During meiosis, cells are particularly vulnerable to damage by radiation or chemicals. Experiments with rats have shown that certain nitroaromatic compounds and dichloroacetyl diamines gradually inhibit spermatogenesis, primarily affecting cells in the meiotic phase. The dichloroacetyl diamines seemed to show particular promise in leaving sexual activity unimpaired and in having low toxicity, reversible effects, and specific effects on the testis. Unfortunately, consumption of alcohol during treatment led to severe vomiting (an Antabuse-like effect).

After meiosis, no further cell division occurs. Each spermatocyte produces four spermatids, which are transformed into mature sperm by the process of *spermiogenesis.* Certain compounds such as the anti-cancer drug Tretamine alter this process in rats. When male rats treated with this drug mated, their sperm appeared normal, but fertilization did not ensue. The term "functional" sterility has been used for the effects of Tretamine and other similar drugs. The compound is stable and effective orally. Investigations using monkeys should provide additional information as to its biological action in primates.

Another target for contraception would be spermatozoa in the epididymis. A variety of drugs have been shown to affect epididymal sperm in rats. Cyproterone acetate, implanted as a capsule, will produce sterility in rats. Treated males were fertile after two months but sterile in three months. The sperm produced during the period of infertility were nonmotile. The rats became fertile two to three weeks after removal of the capsule, which indicated that epididymal sperm were affected. Since cyproterone acetate is an anti-androgen, this observation suggests a role of androgen in sperm nutrition.

Vasectomy and Tubal Ligation

These are relatively irreversible methods of contraception that are being used with increasing frequency. Vasectomy is certainly an easier and safer operation than tubal ligation. Since the sperm contribute little to the volume of seminal fluid, ejaculation is unimpaired. The sperm, however, must be resorbed by the body. Nancy Alexander has shown that in the human, macrophages absorb the sperm; however, in time, antibodies to sperm appear in the blood. Dr. Alexander emphasizes how little we know about the long range effects of vasectomy. Reanastomosis of the ligated vas deferens has been successfully performed; however, comparable attempts at reanastomosis of the oviducts in the female have been disappointing.

Hormonal Contraception: The Pill

The era of hormonal contraception really began with the studies of Rock and Pincus, who treated infertile women with progestins. These progestins had the biological activity of progesterone but possessed 18 carbons instead of 21. The investigators administered derivatives of 19-nortestosterone from day 5 to day 25 of the menstrual cycle; withdrawal bleeding occurred a few days later. They noted that ovulation could be abolished at will for as long as desired by the use of such hormones.

The early preparations of the progestins were contaminated with estrogen. Neither Rock nor Pincus wanted estrogens in the preparations because of their known side effects, such as nausea and weight gain. However, when the progestins were completely purified, and free of estrogen, their effectiveness as contraceptives was lessened, and breakthrough bleeding occurred. Thus estrogen was deliberately added back to the "pill."

Once it was recognized that ovulation could be effectively inhibited by hormones, extensive field studies began. One of the first was conducted in Puerto Rico in 1955 under the direction of Dr. Celso Garcia. The field study used a hormonal preparation called Enovid, which contained 10 mg of norethynodrel (a progestin, 17α-ethinyl-5,10-estren-17β-ol-3-one) and 0.15 mg of mestranol (3-methyl-17α-ethinyl estradiol). This and other field studies showed that if taken regularly as indicated, hormonal contraceptives are essentially 100 percent effective (Table 13–2).

Two methods of hormonal contraception have come into vogue. The combination method uses steroid preparations containing an estrogen and a progestin and are usually given for 21 days followed by a break of 7 days, during which uterine bleeding occurs. The sequential method utilizes estrogen for 14 to 16 days followed by an estrogen-progestin mixture for 5 to 7 days, followed by uterine bleeding. In both methods gonadotropin secretion is suppressed, thus preventing ovulation. In addition, the "pill" prevents the normal maturation of the endometrium and produces cervical mucus hostile to sperm penetration.

As the pill became more widely used, data began to accumulate suggesting certain side effects, primarily related to the dose of estrogen in the preparations. These side effects ranged from discomforts such as nausea, vomiting, weight gain, headaches, and breast soreness to serious complications such as increased incidence of thrombophlebitis. In 1968 two British publications, one from the Committee on Safety of Drugs and the other from the Medical Research Council, cited evidence to show that the risk of death from complications is about six times higher among users of the pill than among nonusers (1.3 vs. 0.2 deaths per 100,000 per year). The risk of death from all causes in pregnancy is 22.8 per 100,000 per year; hormonally, the individual on the pill may be considered a little bit pregnant. The British studies showed an incidence of thromboembolic disease 10 times higher in pill users than in controls; however, the incidence of the disease in the control population cited in the studies was low compared with that in other studies. In 1969 the U. S. Food and Drug Administration released a report stating that although the incidence of thromboembolism *may* be slightly increased by use of the pill, the reported incidence is erroneously high. Nevertheless, it is recommended that the pill not be used by patients with thrombophlebitis, thromboembolic disorders, cerebral apoplexy, or a past history of these disorders. The risk of thromboembolic disease appears to be related to the estrogen content of the pill.

Patients on the pill may rarely give evidence of liver dysfunction. Liver function tests (BSP retention) may be abnormal, or frank jaundice may develop. This is extremely rare, but a history of impaired liver function is considered a contraindication to the use of the pill. Since a mild increase in blood pressure may be induced by estrogens, hypertension constitutes another contraindication. The relationship of estrogens to cancer will be discussed in Chapter Fourteen.

The fear that estrogen may have deleterious effects has prompted the use of less and less estrogen in various proprietary preparations of the pill and even a return to the original idea of Rock and Pincus of a preparation containing only progestin. Continuous administration of progestin abolishes the menstrual cycle if the dose is large enough. To avoid the very high doses of progestin a small amount of estrogen is usually necessary.

In addition to contraception the pill has certain beneficial side effects. Since dysmenorrhea (painful menstruation) occurs only in ovulatory cycles, the use of hormonal therapy relieves or greatly reduces menstrual cramps. Presumably these cramps are due to the effect of progesterone on the uterus. Estrogen causes softening and dilatation of the cervix, but apparently after ovulation the cervix closes and becomes quite spastic, presumably owing to progesterone. This is particularly true in nulliparous women, who have not experienced the cervical dilatation of childbirth. When uterine contractions occur at the onset of menses, crampy pain is felt just above the pubic bone. Dysmenorrhea is influenced by a variety of physiological and psychological events. It is more common and more severe in girls and women who are high-strung and nervous. Genetic factors probably play a role. Dysmenorrhea is not uncommon in women of Mediterranean descent, whereas it is rather rare in girls of Nordic extraction.

About two to three percent of patients receiving hormonal contraceptives have amenorrhea post-treatment. Most of these patients have a history of irregular periods prior to the start of treatment. In general, it is wise to allow the teenager to establish a normal menstrual pattern prior to the use of hormonal contraception.

HORMONES AND SEXUAL IDENTITY

Appropriate hormonal secretion by the gonads and the action of these hormones on the target tissue are major organic factors which determine sexual identity. The hormonal secretion, of course, depends upon structurally and functionally normal gonads; the condition of the gonads in turn depends on the chromosomal arrangement and chromatin pattern. The hormonal secretion also depends upon the presence of the various enzymes and cofactors necessary for hormone synthesis. The action of the sex hormones on target tissues depends upon the presence of the appropriate steroid receptors in these tissues and upon the cellular "machinery" to implement the alterations in the synthesis of nucleic acids and proteins brought about by the steroid-receptor complex. The action of testicular hormones on the target tissues should bring about unequivocal male sexual differentiation of the external genitalia and should stabilize Wolffian ducts induced by testicular hormones. The lack of testicular hormones should bring about female sexual differentiation. The sex of rearing must be determined from the appearance of the external genitalia, the karyotype, and the functional potential of the gonads. Any abnormality which precludes the interaction of appropriate sex hormones and target cells may cause physical and, probably, psychological disturbances in sexual identity.

The final step in sexual identity—the psychological acceptance of the sex of rearing—does not always occur. Even with normal male karyotype, gonadal structure, and differentiation of the genitalia, an individual may not identify himself as a male, or may feel some ambiguity about his male role. After adolescence he may seek medical assistance in changing sex. Transsexual patients often have serious psychiatric disturbances and as a result the condition has been looked upon as a "psychiatric problem." Studies of sexual differentiation of the brain in animals offer an "organic" explanation for transsexual and homosexual patients. The brain is susceptible to androgen effect for only a limited period of time either in fetal or in early postnatal life. If insufficient androgen is available or if the brain cannot respond to androgens (owing to a lack of androgen receptors, perhaps), masculinization of the brain would fail to occur. Thus prenatal hormones probably confer intrinsic sexuality. Kilodny and coworkers have shown that male homosexuals have lower testosterone levels and sperm counts than do "normal" male control subjects. Money and his associates have studied female offspring androgenized in utero. Such offspring exhibit behavior more characteristic of males. This behavior includes preference for male sports, toys, and clothes, a lack of maternal instinct, and greater than average female sexual arousal by visual stimuli. However, none of these offspring showed any predisposition toward lesbianism. Thus the question of how much of sexual identity is imprinted in utero and how much is acquired postnatally remains unanswered.

LIBIDO

Libido, or sexual desire, is dependent in part upon androgens. In the male the androgens are derived from the testis, in the female from the adrenal. The physiological and psychological mechanisms underlying libido are uncertain. There is no doubt that androgens increase the degree of congestion of the clitoris. If the manipulation of the base of the clitoris is important for enjoyment of the sex act, as experts in this field avow, clitoral congestion may play a role in increased libido. Some women treated with progestins that have androgenic effects have noted increased sexual response. Prepubertal females with congenital adrenocortical hyperplasia may have premature or exaggerated sexual desire. As shown by Sutherland and collaborators, adrenalectomy and hypophysectomy produce almost complete loss of female libido, which can be restored by testosterone. The role of estrogens in the sex drive is uncertain. Sexual motivation (lever pressing to admit male) in female rhesus monkeys was increased by administration to the monkeys of either testosterone (0.5 mg per day) or estradiol (0.5 to 10 μg per day), but actual sexual activity was increased only by estradiol.

Women using hormonal contraceptives may experience heightened sexual desire. Since some of the progestins in contraceptive preparations may have certain androgenic properties, increased libido may be explainable on this basis. However, changes in libido can be effected by psychological factors as well. The sex act may be more enjoyable with the elimination of mechanical contraceptive devices, and a more relaxed attitude (no fear of pregnancy) may permit more extended and uninterrupted foreplay.

Far more labile than the female libido is the male libido. The male is generally more susceptible to psychological factors in his sexual activity than is the female. His self-esteem is more closely allied to the sex act, and impotence is far more debilitating psychologically to the male than frigidity is to the female. The sexually aroused female on the pill may frustrate or even render impotent the marginal male. The endocrinologist and gynecologist must be prepared to deal with the psychological as well as the physical aspects of sexual inadequacy.

Libido without gratification leads to frustration. Thus there is a sequence to normal sexual activity: desire, activity, and gratification. Masters and Johnson have catalogued the various physiological reactions of men and women during the sex act. They describe four phases: excitement, plateau, orgasm, and resolution. They define orgasm as the summit of physical and emotional gratification in sexual activity. The various sexual stimuli produce a state of vasocongestion and muscular tension which is released at orgasm. Orgasm can be produced either heterosexually, homosexually, or by masturbation.

Women tend to have their greatest sexual activity at a later age than do men. This is not surprising, for men handle their genitals during urination and thus learn the pleasurable sensations which ensue at an early age. In addition the nature of our society permits greater sexual license at an earlier age for boys than for girls. The advent of effective contraceptives and changing sexual mores will undoubtedly tend to equalize the sexual experiences of the two sexes.

SUMMARY

The attainment of adult sexual function occupies the years of adolescence. The characteristic growth spurt, probably due to GH secretion and the enhanced secretion of androgen precursors by the adrenals, heralds gonadal maturation and the onset of secondary sex characteristics. The target tissues for testosterone or its metabolite dihydrotestosterone include the penis, testis, prostate, seminal vesicle, skin, muscle, bone, kidney, and brain. The tissues respond in different ways: there is an increase in size (penis, testis, muscle) and an increase in function (sex hair growth, sebaceous gland secretion in the skin, secretion by the prostate and seminal vesicles, and erythropoietin production in the kidney). Moreover, there is maturation of the bone and brain. Estrogens stimulate ovarian follicles and the breast, alter the structure and function of endometrial and vaginal cells, and change the distribution of fat in the body. In addition, they probably play a role in bone maturation. Progesterone acts primarily on tissues previously primed by estrogens. It is the "pregnancy" hormone in that it produces and maintains a secretory endometrium in which implantation of the blastocyst can occur. Breasts also are influenced by progesterone.

Any interruption in the pathway from hypothalamus to pituitary to gonad disrupts the process of sexual maturation and function. If this pathway has never functioned normally, the resulting hypogonadism produces primary amenorrhea and lack of breast development in girls and azoospermia with small genitals in boys. Primary disorders of the gonads can produce a similar state of hypogonadism. Often these primary gonadal disorders are due to chromosomal aberrations (gonadal dysgenesis, Klinefelter's syndrome). A failure of target tissue to respond to testosterone can produce "amenorrhea" in a seemingly normal female (testicular feminizing syndrome).

Once sexual maturation occurs, disruption of the hypothalamic-pituitary-gonadal axis can produce secondary amenorrhea in girls and impotence and sterility in males. Primary disorders of gonads after sexual maturation usually involve infectious or space-occupying lesions (cysts, tumors). If such lesions produce excessive amounts of estrogen or androgen, appropriate changes in physical characteristics will ensue. Gonadal tumors producing hormones must be differentiated from androgen-producing and estrogen-producing tumors of the adrenal.

The remarkable physical changes in puberty are mirrored by psychological changes. Androgens, produced in increased quantities in both girls and boys, heighten sexual desire. At the same time the teenager must cope with his or her identity as a male or female. Intra-uterine imprinting of sexual identity by androgens plus a variety of environmental factors determine the completeness of this identity. Failure to identify with the sex of rearing (as seen in homosexuality and transsexuality) creates enormous problems in our present society, where homosexual practices are considered taboo. The legal problems associated with surgical alteration of the sex of an individual are enormous. Thus our society thinks in terms of all or none and can not or will not recognize the individual of ambiguous identity.

The ease with which conception occurs in our present relatively disease-free age brings us to an era of overpopulation and the necessity for control of conception. Numerous devices are available. Of all the reversible methods, hormonal contraception is the most effective; however, it is expensive and requires the motivation to take a pill every day. Abortion, although effective, is even more expensive and is more debilitating psychologically. The abortifacient prostaglandins show promise as a "do it yourself" medication that can be used to induce a menstrual period regularly.

Of all the areas of medicine, it is in the realm of sexual maturation and identity that the most patience and understanding is required. The young adolescent needs assurance and guidance as he or she explores this new world. The physician should be prepared to discuss all aspects of sex with an open mind and to guide the adolescent in coping with the problems of puberty.

SUGGESTED READINGS

Textbook of Endocrinology, edited by Robert Williams, W. B. Saunders Company, Philadelphia, 1974.
Recommended are Chapter 6, "The Testes," by C. A. Paulsen and Chapter 7, "The Ovaries," by G. T. Ross and R. L. Vande Wiele. Both provide excellent up-to-date coverage of the development and function of the gonads. Syndromes of gonadal dysfunction are discussed in detail.

Pediatric and Adolescent Gynecology, Pediatric Clinics of North America, *Vol. 19, No. 3,* Edited by A. Altchek, W. B. Saunders Company, Philadelphia, August, 1972.
Several chapters in this volume are particularly pertinent. Normal sexual maturation in the female, premature thelarche, hirsutism, and amenorrhea are discussed. Abnormalities of sexual function such as gonadal dysgenesis and testicular feminizing syndrome are ably covered. Of special interest, since it is usually not covered in detail in textbooks of endocrinology, is the section dealing with the sexually active teenager. Problems such as rape, adolescent pregnancy, abortion, and contraception are discussed openly, bringing insight to the special problems of adolescence.

Artificial Control of Reproduction (Book 5 of *Reproduction in Mammals*), edited by C. R. Austin and R. V. Short, Cambridge University Press, New York, 1973.
This book deals realistically with the problems of controlling reproduction. The emphasis is on methods to increase productivity of domestic animals and to decrease human overpopulation. A particularly thought-provoking chapter by Roger Short on "Reproduction and Human Society" deals with social and religious attitudes toward contraception from ancient times to the present.

The Pill, Robert W. Kistner, Delacorte Press, New York, 1969.
This book is designed for the lay audience to answer questions about the pill. It traces the history of the pill and its use as a contraceptive. Dr. Kistner has a large clinical practice and has had firsthand experience with the pill from the early days of its use He covers everything from "the pill and your complexion" to "the pill and the Catholic Church." A well-written, well-documented account of oral contraceptives.

PERTINENT LITERATURE REFERENCES

Davidoff, F., and Federman, D. D.: Mixed gonadal dysgenesis. Ped. *52*:725, 1973.

Lipsett, M. B.: Benign masculinizing adrenal adenomas. New England J. Med. *289*:802, 1973.

Rebar R., et al.: Gonadotropin response to synthetic LRF: Dose-response relationship in men. J. Clin. Endocrinol. Metab. *36*:10, 1973.

Root, A. W.: Endocrinology of puberty. J. Pediat. *83*:187, 1973.

Ruf, K. B.: How does the brain control the process of puberty? Z. Neurol. *204*:96, 1973.

Winter, J. S. D., and Faiman, C.: The development of cyclic pituitary-gonadal function in adolescent females. J. Clin. Endocrinol. Metab. *37*:714, 1973.

PART FIVE

THE ADULT

CHAPTER FOURTEEN

Postmaturation and Senescence

Following the completion of growth and the attainment of sexual maturity, a series of cumulative changes occur over the years which inexorably lead to a decreasing capacity for adaptation and a decreasing ability to maintain homeostasis in the face of internal or external stress (senescence). Most of these changes do not become clinically evident until "middle age," but certainly the basic processes begin long before that. For example, a progressive age-related decrease in bone density and mass occurs, and the gradual vertebral compression may result in a decreasing ratio of body length to arm span. The regenerative capacity of articular cartilage decreases with age, and the accumulated insults to joint surfaces, aggravated by excessive weight, make arthritic complaints more common in middle and old age. A sedentary life coupled with the intake of calories in excess of those expended leads to expanded adipose tissue mass. Body weight increases despite a decrease in lean body mass. The functional capacity of various organs declines linearly with age. The most striking difference in types of disorders between youth and adulthood is the shift toward chronic diseases (coronary heart disease, hypertension, peptic ulcer) with advancing age.

The endocrine system is involved either directly or indirectly in many of these changes. Indeed, alterations of endocrine function with age are so predictable that different norms must often be used in assessing endocrine disturbances. Some of the problems of aging which relate to the endocrine system will be discussed to attain a better understanding of the phenomenon of senescence.

CARBOHYDRATE METABOLISM: ADULT ONSET DIABETES

It seems well established that there is a gradual decline with age in the body's ability to utilize glucose. The concentration of glucose in the blood one hour after the ingestion of a standard glucose load increases steadily with age (Figure 14–1). In some surveys the proportion of glucose tolerance tests that were abnormal by accepted standards reached such a high figure (25 percent over the age of 70 in one survey) that the interpretation of such tests in older people is open to question. The incidence of adult onset diabetes mellitus increases with age. Thus it is often difficult to differentiate the age-related decline in glucose tolerance from the glucose intolerance resulting from a genetic diabetic trait.

Most reports have shown that fasting insulin values are not affected by age. Some studies indicate, however, that the amount of insulin secreted after glucose ingestion (during both the early and late phases of insulin secretion) is less in older subjects than in the young. The early insulin release is, of course, an important determinant of glucose tolerance. The response of the β cells to arginine stimulation is also reduced in the older subject. The work by Sherwin and colleagues suggests that peripheral sensitivity to insulin is not altered with age, nor is the metabolic clearance rate or basal secretory rate of insulin. Duckworth and Kitabchi found, however, that a larger proportion of the immunoreactive insulin released after glucose stimulation in older subjects was proinsulin, which is metabolically far less effective than insulin. This plus the decreased secretion of insulin in the early phase of glucose stimulation and the increased total body fat with age may explain the observed decline in glucose tolerance with age.

If we consider diabetes as a syndrome with many causes, then the "diabetes" of aging, as defined by impaired glucose tolerance, represents just one of the many forms of this multifactorial disease. It could be argued that the mild diabetes of the elderly represents a manifestation of the "diabetic gene." This would be hard to prove or disprove for a

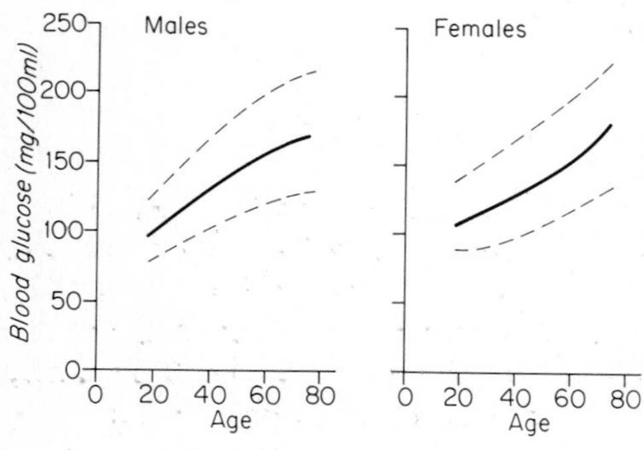

FIGURE 14–1. Relationship between age and blood glucose one hour following a 100 gm oral glucose challenge in males and females in an American community—Tecumseh, Michigan. Solid lines are 50th percentiles; dashed lines are 20th (lower) and 80th (upper) percentiles. (From Epstein, F. H., et al.: Prevalence of chronic diseases and distribution of selected physiological variables in a total community, Tecumseh, Michigan, Am. J. Epidemiol. *81*:307, 1965, as adapted in Smith, D. and Bierman, E., eds., *The Biologic Ages of Man*. Philadelphia: W. B. Saunders Company, 1973, p. 167.)

disease that has no genetic marker and that may manifest itself at any age. Even death at age 90 of a non-diabetic individual does not rule out the presence of the "diabetic gene," for subsequent manifestation of diabetes might have been observed if the individual had lived longer. Thus it is generally assumed that diabetes mellitus is inherited multifactorially with a continuous gradation from normal to abnormal. Undoubtedly hereditary factors are important; however, environmental influences, particularly in adult-onset diabetes, may bring about the onset of clinical disease.

Diabetes mellitus is more than twice as prevalent at age 70 than at age 50. In contrast to the juvenile onset diabetes, diabetes mellitus in the older age group is commonly of a milder, more stable form. Ketosis develops readily in the juvenile diabetic but rarely in the adult form. This is not a "hard and fast" rule, however, and it must be remembered that a differentiation of diabetes into these two forms, although clinically convenient, may bear little relationship to the etiology of the "diabetic syndrome."

Occasionally associated with mild diabetes (or even in the absence of overt diabetes) in individuals over age 60 is the syndrome of *hyperosmolar nonketotic coma.* The onset of symptoms is slow, with a gradual progression to a comatose state. Presumably, some precipitating factor aggravates an already existing diabetic state. Insulin deficiency develops, and the plasma concentration of glucose rises to over 500 mg/100 ml. Characteristically the plasma concentration of bicarbonate and the pH are normal, and no ketonemia occurs. It has been sugested that affected patients secrete enough insulin to produce an antilipolytic effect (enough to prevent ketosis) but insufficient amounts to promote adequate glucose uptake by peripheral tissues. Obviously, any impairment of renal function will prevent excretion of the excess blood glucose and exacerbate the condition. Indeed, dehydration may be a precipitating factor, producing oliguria and a rising blood glucose. Diazide diuretics may precipitate this condition by depressing insulin secretion. Glucocorticoids and catecholamines (stress) are other precipitating factors. Some patients have a history of high intake of carbohydrate, which along with other contributing factors may aggravate an already existing age-related carbohydrate intolerance, precipitating hyperglycemia and coma.

Vascular complications of diabetes mellitus

The diabetic may have microvascular disease of the eye (diabetic retinopathy) or of the kidney (diabetic nephropathy) or arteriosclerotic disease of the large arteries (causing coronary and peripheral vascular occlusive disease) or any combination thereof. The etiology of the vascular disease of diabetes mellitus is unknown. It develops slowly, usually appearing many years after the onset of clinical diabetes. Accordingly, manifestations of vascular complications are most common in the adult who has had diabetes mellitus for many years (juvenile-onset).

Microvascular Disease

The characteristic lesion in diabetic microvascular disease is a thickened capillary basement membrane. Long-term diabetics, regardless of treatment, show this lesion; however, an age-related thickening of the capillary basement membrane has also been described by Williamson. Perhaps this thickening in the capillaries of the aged in some way represents a result of age-related carbohydrate intolerance.

Spiro has studied the glycoprotein of the capillary basement membrane. This glycoprotein contains large amounts of hydroxylysine and hydroxyproline. In addition, it contains glucose, galactose, mannose, hexosamine, sialic acid, and fucose. Spiro has found an increase in hydroxylysine residues in diabetic basement membranes as compared with those from non-diabetics. Disaccharide units are attached at the hydroxylysine residues, and Spiro postulates that the increased availability of glucose and the observed increase in glucosyltransferase activity* in experimental diabetes may explain the altered basement membrane structure. Insulin decreases the activity of glucosyltransferase. Membrane thickening would presumably be greater in tissues that are not dependent upon insulin for glucose uptake (i.e., retina, kidney). However, most investigators agree that there is little positive correlation between the extent of hyperglycemia and the amount of capillary basement membrane thickening.

Thickening of capillary basement membranes has been quantitated in biopsies of skin and muscle with the hope of detecting the *prediabetic* state. Because of variability in results from one biopsy site to another and because of age-related changes in membrane structure, this hope has not been realized. Nevertheless, it seems clear that the basement membrane of capillaries in the muscles of diabetic patients is thicker than that of age- and sex-matched normal subjects. The thickness increases with increased duration of the disease.

Diabetic Retinopathy

This condition is primarily a disease of the capillaries, with thickening of the basement membrane. On examining the retina, tortuosity and congestion of the retinal veins may be noted, followed by the appearance of microaneurysms (small dilatations in the capillaries or arterioles). These microaneurysms appear first in the macular area and in the lateral part of the temporal region. Hemorrhages and serous exudates may develop later. Waxy, hard, lipid-containing exudates are also seen.

New vessels arise and proliferate in response to the chronic microcirculatory deficiency and indicate a worsening of the disease. These new vessels grow forward into the vitreous chamber. They are fragile and

*Glucosyltransferase is the enzyme that attaches glucose to galactose already attached to hydroxylysine.

bleed often; the bleeding stimulates reparative fibrosis. This forward growth of vessels and fibrous tissue into the vitreous is called *retinitis proliferans*. When the fibrous tissue contracts, it often causes retinal detachment, with permanent loss of vision. The occurrence of proliferative changes tends to be more frequent in the juvenile-onset diabetic, but this may be related to the length of time required for the alterations in the retina to occur. It is rare to see retinopathy in patients whose diabetes becomes manifest after age 60.

The progress of retinopathy is erratic: periods of remission and exacerbation occur, and one eye is often more involved than the other. Vision may be lost gradually or suddenly. Twenty years after the initial diagnosis of diabetes mellitus, 80 percent of patients show some evidence of retinopathy, but only 10 percent show proliferative changes.

Diabetic Nephropathy

The kidney is among the most commonly affected organs in the diabetic with microvascular disease. Moreover, the renal involvement is one of the most common causes of death among diabetics, particularly in those patients with onset of disease before age 15. In genetically transmitted diabetes, characteristic thickening of the basement membrane in the renal glomerulus may develop very early—even before glucose intolerance can be demonstrated. The thickening may so progress that the entire glomerulus is replaced by a sheet of amorphous material. The thickening may also appear as nodular masses (described by Kimmelstiel and Wilson) which are characteristic of diabetes mellitus.

The earliest clinical sign of nephropathy is proteinuria, which may be intermittent at first. However, clinically evident nephropathy does not usually appear until 10 to 15 years after the onset of diabetes. Hypoproteinemia and edema develop as a result of the protein loss (nephrotic syndrome). The renal disease is progressive, and the hypertension which ensues eventually causes left ventricular hypertrophy. Sodium retention leads to hypervolemia and cardiac failure. The combination of the nephrotic syndrome and hypertension in a diabetic is known as Kimmelstiel-Wilson disease. With continued progression of the renal disease, uremia develops and death may ensue.

Occlusive Vascular Disease

The medium- to small-caliber arteries of diabetics, especially the coronary and the leg arteries, tend to become occluded. Coronary artery disease tends to occur earlier in the diabetic than in the non-diabetic. The atheromatous changes underlying occlusive vascular disease are indistinguishable from those occurring in non-diabetics but tend to develop earlier and to a greater extent in the diabetic. Over 50 percent of all diabetics eventually die from coronary artery disease. Combined coronary and renal artery disease accounts for nearly 80 percent of all deaths in diabetics.

The elderly diabetic is especially subject to circulatory insufficiencies in the legs. Cold feet, nocturnal cramps in calf muscles, and pain in calf muscles on exercise are frequent complaints. Because of vascular insufficiency healing is slow. Gangrene of the foot, particularly the toes, may develop.

The treatment of occlusive disease is largely preventive. Good diabetic control, normal body weight, and avoidance of trauma to the extremities are indicated. Proper foot hygiene is imperative.

Metabolic complications of diabetes mellitus

Hyperglycemia per se seems to cause certain complications as a result of altered metabolism. In diabetes, glucose cannot be utilized properly by many cells, and alternative pathways of metabolism that are not dependent upon insulin become more active. One of these, the sorbitol pathway, is probably implicated in diabetic cataracts and diabetic neuropathy.

Cataracts

In the older individual, senile cataract has the same incidence in diabetic and non-diabetic patients; however, the progress of the disorder may well be more rapid in the diabetic. Experimentally, hyperglycemia alone can induce cataracts in animals. The lens is an insulin-independent tissue, and in the presence of hyperglycemia large amounts of glucose may enter the lenticular cell and be converted to sorbitol. The latter accumulates within the cell and increases intracellular osmolarity and subsequent water uptake, which promotes cataract formation. This is an analogous situation to the cataract formation that occurs in galactosemics. The enzyme aldose reductase catalyzes the conversion of either glucose or galactose to sorbitol or galactitol. These sugar alcohols are rather poorly transported across cell membranes and thus tend to accumulate within cells when formed in large amounts. Sorbitol accumulation in the lens can be prevented by blocking aldose reductase, thereby limiting cataract formation.

Neuropathies

The sorbitol pathway is very active in diabetic peripheral nerve; large amounts of glucose, sorbitol, and fructose accumulate. This accumulation is directly related to the concentration of glucose in the blood. Sorbitol accumulation in nerve in vitro can be prevented by blocking aldose reductase with tetramethylene glutaric acid. There is some evidence that the sorbitol pathway is operative in the Schwann cell. Apparently, the massive accumulation of sorbitol in the diabetic Schwann cell leads to impaired function. The latter could lead to segmental demyelination, which is found in most diabetics examined postmortem.

The clinical manifestations of diabetic neuropathy are varied. Most commonly, chronic symmetrical sensory neuropathy in the extremities is noted. This involves loss of pain sense before loss of touch and compounds the vascular disease in the legs. The sensory loss is greatest in the peripheral portions and produces the "glove and stocking" loss of sensation. Perforating ulcers develop readily under these conditions. Joints may become swollen and distorted, and they may show painless hypermotility, indicating a Charcot-type degeneration.

Mixed sensory and motor neuropathies can also occur. Weakness in dorsiflexion of the foot may indicate peroneal nerve involvement. Flexion of the hip may be impaired if the femoral nerve is involved. Disturbed function of autonomic nerves may also be noted. Electroneural studies show that conduction rates are decreased in diabetic sensory, motor, and autonomic nerves even before there are any clinical signs of diabetic neuropathy.

TREATMENT OF DIABETES MELLITUS AND ITS COMPLICATIONS IN THE ADULT

Often the adult patient with mild hyperglycemia can be managed by simply restricting dietary calories. Large caloric loads are managed poorly by diabetics; therefore, not only the total daily caloric intake but its distribution must be stressed. Intermittent periods of fasting and feasting should be avoided in the obese diabetic; several small meals a day are preferable to three large meals. The American Diabetes Association currently recommends a roughly normal proportion of carbohydrate (45 to 50 percent), protein (15 percent), and fat. At present, severe restriction of total carbohydrate intake does not seem to be warranted. The obese diabetic should be encouraged to exercise in addition to restricting his caloric intake. Exercise is an excellent means of enhancing glucose utilization without the necessity of increased insulin secretion. Normal individuals actually inhibit insulin secretion during exercise via activation of the sympathetic nervous system. It must be remembered, however, that in diabetics receiving insulin therapy, hypoglycemia may develop with exercise unless calories are provided immediately beforehand. The use of insulin in the therapy of diabetes mellitus was discussed in Chapter Ten.

The Sulfonylureas

When the then new sulfonamide *p*-amino-benzene-sulfonamide-isopropyl thiodiazol was used in German-occupied France during World

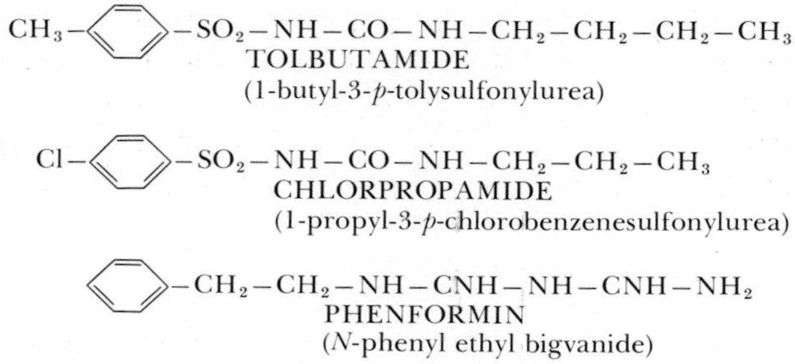

FIGURE 14–2. Representations of three oral antidiabetic compounds.

War II for the control of typhoid fever, hypoglycemia was noted to occur in patients receiving the drug. A single dose of this drug given subcutaneously, intravenously, or orally to a normal fasting dog produced progressive and prolonged hypoglycemia. Such an effect was not demonstrable if the animal had been previously pancreatectomized. Thus the mode of action seemed to involve the release of insulin from the pancreas.

In 1956 German workers experimented with a compound in which the para amino group of a sulfonamide was replaced by a methyl group. Without the amino group the compound was no longer bacteriostatic but still possessed the ability to stimulate insulin secretion. This compound, later called tolbutamide, is a sulfonylurea (Figure 14–2).

The sulfonylureas act on the β cell of the pancreas, stimulating release of insulin. They are therefore useful only to patients with intact β cells. They are rarely used in juvenile-onset diabetes mellitus. Their chief value is in patients who develop diabetes after age 40. Chlorpropamide (Figure 14–2), one of the most useful oral hypoglycemic agents, is poorly metabolized (half-life about 40 hours) and has a long duration of action; thus only one daily dose is required. The use of chlorpropamide is dependent upon renal excretion and is therefore contraindicated in patients with reduced renal function. Tolbutamide, which is carboxylated in the liver to the inactive compound carboxytolbutamide, has a much shorter half-life (three to five hours) and requires two or three doses per day for effective control of hyperglycemia. Even in patients with responsive β cells, about 15 percent do not respond to sulfonylureas (primary failure), and of those who show a good response for a month or more, about 25 percent ultimately escape from control (secondary failure).

The side effects of the sulfonylureas are not inconsequential. Gastrointestinal symptoms may be troublesome. Chlorpropamide potentiates the action of vasopressin and may produce hyponatremia and water intoxication. In some patients who use sulfonylureas, flushing of the face, headache, and tachycardia follow the ingestion of alcohol. The possibility of hypoglycemia due to overdosage or accumulation of the drug must always be considered. Patients who have hypoglycemia and who use oral hypoglycemic agents should be hospitalized and treated with glucose. Because of the long half-life of these compounds, the patient should be observed for at least 48 hours.

Biguanides

Biguanides do not depend upon insulin for their actions. The exact mechanism of action of these compounds is unknown, but two of their major effects are an increased glucose uptake in peripheral tissues and a decreased rate of absorption from the small intestine. Unfortunately, side effects (mostly gastrointestinal) are common. Phenformin (N-phenyl ethyl biguanide, Figure 14–2) has a short duration of action and must be taken several times a day. A sustained release form of phenformin with a long half-life is available for clinical use. One hundred mg per day is considered the maximum dose; above this level gastrointestinal effects (epigastric pain and nausea) become quite frequent.

Cardiovascular Effects of Tolbutamide and Phenformin

In 1961, an eight-year study was initiated under the sponsorship of the National Institutes of Health to determine the long range efficacy of oral hypoglycemic agents vs. insulin in therapy for diabetes mellitus. The two agents included in the investigation were tolbutamide and phenformin. Much to the surprise of the investigators, the results showed an increase (twofold) in cardiovascular-related deaths in patients treated with these oral agents as opposed to the values for patients on insulin therapy or receiving placebos. The study itself has been criticized by many; nevertheless, the justification for the use of oral hypoglycemic agents is now being reviewed carefully. Although we do not know if all hypoglycemic agents are equally hazardous, or even if this hazard is real, most physicians feel that the small benefits derived from the use of the oral hypoglycemic agents do not warrant exposing the patient to the potential hazards of the drugs (most patients in the older age group can be controlled by caloric restriction alone). Certainly there is no evidence to date that these drugs prevent the cardiovascular and neurologic complications of diabetes mellitus. Accordingly, there is no compelling reason for their use in most patients with diabetes.

MINERAL METABOLISM: OSTEOPOROSIS

Osteoporosis is traditionally defined as a condition in which there is a generalized decrease in bone mass. There is a progressive loss in the amount of mineralized tissue; however, the structure of the bone that remains is normal. Osteoporosis may be present but not evident by radiographic studies, since about 30 to 50 percent of mineral must be lost before osteoporosis can be detected with certainty. Ideally, to confirm the diagnosis one should biopsy bone and subject it to chemical and histologic analysis. However, this is not always possible. Osteoporosis often affects the vertebral bodies particularly severely, and their locale is not a very suitable biopsy site.

Osteoporosis develops from about age 30 onward, with its rate of progress increasing with advancing age. Different bones undergo rarefaction at different rates. This wasting of the skeleton with age has raised the question as to whether osteoporosis represents a normal or abnormal phenomenon in the elderly. Is it a disease state or an inexorable accompaniment of senescence?

George Nichols and his coworkers have measured rates of formation and resorption of collagen in bone samples from patients of varying ages. In the younger patients, an approximate balance was noted; in older individuals, the measured resorption rate exceeded the rate of formation. The fact that this osteoporosis begins long before the menopause indicates that estrogen deprivation is not the sole cause of postmenopausal osteoporosis; rather, estrogens may function to delay the process, perhaps by preventing the action of PTH on bone. Indeed, increased secretion of PTH by a previously undetected adenoma may manifest itself in the postmenopausal woman because of increased sensitivity to PTH in the estrogen-deprived state.

In general, the loss of cortical bone begins earlier and progresses more rapidly in women than in men. The rate of loss of trabecular bone from the central skeleton (vertebrae or ilium) is about the same in men and women and about the same as the rate of loss of cortical bone in women (10 percent per decade). Thus bone loss is a nearly universal occurrence in both sexes. Bone morphometry suggests that mean bone formation is normal while mean bone resorption is increased in osteoporosis. However, studies by Meunier and coworkers show no evidence of increased osteoclastic or periosteocytic resorption in senile osteoporosis. They noted a decreased population of marrow cells, which they postulate could reduce the number of osteoblasts formed. Examination of long bones by quantitative radiographic methods reveals a progressive loss of cortical bone mass with age, even though the external transverse diameter of the bone increases. This is due to a slight net positive skeletal balance on the periosteal surface but a more marked negative skeletal balance on the endosteal bone surface.

The cause of the bone loss in osteoporosis is unclear. In a small percentage of patients the concentration of PTH in blood is increased. PTH usually tends to decrease slightly with age; however, in some patients with overt osteoporosis, this normal decline in PTH is not seen, and concentrations of PTH in the blood are significantly higher than in normal subjects of corresponding age. PTH probably plays a causal role in bone loss in these patients. In the vast majority of osteoporotic patients, parathyroid function appears to be decreased, perhaps compensating for the increased rate of calcium release from bone. This may also explain the subnormal intestinal calcium absorption some investigators have noted in osteoporosis. The exact role (if any) of the parathyroid glands in senile osteoporosis remains a mystery.

Postmenopausal osteoporosis

Objective measurements of bone density leave little doubt that bone loss in women accelerates after the menopause. By quantitative microradiography it has been shown that the total extent of resorptive surface in postmenopausal bone is increased; however, histologic analysis reveals that although the extent of active resorptive surface was nearly normal, inactive resorptive surfaces were substantially increased. The active bone-forming surface was decreased. Rasmussen discusses these findings in terms of the bone cell cycle. He suggests that in osteoporosis the activation of new remodeling units continues at a nearly normal rate. Osteoclasts are formed from osteoprogenitor cells; however, they contain fewer nuclei than normal. These osteoclasts probably carry out their normal resorptive function but, after fission to preosteoblasts, the modulation of the latter to osteoblasts is delayed or occurs in reduced numbers. This could explain increased inactive or arrested resorptive surfaces, and the decline in active resorptive surfaces. Thus this theory, like Albright's original theory, suggests that osteoporosis in postmenopausal women results from the failure of osteoblastic activity. Rasmussen calls it an "uncoupling of the normal progression from resorption (osteoclast) to formation (osteoblast) in bone remodeling units."

The incidence of postmenopausal osteoporosis differs in the black and white races. In the United States approximately 25 percent of the white women aged 85 $\pm$ 10 years have clinically evident osteoporosis, whereas it is rare in black women. The bone mass at maturity is greater in the black race than in the white race, and if a steady decrement occurs with age, the black female may have more bone at age 85 than her white counterpart. Similarly, bone mass is greater in men than in women, perhaps explaining some of the sex difference in the incidence of osteoporosis.

The progression of osteoporosis can be followed by maintaining a record of standing body height. The height *gradually* decreases approximately 2 cm from ages 65 to 85 years, owing to degeneration of the intervertebral discs. The progressive kyphoscoliosis produces the characteristic dowager's hump. Spinal osteoporosis manifests itself with pain in the back. Typically compression fractures produce severe back pain coming on after some minor trauma.

Riggs has treated postmenopausal osteoporotic women with a physiologic replacement dose of estrogen and has noted significantly decreased levels of bone resorption and serum calcium but increased PTH. However, the biologic effectiveness of this PTH was impaired by the estrogen. These findings strongly suggest that estrogen exerts its effect by decreasing the responsiveness of bone to endogenous PTH. This effect could occur as a result of direct inhibition of osteoclast function or inhibition of the induction of osteoclasts from osteoprogenitor cells, or as a result of both. In long-term treatment (two to three years) of postmenopausal women with estrogen, Riggs found at first unaltered, then decreased, bone formation. The present evidence suggests that estrogen therapy may be worthwhile for slowing the progressive bone loss in osteoporosis. This effect, together with the desire to control menopausal symptoms, has encouraged the widespread use of estrogen therapy for the menopausal and postmenopausal female.

Secondary osteoporosis

A variety of endocrine disorders are associated with osteoporosis. In addition to endocrinopathies, immobilization and malabsorption syndromes may produce osteoporotic changes in bone. In malabsorption syndromes, defective mineralization may occur also, producing radiographic evidence of osteomalacia. In all forms of osteoporosis, bone resorption exceeds bone formation, regardless of the rate of either process.

Cortisol-induced Osteoporosis

In the description of the syndrome that bears his name, Cushing reported that one of its features was a tendency to spontaneous fracture. Albright subsequently recognized this as due to a form of osteoporosis which he attributed to the antianabolic effects of cortisol. About 40 percent of patients with Cushing's syndrome show radiologic evidence of osteoporosis, with vertebral fractures in 16 percent. With the widespread use of corticosteroid therapy today, the role of cortisol in inducing osteoporosis becomes of some importance.

The studies reported by Jee et al. suggest that there is an effect of cortisol on the activity of bone remodeling units in the mature rat. Small doses caused an increase in the size of the pool of osteoclasts and a decrease in the osteoblast pool. In other studies, cortisol was noted to inhibit the synthesis of bone collagen. Thus the balance of skeletal activity shifts in favor of resorption.

In the studies by Gallagher and coworkers, patients treated with prednisolone for a variety of medical problems had negative calcium balances. Calcium absorption was below the normal mean for calcium intake; however, in most cases urinary calcium was normal relative to intake. The role of cortisol in decreasing calcium absorption by the intestine may explain the tendency of corticosteroids to decrease the concentration of calcium in plasma.

Such hypocalcemia is undoubtedly the signal for the enhanced secretion of PTH in conditions of cortisol excess. The latter may explain the reduced tubular reabsorption of phosphate noted in affected patients. The actual skeletal changes produced by steroids are similar to those seen after PTH administration. In parathyroidectomized animals, cortisol leads to a slight decrease in the size of the osteoblast pool but no longer stimulates the activation of osteoprogenitor cells to osteoclasts. It is possible; therefore, that a factor in the pathogenesis of cortisol-induced osteoporosis may be a secondary hyperparathyroidism.

Hyperthyroidism

The rate of bone turnover is increased in hyperthyroidism. Osteoclastic activity is increased, causing thinning of bone trabeculae and increased porosity of cortical bone and fibrous tissue. Thus histologically there is a resemblance to the condition of bone in hyperparathyroidism; however, the secretion of PTH is decreased in hyperthyroidism.

In hyperthyroidism there is also increased urinary excretion of calcium and decreased absorption of calcium in the intestinal tract. However, there is no indication that there is any failure in the mineralization process associated with hyperthyroidism. All the evidence supports a direct effect of thyroxine on bone cells, with the rate of osteoclast formation exceeding the rate of osteoblast formation.

The treatment of osteoporosis

Where osteoporosis is secondary to an endocrine deficiency state (menopause) or to an excess of hormones (cortisol, thyroid hormone), attention should be directed to rectifying the hormonal imbalance. Unfortunately, there is no good evidence that correction of hormonal imbalance will produce a radiographically detectable increase in bone mass, particularly in adults. Nevertheless, such measures probably prevent or retard further thinning of bone.

Relief of symptoms is not a reliable index of therapeutic efficacy, because in many patients the disorder produces no symptoms of itself; rather, it leads to fracture, most commonly of the vertebral bodies, but also of the upper femur, humerus, distal forearm, and ribs. Thus in caring for the patient with osteoporosis the goal is largely preventive.

Physical exercise within the limitations of the patient should be encouraged; however, any activity which might precipitate vertebral compression (lifting heavy objects) should be avoided. Obese patients should be encouraged to lose weight.

Calcium intake should be maintained at a level of a least 800 mg per day; any amount less than this usually produces negative calcium balance. An excellent way of achieving this intake of calcium is for the patient to drink milk (there is about 1 g of calcium per quart) – preferably skim milk in order to minimize caloric intake. Supplemental calcium is often given in the form of calcium salts; however, prolonged high calcium intake leads to a progressively less positive calcium balance.

Although fluoride has been advocated for the therapy of osteoporosis, its efficacy remains to be established. There is no doubt that low doses of fluoride (less than 10 ppm), as in fluoridated water (which has beneficial effects against dental caries) are harmless; quite possibly, some beneficial effects on bone are achieved. In areas where the drinking water contains large amounts of fluoride (8 to 16 ppm), endemic fluorosis occurs, with abnormalities of the skeleton. Fluorine substitutes for surface hydroxyl ions in the crystal lattice of hydroxyapatite, leading to the formation of fluorapatite crystals. These crystals are larger, less soluble, and less subject to resorption than are the hydroxyapatite crystals. Large doses of fluoride (over 35 mg per day) stimulate bone formation, but the new bone is abnormal. The abnormality is comparable to the mottling of enamel. The bone will not calcify fully. Whether or not intermediate doses would be beneficial in the therapy of osteoporosis remains to be seen. Recent studies suggest that fluoride therapy plus vitamin D and calcium may be beneficial in treating osteoporosis.

Calcitonin has been shown to have rather dramatic effects in cats with osteoporosis induced by low calcium diets; however, the use of this agent in humans has not yielded objective evidence of efficacy.

SEXUAL FUNCTION IN SENESCENCE

The human species is one of the few that outlives its reproductive years. This was not always so, for when the average lifespan was 30 or 40 years, few individuals survived to reach the age of declining fertility. Now an ever increasing percentage of our population has passed the reproductive years. Although the ability to reproduce, particularly in women, declines sharply after age 40, sexual activity may not necessarily be altered.

Male climacteric

A change in any of the organs involved in sexual function in the male – alterations in testicular function, changes in the genital tract and other target tissues of androgens – may contribute to the general decline in sexual function with age. No significant change in testicular weight occurs with age; however, histological alterations have been noted. With aging, new layers of connective tissue are deposited in the basement membranes and capsules of the tubules, thus thickening these structures. This process is deleterious to the formation of sperm and probably underlies the gradual decline in spermatogenesis with aging. Sperm counts in ejaculates from men at various ages suggest a 30 percent reduction in the number of sperm in men in their sixties, with another 20 percent decline in the eighth and ninth decades. Complete cessation of spermatogenesis is rarely observed except in pathologic cases. In general, fertility declines in parallel with the decline in spermatogenic activity. The positive correlation between the relative number of Leydig cells and the spermatogenic activity in each testis supports the concept that androgen secretion is necessary for spermatogenesis.

Paralleling the decline in the number of Leydig cells is a fall in plasma testosterone concentration after about the age of 50. The mean value for subjects 80 to 90 years of age is about 40 percent of that in subjects under age 50; however, the variability is great. Some elderly men have normal amounts of plasma testosterone; others have values as low as those in normal women. The decline in testosterone values with age is due to diminished testosterone production. This decreased production, coupled with the age-related increase in the concentration of sex hormone binding globulin, results in less "free" testosterone in the blood for action on target tissues. The metabolic clearance rate of testosterone also declines with age.

The accessory sex glands are largely dependent upon androgens for their function. As a result, atrophic changes in these glands are not unusual in the elderly male with impaired testicular function. Tubular atrophy of the prostate is often noted at about 45 to 50 years of age; in subsequent years the prostatic muscles atrophy and fibrosis occurs. There is a decline in the activity of many of the enzymes secreted by prostatic cells, such as fibrinolysin and acid phosphatase.

Hypertrophy of the prostate is a common disorder in older men and is considered to be the result of chronic stimulation of this gland by testosterone, since this condition is not found in castrated males. Carcinoma of the prostate is the second most common form of cancer in men in the United States, and most patients with this disorder are over 70 years of age. Androgens have been implicated in the etiology of prostatic cancer; therapy therefore involves orchiectomy and/or estrogen treatment. The risk of gynecomastia and of increased mortality from cardiovascular disease with estrogen therapy has caused many investigators to advocate castration alone. Other forms of therapy for patients with recurrence of disease include adrenalectomy (to eliminate the adrenal androgens) and hypophysectomy (prolactin may play a role in prostatic growth).

Dihydrotestosterone induces growth in prostatic tissue, and the conversion of testosterone to dihydrotestosterone in this tissue has been well documented. Recent evidence suggests that the concentration of dihydrotestosterone in carcinomatous prostatic tissue is greater than that found in benign prostatic hypertrophy, which, in turn, is greater than that found in normal prostatic tissue. The role of the hormonal milieu in the onset of carcinomatous changes in target tissues has received much attention. The significance of estrogens and androgens in the control of the onset of cancer of the breast and prostate, respectively, has caused some investigators to speak of these hormones as *cocarcinogens* or as *promoters of carcinogenesis* in their target tissues (p. 419).

It is obvious from the foregoing that there is no sudden decline in reproductive physiology in men comparable to the menopause in women. Some men do have symptoms suggestive of a male climacteric; these symptoms include loss of potency and libido, flushes, tachycardia, emotional instability, and vertigo. Such a climacteric, which is *not* found in most men, is rare before age 60.

Wide individual variations in sexual interest and drive make it difficult to assess the role of androgens in the sexual activity of older males. Surveys generally agree that coital frequency decreases with age; however, sexual behavior in both elderly men and women seems to be more closely related to their prior sexual habits than to any alteration in androgen production. The regularity and frequency of sexual and coital experiences during mature life influence greatly the sexual adequacy and general physiologic competence of older persons. The reaction patterns of erection and ejaculation are slowed with advancing age, especially after age 60. The vasocongestive response of the scrotum and testicles is reduced in older men, and penile erection is more difficult to achieve. The intensity of orgasmic experience is reduced in both sexes. Despite these physiologic limitations with age, the studies by Masters and Johnson indicate that in the absence of pathology, the major determinants of sexual adequacy in later years are psychodynamic in nature.

THE MENOPAUSE

The menopause represents permanent cessation of menstruation and occurs whenever the ovaries are depleted of ova and hormone-producing follicular cells. The woman in effect becomes relatively estrogen-deficient; this usually occurs sometime between the ages of 48 and 52. The climacteric (change of life) refers to the perimenopausal years, when a syndrome of endocrine, somatic, and psychic changes of varying degree may occur.

Specific changes in the ovary have been observed as early as 30 years of age, when the relative and absolute weights of the ovaries begin to decline. The weight loss is accompanied later by a progressive and generalized atrophy, proliferation of fibrous tissue, a tendency to form follicular cysts, and various degrees of vascular sclerosis. In the human female (and most other mammals), the ovarian reserve of primordial follicles established at birth is dramatically diminished by the time of puberty. The rate of decline in oocytes appears to follow an exponential curve. Although the loss of oocytes appears to be intrinsic to the ovary, extrinsic factors may influence the process. In the mouse, hypophysectomy decreases the rate of oocyte loss.

The number of follicles that mature and ovulate also falls progressively. The number of growing follicles decreases steadily from childhood to the premenopausal period, but the number of graafian follicles is relatively constant up to age 40 and diminishes significantly in the next five years. Follicular cysts are often found in ovaries of women during the years just prior to the menopause. Active corpora lutea are very rare at this time. Even when mature follicles are present after the menopause, they show clear signs of degeneration and disappear completely during the late fifties.

The decreased formation of corpora lutea begins in the premenopausal years and may account, in part, for the lower incidence of pregnancy and the increasing frequency of miscarriages in premenopausal women. Indirect evidence suggests that ova released during the immediate premenopausal and menopausal years may have diminished viability and perhaps increased frequency of chromosomal aberrations. Ova recovered from the uterus of menopausal women and old animals appear grossly abnormal. Transplanting such ova to uteri of young animals shows that their ability to develop normally is significantly impaired.

Clinical and Laboratory Findings

Several years before the cessation of menstruation there is a decrease in the responsiveness of the ovary to gonadotropins. In this period the mean concentrations of FSH and LH in plasma are increased over values found in younger women. Concomitantly, the circulating levels of estrogens and progesterone are decreased. Decreased progesterone production is one of the earliest changes and reflects the increasing frequency of anovulatory cycles prior to menopause. There is a decline in both the production rate and the metabolic clearance rate of estrogens in the perimenopausal period, a situation analogous to that of testosterone in the aging male. An important sign of the imminence of the menopause, of course, is the onset of menstrual irregularities. Eventually all cyclic functions of the ovary cease, and concentrations of circulating gonadotropins remain high.

Various target tissues manifest estrogen deprivation in menopausal women. The uterus reaches its maximum weight at about age 30 and then undergoes a 53 percent loss of weight by age 50. This reduction is accompanied by a 61 percent decline in collagen and a 44 percent decline in elastin content. The vaginal walls undergo shrinkage and thinning. In some postmenopausal women, the vagina becomes paper-thin and decreases to about half its previous length and width. Just before the menopause, there is a decrease in the number of cornified cells seen in the preovulatory phase of the normal menstrual cycle. In the menopause, only precornified cells and transitional epithelium are noted in vaginal smears. The external genitalia show gradually increasing atrophic changes. There is a loss of subcutaneous fat of the labia majora. The labia minora and clitoris diminish in size. The breasts typically become flaccid. The alveoli gradually disappear, and the ducts diminish in size. The size and erectibility of the nipples diminish. Some of these changes represent the results of both estrogen deprivation and senescence.

Certain signs and symptoms are characteristic of the menopausal period. A considerable number of women (20 to 60 percent in surveys) have hot flashes and other vasomotor symptoms. The pathophysiology of the vasomotor instability is unknown; however, almost all women show a favorable response to estrogen therapy. Treatment with estrogens will also relieve the genital atrophy characteristic of the menopause. Other symptoms of the menopause include irritability, depression, and insomnia.

The only laboratory finding characteristic of the menopause is elevation of the concentrations of gonadotropins in blood and urine. The normal daily premenopausal production of estradiol in the menstrual cycle varies from 50 to 500 μg. Estrone, a much weaker estrogen, can be formed by the peripheral conversion of adrenal (or ovarian) androstenedione. Such estrone may be produced after the menopause in clinically significant amounts and may occasionally cause postmenopausal bleeding. Indeed, it has been reported that the conversion of plasma androstenedione to estrone averages 2.8 percent in postmenopausal women compared to a figure of 1.3 percent in premenopausal women. This increased conversion of circulating precursors to estrogen with advancing age has also been observed in male subjects.

Heart Disease and Breast Cancer

Certain disorders may be associated with estrogen deficiency. For example, the incidence of coronary heart disease in women increases markedly following the menopause. The ratio of coronary disease mortality rates in males and females shows a marked decrease beginning in the fifth decade of life and reaches unity in the ninth decade of life. Such a change, of course, could be due to a decline in the male mortality rate or to an increase in the female mortality rate. As yet, no clear-cut protective effect of estrogens against coronary artery disease has been demonstrated. In fact, males on estrogen therapy (for carcinoma of the prostate) have been shown to have *increased* mortality from cardiovascular disease.

The role of estrogens in postmenopausal osteoporosis has been discussed, as has the role of estrogen in thromboembolic disease. The increased incidence of breast cancer with age until the fifth decade and the decline thereafter suggested to many investigators that estrogens may influence the onset of breast cancer. The incidence of breast cancer is greater in women who have never borne children or who delay child-bearing. The risk of breast cancer increases with age at first parturition: women whose first pregnancy occurs after age 35 have three times the risk of breast cancer as do those who deliver their first child before age 18. The explanation for this phenomenon is unknown, but repeated growth of breast tissue under the influence of sex hormones without the natural events of pregnancy and lactation following may be involved. Menstruation is not a "natural" phenomenon, because under normal circumstances the primate female is either pregnant or lactating. Women who have never or rarely menstruated (as in primitive tribes) and who have their children early rarely manifest breast cancer. There may, of course, be genetic differences which could explain many of these findings. There seems no doubt of a familial tendency to breast cancer; a close relative of a woman with breast cancer has a significantly increased risk (over that of the general population) of developing this disorder.

The incidence of breast cancer is lower in women who have an early artificial menopause than in women who experience normal menopause. Perhaps of even greater import is the reported cancer of the breast in men treated with estrogens for prostatic cancer and in transsexuals given estrogen. The incidence of breast cancer in men is normally quite low. Thus the relationship of estrogen to breast cancer is suggestive, but as yet no definite evidence of a causal (or protective) role has been reported.

Some mammary carcinomas are hormone-dependent. Recently, investigators have attempted to differentiate these tumors from those not dependent on hormones by looking for hormone receptors in the carcinomatous breast tissues. Estradiol receptors (p. 99) were found in the estrogen-responsive tumors but not in those tumors growing autonomously. Approximately two thirds of primary breast cancers contain estrogen receptors, but in patients with metastatic disease only about 30 percent have a remission of disease after oophorectomy. Presumably, the population of cancer cells in some tumors is mixed, some containing estrogen receptors, some not. Oophorectomy might eliminate those cells which require estrogen, but the cells which lack receptors could continue to proliferate.

Estrogen induces the release of prolactin, which in turn may enhance tumor growth. Clearly, the total hormonal milieu may be critical for the survival and spread of hormone-sensitive tumors. Many investigators would categorize estrogens (and perhaps androgens) as *cocarcinogens,* capable of priming the tissue for subsequent anaplastic changes. An estrogen-induced renal cell adenoma and adenocarcinoma in hamsters has been studied intensively with this theory in mind.

Estrogen Therapy in the Menopause

There is controversy regarding the advisability of treating all menopausal women with estrogen. Thousands of middle-aged women look upon estrogens as the panacea for senescence. The premenopausal woman all too often believes that these hormones will prevent the dreaded symptoms of the menopause and the associated facial wrinkling, drooping breasts, muscular weakness, and diminished libido. The physician may want to prescribe estrogens in the hope of possibly retarding osteoporosis or arteriosclerosis.

Do all women need estrogens after the menopause? Analysis of estrogens in urine and blood in one study showed that estrogen values in patients during the first year after cessation of menses were not appreciably diminished from those obtained during the normal menstrual cycle. Vaginal smears during early menopause (ages 45 to 60) showed excellent cornification in 25 percent of patients. Even in late menopause (ages 61 to 85), a high degree of cornification is seen in about five percent of patients. Thus not *all* postmenopausal women appear to be estrogen-deficient.

However, an estrogen-deficient postmenopausal woman cannot expect estrogen administration to give her youthful breasts and smooth skin. The aging of these tissues is related to other factors and not simply to hormonal balance. Certainly the evidence for the value of estrogens in preventing coronary artery disease is circumspect, and the association of estrogen deprivation with osteoporosis remains just that—an association.

When is estrogen therapy advisable in the postmenopausal woman? Estrogens are efficacious in relieving vasomotor symptoms (hot flashes, sweats, insomnia) and in preventing atrophic changes of the vaginal and urethral epithelia, which may result in painful intercourse and urination respectively.

The disadvantages of estrogen therapy in the postmenopausal woman should be considered. Fibroids may grow suddenly during estrogen therapy. Endometrial bleeding may occur if excessive amounts of estrogen are given. The physician must *never* assume that bleeding in the postmenopausal woman is due to excessive estrogen therapy. Half the patients who bleed in the postmenopausal period have been found to have cancer of the genital tract. Estrogen induces cellular growth of the endometrium. Hyperplasia of the endometrium is potentially malignant in about 10 percent of cases.

Relative contraindications to the use of estrogens include liver disease, cystic disease of the breast, thromboembolic disease, and fibroid tumors of the uterus. They are also contraindicated in any patient with breast or uterine cancer or with a history of such disorders. Women who might be pregnant should not receive stilbestrol, since female offspring of women treated with stilbestrol during pregnancy have been shown to have an increased incidence of adenocarcinoma of the vagina. Breakthrough bleeding in women using estrogens suggests an abnormality within the uterus (hyperplasia, polyp, fibroid) and should be thoroughly investigated.

LIPID METABOLISM: OBESITY, ATHEROSCLEROSIS

OBESITY

Acquired obesity is a hallmark of middle age ("middle age spread"). In contrast to lifelong obesity, which is characterized by adipose cells of increased number and size, acquired or adult-onset obesity is usually associated with hypertrophy of adipose cells. Obesity leads to morbidity because of its aggravating effect on a variety of other disorders, such as hypertension, diabetes mellitus, atherosclerosis, and osteoarthritis. It is the single most common preventable factor associated with excess mortality and morbidity in the middle-aged group.

Obese individuals have a much higher incidence of diabetes mellitus than those of normal weight. Both conditions have an increased prevalence in old age, and one might postulate that the same surfeit of calories is responsible for both obesity and the clinical manifestation of the diabetic genotype. Neel has linked the environmental and hereditary components of both conditions in a hypothesis suggesting that they were of survival value to primitive man ("thrifty genotype"). Primitive man ate a huge meal after a successful hunt, but he had to be able to sustain long periods of fasting. The conditions in primitive times required hard physical work, with the overall availability of food a restricted and an irregular affair. As energy is more efficiently stored as fat (nine calories per gram in contrast to four calories per gram of carbohydrate or protein), the man who was able to store his excess calories in adipose tissue probably was at an advantage.

Present-day conditions of essentially unrestricted availability of food throughout the year and greatly reduced need for physical activity would require readaptation. The diabetic genotype, according to Neel, represents failure of adaptation to a relatively sudden transition to a sedentary existence with an abundance of food. This hypothesis is supported by studies with experimental animals in which dietary manipulation was used to accelerate or delay β cell hyperplasia and manifestations of diabetes mellitus. It appears, then, that the increased incidence of obesity and diabetes mellitus with age may be linked with and reflect a surfeit of calories in a population with increasingly limited physical activity.

ATHEROSCLEROSIS

Dietary factors, especially carbohydrate and lipid factors, may influence the development of atherosclerosis. The major cause of death in most socioeconomically advanced countries is arterial failure, the most predominant form of which is arteriosclerosis (vascular degeneration leading to progressive thickening and loss of resiliency of the arterial wall). One type of arteriosclerosis is atherosclerosis, characterized by atheromas, or plaques, of fatty material in the intima and increased connective tissue in the subintimal layers of the arterial wall. This form of arteriosclerosis, which is the underlying cause of most coronary heart disease and cerebrovascular disease, may affect, among other vessels, the aorta, the coronary arteries, and the cerebral arteries.

The intima is the primary focus of the atherosclerotic process. The thickness of the intima increases with age owing to proliferation of smooth muscle cells. The thickening is particularly pronounced at sites of arterial branching. The first fatty streaks (regarded by many pathologists as an early stage of atherosclerosis) appear in the first decade of life. Lipid deposition begins in the aorta in the first decade of life, in the coronary arteries in the second decade, and in the cerebral arteries in the third decade. The pathogenesis of atherosclerosis has been the subject of much controversy, and several theories have been put forward. Since the atherosclerotic process tends to be focal rather than generalized, local factors which affect the arterial wall may be important in its etiology. Turbulent blood flow could "injure" the vessel wall and alter the permeability of the intima to constituents of the blood. Experimental injury or removal of the arterial endothelium promotes proliferation of smooth muscle cells, possibly because nutrients needed for cell proliferation become more readily available when the endothelial barrier is removed. In short, then, injury to the vessel wall may represent one of the predisposing factors to atherosclerosis. Another etiologic factor might be an abnormality of lipid metabolism that predisposes to high levels of circulating lipids which gradually are deposited in various arteries. Another factor might be abnormalities in proteins (collagen, elastin) of the arterial wall that predispose to lipid deposition and subsequent calcification. Is there any evidence to bear on these theories?

The arterial wall contains phospholipids, triglycerides, free cholesterol, and cholesterol esters. In the young, healthy aorta, phospholipids predominate, and the least prominent are the cholesterol esters. With increasing age, *all* lipids increase in the intima, but cholesterol esters increase the most. At age 65, in vessels free of atherosclerosis, cholesterol esters are the major lipids, whereas the percentage of phospholipid declines to about one half the value in young aortae. In addition, the composition of cholesterol esters changes, with increased linoleic acid (unsaturated) and decreased palmitic acid (saturated).

During atherogenesis, cholesterol, cholesterol esters, and phospholipids increase in concentration in the vessel walls, whereas triglycerides decrease. Most of these excess lipids found in atherosclerotic arteries are not synthesized locally in the cells of the wall, but come from the blood. There is extensive epidemiologic evidence now supporting a correlation between abnormally high amounts of circulating lipids and atherosclerosis. To support this correlation, laboratory studies have shown that lesions resembling the fatty streaks in the human can be induced in various animals by feeding them excessive amounts of cholesterol. Thus circulating lipids undoubtedly contribute to the atherosclerotic process. In addition, certain structural features are important. The first lipid accumulation almost invariably appears in those spots of the human aorta and coronary arteries that show signs of injury and thickening. Animal studies also support the view that injury to the arterial wall predisposes to lipid deposition.

Fibers (elastic and collagenous) and ground substance (mucopolysaccharides) comprise the major extracellular components of the arterial wall. Collagen increases with the severity of the atherosclerotic lesion, whereas mucopolysaccharides tend to decrease. Time-dependent changes in collagen may predispose to the accumulation of lipid material, and the age-dependent increase in calcium in the media may predispose to calcification of atherosclerotic plaques. Thus the structure of the arterial wall, which undoubtedly changes with age as structural proteins undergo further cross-linking, may play a role in the advancement of the atherosclerotic process.

Genetic factors undoubtedly influence the progress of the disorder, because the age of onset and the severity of the clinical manifestations of the disease differ from one individual to another. Genetic differences in the blood clotting mechanism may be important, for atherosclerosis has been linked with the formation of thrombi. Hypertension may potentiate atherosclerosis, and heredity probably is important as one of the etiologic factors of hypertension. There is a direct relationship between the degree of hypertension and the extent of atherosclerotic heart disease. Presumably, increasing blood pressure heightens the permeability of the intima and thus influences the metabolism of arterial cells. Experimental hypertension increases the content of sulfated mucopolysaccharide in the aorta. Familial types of hyperlipoproteinemia are linked with a predisposition to atherosclerosis. Perhaps most interesting of all is the high incidence of atherosclerosis in patients with diabetes mellitus. The significance of this association is further underscored by the observation that non-diabetic individuals from diabetic families show a higher incidence of atherosclerosis than those from normal parents.

Endocrine regulation of lipid metabolism

Abnormal amounts of circulating lipids are found in several endocrine disorders. Of particular interest are the effects of insulin and thyroid hormone on the pathways involved in the synthesis and breakdown of these lipids. The major lipids in normal human plasma are cholesterol esters, phospholipids, triglycerides, cholesterol, and free fatty acids. The latter are transported bound to albumin. Oxidation of fatty acids is a major source of energy in the normal individual and even more so in the diabetic, whose utilization of glucose is impaired. In an insulin-deficient state, lipogenesis is decreased and lipolysis is increased. A hormone-sensitive lipase in both liver and adipose tissue is activated by a cyclic AMP-protein kinase. Hormones such as epinephrine and glucagon stimulate adenyl cyclase, which increases the concentration of cyclic AMP in the cell. Thus in a situation analogous to that of glycogen breakdown, the hydrolysis of triglyceride is enhanced by specific hormones. Insulin acts to diminish the amount of cyclic AMP in the cells, probably by stimulating phosphodiesterase (see Figure 10–2). Methyl xanthines such as caffeine inhibit phosphodiesterase, thereby increasing the amount of cyclic AMP in the cell. It is interesting that drinking coffee, for example, causes elevation of plasma free fatty acids.

Insulin is highly involved in the formation of triglycerides, which are composed of glycerol and fatty acids. Both of these can be formed in the liver and adipose cell if glucose is available (Figure 14–3). The transport of glucose, though, is impaired in nonhepatic cells in the insulin-deprived state. Even though glycerol and fatty acid synthesis in diabetic adipose tissue is impaired, another source of these substances might be the circulating triglyceride. If the triglyceride could be hydrolyzed in adipose tissue before entering the cell, and could subsequently be formed anew and stored within the adipose cell, lipogenesis could continue. Under normal circumstances this is exactly what occurs. Triglyceride circulates in the plasma "packaged" with cholesterol esters and surrounded by a protein shell containing phospholipids and free cholesterol. Some of this triglyceride is dietary in origin. It is hydrolyzed in the intestinal tract (by pancreatic lipases), absorbed, and then formed anew in the mucosal cell, finally appearing in the lymph and subsequently in the plasma as *chylomicrons* (Figure 14–3).

These circulating lipoprotein particles contain 81 percent triglyceride, 10 percent cholesterol, 7 percent phospholipid, and about 2 percent protein. The proteins coating the lipid particles *(apoproteins)* are important determinants of the stability and ultimate fate of the particles. In particular, certain apoproteins of the C family stimulate and others inhibit lipoprotein lipase (LPL), the enzyme that hydrolyzes triglyceride circulating in the blood. Most tissues can hydrolyze the triglycerides of chylomicrons by the LPL located on the endothelial walls of capillaries supplying the tissues. This enzyme is formed in adipose tissue but only in the presence of glucose and insulin. Fat cells can also release the enzyme in the presence of glucose and insulin. Presumably, the released enzyme becomes attached to the vasculature and can be released from the vessel wall by heparin (made in mast cells). A standard test for lipoprotein lipase is the measurement of lipolytic activity in the blood of the patient after heparin administration. This value is referred to as post-heparin lipolytic activity (PHLA). A hereditary disorder in which

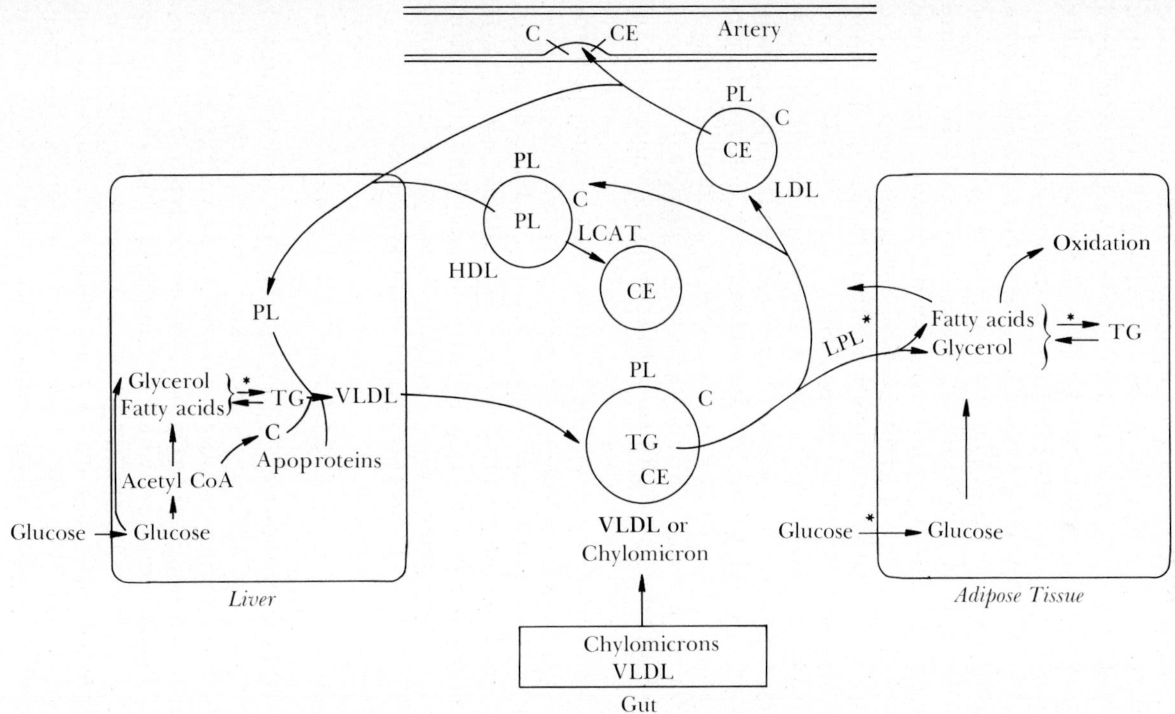

FIGURE 14–3. Biosynthesis and metabolism of plasma lipoproteins. The asterisk (*) denotes those enzymes or reactions that are stimulated by insulin. Abbreviations used are: C = cholesterol; CE = cholesterol ester; HDL = high density lipoprotein; LCAT = lecithin:cholesterol acyltransferase; LDL = low density lipoprotein; LPL = lipoprotein lipase; PL = phospholipid; TG = triglyceride; VLDL = very low density lipoprotein. The apoproteins, which are located on the surface of the lipoprotein particle, are not shown.

there is a deficiency of LPL is characterized by very slow clearing of chylomicrons from the circulation. Chylomicrons are the least dense of the plasma lipoproteins forming particles sufficiently large (0.075 to 1 μm in diameter) to be seen in a dark-field microscope and to cause turbidity of the plasma. The normal clearance of chylomicrons from the blood is rapid, the half-time of disappearance being only a few minutes.

Other circulating triglycerides are formed in the liver (from glycerol and fatty acids synthesized in the liver) and to a much lesser extent in the intestine. In the liver these triglycerides are combined with phospholipids, cholesterol, and apoproteins in the Golgi apparatus and secreted as very low density lipoproteins (VLDL). The intestine utilizes dietary or biliary fatty acids for triglyceride synthesis. It also secretes VLDL (Figure 14–3). These lipoproteins are rich in triglyceride, and the triglyceride can serve as a substrate for LPL. Thus both chylomicrons and VLDL are lipoproteins composed largely of triglyceride that circulate in the blood and are readily cleared in normal tissues. During this clearing process, the triglyceride is hydrolyzed by LPL (the synthesis and release of which in adipose tissue is dependent upon glucose and insulin). Lipoprotein particles remain, containing cores composed largely of cholesterol esters (low density lipoprotein, LDL) or phospholipids (high density lipoprotein, HDL). These various lipoproteins can be distinguished from one another by their density in the ultracentrifuge or by their migration on electrophoresis (Table 14–1).

An increased concentration of one or more of the plasma lipoproteins constitutes *hyperlipoproteinemia*. For example, type I hyperlipoproteinemia is due to impaired activity or synthesis of LPL. It can be hereditary (as mentioned) or the result of severe insulin deficiency. Type II hyperlipoproteinemia is characterized by an abnormally high concentration of plasma β lipoproteins (LDL), essentially an excess of circulating cholesterol derived from the diet or from hepatic synthesis.

Cholesterol

Hepatic synthesis of cholesterol is regulated by hormonal control of the rate-limiting step in the biosynthetic path as well as by product inhibition. The rate-limiting step, the conversion of β-hydroxy-β-methyl glutaryl CoA to mevalonic acid (Figure 2–4), is catalyzed by hydroxymethylglutaryl CoA reductase, which is stimulated by insulin. Any β-hydroxy-β-methyl glutaryl CoA not converted to mevalonic acid can be converted to ketone bodies for use as a metabolic fuel. Thus it is not surprising that during starvation cholesterol formation is decreased (decreased insulin) and that in the fed state its synthesis is increased (increased insulin). A further regulation, and perhaps the more important one, is the inhibition of hydroxymethylglutaryl CoA reductase by cholesterol in the liver. This negative feedback in liver probably explains the fact that diabetics show no consistent abnormality in the amount of

TABLE 14–1. The Classes of Lipoproteins in Human Plasma*†

FLOTATION RATE (DENSITY)	DESIGNATION (ELECTROPHORETIC MOBILITY)	SOURCE	MAJOR APOPROTEINS	MAJOR LIPIDS "CORE"/"SURFACE"	DIRECT ENZYMIC ATTACK BY
$S_f > 400$	CHYLOMICRONS	GUT	APO C,B,A	TG/UC,PC	LPL
S_f 20 - 400	VLDL (PRE β)	LIVER, GUT	APO C,B	TG/UC,PC	LPL
(1.006 g/ml)					
S_f 0 - 20	LDL (β)	PLASMA CHYLOMICRONS, VLDL, OTHER ?	APO B	CE/UC,PC,S	LCAT (?)
(1.063 g/ml)					
$F_{1.20}$ 0 - 9	HDL (α_1)	PLASMA CHYLOMICRONS ? LIVER, OTHER ?	APO A,C	PC/UC,PC	LCAT
(1.21 g/ml)					
	ALBUMIN APOPROTEINS	LIVER, ?	APO A	FFA, LYSO PC	

*Apo A-C = apoprotein A-C; TG = triglyceride; UC = unesterified cholesterol; CE = cholesterol ester; PC = phosphatidylcholine (lecithin); LYSO PC = lysolecithin; S = sphingomyelin; FFA = free fatty acid; LPL = lipoprotein lipase; LCAT = lecithin:cholesterol acyltransferase.

†From Williams, R., ed. *Textbook of Endocrinology*. Philadelphia: W. B. Saunders Company, 1974, p. 901.

circulating cholesterol. Apparently, there is no negative feedback control of the enzyme in intestinal mucosa.

In man, endogenous synthesis of cholesterol (liver and intestine) yields about 1.0 g of cholesterol per day. Approximately 0.3 g of cholesterol is absorbed via the intestine each day (even if intake is much larger). Clearly, endogenous production of cholesterol far outweighs the dietary component that is absorbed, and intake would have to be less than 300 mg per day to affect the circulating levels of cholesterol. These data become of some significance in view of recent prospective studies in the United States showing that the probability that a person aged 49 to 59 years will develop ischemic heart disease within 12 years is directly related to his or her plasma cholesterol concentration.

The major carrier of cholesterol in the plasma is LDL (β-lipoprotein). The concentration of cholesterol in the plasma depends not only upon the amount of cholesterol absorbed and synthesized but also on the rates at which the various lipoproteins enter and leave the plasma. For example, in hypothyroidism the rates of LDL formation and clearance from the plasma are slowed. The clearance rate is particularly impaired, and the net effect of the thyroid-deprived state is an increase in the circulating level of LDL, with a concomitant increase in the concentration of cholesterol in the plasma. Thyroid hormone is also important for the normal activity of LPL. Low LPL activity favors accumulation of triglyceride, leading to hypertriglyceridemia. In hypothyroidism the majority of patients are hyperlipidemic, with increased pre-β or β lipoproteins, or both.

Thyroid hormones appear to stimulate virtually all aspects of lipid metabolism. In general, degradation is affected more than synthesis; consequently, the concentration of lipid in plasma is inversely related to the concentration of thyroid hormone. In adipose tissue thyroid hormones increase lipolysis both by directly stimulating adenyl cyclase and by sensitizing the tissue to other lipolytic hormones such as catecholamines, GH, glucocorticoids, and glucagon. Oxidation of free fatty acids is also increased and may account for some of the calorigenic action of thyroid hormone.

The familial form of hypercholesterolemia is thought to be due to an inherited defect in LDL catabolism. The homozygote has about twice the plasma LDL and cholesterol concentrations of the heterozygote. Both develop xanthomas, or cholesterol deposits, producing arthritis and premature coronary, cerebral, and peripheral, vascular disease. Treatment can effectively lower the concentration of cholesterol and LDL in plasma for long periods of time. Most physicians recommend a diet high in unsaturated fats and low in cholesterol and saturated fats. The rationale for the increase in dietary unsaturated fats is still unclear. Ordinarily, an animal fat diet has a ratio of polyunsaturated fatty acids to saturated fatty acids of 0.2. With the addition of polyunsaturated fats and the reduction of animal fat, the ratio can be raised to 2.0. It is believed by some that the configuration of the unsaturated fatty acids to which cholesterol is esterified in LDL requires greater space, thereby reducing the amount of cholesterol in a given LDL particle. Certainly unsaturated fats appear to lower blood cholesterol concentration; however, there is disagreement as to where the cholesterol goes. The results of one study suggested that the cholesterol enters the slowly exchanging pools of the body, which could include the blood vessel walls. The results of another study were compatible with the hypothesis that increased bile salt excretion accounted for the decreased blood cholesterol. Approximately half of the cholesterol eliminated from the body is normally excreted in the feces after conversion to bile salts.

The greater part of total plasma cholesterol is found in the esterified form. In general, free cholesterol in plasma exchanges readily with the cholesterol in tissues and in other plasma lipoproteins, whereas the cholesterol esters do not exchange freely. Although the core of HDL is composed primarily of phospholipid (Figure 14–3), some cholesterol ester may be formed in HDL as a result of a transesterification reaction in plasma between cholesterol and the fatty acid in position two of lecithin (Figure 14–4), catalyzed by lecithin:cholesterol acyltransferase (LCAT). This enzyme is synthesized in the liver and then secreted into

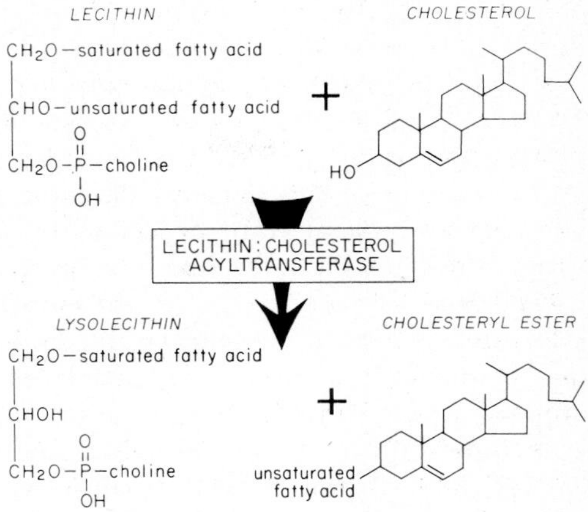

FIGURE 14–4. Principal reaction catalyzed by lecithin:cholesterol acyltransferase. (From Glomset, J. A.: J. Lipid Res. *9*:155, 1968, as presented in Williams, R., ed. *Textbook of Endocrinology*. Philadelphia: W. B. Saunders Company, 1974, p. 902.)

the circulation. It is responsible for the formation of virtually all the cholesterol esters in the plasma.

Although LCAT acts for the most part to esterify the cholesterol of HDL, it affects VLDL and LDL also. The direct catalysis of exchange in HDL promotes non-enzymatic transfers of lipid between HDL and VLDL or LDL. In addition, the enzyme can catalyze the esterification of LDL cholesterol to a certain extent. Presumably, the principal function of the LCAT reaction is to regulate the level of unesterified cholesterol and lecithin in plasma lipoproteins and plasma membranes. Since free cholesterol exchanges readily but cholesterol ester does not, by keeping down the amount of free cholesterol circulating in the plasma, one might expect that less cholesterol would accumulate in tissues and membranes. These concepts are unproven but may bear very directly on the accumulation of cholesterol and its esters in atherosclerosis.

Dietary therapy alone often is not sufficient to reduce to normal values the plasma concentration of cholesterol in hypercholesterolemia. Drugs which reduce the production of triglyceride by the liver (chlorophenoxyisobutyric acid, clofibrate, nicotinic acid) and agents which bind bile acid (cholestyramine) may be useful in lowering the concentration of cholesterol in plasma.

Triglyceride

Type III hyperlipoproteinemia represents a rare disorder of the conversion of VLDL to LDL. An intermediate accumulates to great excess and even appears in the VLDL fraction. Because this intermediate shares properties of both VLDL and LDL, it appears on electrophoresis as a broad β band. Both plasma triglyceride and cholesterol are elevated in the type III disorder. The disorder also increases the likelihood of coronary heart disease.

Type IV hyperlipoproteinemia seems primarily to result from an excess of triglyceride. This excess may be due to overproduction or impaired removal of triglyceride. A high carbohydrate diet may produce an increase in serum triglyceride concentration because the liver converts excess carbohydrate, especially fructose, to triglycerides. Carbohydrates differ in their tendency to be incorporated into triglyceride. A correlation between the increased consumption of sucrose and atherosclerosis has been demonstrated by Yudkin and Roddy. Foods that contain primarily glucose as the carbohydrate constituent (starch, for example) cause less hypertriglyceridemia than do fructose foods. Individuals undoubtedly manifest different sensitivities to a given carbohydrate load. Almost all will develop hypertriglyceridemia when the caloric intake is 80 to 90 percent carbohydrate. Some, however, manifest hypertriglyceridemia even with a much smaller carbohydrate intake.

Any condition in which the concentration of insulin in the blood is increased will favor VLDL formation in the liver. For example, in obesity the pancreas secretes additional insulin (in response to insulin resistance), and this excess insulin stimulates VLDL formation in the liver. The amount of this lipoprotein (pre-β) in the plasma is increased. This, then, represents a form of overproduction lipemia, as does the example of high carbohydrate intake. A lack of insulin, which is needed for LPL activity, can impede removal of the triglyceride in VLDL, and lipemia may result. The "removal" type of lipemia is commonly seen in diabetics. Severe insulin deficiency (as in poorly controlled diabetics) may so impair the hydrolysis of triglyceride that chylomicrons accumulate (type I hyperlipoproteinemia). The accumulation of both chylomicrons and VLDL (type I plus type IV) in the plasma has been called type V hyperlipoproteinemia. With insulin therapy the condition of the poorly controlled diabetic will revert to type IV hyperlipoproteinemia.

All of the hyperlipoproteinemias except type I predispose to atherosclerosis. With all the associated factors which have been linked to atherosclerosis and coronary heart disease, it is difficult to unravel the etiology of the atherosclerotic process. One of the more reasonable delineations of a possible sequence leading to atherosclerotic plaque formation has been offered by Ross and Glomset. They postulate that the initial event is injury to the vessel wall, especially at sites with high shear rates, such as the bifurcation of the aorta. This injury may be due to any one of a number of factors, including hypertension, smoking, or hyperglycemia. Smooth muscle cells from the arterial media migrate into the intima, forming the matrix for the future atherosclerotic plaque. Whole lipoprotein particles pass by transudation through the injured endothelium into this matrix. Apoproteins have been found in the luminal wall, a discovery which supports the possibility of such transudation of lipoprotein particles. Eventually, the fatty acids, glycerol, protein, and phospholipids are metabolized, leaving behind the scar of collagen matrix and cholesterol esters.

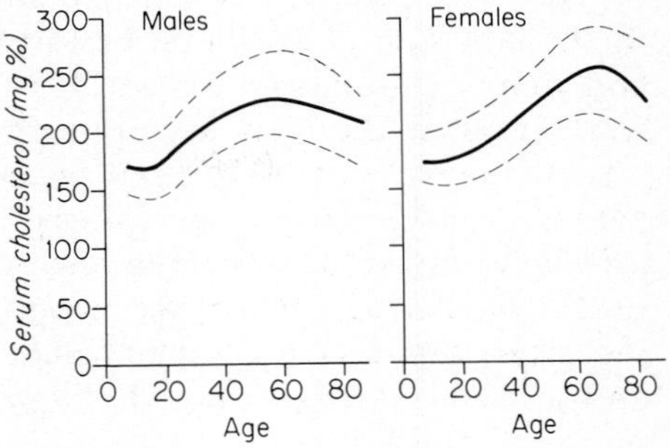

FIGURE 14–5. Relationship between age and serum cholesterol concentration in males and females in an American community—Tecumseh, Michigan. Solid lines are 50th percentiles; dashed lines are 20th (lower) and 80th (upper) percentiles. (From Epstein, F. H., et al.: Prevalence of chronic diseases and distribution of selected physiological variables in a total community, Tecumseh, Michigan. Am. J. Epidemiol. *81*:307, 1965, as adapted in Smith, D. and Bierman, E., eds. *The Biologic Ages of Man.* Philadelphia: W. B. Saunders Company, 1973, p. 167.)

Aging and Atherosclerosis

The process of atherosclerosis in the older population might well be exacerbated by the increasing levels of cholesterol-rich and triglyeride-rich plasma lipoproteins with age (Figure 14–5). It is tempting to relate this rise in lipids in the blood to the gradual decline of glucose tolerance with age. When glucose utilization is impaired, the concentrations of free fatty acids, phospholipids, cholesterol, and triglyceride in the blood rise. The substrate for the synthesis of these lipids in the liver is glucose, which can enter the hepatic cell readily even with a relative lack of insulin because of the effect of glucose concentration on the activity of either hexokinase or glucokinase (see discussion of K*m* values, p. 228). The lipids within these circulating lipoproteins can be deposited in injured vessel walls (Figure 14–3).

HYPERTENSION

Just as body weight, serum cholesterol content, and blood glucose level following an oral glucose challenge increase with age, likewise blood pressure rises (Figure 14–6). According to the statistics compiled

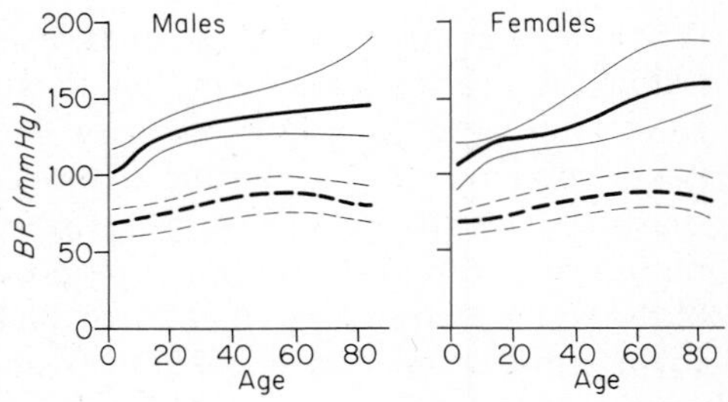

FIGURE 14–6. Relationship between age and systolic (upper, solid lines) and diastolic blood pressure (BP) (lower, dashed lines) in males and females in an American Community—Tecumseh, Michigan. Heavy lines are 50th percentile; lighter lines are 20th (lower) and 80th (upper) percentiles. (From Epstein, F. H., et al.: Prevalence of chronic diseases and distribution of selected physiological variables in a total community, Tecumseh, Michigan. Am. J. Epidemiol. *81*:307, 1965, as adapted in Smith, D. and Bierman, E., eds. *The Biologic Ages of Man.* Philadelphia: W. B. Saunders Company, 1973, p. 166.)

by insurance companies, approximately 10 percent of the population of the United States have blood pressures greater than 140 mm Hg systolic and 90 mm Hg diastolic by the age of 40 to 50. Many of these "hypertensives," however, remain asymptomatic.

Blood pressure is affected by a variety of factors, including blood volume, cardiac output, peripheral resistance, and the elasticity of the arterial walls. An alteration in one or more of these parameters may induce hypertension. Changes in peripheral resistance are mediated by the arterioles, vessels of small caliber with much more smooth muscle and less elastic tissue than the larger arteries. The smooth muscle of these vessels is innervated mainly by adrenergic (sympathetic) nerve fibers that function as constrictors. Small changes in the degree of constriction result in alterations of arteriolar caliber and bring about large changes in total peripheral resistance. In the aged, the vessel caliber and elasticity may already be compromised by arteriosclerotic lesions, and the arteriosclerotic process may, in part, be the cause of the age-related increase in blood pressure. This same process within the vessels of the kidney may lead to increased release of renin and subsequent elevation of angiotensin levels in the blood.

In assessing hypertension, one should be aware of genetic, racial, and environmental factors that may contribute to the disease. For example, hypertension occurs earlier and in a higher percentage of blacks than in white or Indian populations. Women develop hypertension more frequently than men but seem to tolerate it better. In the individual, the early morning pressure on awakening (basal blood pressure) is lower than during subsequent hours of the day. Sitting or standing generally raises diastolic pressure, whereas exercise or hypoxia raises both systolic and diastolic pressures. A high salt intake may predispose to hypertension. Certain primitive tribes have been discovered in which the incidence of hypertension is extremely low. A study of their diet revealed a markedly lower salt intake than that in populations with a high incidence of hypertension.

Although the blood pressure tends to rise with age in all individuals, elevated blood pressures occur earlier and remain higher in relatives of hypertensives than in relatives of non-hypertensives. Blood pressures consistently greater than 140 mm Hg systolic and/or 90 mm Hg diastolic are considered elevated and abnormal in young adults. There is no question that a longer life is associated with blood pressures considerably below the average, and a higher mortality is associated with hypertension. If only the systolic pressure is elevated, peripheral resistance may be normal or low, and cardiac output may be increased. Increased diastolic pressure reflects an increase in peripheral resistance. In the initial phases of hypertension, the blood pressure may be labile, sometimes elevated, sometimes normal. This "labile" hypertension may continue for months or even years. There is no evidence of vascular changes on examination of the patient. It has been suggested that abnormal tone of the sympathetic nervous system may account for the condition. Such labile hypertension tends to develop into persistent or fixed hypertension.

The most common disorder associated with systolic hypertension is arteriosclerosis of the aorta and its main branches. In patients in the older age group, there is a high incidence of systolic hypertension associated with loss of elasticity of the aorta secondary to arteriosclerosis. This type of systolic hypertension is due to increased arterial rigidity and is quite different from the diastolic hypertension in which arteriolar constriction is of paramount importance. There is no evidence that generalized arteriosclerosis produces diastolic hypertension except when renal artery stenosis or essential hypertension is involved. Other causes of high cardiac output and systolic hypertension are severe anemia, thyrotoxicosis, beriberi, Paget's disease, and arteriovenous fistula.

The diastolic blood pressure represents the residual impelling force in the circulation during cardiac diastole. It reflects the extent of arteriolar constriction. Elevated diastolic blood pressure for which there is no etiologic factor is termed *essential hypertension*. The vast majority (90 to 95 percent) of hypertensive patients are in this category. However, more and more types of hypertension are being discovered that are reversible through specific treatment; as a result, the high percentage of individuals classified as having "essential hypertension" is decreasing and hopefully will disappear in time. The most important entities to diagnose, since they are curable, are the endocrine disorders producing hypertension. We may group these disorders into those due to excessive secretion of (1) catecholamines, (2) renin-angiotensin, or (3) mineralocorticoids.

CATECHOLAMINES

Catecholamines are produced by the central nervous system, the postganglionic neurons, and the chromaffin cells of the adrenal medulla. There is little if any epinephrine in the central nervous system, where the major catecholamines are dopamine (found in tracts from the upper brain stem to basal ganglia and some limbic forebrain structures and in intrahypothalamic neurons terminating in the median eminence) and norepinephrine (found in tracts from the lower brain stem which ascend to the hypothalamus, limbic forebrain, forebrain, telencephalon, and cerebellum, and descend in the spinal cord). The postganglionic sympathetic neurons contain norepinephrine. Some dopamine is found in cells within the sympathetic ganglia. The adrenal medulla contains primarily epinephrine but also has some dopamine and norepinephrine, present as precursors of epinephrine.

Wurtman uses the term "neuroendocrine transducer" for substances such as acetylcholine, the catecholamines, melatonin, the neurohormones oxytocin and vasopressin, and the releasing factors which are released from neurons in response to stimuli. Neurons in the supraoptic and paraventricular nuclei respond to stimuli and release oxytocin and vasopressin. Similarly, the neurons of the hypothalamus secrete their specific releasing factors. The adrenal medullary cells are also dependent upon neural imput (acetylcholine) for release of catecholamines. If the adrenal gland is transplanted to another area of the body, the cortex, but not the medulla, continues to function. The pineal gland provides another example of neuroendocrine transduction. When adrenergic nerves in the gland are stimulated, they release norepinephrine, which brings about the release of melatonin from the gland. Similarly, adrenergic nerve endings in the juxtaglomerular apparatus of the kidney release norepinephrine, which in turn brings about the secretion of renin. The importance of these neuroendocrine transducers cannot be over-emphasized, for they form a bridge between neural and endocrine control systems.

The catecholamines are protected from degradation by storage in an inactive, protein-bound form in vesicles in the cells in which they are produced. For example, norepinephrine is localized within specific vesicles in the sympathetic nerve endings. Upon activation of these cells, the catecholamines are released from the vesicles as the free amines. After release and action the molecules are recaptured and stored again in the vesicles. The catecholamine content of adrenergic neurons remains remarkably constant despite considerable variation in the activity of the sympathetic nerves.

Excessive amounts of catecholamines are produced by tumors of chromaffin tissue such as *pheochromocytomas.* Although rare (less than 0.5 percent of hypertensive patients have such tumors), this form of hypertension is curable and should be considered whenever symptoms of excessive adrenergic stimulation are present. These symptoms are mediated by α and β receptors. For example, β receptors in general mediate the vasodilator effects of epinephrine and α receptors the vasoconstrictor effects (Table 14–2). Small doses of epinephrine (0.1 μg/kg) may cause the blood pressure to fall below normal owing to the greater sensitivity of the vascular β receptors. Higher doses stimulate the α receptors, and the blood pressure rises. The cardiac effects of epinephrine (myocardial stimulation and increased heart rate) may also contribute to the pressor effect. Norepinephrine acts predominantly on α receptors and has little action on β receptors, except in the heart. Thus it too produces a rise in the blood pressure. Whereas small doses of epinephrine produce vasodilatation, small doses of norepinephrine do not. Isoproterenol, a sympathomimetic drug, has a powerful action on β receptors and almost no action on α receptors. Its main actions, therefore, are on the heart, the smooth muscle of bronchi, skeletal muscle vasculature, and the alimentary tract (Table 14–2). Both epinephrine and isoproterenol have similar calorigenic actions.

Clearly, symptoms of excessive adrenergic stimulation due to excess catecholamines are often varied and depend in large part on the relative amounts of epinephrine and norepinephrine secreted by the tumor. Norepinephrine constitutes 10 to 18 percent of the catecholamine con-

TABLE 14–2. Effects of Catecholamines**

	Receptor	Predominant Physiologic or Pharmacologic Effects	Predominant in vivo Response
Circulatory Effects			
Heart			
Sinus node	β	↑ Rate	↑ Cardiac output
Junctional tissue	β	↑ Conduction velocity	
Myocardium	β	↑ Contractility	
Arteries			
Renal	α	Vasoconstriction	
Splanchnic	α	Vasoconstriction	↓ Local blood flow
Subcutaneous	α	Vasoconstriction	↑ Systemic blood pressure
Mucosa	α	Vasoconstriction	
Cerebral	*	Minimal direct effect	No change in cerebral flow
Coronary	*	Minimal direct effect	↑ Coronary flow (indirect effect)
Skeletal muscle	β	Vasodilation	↑ Local blood flow ↓ Systemic blood pressure
Veins	α	Vasoconstriction	↑ Venous return ↑ Cardiac output
Juxtaglomerular apparatus	β	↑ Renin secretion	↑ Na^+ reabsorption ↑ Blood pressure
*Metabolic Effects**			
Liver	*	↑ Glycogenolysis	↑ Blood glucose
	*	↑ Gluconeogenesis	↑ Blood glucose
Muscle	β	↑ Glycogenolysis	↑ Blood lactate
	β	↓ Glucose utilization	↑ Blood glucose
Pancreas†	α	↓ Insulin secretion	↑ Blood glucose
Adipose tissue	β	↑ Lipolysis	↑ Blood FFA
GI tract			
Gastric glands	α, β	↓ Secretion	↓ Gastric acidity, volume
Gastric smooth muscle	β	Relaxation	
Intestinal smooth muscle	α, β	Relaxation	↓ Motility
Intestinal sphincter	α	Contraction	
Lung			
Bronchial smooth muscle	β	Relaxation	Bronchodilation
Urinary bladder			
Detrusor muscle	β	Relaxation	Inhibits micturition
Trigone, sphincter	α	Contraction	
Eye			
Iris, radial muscle	α	Contraction	Mydriasis
Ciliary muscle	β	Relaxation	Accommodation
Uterus			
Myometrium	α	Contraction	Depends on hormonal milieu
Skin			
Pilomotor muscle	α	Contraction	Piloerection
Sweat glands	α	Secretion	"Adrenergic" sweating

↑ = Increased. ↓ = Decreased.
*Characterization with regard to receptors is not clearly defined
†β-receptor effect is to increase insulin secretion, but α effect predominates in vivo
**From Bondy, P., and Rosenberg, L. *Duncan's Diseases of Metabolism, Vol. 2: Endocrinology.* Philadelphia: W. B. Saunders Company, 1974, p. 1190.

tent of the human adrenal medulla, but in some pheochromocytomas this value may reach as much as 97.

Symptoms of pheochromocytoma commonly include hypertension, sweating, flushing, palpitations, tachycardia, and postural hypotension. These symptoms are frequently episodic, suggesting bursts of catecholamine secretion; however, sustained hypertension is the single most common manifestation of the disease. Headache is a frequent symptom, and signs of hypermetabolism may suggest a diagnosis of thyrotoxicosis. Hyperglycemia is common and may suggest the presence of diabetes mellitus.

The activity of tyrosine hydroxylase in the tumor cells per unit weight is higher than that in normal adrenal medullary cells. Consequently, more catecholamines are synthesized. Catecholamines, however, seem less effective in inhibiting tyrosine hydroxylase activity in tumor cells than in normal cells. Large amounts of catecholamines are stored in the tumor, and even slight manipulation of the tissue (for example, in examining the patient's abdomen either before or during surgery) may cause a sudden release of these hormones, with a rapid rise in blood pressure.

Pheochromocytomas are most often solitary tumors of the adrenal. In recent years, familial forms of these tumors have been described, often as part of a multiple endocrine syndrome. The diagnosis depends upon the symptomatology and the results of chemical tests. Free catecholamines, VMA, or total metanephrines, may be measured in the urine. Certain adrenergic blocking agents inhibit responses to adrenergic nerve activity and to epinephrine. The effect is on the target cell. One such α-blocker, *phentolamine* (Regitine), is used in the diagnosis of pheochromocytoma. Phentolamine is administered intravenously to the patient and the blood pressure is measured every 30 seconds for three minutes and then every minute for an additional seven minutes. Hypertension due to increased circulating catecholamines will decrease, with a maximal response after two to three minutes and lasting 10 minutes. During the performance of such a test (Regitine test), norepinephrine should be immediately available should severe hypotension occur. If the diagnostic tests suggest a pheochromocytoma, an attempt to localize the tumor can be made using arteriography (the tumor is vascular and often will show a "blush" during the capillary phase of arteriography). Angiography and operative removal of the tumor should be preceded by administration of an α-adrenergic blocking agent to prevent a sudden rise in blood pressure during manipulation of the tumor.

Renin-Angiotensin

The regulation of renin release and the role of renin in electrolyte homeostasis was discussed in Chapter Nine. Renal receptors "sense" diminished blood volume and/or concentration of sodium and respond by stimulating the release of renin. The increased release of renin causes formation of more angiotensin II, a powerful vasopressor hormone that helps regulate blood pressure. Angiotensin II also stimulates the synthesis and release of aldosterone from the adrenal gland. In addition to the "volume sensors" in renal afferent arterioles and the "sodium sensors" in the macula densa, changes in sympathetic tone (catecholamines) and in potassium balance can also alter renin release. Beta receptors in the juxtaglomerular apparatus respond to catecholamines by increasing renin secretion (Table 14–2). Loss of potassium can stimulate renin release directly. An indirectly decreased concentration of potassium in the blood diminishes aldosterone secretion, permitting sodium loss in the kidney, which in turn stimulates renin release.

A variety of hypertensive states are associated with increased plasma renin activity and secondary aldosteronism. Among these would be included renal parenchymal disease and renin-secreting tumors. Acute hypertension with rapid development of disseminated arteriolar necrosis can be induced in rats by applying clips to both renal arteries. Crude saline extracts of rat kidneys can be administered to nephrectomized rats to produce the same results—indicating that the vascular lesions are due to some substance released from kidney tissue. Similar vascular lesions can be produced by infusing either renin or angiotensin II into nephrectomized rats. From such experiments it has been concluded that the hypertension resulting from kidney disease is secondary to the release of renin from degenerating kidney tissue with the subsequent formation of large amounts of angiotensin. It appears that malignant hypertension is attributable to a primary kidney defect resulting in inappropriate release of excess renin. If just one kidney is involved, nephrectomy may alleviate the hypertension; however, vascular damage that has already occurred is irreversible.

Laragh has attempted to establish whether or not the renal-adrenal axis is abnormal in patients with essential hypertension. Using urinary sodium excretion as an index of sodium balance, he has studied the plasma renin activity and the urinary excretion of aldosterone under various conditions of salt intake. After a "salt load" in the normal individual, both plasma renin activity and urinary aldosterone excretion decrease as sodium excretion increases (see Chapter Nine for a discussion of the regulation of aldosterone secretion). The relationship of each to sodium excretion is similar and suggests that the response of aldosterone secretion to changes in sodium balance is mediated by changes in renin activity. In many patients with essential hypertension (57 percent), this relationship between renin and aldosterone is appropriate and normal (normal renin essential hypertension); however, the level of renin is inappropriate for the degree of hypertension (increased blood pressure should decrease renin release). In some patients (16 percent), plasma renin activity was high but appropriately related to aldosterone excretion (high renin essential hypertension). These patients often respond well to propranolol (which blocks renin release, as will be discussed).

Laragh has described a third group of patients with low renin essential hypertension (about 30 percent of all patients with essential hypertension), in which the plasma renin concentration is below normal. The urinary aldosterone excretion in such patients might be appropriately low or inappropriately normal or high. These patients manifest chronic volume expansion. There is some evidence that vascular receptors for angiotensin II can vary their activity in relation to sodium balance. Thus on a high salt diet an increased sensitivity of vascular receptors to angiotension could result in hypertension even in the presence of low aldosterone and low renin. The low aldosterone may not truly reflect the level of circulating mineralocorticoids. Deoxycorticosterone and 18-hydroxydeoxycorticosterone may be formed in large amounts. These ACTH-dependent mineralocorticoids have been found in increased amounts in some patients with low renin essential hypertension. Normal or high levels of aldosterone associated with low renin values may point to an adrenal disorder.

As can be seen, the measurement of plasma renin activity, urinary aldosterone excretion, and sodium balance may be helpful in characterizing various subgroups of essential hypertension. Laragh believes such a breakdown may have prognostic value. In his view, predominantly vasoconstrictor hypertension is largely renin-induced and is more likely to be associated with vascular injury (malignant hypertension). On the other hand, predominantly "volume" hypertension is secondary to sodium and water retention (for example, aldosteronism). The low renin group of essential hypertensives would fall into this category; these patients appear to have significantly lower incidence of heart attacks or strokes than do patients with either normal or high renin values.

MINERALOCORTICOIDS

The synthesis and release of aldosterone is regulated primarily by angiotensin II and the plasma concentration of potassium (see Chapter Nine). Thus any condition of increased renin release will usually be accompanied by increased plasma concentration of aldosterone (secondary aldosteronism). Exceptions to this general rule would be conditions of adrenal cortical insufficiency and conditions of potassium loss (diarrhea, renal potassium loss, thiazide diuretics).

Aldosterone and other mineralocorticoids do not have a direct effect on blood pressure. Rather, these agents alter sodium absorption, bringing about a significant increase in exchangeable sodium and extracellular fluid volume. Reduction in sodium intake can prevent the development of this "volume" hypertension. Hypertension is seen in most patients with Cushing's syndrome, probably because of increased steroid synthesis (including the mineralocorticoid deoxycorticosterone) secondary to excess ACTH stimulation of the adrenal glands. Aldosterone secretion is usually normal or low in Cushing's syndrome. Hypersecretion of other mineralocorticoids (for example, 18-hydroxydeoxycorticosterone) or ingestion of mineralocorticoid-like substances (ammonium glycyrrhizate in licorice) may also induce hypokalemia, suppressed plasma renin activity, and hypertension.

Measurement of the concentration of potassium in the serum may be very helpful in differentiating adrenal vs. nonadrenal causes of hypertension. Hypokalemia in a patient with hypertension should immediately raise the possibility of excess mineralocorticoid production. If the aldosterone secretion rate is low, however, one must suspect (1) the recent use of thiazide diuretics, (2) diarrhea, or (3) the excess production of another mineralocorticoid as the cause of the hypokalemia. If the concentration of serum potassium is normal, the likelihood of aldosteronism is small (although possible if the patient were on a low sodium diet).

Laragh has integrated the various factors involved in the regulation of blood pressure (Figure 14–7). Blood pressure is maintained by agents affecting the constriction of vessels (angiotensin II) and the blood volume (aldosterone, sodium intake). Either of the agents or any combination may cause an elevation of the blood pressure. For example, a high salt diet might increase the amount of sodium in body fluids (sodium gain), which in turn would increase blood volume and increase the

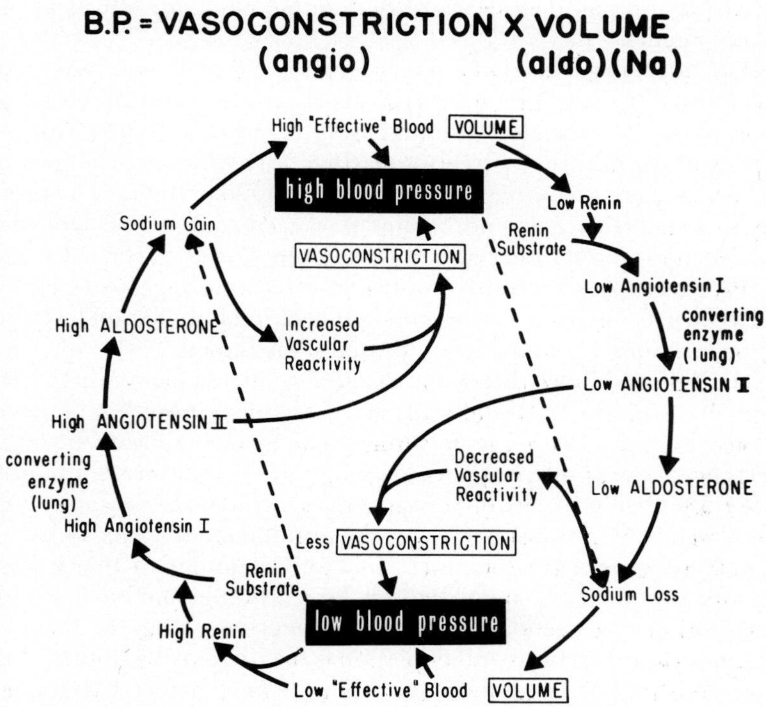

FIGURE 14–7. The renin-angiotensin-aldosterone system and sodium-volume-blood pressure homeostasis. (From Williams, R., *ed. Textbook of Endocrinology.* Philadelphia: W. B. Saunders Company, 1974, p. 949.)

vascular reactivity to angiotensin II, both factors raising the blood pressure. This increased pressure is sensed in the kidney, which decreases its release of renin, thus lowering angiotensin II and aldosterone, thereby favoring sodium loss. The ensuing decrease in both blood volume and vascular reactivity would restore the blood pressure to normal. Although not shown in Figure 14–7, potassium also helps regulate blood pressure by direct effects on renin release and aldosterone synthesis and release.

TREATMENT OF HYPERTENSION

The number of hypertensive individuals in the adult population precludes an elaborate investigation for each patient. As a practical measure, the Task Force on Hypertension of the National Blood Pressure Education Program recommends *elaborate* investigative studies only if treatment fails to control blood pressure. In general, drugs used in therapy for hypertension attempt to decrease sympathetic tone or to counteract the effects of mineralocorticoids. One might anticipate that an α-adrenergic blocking agent would be therapeutically useful in the hypertensive patient; however, results with such agents have been disappointing. Since β receptors are unaffected by α-blocking agents, reflex tachycardia and palpitations are added to the other side effects of the α-blocking agents.

Beta-adrenergic blocking agents, such as propranolol, have proved to be of use in the treatment of hypertension. The effect on blood pressure is probably mediated by decreasing renin secretion. Propranolol has proved useful also in treating cardiac arrhythmias or angina pectoris, which may accompany hypertensive vascular disease. The major danger of such a drug would be impaired cardiac function; blocking of the β receptors would decrease the heart rate and the force of contraction. Propranolol is therefore contraindicated in congestive heart failure. Because bronchial smooth muscle relaxation is mediated by β receptors, propranolol is also contraindicated in asthmatics.

Another and more direct approach to reducing sympathetic tone is to impair synthesis or uptake of the catecholamines. The Rauwolfia alkaloids interfere with the intraneuronal storage of catecholamines. Reserpine, for example, appears to antagonize competitively the uptake of norepinephrine by chromaffin granules. It may act on some "amine carrier" involved in transport across the granule membrane. Thus, in effect, reserpine depletes the stores of catecholamines in many organs, including brain, heart, blood vessels, and adrenal medulla. Reduced concentration of catecholamines can be detected within an hour after reserpine administration, and depletion is maximal by 24 hours. Most of the catecholamines are catabolized within the neuron by monoamine oxidases. The depletion of catecholamines in the brain may explain the known effect of Rauwolfia alkaloids on the central nervous system. They have a calming effect; with high doses over a prolonged time, extrapyramidal effects may be noted. Even small doses of reserpine can produce psychic depression sometimes severe enough to require hospitalization or to result in suicide. Other side effects include abdominal cramps, diarrhea, and increased gastric acidity. Small doses of reserpine may be useful in mild hypertension; however, it must be remembered that reserpine has a very long half-life and is potentially dangerous. A recent study suggests that women over the age of 50 receiving reserpine-like drugs may run a greater risk of developing breast cancer.

Guanethidine is a postganglionic sympathetic blocker that brings about a slow, prolonged depletion of catecholamines which are largely metabolized by monoamine oxidase prior to their release. It is the most potent antihypertensive agent available today. It is used for those patients who maintain elevated diastolic pressures even after therapy with other antihypertensive agents. It lowers blood pressure through decreasing cardiac output and venous return, with little or no decrease in peripheral resistance. Secondary to the decrease in cardiac output is a decrease in renal blood flow and glomerular filtration rate. This latter effect must be borne in mind particularly if the drug is used in combination with the thiazides, which produce similar effects on renal hemodynamics. Guanethidine causes bradycardia through blockade of sympathetic impulses to the sinoatrial node. Better effects are obtained when the drug is used in combination with diuretics or hydralazine.

The synthesis of catecholamines can be blocked by inhibiting any one of the enzyme steps in the biosynthetic pathway. Methyldopa is an effective competitive inhibitor of dopa decarboxylase and is currently widely used as an antihypertensive agent. Dopa decarboxylase can catalyze the conversion of α-methyl dopa to α-methyl dopamine, which in turn is converted by dopamine β-oxidase to the "false transmitter" α-methyl norepinephrine. The latter is somewhat less potent than norepinephrine and replaces it in the adrenergic terminals. Its release by nerve impulses produces reduced responses; however, its role as a false transmitter does not appear to be the major target of the hypotensive action of methyldopa. Urinary excretion of catecholamines and their metabolites is not altered very much by antihypertensive doses of methyldopa in man. The hemodynamic characteristics of the antihypertensive effect of methyldopa appear to differ significantly from those of an adrenergic blocking agent. For these and other reasons, the exact mechanism of the hypotensive effect of methyldopa remains unclear.

Methyldopa is useful in treating patients with moderate hypertension. The hemodynamic effects approach the ideal, with only a slight fall in cardiac output but a significant fall in peripheral resistance. Since renal vascular resistance is also reduced, this drug is of special value in the treatment of patients with renal insufficiency. Side effects are few.

Drowsiness may occur early in therapy but usually disappears later. Rarely, mental depression and Parkinsonian symptoms may occur. Galactorrhea and anemia have also been reported.

In general, hypertension can be controlled by judicious use of the antisympathetic drugs described together with a diuretic. Diuretics are agents that increase the rate of urine formation. The benzothiadiazide (thiazide) diuretics decrease extracellular fluid and plasma volumes, cardiac output, and total exchangeable sodium and potassium. These natriuretic and diuretic effects appear to be dependent primarily upon the ability of the thiazides to block the reabsorption of sodium in the distal tubules of the kidney. After prolonged thiazide therapy, the plasma volume and total body sodium return to normal, but peripheral resistance is by then definitely decreased. The mechanism of the hypotensive action, therefore, is unclear, but in any event the diuretic thiazides relax peripheral vascular smooth muscle. This lowering of blood pressure is modest and occurs only in hypertensive individuals. When used alone, the thiazides are rarely sufficient to control severe hypertension, but in combination with other agents, excellent control of blood pressure is often possible. This synergism of thiazides with other antihypertensive agents has made them the most popular and most prescribed of the antihypertensive drugs. Hypokalemia frequently develops, however, during thiazide therapy and may require potassium supplementation.

Spironolactone enhances urinary excretion of sodium and water by interfering with the action of aldosterone at the distal tubule. Spironolactone produces a selective effect similar to that of the thiazides in reducing the blood pressure of hypertensive patients but not of normotensive patients. In combination with thiazides, an even greater reduction of blood pressure can be attained. In addition, potassium loss is reduced by spironolactone.

There is a high incidence of coronary artery disease among hypertensive patients, especially those over the age of 50. The existence of such disease should be ascertained prior to initiating antihypertensive therapy. In patients with heart disease, reserpine, methyldopa, and the thiazide diuretics are the drugs of choice, since they reduce cardiac output to a lesser degree than do other antihypertensive agents.

In patients with renal insufficiency secondary to hypertension, it is important to use drugs that will not reduce renal blood flow. There may actually be an increase in renal blood flow with either methyldopa or hydralazine (Apresoline, a phthalazine derivative with cardiovascular effects including decreased blood pressure and peripheral resistance and increased heart rate, stroke volume, and cardiac output); unfortunately this increase is usually temporary and is not accompanied by any increase in glomerular filtration rate. In general, in order to avoid severe complications, the greater the degree of renal insufficiency, the less vigorous one should be in lowering blood pressure.

Cerebral vascular disease is another complication of long-standing hypertension. Headaches, dizziness, and cerebral hemorrhage may be alleviated or prevented by hypotensive agents; however, too great a reduction in blood pressure may lead to cerebral thrombosis or ischemia.

Another form of antihypertensive therapy which is of investigative interest is the use of prostaglandins. One of the original physiologic manifestations of the prostaglandins described by Von Euler in the early thirties was their marked depressor effect, which in dogs was characterized by a dramatic lowering of peripheral resistance. Apparently, prostaglandin E_1 lowers blood pressure mainly by actions independent of the catecholamines, through its smooth muscle relaxing properties in the peripheral vascular bed. Similar effects are noted on respiratory, gastrointestinal, and uterine smooth muscle.

Prostaglandin A compounds are formed in the kidney and may play an important role in regulating blood pressure. Prostaglandin A_2 has a potent natriuretic action in vivo and reduces blood pressure by direct peripheral arteriolar dilatation. A baroreceptor-mediated reflex increases the heart rate, leading to an elevation in cardiac output. This effect appears to be primarily in the splanchnic vascular bed. Prostaglandins have just begun to be available for clinical use and are being used in obstetrics. Their potential use as antihypertensive agents has yet to be fully explored.

Some individuals with chronic hypertension develop vascular disease, others never develop any significant ischemia. Overall, atherosclerotic lesions in the large arteries of the brain, heart, and kidney directly or indirectly constitute the most common cause of death in people over 65 years of age in Westernized societies. Progressive changes associated with chronic hypertensive disease culminate in this age group in the form of congestive heart failure, myocardial infarction, stroke, and nephrosclerosis.

STRUCTURAL CHANGES WITH AGE

Surrounding the cells and holding them together are the structural proteins and mucopolysaccharides. Changes in these extracellular components occur with age, suggesting to some investigators that the aging process itself may be related to these changes. In particular, the "aging" of collagen has been studied. It is not unrealistic to attribute some importance to this ubiquitous molecule which constitutes as much as one third of the total protein of the body.

Collagen is the most abundant protein in the animal kingdom. Within tissues collagenous fibers are made up of microfibrils. These microfibrils may be arranged differently in each tissue. For example, in tendons, which must accommodate a high tensile strength applied along the longitudinal axis, the microfibrils are closely packed in a parallel manner. Under the electron microscope one can see an axial repeating period of 640 to 700 Å. Glycine makes up one third of the total amino acid residues of collagen, and proline and hydroxyproline about one fourth. There is no tryptophan or cystine and very little tyrosine. One of the characteristics of collagen is its shrinkage temperature, the temperature at which the collagen fiber shrinks and changes to an amorphous structure. The shrinkage temperatures of different collagens are functions of the amount of cross linkage between adjacent fibers.

Collagen is produced by fibrocytes, primarily, but also by smooth muscle cells. The polypeptide chains are assembled on ribosomal aggregates as *protocollagen,* containing frequent sequences of Gly-X-Pro. It is this sequence which confers a helical conformation on the polypeptide chains. Specific prolyl residues (the third amino acid of a triplet starting with glycine, Figure 14–8) are enzymatically hydroxylated, catalyzed by the enzyme *peptidyl proline hydroxylase,* which requires α-ketoglutarate, ascorbic acid, Fe^{++}, and K^{+} as cofactors. The manner in which molecular oxygen and the cofactors interact in the hydroxylation reaction is not known. Approximately half the proline residues become hydroxylated. Another enzyme, *peptidyl lysine hydroxylase,* catalyzes the hydroxylation of a few lysyl residues in the molecule, for the most part also located in the third position of the collagen triplet. Hydroxylations occur on nascent α chains prior to release from ribosomes.

The process of attaching carbohydrate to collagen (glycosylation) involves the transfer of glucose from UDP-glucose to collagen. The enzyme catalyzing this transfer is *glucosyl transferase.* In addition, a *galactosyl transferase* attaches a galactose molecule to collagen. The carbohydrate moieties are attached mainly to the hydroxyl group of the N-terminal hydroxylysine residue in the α_1 chains. They exist as monosaccharide units (galactosyl hydroxylysine) or as disaccharide units (glycosylgalactosyl hydroxylysine). The collagen molecule of a vertebrate is composed of three polypeptide chains arranged in a triple helix (Figure 14–8). Two of these chains, α_1 chains, appear to be identical, while the other (α_2 chain) is different. The collagen of cartilage, however, consists of three identical α chains. The α chains of collagen associate to form a large precursor molecule of about 360,000 molecular weight (*procollagen*). The latter is converted to *tropocollagen* by the enzyme *procollagen peptidase* (Figure 14–18), either within the cell or after secretion from the cell. The polymerization of the tropocollagen molecules into microfibrils then takes place. The microfibrils (44 Å in diameter) polymerize further to form collagen fibrils (150 to 1300 Å in diameter).

The first step in the extracellular formation of cross links in collagen is the oxidation of protein-bound lysine residues. Soluble collagens contain a lysyl residue in the fifth or ninth position from the N-terminal end. This lysyl residue is oxidized by a specific enzyme, *lysyl oxidase,* to give α-amino adipic acid-δ-semialdehyde (allysine). Some chains contain hydroxylysyl residues which can also undergo oxidation. Copper is a

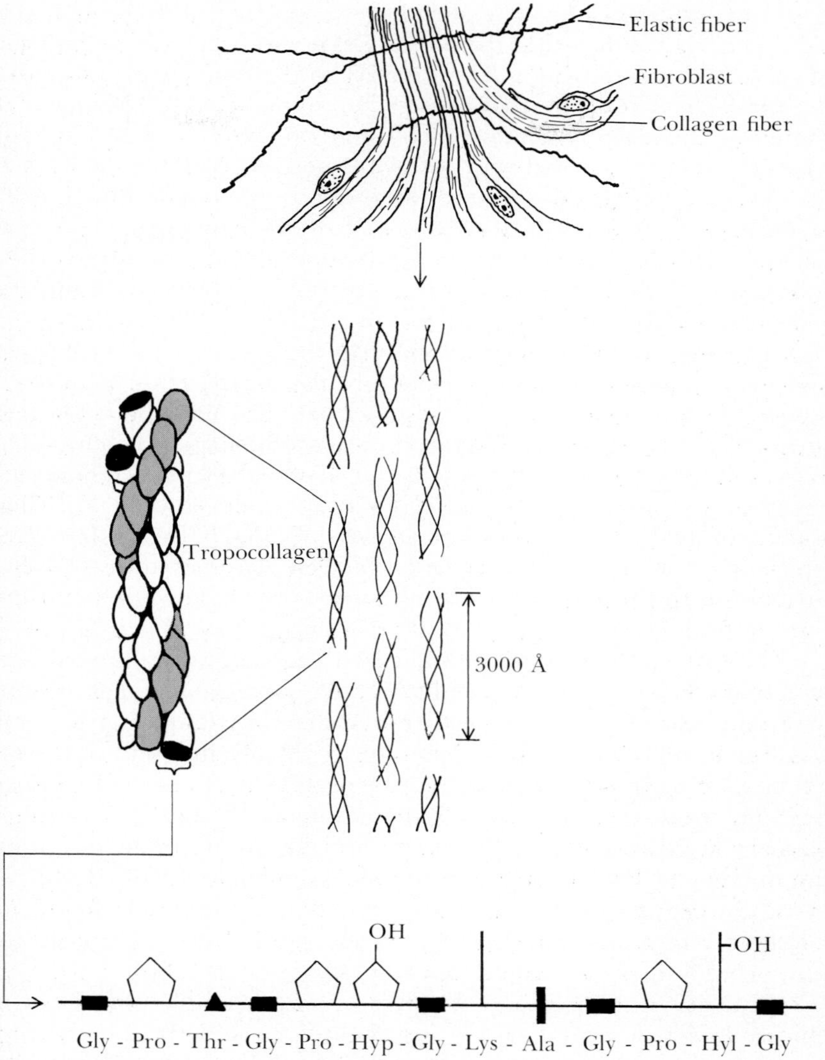

FIGURE 14–8. Structure of collagen fiber showing individual tropocollagen units in staggered array. A hypothetical amino acid sequence for one of the α chains is depicted schematically.

cofactor for lysyl oxidase. The second step in the formation of cross links is the condensation of two aldehydes, via aldol condensation, to form an α, β-unsaturated aldehyde. This aldol condensation in collagen is a spontaneous reaction. The cross links in elastin are formed in much the same way as those in collagen.

Collagen solubility decreases with age, and this decrease has been related to increased cross linking. With advancing age, the number of cross linkages increases. The shrinkage temperature of collagen from old rats is higher than that from young rats and is probably a reflection of increased cross linkage. The capacity to degrade collagen seems to decline with increasing cross linkage. In young rats, for example, the chemically insoluble fraction of collagen can be effectively degraded when the rats are treated with cortisol, whereas in older rats glucocorticoid treatment does not restore the reduced capacity of the animal to degrade collagen. This greater resistance of older collagen to enzymatic degradation may also be due to a decrease in the amount or activity of collagenase. It has been shown that cortisol is capable of stimulating collagenase activity in young but not in old rats.

A marked reduction in the volume of the ground substance in relation to the collagen content of tissue is also a typical consequence of aging. This decrease in ground substance has been attributed to its faster turnover (days, weeks) as compared to that of collagen (much longer). The replacement of elastin fibers by the less flexible collagen fibers with age accounts for the decreased elasticity of senile skin. Total collagen content of the heart increases with age, as does that of the cardiac valves, which therefore become more rigid. Collagen increases in vessel walls in proportion to the severity of the atherosclerotic lesion, whereas mucopolysaccharides decrease.

Changes in the ground substance with age may affect the basement membranes of the capillaries, reducing their permeability. For example, over one fifth of the amino acid residues of the glomerular basement membrane of the normal human consist of glycine, and substantial amounts of hydroxylysine and hydroxyproline are present. In diabetes mellitus, there is an increase in the covalently bound glucose in the glomerular basement membrane, presumably owing to an increase in the number of hydroxylysyl residues with attached carbohydrate. The extra glucose increases the bulk of the non-protein side chains and might interfere with the packing of the membrane molecules, thus producing a thicker, "leakier," membrane.

Synthesis of the carbohydrate components of glycoprotein from glucose is not dependent upon insulin and therefore can occur more readily in the insulin-deprived state in those tissues not totally dependent upon insulin for glucose uptake. The enzyme that links glucose to hydroxylysine residues in collagen, glucosyl transferase, increases in activity in insulin-deficient states and can be decreased to normal with insulin therapy. It is easy to imagine the far-reaching effects of altered membrane structure on membrane function. Such effects can be noted in patients with diabetes mellitus but may also be present to some extent in the aged individual with glucose intolerance.

A loss of mucopolysaccharides of connective tissue occurs with age. For example, the skin of a three-month-old human fetus has 20 times the amount of mucopolysaccharide as does the adult human skin. Aorta and myocardium also show a diminished amount of mucopolysaccharide with age. A shift from the synthesis of chondroitin sulfate and very little keratosulfate to more keratosulfate synthesis occurs with age.

It is now well established that most, if not all, mucopolysaccharides include a protein portion which is attached covalently. The polysaccharide chain of the mucopolysaccharide is synthesized from sugar nucleotide precursors. For example, UDP-glucuronic acid and UDP-N-acetyl glucosamine are precursors for hyaluronic acid, and UDP-glucuronic acid and UDP-N-acetyl galactosamine are precursors for chondroitin sulfate. Sulfation apparently occurs by the direct transfer of a sulfate group from PAPS to the appropriate sites on the mucopolysaccharide.

From the preceding discussion, we can see that there is a tendency for connective tissue changes in old age to result in increased cross linking, stiffness, and loss of elasticity. These changes are clearly important in skin and arteries, and, in so far as they impair the diffusion of metabolites from the circulation to cells, impaired organ function would be expected. Thickening of basement membranes occurs with age and in diabetes mellitus and suggests a relationship between glucose metabolism and structural characteristics of membranes.

One other interesting aspect of aging is the accumulation in cells of substances that are not metabolized and may, in fact, be harmful. A fluorescent pigment called "lipofuscin" is deposited in cells that turn over very slowly, such as brain cells and heart muscle cells. The pigment may occupy as much as five percent of the volume of the heart muscle cell. The deposition of this pigment may play some role in the decreased functional capacity of certain cells and tissues with age.

NEOPLASTIC DISORDERS

The incidence of many cancers increases with age. Indeed, approximately half of all cancer deaths occur over age 65. Does this represent a failure of the cell to respond to normal controls of growth? The hallmark of most anaplastic tumors is rapid growth, and one of the major regulators of growth is cyclic AMP, which in turn may be regulated by hormones. As the adenyl cyclase system is located in the cell membrane, changes in membrane structure and function with age could alter this system. Is their any evidence for changes in adenyl cyclase activity with age?

In the rat, adenyl cyclase activity of the heart, lung, liver, and skeletal muscle decreases with maturation. Catecholamine-induced lipolysis (mediated by cyclic AMP) decreases progressively with age in man and rat. Age-dependent decreases in sensitivity to hormones occur also with respect to insulin, GH, and ACTH. Part of this altered sensitivity may be due to changes in the adenyl cyclase system with age. The role of cyclic nucleotides in the genesis of cancer is being actively investigated.

Many of the tumors and malignancies occurring in the older population involve tissues responsive to hormones as exemplified by the high incidence of carcinoma of the breast in women and prostatic neoplasia in men. It is well known that carcinoma of the breast may sometimes be aggravated by estrogen. This effect may be due in part to the direct growth-promoting action of estrogen on breast tissue and in part to the estrogen-stimulated release of prolactin, which also stimulates tumor growth. Adrenalectomy, oophorectomy, and/or hypophysectomy are used to retard the progress of the disease. Carcinoma of the prostate is also influenced by the hormonal milieu. Androgens may aggravate the carcinoma, whereas orchidectomy and/or estrogen may bring prolonged and often remarkable benefit.

Certain tumors arising in nonendocrine tissue produce hormones. One of the commonly seen conditions of this sort is called the "ectopic ACTH syndrome." The vast majority of the ACTH-producing tumors in this syndrome are found in either bronchogenic carcinoma, thymic carcinoma, or pancreatic carcinoma. Cushing's syndrome may be the first manifestation of the neoplasm, or, conversely, the symptoms of Cushing's syndrome may develop after neoplastic disease has been diagnosed. Classical signs of Cushing's syndrome do not always develop, even though plasma ACTH concentration is high. The ACTH produced by the tumors is similar to pituitary ACTH.

A great variety of nonendocrine neoplasms are capable of producing hypercalcemia. In most cases, this is due to bone metastases, but in some, hypercalcemia develops in the absence of bone metastases. Although there is no evidence of hyperparathyroidism, a substance identical to PTH has been isolated from some of these tumors. Other tumors have a substance immunologically different from PTH but physiologically similar to it.

Some nonendocrine tumors produce hypoglycemia, and it has been postulated that an insulin-like substance may be produced by such tumors, or that over-utilization of glucose by the neoplastic tissue predisposes to hypoglycemia. Still other tumors (generally renal) cause polycythemia (an increase in the absolute number of red cells in the blood). The polycythemia appears to be a response to an "erythropoietin-like" material found in the tumor. The kidney is the major site of production of erythropoietin. Renal tumors, cysts, or hydronephrosis have been associated with polycythemia and increased erythropoietin production for many years; it is not surprising, therefore, that renal carcinoma should also be associated with polycythemia.

Cerebellar hemangiomas have been found in several patients with polycythemia. The cystic fluid within many of these tumors contains an erythropoiesis-stimulating factor. Several other neoplasms have been associated with polycythemia. Many cases of hepatoma with polycythemia have been reported in which elevated concentrations of erythropoietin in the blood were present.

Biologically active materials may be formed by enterochromaffin cells derived from neuroectoderm and migrating to various sites in the primitive alimentary tract. Tumors composed of these enterochromaffin cells are called *carcinoid tumors* and may be found throughout the gastrointestinal tract, bronchus, gallbladder, and ducts of the pancreas. These cells usually produce large amounts of serotonin, but histamine, catecholamines, prostaglandins, and vasoactive peptides have been isolated from these tumors also. Peptides resembling ACTH, MSH, and insulin have also, on occasion, been produced. Thus the clinical features of this condition can vary considerably. Most typically, vasomotor phenomena (flushes) are noted and are probably due to a group of vasodilator peptides. On stimulation with catecholamines or alcohol, the enzyme *kallikrein* is released from the carcinoid tumor and catalyzes the conversion of *kininogen* in plasma to *lysyl-bradykinin*. The latter is split to *bradykinin* by a plasma aminopeptidase. Both lysyl-bradykinin and bradykinin are potent vasodilators. Other features of the *carcinoid syndrome* include bronchial constriction, lesions of the valves of the heart, and diarrhea. The exact role of serotonin, or some other product of the tumor, in the production of these features is unknown.

PROGERIA

In order to better understand senescence, many investigators have sought models of the aging process. One such model may be the disorder progeria (premature aging). This rare disorder was first reported in the late nineteenth century by Hutchinson and Gilford, and the original description presented a clinical picture of "immaturity upon which was descended the blight of premature senility." Progeric children characteristically appear normal at birth (although often born slightly premature and with birth weights in the lower normal range). At approximately one year of age, the disorder begins to manifest itself as a failure to gain in weight and to grow normally. Presumably, progeric children grow normally in utero, but postnatally they cope less well. Subcutaneous fat begins to disappear, and it has been assumed that it is the utilization of this fat for energy which permits the progeric child to continue to grow (but subnormally) for a few years after birth. These children usually attain a height age of about three years and a weight age of about five years. Hair falls out, and by about age two or three the child is completely bald. The skin becomes increasingly dry and loses its elasticity, resembling senile skin. Certain peculiarities of the skeletal system give a characteristic appearance and gait. The relatively normal-sized cranium plus hypoplasia of the mandible and maxilla give a bird-headed appearance. The clavicles, which are normal at birth, become progressively replaced by fibrous tissue and are strikingly hypoplastic. Bilateral coxa valga gives a horse-riding stance and a peculiar gait, and widespread flexion deformities give the appearance of senility and debility.

Children with progeria develop severe atherosclerosis, which usually leads to coronary heart disease and death at an early age (mean age at death: 16). On investigation, these children manifest insulin resistance but no other evidence of endocrine abnormality. Hypercholesterolemia and hyperlipoproteinemia (LDL) have been reported in some patients. The collagen isolated from progeric skin shows evidence of being highly cross-linked as measured by shrinkage temperature (increased) and solubility (higher percentage of insoluble collagen). Similar characteristics are found in the collagen isolated from skin of old individuals. Lipofuscin (the age pigment) has been found in myocardium and other organs in two patients with progeria.

Cultured fibroblasts from progeric children exhibit reduced growth potential, with fewer generations of cells as compared to cultures containing fibroblasts from normal children. Hayflick has shown that the number of cell replications in cultures of fibroblasts from aged individuals is far fewer than in comparable cultures of fibroblasts from young or embryonic tissues. Danes has shown that progeric fibroblasts have decreased mitotic potential and less DNA synthesis than controls. More recently, Goldstein has reported the lack of HL-A antigens in progeric fibroblasts in culture. These antigens are the histocompatibility antigens by which cells recognize one another. Presumably, cells lacking such antigens or with different (undetectable) antigens would not be recognized as "self" and would be destroyed. Such studies of cultured fibroblasts indicate that the metabolic potential of these cells, whether it be for mitosis or for synthesis of proteins, is grossly impaired. Nonetheless, wound healing in progeric patients is normal, and their response to infection is similar to that of normal children.

Removal of the thymus gland in newborn mice, or administration of ACTH (which decreases the amount of thymic tissue via glucocorticoids) can produce a "wasting" disease called runt syndrome. Mice homozygous for the "nude" gene are hairless, retarded in growth, and have hypoplastic or absent thymus glands. Such animal studies suggest that thymic function in early life may be important in normal growth and development. The thymus gland has been found at autopsy in several patients dying of progeria; however, whether the gland actually functions in progerics is unknown.

The composite picture of the child with progeria is strikingly similar to that of accelerated aging, with cessation of growth, severe arteriosclerosis and atherosclerosis, coronary heart disease, insulin resistance, highly cross-linked collagen, and decreased cellular growth potential. Even more striking is the anthropomorphic resemblance of the progeric child to an old man (Figure 14–9). It has been noted that progeric children look more like one another (or very elderly individuals) than like their sibs. The aberrations of metabolism that bring about this condition are unknown but may well be related to the metabolic derangements which at present are considered to play a possible role in senescence. Among these should be listed (1) cell death (programmed decrease in mitotic potential with age), (2) altered nucleic acids and/or structural proteins (cross linking of DNA, collagen, elastin), (3) autoimmunity

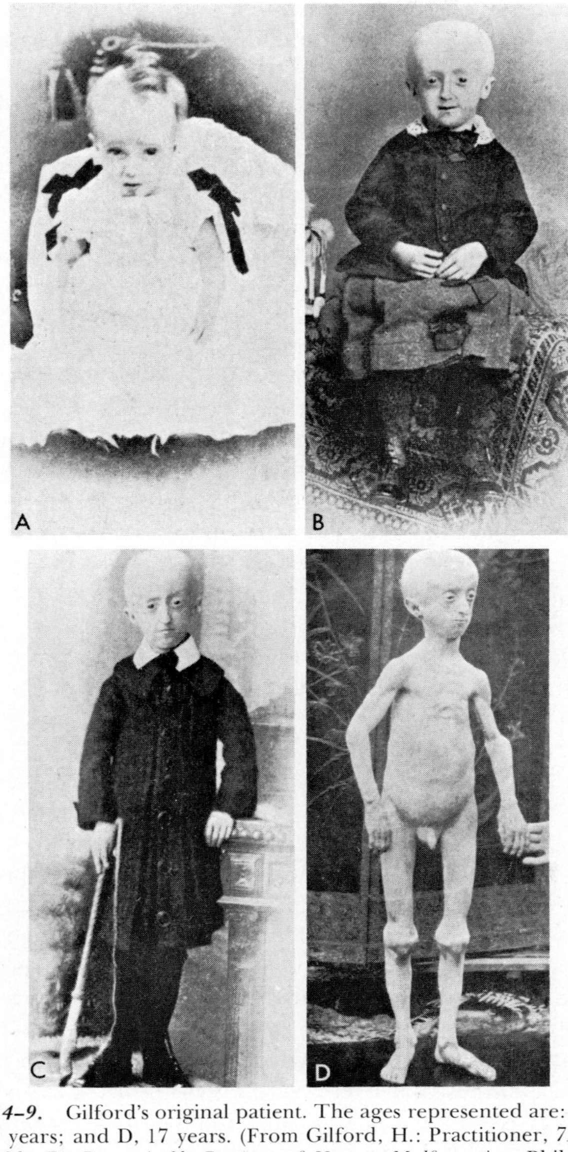

FIGURE 14–9. Gilford's original patient. The ages represented are: A, 1½ years; B, 7 years; C, 12 years; and D, 17 years. (From Gilford, H.: Practitioner, *73*:188, 1904; reprinted in Smith, D. *Recognizable Patterns of Human Malformation*, Philadelphia, W. B. Saunders Company, 1970, p. 75.)

(decreased immunologic competence to recognize self—related to HL-A surface antigens), (4) diminished carbohydrate tolerance with age (insulin resistance, with resulting diabetogenic syndrome), (5) diminished lipid tolerance with age (hypercholesterolemia, hyperlipoproteinemia with atherosclerosis), and (6) errors in transcription and translation, producing abnormal proteins (abnormal insulin?, abnormal HL-A antigens?).

It is in the aged individual that we see the culmination of hundreds, perhaps thousands, of minute deviations from "normal." It is discouraging for the physician who wants to make the sort of diagnosis that is possible with the young child or adult, for it is rare to find a *single* disorder in the elderly patient; moreover, because of alterations in mental function with age, the history may be unreliable. The endocrine system appears to be functioning normally for the most part, but our criteria for function are gross at best. Even a small deviation in synthesis, action, metabolism, or excretion of a single hormone could have wide ramifications in the economy of the body. The intermingling of the effects of the various hormones provides a remarkably tight regulation of metabolism. It is difficult to think of a single pathway of metabolism that is not carefully regulated by an interaction of hormones, usually at the rate-limiting step for that pathway. In an increasingly rigid system (senescence), a slight perturbation (a very slight decreased response of the β cell to glucose, for example) will be felt far more widely than in a system where compensatory controls are rapidly called into play. It is this inexorable decline in adaptability which renders the aging organism increasingly vulnerable to irreversible cell loss and death. The mystery of the origin of life is no more puzzling than the riddle of the origin of death.

SUMMARY

The disorders associated with the post-maturity years become chronic and involve certain characteristic systems. Metabolically there seems to be an increasing intolerance for calories, glucose, salt, and cholesterol, with a resulting increase in the incidence of obesity, diabetes mellitus, hypertension, and atherosclerosis. These disorders frequently coexist in the patient. Other factors exacerbate these conditions, and in turn these disorders affect other medical conditions.

The metabolic alterations may themselves generate (or be generated by) structural changes that occur with age. The progressive accumulation of highly cross-linked collagen and the loss of elastin and mucopolysaccharides brings about a rigidity of structural elements which may impair vascular function (distensibility) and permeability (membranes). The decreased adaptability of the aged and the possible increased errors in protein synthesis may predispose to a variety of processes, including neoplastic and/or autoimmune disease.

The disorder progeria includes many if not all of the characteristics of the aged individual. It has been proposed as a convenient model for the study of the aging process in the normal individual, whose early development encompasses a period of growth and differentiation, followed by maturation, as we have seen. After cessation of growth and maturation, a process of decline begins as the accumulated insults of the years manifest themselves. Although it may be convenient to think in terms of these periods of development, it is important to remember that the lifespan of an individual is a continuum, with modulations occurring at each step along the way. Undoubtedly some of these modulations are instigated by the endocrine system. The obvious importance of circulating substances which can regulate metabolism suggests that at all phases of development the endocrine system plays a key role.

SUGGESTED READINGS

Atherosclerosis, edited by M. D. Altschule, in Medical Clinics of North America, *58*:2, 1974.
Discussions by experts in the field comprise this volume covering various facets of the etiology and manifestations of atherosclerosis. A chapter on "Hyperlipidemia and Coronary Artery Disease," by P. T. Kuo, and a chapter on "The Etiology of Atherosclerosis," by M. D. Altschule, are particularly interesting and pertinent.

"Catecholamines and the Adrenal Medulla," R. J. Levine and L. Landsberg, in *Duncan's Diseases of Metabolism,* edited by Philip K. Bondy and Leon E. Rosenberg, Philadelphia, W. B. Saunders, July, 1974.
A very informative discussion of the synthesis, storage, release, and metabolism of the catecholamines. Pheochromocytoma is discussed, as are the various sympathomimetic drugs used in medicine. Of particular interest are the descriptions of α and β receptor effects and the role of blocking agents in the treatment of hypertension.

"Disorders of Connective Tissues," Paul Bornstein, In *Duncan's Diseases of Metabolism,* edited by Philip K. Bondy and Leon E. Rosenberg, Philadelphia, W. B. Saunders, 1974.
An excellent description of the synthesis and physical properties of collagen, elastin, and mucopolysaccharides. Diseases illustrating abnormalities of metabolism of structural proteins are presented. A small section on the alterations of connective tissue with age is very appropriate.

SELECTED REFERENCES FROM THE LITERATURE

Beisswenger, P. J. Specificity of the chemical alteration in the diabetic glomerular basement membrane. Diabetes *22*:744, 1973.

Hughes, R. C. Glycoproteins as components of cellular membranes. Progr. Biophys. Mol. Biol. *26*:191, 1973.

Laragh, J. H. Vasoconstriction-volume analysis for understanding and treating hypertension. The use of renin and aldosterone profiles. Am. J. Med. *55*:261, 1973.

Lee, J. B. Hypertension, natriuresis and the renomedullary prostaglandins: an overview. Prostaglandins *3*:551, 1973.

McGuire, W. L. et al. Hormone dependence in breast cancer. Metabolism *23*:75, 1974.

Miller, E. J. and Matukas, V. J. Biosynthesis of collagen. Fed. Proc. *33*:1197, 1974.

Robert, B. and Robert, L. Aging of connective tissue. Triangle *12*:163, 1973.

Singal, D. P. and Goldstein, S. Absence of detectable HL-A antigens on cultured fibroblasts in progeria. J. Clin. Inv. *52*:2259, 1973.

Soloff, L. A., Rutenberg, H. L., and Lacko, A. G. Serum cholesterol esterification in patients with coronary heart disease. Am. Heart J. *85*:153, 1973.

INDEX